D1521466

Autism

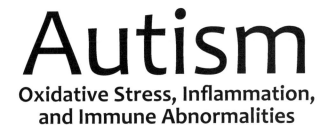

Autism
Oxidative Stress, Inflammation, and Immune Abnormalities

Edited by
Abha Chauhan
Ved Chauhan
W. Ted Brown

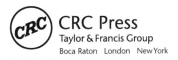

CRC Press
Taylor & Francis Group
Boca Raton   London   New York

CRC Press is an imprint of the
Taylor & Francis Group, an **informa** business

CRC Press
Taylor & Francis Group
6000 Broken Sound Parkway NW, Suite 300
Boca Raton, FL 33487-2742

Library of Congress Cataloging-in-Publication Data

Autism : oxidative stress, inflammation, and immune abnormalities / edited by Abha
Chauhan, Ved Chauhan, and Ted Brown.
    p. ; cm.
Includes bibliographical references and index.
ISBN 978-1-4200-6881-8 (hardcover : alk. paper)
    1. Autism--Pathophysiology. 2. Oxidative stress. 3. Inflammation. 4.
Neuroimmunology. I. Chauhan, Abha, 1957- II. Chauhan, Ved. III. Brown, Ted, 1946-
    [DNLM: 1. Autistic Disorder--etiology. 2. Inflammation. 3. Oxidative Stress. WM
203.5 A93805 2010]

    RC553.A88A8726 2010
    616.85'882--dc22   2009024353

Visit the Taylor & Francis Web site at
http://www.taylorandfrancis.com

and the CRC Press Web site at
http://www.crcpress.com

This book is dedicated to the children and adults who have Autism spectrum disorders, to the family members and health care professionals who provide care for them, and to the scientists and sponsoring agencies devoted to research on autism and related disorders.

Contents

Contents

Preface

Autism spectrum disorders (ASD) are a group of behaviorally defined neuro-developmental disorders characterized by deficits in social interaction; impairments in verbal and nonverbal communication; and restricted, stereotyped patterns of behaviors and interests. In 2007, the Centers for Disease Control and Prevention issued an "autism alarm," with 1 in 150 children estimated to be affected by ASD. Epidemiological studies suggest that more than 1.5 million people in the United States are affected with this disorder. Autism is the most severe disorder in the broad spectrum of pervasive developmental disorders (PDDs), which also include Asperger's syndrome, Rett's disorder, childhood disintegrative disorder, and PDD-not otherwise specified. Within this spectrum, there are variations in the severity, level of cognitive functioning, the presence or absence of associated medical conditions such as seizures or other neurological disorders, and whether or not there is a history of regression from apparent normal development. Currently, there is no biochemical or genetic marker to support the behavioral diagnosis of autism.

Autism is a heterogeneous disorder, both etiologically and phenotypically. While the cause of autism remains elusive, autism is considered a multifactorial disorder that is influenced by genetic, epigenetic, and environmental factors. Accumulating evidence from our studies and that of other groups suggests that oxidative stress may be a common feature in autism linking the mechanism through which the environmental factors exert their deleterious effects with the purported genetic alterations in autism. The oxidative stress and intracellular redox imbalance can be induced or triggered in autism by prenatal or postnatal exposure to certain environmental factors such as heavy metals, viruses, bacterial infections, air pollutants, toxins, valproic acid, thalidomide, terbutaline, retinoic acid, and ethanol. Genetic factors can also modulate the threshold for vulnerability to oxidative stress in autism. In addition to behavior impairments, some individuals with autism may have a higher prevalence of gastrointestinal (GI) disturbances. Several studies suggest that inflammatory phenomena, immune dysregulation, and certain autoimmune risk factors may also contribute to the development and pathogenesis of autism. The chapters in this book provide a comprehensive overview of neuropathological abnormalities, genetics, oxidative stress, inflammation, immune dysfunction, aberrant cellular signaling, gene–environment interactions, diagnostic tools, and treatment in autism.

In Chapter 1, Jerzy Wegiel and colleagues review neuropathological changes in autism contributing to the clinical phenotype. These changes include (a) pathological acceleration of brain growth in early childhood, (b) developmental heterochronicity with different rates of growth for different brain regions/structures, (c) brain structure–specific delay of neuronal growth in early childhood and partial correction of cell size in late childhood/adulthood, and (d) regional cytoarchitectonic abnormalities with consistent changes of structure of minicolumns, and variable topography and severity of dysplastic changes and ectopias. These developmental abnormalities are paralleled by signs of metabolic changes with modified expression and processing of β-amyloid precursor protein, enhanced turnover of cell organelle and pigment accumulation, as well as oxidative stress.

Under normal conditions, a dynamic equilibrium exists between the production of reactive oxygen species (ROS) and the antioxidant capacity of the cell. Oxidative stress occurs when ROS levels exceed the antioxidant capacity of a cell. These ROS are highly toxic and oxidize vital cellular components such as lipids, proteins, and DNA, thus causing cellular damage and subsequent cell death via apoptosis or necrosis. Oxidative stress is known to be associated with premature aging of cells and can lead to inflammation, damaged cell membranes, autoimmunity, and cell death. In this book, several chapters present evidence that support the concept of oxidative stress in autism.

The brain is highly vulnerable to oxidative stress because of its limited antioxidant capacity, higher energy requirement, and high amounts of unsaturated lipids and iron. Based on immunocytochemical and biochemical studies, in Chapter 2, Xiongwei Zhu and colleagues demonstrate lipid-derived oxidative protein modifications in postmortem brain samples from autistic subjects and suggest carboxyethyl pyrrole (CEP) and iso[4]levuglandin E_2 protein adducts as possible oxidative stress markers for the autistic brain. From a structural perspective, their findings suggest that axons of cholinergic neurons in the white matter are the primary site of oxidative damage. At the molecular level, they have identified neurofilament heavy chain to be the major target for CEP-modification. In Chapter 3, Elizabeth Sajdel-Sulkowska reviews the evidence of oxidative stress–related protein and DNA modifications in autism, and discusses data supporting altered neurotrophin signaling in autism and the possible association between oxidative stress and altered neurotrophin expression. These findings not only support the notion that brain oxidative stress plays an important role in autism but also warrant future in-depth mechanistic studies to provide new targets for therapeutic intervention.

The genetics underlying autism is highly complex, with estimates of heritability at greater than 90%. While no single gene has been found to be associated with autism, multiple genes and interactions between genetic and environmental factors have been postulated in autism. In Chapter 4, Ted Brown reviews this subject. The association of single-gene disorders, such as fragile X syndrome with autism, and the role of copy number variations, noncoding RNAs, parental age, and prenatal environmental stressors, such as exposure to hurricanes in autism, are discussed in this chapter.

Reactive oxygen and nitrogen species are generated endogenously during oxidative metabolism and energy production by mitochondria in the cell. While oxidative phosphorylation in the mitochondria generates superoxide anions, the enzymatic oxidation of biogenic amines by monoamine oxidase (MAO) in mitochondrial outer membrane produces H_2O_2. A functional polymorphism in the monoamine oxidase A (MAOA) promoter region has been reported to be associated with the severity of autism. MAOA catalyzes the oxidation of amine-containing neurotransmitters, such as serotonin and norepinephrine. Several studies suggest that serotonin function is abnormal in autism. In Chapter 5, Ira Cohen reviews evidence on maternal depression and a polymorphism in the MAOA gene affecting the severity of autism using a PDD behavior inventory (PDDBI). He also discusses the advantages of using the PDDBI.

In Chapter 6, Maria Dronca and Sergiu Paşca present evidence for the involvement of paraoxonase 1 (PON1) in the pathogenesis of ASD. PON1, an esterase/lactonase enzyme, plays an important role in hydrolyzing pesticides, protecting against oxidative stress, and modulating the immune/inflammatory response. First, the authors review the general biochemical properties of PON1, with the recent biochemical and genetic studies indicating impaired PON1 status in ASD and the literature suggesting a correlation between pesticide (mainly organophosphates) exposure and neurodevelopmental delays or neuropsychiatric conditions. Second, the authors describe several gene × environment models for autism, which include PON1: organophosphates exposure × reelin × PON1 and organophosphates exposure × acetylcholine receptor (AchR) × PON1. Finally, they illustrate how PON1 could contribute to the aberrant immune response and abnormal redox status in autism. They also discuss how these disturbances could affect the PON1 status and further increase the susceptibility to various environmental neurotoxic agents during neurodevelopment.

Sulfur metabolism serves a number of critical roles, including the maintenance of cellular redox status and support for several methylation reactions. Methylation capacity is reduced during oxidative stress, affecting many processes such as epigenetic regulation of gene expression, which is critical for development, as well as dopamine-stimulated phospholipid methylation, which is involved in the synchronization of neuronal firing. The unique features of sulfur metabolism in the brain make it highly vulnerable to heavy metals, which bind with high affinity to thiol and selenocysteine oxidoreductases and interfere with redox regulation. Methionine synthase (folate and vitamin B12–dependent enzyme) plays a key role as a monitor of cellular redox status and as a regulator of the flux of homocysteine through transsulfuration to glutathione synthesis. Levels of methionione synthase mRNA are significantly lower in brain samples from autistic subjects, reflecting an adaptive response to neuroinflammation and oxidative stress. These factors allow the formulation of a "redox/methylation hypothesis of autism," described by Richard Deth in Chapter 7, which outlines a molecular mechanism whereby heavy metals promote oxidative stress and impaired methylation, leading to disrupted development and autism.

In Chapter 8, George Wagner and colleagues describe novel models of autism in which mice are exposed either pre- or post-natally to toxicants such as valproic acid and methylmercury. The early toxicant exposure results in neurodevelopmental deficits in mice that are analogous to deficits observed in humans affected by autism. Evidence that oxidative stress is involved in autism is provided by the ability of pretreatment with antioxidants (trolox, a water-soluble vitamin E derivative) to fully protect the developing mice against the neurobehavioral deficits induced by these toxicants. These observations are discussed in the context of autism prevention.

In Chapter 9, Woody McGinnis and colleagues discuss an interesting hypothesis for the unexplained phenomenon of regression in autism. In their model, visceral dysfunction in autism occurs in conjunction with lost phonation and social function because of selective toxicant effects on a relatively minute region of the brainstem, which is known to remain permeable to a broad class of neurotoxins after the closure of the blood–brain barrier elsewhere. By converging on the same site and sharing oxidative modes of injury, these toxins may act independently, additively, or sequentially to result in autistic regression.

In Chapter 10, Ved Chauhan and I review evidence that ASD are associated with abnormalities in lipid metabolism, membrane-associated proteins, and signal transduction. Phospholipids and their lipid raft domain play important roles in cellular signaling, and phosphoinositides are major signaling molecules in G protein–coupled receptor signaling. We discuss our findings on altered levels of amino-glycerophospholipids in the membrane, increased peroxidation of lipids, decreased membrane fluidity, increased activity of phospholipase A_2 (lipid-metabolizing enzyme), and altered activities of protein kinase C and protein kinase A in autism, suggesting that membrane signaling may be affected in autism. We also review the evidence of an association of the phosphatidylinositol 3-kinase gene in autism, altered brain levels of Bcl2 and p53 (involved in apoptosis), altered levels of cytokines and inflammation and mutational changes in the proteins involved in cell signaling such as neuroligins, Pten, SHANK3, Wnt, reelin, and voltage-dependent calcium channels, all suggesting impairment in signal transduction in autism. These abnormalities in the signal system may account for some of the structural changes and cognitive deficits in the brains of individuals with autism.

Mitochondria play a major role in ROS generation and cytosolic calcium sequestration, and a primary defect in mitochondrial electron transport and oxidative phosphorylation impairs both processes. Conversely, abnormal calcium signaling will secondarily perturb these mitochondrial functions, as the mitochondria have recently been shown to participate with the endoplasmic reticulum in this important process that governs a wide array of cellular functions. In Chapter 11, Jay Gargus presents a genetic scheme as the basis for the elevated levels of ROS observed in autism, which integrates earlier observations of genetic and functional mitochondrial dysfunction in autism with newer observations of defects in calcium signaling in the disease. Recently, Timothy syndrome, a rare monogenic form of autism, was shown to be a channelopathy caused by a mutation in a calcium channel. In addition, diseases comorbid with autism, such as migraine and seizures, share a channelopathy pathogenesis, strengthening the notion that defects in calcium signaling may be a cardinal aspect of the disorder that may represent a target for novel therapeutics.

Some parents of autistic children report frequent infection, prolonged illness, or chronic sinopulmonary symptoms, which are suggestive of immune abnormalities in autism. Emerging evidence from several independent research groups indicates the role of the immune system and inflammation in the pathogenesis and pathophysiology of ASD. Increased oxidative damage and/or mitochondrial dysfunction can also lead to inflammation because oxidative stress serves as a major upstream component in the signaling cascade involved in the activation of redox-sensitive transcription factors and pro-inflammatory gene expression resulting in an inflammatory response.

Recently, it has become evident that the neuroimmune network is crucial for immune homeostasis and the function of the central nervous system (CNS). In Chapter 12, Carlos Pardo-Villamizar and Andrew Zimmerman review the findings on the activation of neuroglia and the neuroimmune system, as evidenced by neuroinflammation in brains, reactive astrogliosis, activated microglia, and cytokine abnormalities. They also discuss the role of the maternal immune environment and immunogenetic factors in autism.

Innate immunity plays a key role in the neuroimmune network. However, the role of innate immunity in the onset and progression of ASD is not well understood. In Chapter 13, Harumi Jyonouchi reviews immune abnormalities reported in children with ASD, following an overview of innate immunity in the GI tract and the CNS. Finally, the possible impact of innate immunity on neuroimmune interactions in autistic children is discussed. In Chapter 14, Paul Ashwood and colleagues review cell-mediated immune response, autoimmunity, cytokine abnormalities, gut inflammation, and GI dysfunction and suggest a relationship between GI-related immune dysfunction and autistic behaviors. Abnormal immune responses may predispose individuals to frequent infections, adverse reactions to benign environmental factors, and possibly autoimmune conditions, leading to increased oxidative stress.

Oxytocin (OT) is known to be dysregulated in some autistic children. In Chapter 15, Martha Welch and Benjamin Klein offer the hypothesis that autism arises from the dysregulation of a unified gut/brain system rather than originating in the brain alone. They postulate that autism stems from physiological stress, including oxidative stress, which, if unmodulated, triggers a cascade of adverse interrelated autonomic, endocrinological, neurological, and immunological reactions. They review evidence that dysregulated OT levels and signaling pathways downstream of the oxytocin receptor combined with oxidative stress in the gut may dysregulate a unified gut/brain network and be involved in the pathogenesis of a subset of autism. They also discuss a chain of possible cellular events in gut Paneth cells, involving ROS, β-catenin, matrix metalloproteinase-7, prodefensin, and defensin, which could impact various ion channels in enteric neurons and ultimately influence behavior. A possible mechanism for dysregulation of gut/brain signaling under conditions of abnormal OT levels during a time window critical for newborn development is discussed and compared with the same mechanism when modulated by adequate OT levels in normal newborns. Finally, they discuss possible early therapeutic interventions aimed at the OT-related mechanism postulated in this chapter.

Cytokines play an important role in the regulation of inflammatory responses and are involved in the regulation of both innate and acquired immunities. They are often encoded by highly polymorphic genes. Some of these polymorphisms are responsible for quantitative interindividual differences in cytokine production, thereby influencing the relative strength of immune responses. In the last 10 years, evidence has accumulated that increased levels of some pro-inflammatory cytokines are present in the peripheral blood mononuclear cells of children with ASD. In Chapter 16, Fabián Crespo and colleagues suggest that there are phenotypes of the immune system that are predisposed to stronger or weaker inflammatory immune responses, and these phenotypes can manifest from several different combinations of genotypes of different cytokine genes with variable expressions. They propose that certain expression polymorphisms in key cytokine genes may contribute to the etiology or the emergence of autism by predisposing individuals carrying those genotypes (or their mothers) to altered immune activation to certain antigens. The authors also suggest that the maternal immunogenetic makeup may be associated with the fetal pathogenesis of ASD since cytokines are able to cross the placenta.

In Chapter 17, William Johnson and colleagues discuss alleles of maternal genes that act in the mother to contribute to the phenotype of their affected offspring. These alleles most likely act in the mother during pregnancy to modify the development of the embryo or fetus, for example, brain development in the affected children. Of the 34 reports so far of these maternal alleles, nearly all were in neurodevelopmental disorders, including autism. *HLA-DR4* was originally suspected of being a maternally acting gene allele for autism because its allele frequency was increased in individuals with autism and their mothers, but not their fathers. This has now been confirmed by a case–parent study design. *HLA-DR4* may act in autism by affecting synapse development, by a mechanism including oxidative stress, by a combination of these, or by an as-yet-unknown mechanism.

Chapter 18 is a commentary by Martha Herbert. On the basis of active pathophysiological processes, such as oxidative stress and inflammation in autism, she discusses that the classical autism model, which frames ASD as a genetically determined developmental disorder of the brain whose main manifestation is behavioral alterations, does not predict persistent pathophysiological disturbances in autism. Herbert describes a pathophysiology-centered model of autism, in which it is argued that ASD is not only developmental but also a chronic condition based on active pathophysiology; is not only behavioral but also has somatic and systemic features; is not only genetic but also environmental; and is not a static encephalopathy but is a dynamic, recalcitrant encephalopathy.

The history of the treatment of autism has been dominated by a technical approach mostly highlighted by applied behavior analysis and, to a lesser extent, by psychopharmacology. In Chapter 19, Eric London proposes the utility of using the biopsychosocial method elaborated by George Engel as a conceptual way to treat autism. The implications of these concepts for both research and clinical works are discussed.

I would like to express my gratitude to my coeditors, Drs. Ved Chauhan and Ted Brown, for their help in the review process, and to all the contributors for their chapters. My sincere thanks to CRC Press/Taylor & Francis Group, especially Barbara Norwitz, Patricia Roberson and Jennifer Smith, for their support in compiling and publishing this book. I hope that it will stimulate hypothesis-driven research and be a valuable reference source not only to scientists in the laboratory but also to clinicians and caregivers in the field of autism and related disorders.

Abha Chauhan, PhD

Head, Developmental Neuroscience Laboratory
New York State Institute for Basic Research in Developmental Disabilities
1050 Forest Hill Road
Staten Island, New York 10314, U.S.A.

Tel: 718-494-5258; *Fax*: 718-698-7916
Email: abha.chauhan@omr.state.ny.us

Editors

Abha Chauhan, PhD, is the head of the Developmental Neuroscience Laboratory at the New York State Institute for Basic Research in Developmental Disabilities (IBR), Staten Island, New York.

As a National Science Talent Scholar, Dr. Chauhan received her BS (chemistry honors) in 1976 from the University of Delhi, her MS (biochemistry) in 1978 and her PhD in 1982 from the Department of Biochemistry, Postgraduate Institute of Medical Education and Research, Chandigarh, India. From 1983 to 1984, she worked as a research associate in the Department of Biochemistry at the Mount Sinai School of Medicine, New York. Dr. Chauhan then joined the Department of Neurochemistry at IBR, where she has over 60 publications in the fields of membrane biochemistry, signal transduction, Alzheimer's disease, and autism.

Currently, Dr. Chauhan's major interest is to investigate the biochemical and immunological changes associated with autism in blood samples, lymphoblast cell cultures, and postmortem brain samples, particularly as they relate to markers of oxidative stress, inflammatory response, and the function of the immune system. She is also studying the relationship, if any, between these abnormalities and low- or high-functioning autism groups, as well as the severity of behavior deficits and neuropathological abnormalities in autism. She has been awarded research grants as a principal investigator from the Department of Defense, Autism Speaks, and the Autism Research Institute for her work on autism.

In 2008, Dr. Chauhan served as the guest editor of the "Special Issue on Autism Spectrum Disorders" of the *American Journal of Biochemistry and Biotechnology* (April 2008). She also organized and chaired a colloquium on "Oxidative Stress and Inflammation in Autism Spectrum Disorders" at the American Society for Neurochemistry Meeting in 2009.

Ved Chauhan, PhD, is the head of the Cellular Neurochemistry Laboratory at the New York State Institute for Basic Research in Developmental Disabilities (IBR), Staten Island, New York.

Dr. Chauhan received his MS (biochemistry) in 1975 and his PhD (biochemistry) in 1980 from the Postgraduate Institute for Medical Education and Research, Chandigarh, India. After working as a research associate for two years in the Department of Biochemistry at the University of Southern California, Los Angeles, he joined IBR as a research scientist in 1983.

Dr. Chauhan has published more than 70 research articles in peer-reviewed journals. His work includes but is not limited to phospholipid methylation, calcium traversal across bilayers, the role of phosphoinositides in the activation of protein kinase C, lipid and amyloid β-protein interactions, hydrophobic domain formation by fibrillar amyloid β-protein and its regulation by gelsolin, and membrane abnormalities and cellular signaling in autism.

Dr. Chauhan is a member of the editorial board of the *International Archives of Medicine*, an associate editor of the *Journal of Alzheimer's Disease*, and an associate editor of the "Special Issue on Autism Spectrum Disorders" of the *American Journal of Biochemistry and Biotechnology* (April 2008). He has organized and chaired several national and international symposia on autism.

W. Ted Brown, MD, PhD, is the director of the New York State Institute for Basic Research in Developmental Disabilities (IBR), the chairperson of IBR's Department of Human Genetics, and the director of IBR's George A. Jervis Clinic. He is a fellow of the American College of Medical Genetics and an adjunct professor at the State University of New York-Downstate Medical Center in Brooklyn.

Dr. Brown received his BA in 1967, his MA in 1969 and his PhD in biophysics in 1973 from The Johns Hopkins University, Baltimore, Maryland. He received his MD from Harvard Medical School (cum laude) in 1974. He trained in internal medicine in New York City, undertook a fellowship in clinical genetics, and was appointed as an assistant professor of medicine at the New York Hospital-Cornell University Medical Center in 1978. He began research into premature aging syndromes and Down syndrome while on the Cornell Medical School Faculty, and was an attending physician at New York Hospital and a faculty member of Rockefeller University. In 1981, he became the chairperson of the Department of Human Genetics at IBR. In 1991, he was appointed the director of IBR's Jervis Clinic, and in 2005, he became the director of IBR.

Dr. Brown is the author of more than 300 publications. At IBR, his initial research was on Down syndrome genes. He then focused his research on the fragile X syndrome, which was then newly recognized and is now considered the most common inherited cause of mental retardation. At IBR, he established a DNA diagnostic and molecular laboratory and developed a screening and prenatal testing program for fragile X. He was the first to discover a relationship between autism and the fragile X syndrome. His work on fragile X has ranged from clinical studies relating to phenotype, to family inheritance studies, to mouse model development, and to basic molecular research. His current research focuses on autism genetics and the fragile X syndrome. Dr. Brown is also a recognized world authority on progeria, a rare and tragic disease that afflicts young children with premature aging. He was instrumental in the discovery of the genetic mutation that causes this disease.

Dr. Brown serves on the editorial board of the *American Journal of Intellectual and Developmental Disability*. He has served on the scientific advisory board for Cure Autism Now, the Progeria Research Foundation, and the National Fragile X Foundation.

Contributors

Paul Ashwood, PhD
Department of Medical Microbiology
and Immunology

and

M.I.N.D Institute
University of California at Davis
Davis, California

Tapan Audhya, PhD
Division of Endocrinology
Department of Medicine
New York University School
of Medicine
New York, New York

and

Vitamin Diagnostics Laboratory
Cliffwood Beach, New Jersey

Teresa Wierzba Bobrowicz, MD, PhD
Department of Neuropathology
Institute of Psychiatry and Neurology
Warsaw, Poland

W. Ted Brown, MD, PhD
Department of Human Genetics
New York State Institute for Basic
Research in Developmental
Disabilities
Staten Island, New York

Steven Buyske, PhD
Departments of Statistics and Genetics
Rutgers University
New Brunswick, New Jersey

Manuel Casanova, MD
Department of Psychiatry
and Behavioral Sciences
University of Louisville
Louisville, Kentucky

Abha Chauhan, PhD
Department of Neurochemistry
New York State Institute for Basic
Research in Developmental
Disabilities
Staten Island, New York

Ved Chauhan, PhD
Department of Neurochemistry
New York State Institute for Basic
Research in Developmental
Disabilities
Staten Island, New York

Michelle A. Cheh, PhD
Department of Neuroscience
Rutgers University
New Brunswick, New Jersey

Ira L. Cohen, PhD
Department of Psychology
New York State Institute for Basic
Research in Developmental
Disabilities
Staten Island, New York

Fabián Crespo, PhD
Department of Anthropology

and

Department of Psychiatry
and Behavioral Sciences
University of Louisville
Louisville, Kentucky

Richard C. Deth, PhD
Department of Pharmaceutical
Sciences
Northeastern University
Boston, Massachusetts

Maria Dronca, PhD
Department of Medical Biochemistry
Iuliu Haţieganu University
    of Medicine and Pharmacy
Cluj-Napoca, Romania

Stephen M. Edelson, PhD
Autism Research Institute
San Diego, California

Amanda Enstrom, PhD
Department of Medical Microbiology
    and Immunology

and

M.I.N.D Institute
University of California at Davis
Davis, California

Teresa A. Evans, BS
Department of Pathology
Case Western Reserve University
Cleveland, Ohio

Rafael Fernandez-Botran, PhD
Department of Pathology
    and Laboratory Medicine
School of Medicine
University of Louisville
Louisville, Kentucky

J. Jay Gargus, MD, PhD
Department of Physiology and
    Biophysics

and

Division of Human Genetics
Department of Pediatrics
School of Medicine
University of California, Irvine
Irvine, California

Alycia K. Halladay, PhD
Department of Psychology

and

Department of Pharmacology
    and Toxicology
Rutgers University
New Brunswick, New Jersey

Martha R. Herbert, MD, PhD
Department of Pediatric
    Neurology
Massachusetts General Hospital
Harvard Medical School
Charlestown, Massachusetts

Humi Imaki, PhD
Department of Developmental
    Neurobiology
New York State Institute for Basic
    Research in Developmental
    Disabilities
Staten Island, New York

William G. Johnson, MD
Department of Neurology

and

Center for Childhood Neurotoxicology
    and Exposure Assessment
Robert Wood Johnson
    Medical School
University of Medicine and
    Dentistry of New Jersey
Piscataway, New Jersey

Harumi Jyonouchi, MD
Department of Pediatrics
University of Medicine and
    Dentistry of New Jersey
Newark, New Jersey

Benjamin Y. Klein, MD
Division of Developmental
  Neuroscience
Department of Psychiatry

and

Department of Pathology and Cell Biology
Columbia University Medical Center
New York, New York

Izabela Kuchna, MD, PhD
Department of Developmental
  Neurobiology
New York State Institute for Basic
  Research in Developmental
  Disabilities
Staten Island, New York

George H. Lambert, MD
Department of Pediatrics

and

Center for Childhood Neurotoxicology
  and Exposure Assessment
Robert Wood Johnson
  Medical School
University of Medicine and
  Dentistry of New Jersey
Piscataway, New Jersey

Eric London, MD
Department of Psychology
New York State Institute for Basic
  Research in Developmental
  Disabilities
Staten Island, New York

Shuang Yong Ma, MD, PhD
Department of Developmental
  Neurobiology
New York State Institute for Basic
  Research in Developmental
  Disabilities
Staten Island, New York

Woody R. McGinnis, MD
Autism House of Auckland
Autism New Zealand, Inc.
Auckland, New Zealand

Veronica M. Miller, PhD
Wadsworth Center for Laboratories
  and Research
New York State Department of Health
Albany, New York

Xue Ming, MD, PhD
Department of Neuroscience
University of Medicine and
  Dentistry of New Jersey
Newark, New Jersey

Meghan Mott, MS
Department of Psychiatry
  and Behavioral Sciences
School of Medicine
University of Louisville
Louisville, Kentucky

Christina R. Muratore, BS
Department of Pharmaceutical
  Sciences
Northeastern University
Boston, Massachusetts

Krzysztof Nowicki, MD
Department of Developmental
  Neurobiology
New York State Institute for Basic
  Research in Developmental
  Disabilities
Staten Island, New York

Carlos A. Pardo-Villamizar, MD
Division of Neuroimmunology
  and Neuroinfectious Disorders
Department of Neurology
Johns Hopkins University School
  of Medicine
Baltimore, Maryland

Sergiu P. Paşca, MD
Center for Cognitive and Neural Studies
Cluj-Napoca, Romania

George Perry, PhD
College of Sciences
University of Texas at San Antonio
San Antonio, Texas

and

Department of Pathology
Case Western Reserve University
Cleveland, Ohio

Marianne Polunas, MS
Department of Pharmacology
    and Toxicology
Rutgers University
New Brunswick, New Jersey

Kenneth R. Reuhl, PhD
Department of Pharmacology
    and Toxicology
Rutgers University
New Brunswick, New Jersey

Elizabeth M. Sajdel-Sulkowska, DSc
Department of Psychiatry
Harvard Medical School

and

Department of Psychiatry
Brigham and Women's Hospital
Boston, Massachusetts

Robert G. Salomon, PhD
Department of Chemistry
Case Western Reserve University
Cleveland, Ohio

Lonnie Sears, PhD
Department of Pediatrics
University of Louisville
Louisville, Kentucky

Mark A. Smith, PhD
Department of Pathology
Case Western Reserve University
Cleveland, Ohio

Edward S. Stenroos, BS
Department of Neurology

and

Center for Childhood Neurotoxicology
    and Exposure Assessment
Robert Wood Johnson
    Medical School
University of Medicine and
    Dentistry of New Jersey
Piscataway, New Jersey

Christopher Tillquist, PhD, MPH
Department of Anthropology
University of Louisville
Louisville, Kentucky

George C. Wagner, PhD
Department of Psychology
Rutgers University
New Brunswick, New Jersey

Judy Van de Water, PhD
Division of Rheumatology, Allergy
    and Clinical Immunology
Department of Internal Medicine

and

M.I.N.D Institute
University of California at Davis
Davis, California

Jarek Wegiel, MS
Department of Developmental
    Neurobiology
New York State Institute for Basic
    Research in Developmental
    Disabilities
Staten Island, New York

Jerzy Wegiel, VMD, PhD
Department of Developmental
  Neurobiology
New York State Institute for Basic
  Research in Developmental
  Disabilities
Staten Island, New York

Martha G. Welch, MD
Division of Developmental
  Neuroscience
Department of Psychiatry

and

Department of Pathology and Cell Biology
Columbia University Medical Center
New York, New York

Thomas Wisniewski, MD, PhD
Department of Psychiatry
New York University School
  of Medicine
Silberstein Aging and Dementia
  Research and Treatment Center
New York, New York

Carrie L. Yochum, MS
Department of Psychology
Rutgers University
New Brunswick, New Jersey

Xiongwei Zhu, PhD
Department of Pathology
Case Western Reserve University
Cleveland, Ohio

Andrew W. Zimmerman, MD
Department of Neurology
  and Developmental Medicine
Kennedy Krieger Institute
Baltimore, Maryland

and

Departments of Neurology and
  Psychiatry and Behavioral
  Sciences
Johns Hopkins University School
  of Medicine
Baltimore, Maryland

1 Type, Topography, and Sequelae of Neuropathological Changes Shaping Clinical Phenotype of Autism

Jerzy Wegiel,[1,]* Thomas Wisniewski,[2] Abha Chauhan,[3] Ved Chauhan,[3] Izabela Kuchna,[1] Krzysztof Nowicki,[1] Humi Imaki,[1] Jarek Wegiel,[1] Shuang Yong Ma,[1] Teresa Wierzba Bobrowicz,[4] Ira L. Cohen,[5] Eric London,[5] and W. Ted Brown[6]

Departments of [1]Developmental Neurobiology, [3]Neurochemistry, [5]Psychology, and [6]Human Genetics, New York State Institute for Basic Research in Developmental Disabilities, Staten Island, NY 10314, USA

[2]Department of Psychiatry, New York University School of Medicine, Silberstein Aging and Dementia Research and Treatment Center, New York, NY 10016, USA

[4]Department of Neuropathology, Institute of Psychiatry and Neurology, Warsaw, Poland

CONTENTS

* Corresponding author: Tel.: +1-718-494-5231; fax: +1-718-982-4856; e-mail: J_Wegiel@msn.com

1.1   INTRODUCTION

The aim of this chapter is to identify the type, topography, and sequelae of neuro-pathological changes that contribute to the clinical phenotype of autism. Results of recent magnetic resonance imaging (MRI) and postmortem neuropathological and stereological studies of autism brain suggest a dynamic model of sequential subdivision of age- and brain-specific structural and functional changes. Acceleration of brain growth in the first year of life and deceleration in the second and third years appear to play a pivotal role in the onset of clinical signs of autism (Courchesne and Pierce, 2005b; Courchesne et al., 2001, 2003; Dawson et al., 2007; Dementieva et al., 2005; Gillberg and de Souza, 2002; Redcay and Courchesne, 2005). The range of deviation from the normal trajectory of brain growth may be a factor determining the severity of the disease (Courchesne et al., 2003). Developmental heterochronicity (differential rates of growth of various brain regions compared to controls), resulting in selective overgrowth of some brain regions, appears to be a key factor determining topography and brain region–specific type of cytoarchitectonic changes (Carper and Courchesne, 2005; Carper et al., 2002; Courchesne et al., 2001; Hazlett et al., 2005; Sparks et al., 2002). Topographic developmental heterochronicity may result in impairment of both local and global connectivity, leading to local overconnectivity and impairment of long-distance connectivity (Baron-Cohen, 2004; Casanova et al., 2006; Courchesne and Pierce, 2005a). Stereological studies have revealed neuronal developmental heterochronicity in early childhood, resulting in selective developmental delay of the growth of neurons in some subcortical structures and the cerebellum during the most critical stage of development of social behaviors and communication skills (Wegiel et al., 2008). Distortions of brain and neuronal development are reflected in abnormal cortical minicolumn organization (Casanova et al., 2002, 2006), local dysgenesis, and ectopias (Bauman and Kemper, 1985; Bauman et al., 1997; Kemper and Bauman, 1993, 1998). These complex developmental abnormalities appear to lay the foundation for secondary and tertiary metabolic, structural, and functional changes, including seizures and risk of sudden unexpected death; signs of oxidative stress, early and enhanced accumulation of products of cell organelle degradation with lipofuscin deposition; modified processing of β-amyloid precursor protein with accumulation of truncated amyloid beta; and other as of yet unidentified changes. Secondary pathologic changes appear to be indicators of the susceptibility of abnormally developing neurons to further modifications during cell maturation and aging. The pattern of morphological changes emerging from these multidisciplinary studies appears to represent a major trend. However, modifications of the course of disease and subpatterns of developmental changes result in a broad spectrum of morphological and clinical interindividual differences.

1.2 CLINICAL, ETIOLOGICAL, AND NEUROPATHOLOGICAL DIVERSITY IN AUTISM

Autism is the prototype of a pervasive developmental disorder (PDD) and is characterized by (a) qualitative impairments in reciprocal social interactions, (b) qualitative impairments in verbal and nonverbal communication, (c) restricted repetitive and stereotyped patterns of behavior, interests, and activities, and (d) onset prior to the age of 3 years. PDD also includes childhood disintegrative disorder, Asperger's disorder, Rett syndrome, and pervasive developmental disorder—not otherwise specified (PDD-NOS). The common features of all these disorders are qualitative deficits in social behavior and communication (American Psychiatric Association, 2000).

1.2.1 CLINIC

In most cases (90%–95%), it is not presently possible to detect a known or specific etiology. These cases are referred to as idiopathic or nonsyndromic autism (Boddaert et al., 2009; Gillberg and Coleman, 1996). In 6% (Fombonne, 2003), 5% (Tuchman et al., 1991), or 10% (Rutter et al., 1994) of cases, autism was diagnosed in association with other disorders. About 30% of children with idiopathic autism have complex autism, defined by the presence of dysmorphic features, microcephaly and/or a structural brain malformation (Miles et al., 2005). About 70% of children with autism have essential autism, defined by the absence of physical abnormalities. For most children, the onset of autism is gradual. However, a multisite study revealed significant regression at ages of 18 to 33 months (regressive autism) in about 13.8% (Colorado) to 31.6% (Utah) of autistic subjects (Department of Health and Human Services, 2007). Moreover, the manifestations of autism vary greatly, depending on developmental level and chronological age of the affected individual. The majority of patients exhibit serious social and communicative impairments throughout life but some improve enough to be able to live relatively independently as adults. In 44.6% of children, autism is associated with cognitive impairment (defined as having intelligence quotient scores of <70; Department of Health and Human Services, 2007). Expressive language function in individuals with autism may vary from mutism to verbal fluency (Rapin, 1996; Stone et al., 1997; Wetherby et al., 1998). Sensorimotor deficits also show significant interindividual differences, with more frequent and severe impairments of gross and fine motor function (motor stereotypes, hypotonia, limbic apraxia) in subjects with lower IQ (Rogers et al., 1996). Hand mannerisms and body rocking are reported in 37% to 95% of individuals with autism (Lord and Rutter, 1995; Rapin, 1996; Rogers et al., 1996), whereas preoccupation with sensory features of objects, abnormal responsiveness to environmental stimuli, or paradoxical responses to sensory stimuli are seen in 42% to 88% of people with autism (Kientz and Dunn, 1997). Epilepsy is a comorbid complication, occurring in up to 33% of individuals with autism (Tuchman and Rapin, 2002).

1.2.2 Etiology

The clinical diversity of autism reflects the etiologic heterogeneity of this disorder. Genetic factors; pre-, peri-, and postnatal pathological factors; and concurrent diseases may contribute to autism (Muhle et al., 2004; Newschaffer et al., 2002; Rutter et al., 1994). About 5% to 10% of cases are associated with several distinct genetic conditions including fragile X syndrome, tuberous sclerosis, phenylketonuria, Rett syndrome, and chromosomal anomalies such as Down syndrome (DS) (Folstein and Rosen-Scheidley, 2001; Fombonne, 2003; Smalley et al., 1988; Yonan et al., 2003). Autism spectrum disorders (ASDs) in people with DS have been described in several reports (Ghaziuddin et al., 1992; Howlin et al., 1995; Prasher and Clarke, 1996; Wakabayashi, 1979), and the prevalence of autism in boys with DS was estimated as at least 7% (Kent et al., 1999). The prevalence of autism in the fragile X syndrome is estimated as 15%–28% (Hagerman, 2002). Cytogenetic abnormalities (partial duplications, deletions, inversions) in the 15q11-q13 region account for 1% to 4% of autism cases (Cook, 1998; Gillberg, 1998). Several potential candidate genes have been identified in both autosomes and X chromosomes, including the tuberous sclerosis gene on chromosomes 9 and 16; serotonin transporter on chromosome 17; gamma-aminobutyric acid receptor-beta 3 on chromosome 15; neuroligins on the X chromosome (see Vorstman et al., 2006); and possibly *PTEN* on chromosome 10 (Butler et al., 2005). Modifications in the tryptophan hydroxylase gene may play a modest role in autism susceptibility (Coon et al., 2005).

1.2.3 NEUROPATHOLOGY

While knowledge of the clinical and genetic factors in autism is based on examination of thousands of patients, postmortem neuropathological studies are based on reports of a very small number of brains. A review by Palmen et al. (2004) revealed that between 1980 and 2003, only 58 brains of individuals with autism have been examined, and results of only a few neuropathological and stereological studies were published. Usually, neuropathological reports and morphometric reports were based on evaluation of one or several brains. Due to the broad age spectrum and the etiological and clinical diversity in autism, the pattern of neuropathological changes reported is incomplete and often inconsistent. As a result, the morphological markers and neuropathological diagnostic criteria of autism have not yet been established (Lord et al., 2000; Pickett and London, 2005). In the past, the contribution of postmortem studies to the detection and characterization of neuropathological changes and mechanisms leading to structural and functional manifestations of autism was limited because of (a) the deficit of autism brains, resulting in a lack of statistical power, (b) the lack of efficient mechanisms for sharing the limited tissue resources, (c) the lack of complex studies of the dynamic of changes during the life span, (d) the infrequent application of unbiased morphometric methods to detect quantitative differences, and (e) the averaging of results from subjects with different clinical and morphological manifestations of autism. Heterogeneity within the autism spectrum is the major obstacle to autism research at all levels (Newschaffer et al., 2002), including neuropathological studies and attempts at detection of clinicopathological correlations. Recent evidence of genetic fractionation of social impairment, communication difficulties, and rigid and repetitive behaviors indicates that heterogeneity in ASD could be an unavoidable consequence of the contribution of nonoverlapping genes. If different features of autism are caused by different genes associated with different brain regions and related to different core cognitive impairments (Happe et al., 2006), it seems likely that many brain networks are involved in the pathology of autism. The diversity of neuropathological findings and the commonly reported inconsistencies in regional findings correspond to developmental impairments in many interacting brain networks and to expansion from "local" abnormalities to "nonlocal" effects of the emerging cognitive system. In spite of these limitations, "localizing" models are still the main approach to the identification of pathological changes as a component of the structural and functional abnormalities of the networks (Müller, 2007).

The possibility that autism is associated with neuropathological changes was explored in the first studies reported between 1980 and 1989 (Bauman and Kemper, 1985; Courchesne et al., 1987, 1988; Damasio et al., 1980; Gaffney et al., 1987; Hashimoto et al., 1989, 1993; Murakami et al., 1989; Ritvo et al., 1986). Expansion of these studies through examination of larger cohorts and application of stereology, functional and structural MRI, and biochemistry resulted in the identification of several major forms of pathology contributing to the clinical phenotype including abnormal acceleration of brain growth in early childhood (Redcay and Courchesne, 2005), delay of neuronal growth (Wegiel et al., 2008), changes in brain cytoarchitecture (Bailey et al., 1998; Bauman and Kemper, 1985; Casanova et al., 2002, 2006), metabolic modifications with abnormal amyloid precursor protein (APP) processing (Bailey et al., 2008; Brown et al., 2008; Sokol et al., 2006), enhanced oxidative stress (reviewed in Chauhan and Chauhan, 2006), and turnover of cell organelle with pigment accumulation and glial activation (Lopez-Hurtado and Prieto, 2008).

1.3   DEREGULATION OF BRAIN GROWTH IN EARLY CHILDHOOD

The major measures of age-related changes are head circumference, MRI-based volumetry of the brain and brain structures, and postmortem brain weight and volume of brain subdivisions. Between 1990 and 2000, several groups reported increased head circumference (Bailey et al., 1995; Bolton et al., 1995; Davidovitch et al., 1996; Fidler et al., 2000; Fombonne et al., 1999; Lainhart et al., 1997; Miles et al., 2000; Steg and Rapoport, 1975; Stevenson et al., 1997), whereas MRI-based studies revealed increased brain volume (Piven et al., 1995, 1996). According to Fombonne et al. (1999), the prevalence of macrocephaly in autism is about 20%. In a report by Bailey et al. (1998), four of six subjects with autism 4 to 24 years of age had macrocephaly. Increased brain weight was reported in postmortem studies by Bailey et al. (1993) and Kemper and Bauman (1998). Increase in the volume was regional and not generalized, with the greatest enlargement in the occipital and parietal lobes (Filipek, 1996; Filipek et al., 1999; Piven et al., 1995, 1996). However, in several studies, an increase in brain size was not detected (Garber and Ritvo, 1992; Haznedar et al., 2000). Inconsistency in detection of abnormal head and brain size can be associated with interindividual differences, the age of examined individuals, and the methods applied. Courchesne et al. (2003) integrated their work and that of other researchers into the concept of four phases of modified brain growth, described below.

At birth, the head circumference of neonates later diagnosed with autism is normal or slightly less than that observed in normally developing children (Courchesne et al., 2003; Dawson et al., 2007; Dementieva et al., 2005; Dissanayake et al., 2006; Gillberg and de Souza, 2002; Hazlett et al., 2005; Lainhart et al., 1997; Mason-Brothers et al., 1990; Stevenson et al., 1997). Slight undergrowth is independent of body growth and may be a reflection of prenatal neural developmental defects corresponding to pathology detected in postmortem studies of the brains of autistic adults (Bailey et al., 1998; Casanova et al., 2002; Courchesne et al., 2003; Kemper and Bauman, 1998). In only 5% of neonates diagnosed later as autistic was the head circumference more than that in normally developing infants (Courchesne et al., 2003; Dementieva et al., 2005).

In the second phase, by 1 or 2 years of age, a rapid and large increase in head circumference distinguished children diagnosed later with autism from normally developing children (Courchesne et al., 2003; Dawson et al., 2007; Dementieva et al., 2005; Dissanayake et al., 2006; Hazlett et al., 2005). Ninety percent of 2- and 3-year-old children with autism had brain volumes larger than those of control children (Courchesne at al., 2001). According to Dawson et al. (2007), a period of exceptionally rapid head growth is limited to the first year of life, and head growth decelerates after 12 months of age. Acceleration of growth in head circumference appears to begin at about 4 months (Courchesne and Pierce, 2005a; Gillberg and de Souza, 2002; Redcay and Courchesne, 2005). Using meta-analysis based on evaluation of head circumference converted to brain volume, brain volume measured from MRI, and brain weight from postmortem studies, Redcay and Courchesne (2005) revealed that brain size increases from 13% smaller than in control subjects at birth to 10% larger than in control infants at 1 year, but only 2% greater by adolescence. The greater growth rate of head circumference in the first year, and its return to normal rates thereafter, is not accounted for by an overall growth in stature. Studies of behavioral development in infants later diagnosed with autism suggest that the period of acceleration of head growth precedes and overlaps with the onset of behavioral changes, and that the period of deceleration coincides with a period of behavioral decline or worsening of symptoms in the second year of life (Dawson et al., 2007). Coincidence of acceleration of brain growth rate with onset and worsening of clinical symptoms may indicate that structural developmental changes critical for a lifelong phenotype occur in early infancy. Acceleration of brain growth in the first year and deceleration in the second year of life suggest that failure of the mechanism controlling brain growth in the first year of life plays an essential role in the onset of clinical features of autism. Identification of these mechanisms may lead to conceptualization of early preventive treatments.

In the third phase, of 2 to 4 years, the overall rate of brain growth slows but is still 10% more than in normally developing children (Carper et al., 2002; Courchesne et al., 2001; Hazlett et al., 2005; Sparks et al., 2002). In 4- to 5-year-old autistic children, MRI-based estimated brain volume is 1350 mL, whereas in normally developing children, a comparable volume (1360 mL) is reached about 8 years later. In postmortem studies, the brain weight of 3- to 5-year-old autistic males was 15% higher (1451 g) than in control males of this age (1259 g) (Redcay and Courchesne, 2005).

In the fourth phase, the volume of the brain decreases, and this trend extends from middle/late childhood through adulthood. Head (Aylward et al., 2002) or brain enlargement (Bailey et al., 1998; Hardan et al., 2001; Lainhart et al., 1997; Piven et al., 1995, 1996) has also been observed in studies of older populations of autistic individuals. However, by adolescence and adulthood, the average size of the brain is only 1% to 3% greater in autistic than in control cohorts (Redcay and Courchesne, 2005).

Moreover, the pattern of brain growth reflects the severity of clinical manifestation of autism (Courchesne et al., 2003). Among infants who have the more severe form of autism, 71% showed increases during their first year of more than 1.5 S.D., with 59% showing increases between 2.0 and 4.3 S.D. In children with a less severe form of autism, PDD-NOS, acceleration of brain growth is observed later, and the increase is less pronounced. Later onset and slower rate of progression of autism appear to be associated with a better outcome.

1.3.1 DEVELOPMENTAL HETEROCHRONICITY

Developmental heterochronicity studies indicate that autism is a disorder involving a transient period of pathological acceleration of brain growth. Developmental heterochronicity, with different rates of growth for different brain regions/structures, appears to be the second major factor contributing to the clinical phenotype. MRI studies showed that overgrowth of the frontal and temporal lobes and amygdala, brain regions that are involved in cognitive, social, and emotional functions as well as language development, is synchronized with brain overgrowth in 2- to 4-year-old autistic children in contrast to a different rate of growth of the occipital cortex (Carper and Courchesne, 2005; Carper et al., 2002; Courchesne et al., 2001; Hazlett et al., 2005; Sparks et al., 2002). The reduced size of the body and posterior subregions of the corpus callosum noted in subjects with autism may indicate disproportions in brain subregions development (Piven et al., 1997b). The cellular and molecular basis for transient acceleration of brain growth and enhanced growth of some brain regions is not known, but Courchesne et al. (2003) proposed that the observed pattern is associated with an excessive number of neurons, enhanced rate of growth of size of neurons, and increased number of minicolumns as well as excessive and premature expansion of the dendritic tree.

1.3.2 FUNCTIONAL CONSEQUENCES OF ABNORMAL BRAIN DEVELOPMENT

Using a computational model analogue of autism, Cohen (2007) has argued that an interaction between stochastic and above-average or "excessive" numbers of neural connection factors has implications for understanding the disorder. In particular, a relative excess of connections could lead to enhanced recognition of complex patterns in the environment. In Cohen's chapter, it was noted that if large and complex brains are in part familial (Courchesne et al., 2003; Fidler et al., 2000), and brain size is heritable (Pfefferbaum et al., 2000) and positively correlated with IQ (Pennington et al., 2000), then behavioral outcomes both within and across generations of family members could result in (a) individuals who may be unusually gifted in their ability to handle complex nonlinear problems such as mathematics or computer science, (b) individuals with autism, or (c) individuals with a combination of autism or autistic-like behavior and giftedness (many typical Asperger's cases). These trends are detected among relatives of subjects with autism (Folstein and Rutter, 1988).

The effect of an abnormal trajectory of brain development observed in autism are well-validated characteristics of the learning style of children with autism, including (a) greater attention to idiosyncratic than socially relevant stimuli, (b) stimulus overselectivity or a lack of drive for central coherence, (c) problems with acquiring fuzzy concepts, (d) development of savant skills, (e) problems with generalization of previously acquired skills, (f) rigidity and resistance to change, (g) social and communication deficits, and (h) difficulty in learning complex higher-order concepts (Cohen, 2007).

1.4 CORTICAL AND SUBCORTICAL NEUROPATHOLOGY

1.4.1 CORTICAL DYSGENESIS, LAMINATION DEFECTS, MIGRATION DISTURBANCES

The fundamental characteristics of the neuropathological changes described by Kemper and Bauman (1993, 1998), Bauman and Kemper (1985, 1996), and Bauman et al. (1997) suggest three major neuropathologies in the brain of people with autism: (a) curtailed development of neurons in the structures that are substrates for memory and emotions—the entorhinal cortex, hippocampus, subiculum, anterior cingulate gyrus and mamillary body; (b) a congenital decrease in the number of Purkinje cells in the cerebellum; and (c) age-related differences in cell size and number of neurons in the cerebellar nuclei and in the inferior olivary nucleus. Microdysgenesis is represented by increased neuronal density in the cortical layer, clustering of cortical neurons, disorganization of cortical layers, neuron cytomegaly, ectopic neurons, and nodular heterotopias. A detailed study of serial sections from the brain of a 29-year-old man with autism revealed reduced neuronal size and increased cell-packing density (Bauman and Kemper, 1985), both features of an immature brain (Friede, 1975). Cell-packing density was increased by 66% in the hypothalamus and mamillary body, and by 54% in the medial septal nucleus, with smaller nerve cells. The reduced size of neurons and the selective increase in cell-packing density were seen in central (40%), medial (28%), and cortical nuclei (35%). Atrophy of the neocerebellar cortex, with marked loss of Purkinje cells and, to a lesser extent, of granule cells, was present in gracile, tonsil, and inferior semilunar lobules. Changes were not detected in the anterior lobe or the vermis. Reduced numbers of cells were noticed in fastiglial, globose, and emboliform nuclei, and cells were small and pale. The dentate nucleus was distorted. Retrograde neuronal loss in the inferior olive related to neuronal loss in cerebellar cortex was not found, but olivary neurons were small and pale. Brain cytoarchitecture abnormalities were not associated with gliosis. In a 21-year-old female with autism, Rodier et al. (1996) found that the brain was smaller than a control brain, and the length of facial nerve nucleus was less than 500 μm as compared to 2610 μm in the control subject.

1.4.2 Brain Structure–Specific Delay of Neuronal Growth

The reduced size of neurons and their nuclei in the cortex of autistic subjects reported by Casanova et al. (2006) could be an indicator of reduced or impaired functional connectivity between distant cortical regions (Casanova et al., 2006; Just et al., 2004; Koshino et al., 2005). Our ongoing studies of series of brains from age-matched autistic and control subjects (Wegiel et al., 2008) indicate that reduced size of neurons is a brain structure–specific marker. In 4- to 7-year-old autistic children, Purkinje cells were smaller by 38%. Neurons in the dentate nucleus were reduced by 26%; in the amygdala, by 24%; in the nucleus accumbens, by 41%; in caudate, by 20%; and in the putamen, by 27%. Neurons in the nucleus of the facial nerve and the nucleus olivaris did not show a significant difference from controls. The second significant feature of the pattern of neuronal size abnormalities is the partial or complete correction of the size of neurons (for example, in the nucleus accumbens) observed in late childhood or adulthood. This study indicates that the delay of growth of neurons is the most consistent pathology detected in the brains of examined people with autism. Pathology is brain structure–specific. Changes may range from no delay to severe developmental delay. The youngest examined children (4 to 7 years old) show the most severe deficit in the volume of the neuronal body and nucleus. Partial correction of cell volume is observed in late childhood and adulthood, which indicates that brain structure and function undergo modifications during the life span. The study of basal ganglia and cerebellum supports the hypothesis that clinical manifestations of autism are the result of regional neuronal maldevelopment.

One may assume that mechanisms regulating growth of the neuron in early childhood are the target of factors that are the cause of autism. The result of deregulation of these mechanisms could be (a) significantly delayed growth of neuronal body, nucleus, dendritic tree, spines, and reduced number of synapses and (b) functional deficits corresponding to these structural developmental delays. These abnormalities of very early childhood might be the major contributor to clinical deficits that are the basis for the clinical diagnosis of autism at the age of 3 years.

1.4.3 MINICOLUMNAR ABNORMALITIES IN AUTISM

The next significant contribution to detection of neocortical developmental pathology is the result of studies of minicolumns by Casanova's group (Buxhoeveden and Casanova, 2002; Casanova et al., 2002, 2006). Malformations of cortical development are observed in heterogeneous disorders caused by abnormalities of cell proliferation, apoptosis, cell migration, cortical organization, and axon pathfinding (Hevner, 2007). Clinically malformations of cortical development are significant causes of mental retardation, seizures, cerebral palsy, and neuropsychiatric disorders (Barkovich et al., 2005; Guerrini and Marini, 2006; Sarnat and Flores-Sarnat, 2004). Minicolumns are considered a basic architectonic and functional unit of the human neocortex (Buxhoeveden and Casanova, 2002; Casanova et al., 2002). Increased neuron density by 23%, reduced size of neurons in minicolumns, and a concomitant increase in the total number of minicolumns appears to illustrate the bias of local rather than global information processing (Casanova et al., 2002, 2006), resulting in a "hyper-specific brain" (McClelland, 2000). Synchronization of interactions requiring the involvement of distant brain regions is impaired in autism as a result of developmental connectivity deficits (underconnectivity) of smaller neurons (Just et al., 2004; Koshino et al., 2005; Zilbovicius et al., 1995). Structural imaging studies also suggest the overrepresentation of short association fibers in autism, with a regional increase in the volume of white matter (Herbert et al., 2004) favoring the local information processing observed in autistic subjects (Happe, 1999).

1.5 NEURONAL OXIDATIVE STRESS AND METABOLIC CHANGES

An increasing body of evidence suggests that the abnormal rate of development of neurons and neuronal networks in early infancy is followed by metabolic changes, with signs of oxidative stress, enhanced autophagocytosis, and lipofuscin accumulation, leading to early selective neuronal structural and functional changes.

1.5.1 OXIDATIVE STRESS IN AUTISM

Oxidative stress is known to be associated with premature aging of cells and can lead to inflammation, damaged cell membranes, autoimmunity, and cell death. The brain is highly vulnerable to oxidative stress due to its limited antioxidant capacity, higher energy requirement, and high amounts of unsaturated lipids and iron (Juurlink and Peterson, 1998). The brain makes up about 2% of body mass but consumes 20% of metabolic oxygen. The vast majority of energy is used by the neurons (Shulman et al., 2004). Glutathione (GSH) is the most important antioxidant for detoxification and elimination of environmental toxins. Due to the lack of glutathione-producing capacity by neurons, the brain has a limited capacity to detoxify reactive oxygen species (ROS). Therefore, neurons are the first cells to be affected by the increase in ROS and shortage of antioxidants and, as a result, they are most susceptible to oxidative stress. Antioxidants are required for neuronal survival during the early critical period (Perry et al., 2004). Children are more vulnerable than adults to oxidative stress because of their naturally low glutathione levels from conception through infancy (Erden-Inal et al., 2002; Ono et al., 2001). The risk created by this natural deficit in detoxification capacity in infants is increased by the fact that some environmental factors that induce oxidative stress are found at higher concentrations in developing infants than in their mothers, and accumulate in the placenta.

Accumulating evidence from our and other groups suggests increased oxidative stress in autism (reviewed in Chauhan and Chauhan, 2006). Lipid peroxidation is a chain reaction between polyunsaturated fatty acids and ROS, producing lipid peroxides and hydrocarbon polymers that are both highly toxic to the cell. We have reported that levels of malondialdehyde (MDA), a marker of lipid peroxidation, are increased in the plasma from children with autism (Chauhan et al., 2004). Other studies on erythrocytes (Zoroglu et al., 2004) and urine samples (Ming et al., 2005) have also indicated increased levels of lipid peroxidation markers in autism, thus confirming an increased oxidative stress in autism. Recent studies with the postmortem brain samples from autism and control subjects have provided further evidence on increased oxidative stress in autism. Increased levels of lipid-derived oxidative protein modifications, i.e., carboxyethylpyrrole and iso[4]levuglandin E_2–protein adducts, and heme-oxygenase-1 (an inducible antioxidant enzyme) have been reported in the autistic brain, primarily in the white matter (Evans et al., 2008). Sajdel-Sulkowska et al. (2008) have reported elevated levels of 3-nitrotyrosine (a specific marker for oxidative damage to proteins) in the cerebella of subjects with autism. In addition, we have observed increased lipid peroxidation in cerebellum and temporal cortex of brain in autism (Chauhan et al., 2009). MDA levels were significantly increased by 124% in the cerebellum, and by 256% in the temporal cortex in autism as compared to control subjects.

1.5.2 Lipofuscin in Autism

Lopez-Hurtado and Prieto (2008) revealed a significant increase in the number of lipofuscin-containing cells in the brain of 7- to 14-year-old autistic subjects (by 69% in area 22, 149% in area 39, and 45% in area 44). The increase in the number of lipofuscin-containing cells was paralleled by neuronal loss and glial proliferation. Lipofuscin accumulation is a component of aging (Brunk and Terman 2002a,b; Brunk et al., 1992; Szweda et al., 2003), the neurodegeneration observed in Alzheimer's (Stojanovic et al., 1994) and Parkinson's diseases (Tórsdóttir et al., 1999), developmental syndromes such as Rett syndrome (Jellinger et al., 1988), and autism (Lopez-Hurtado and Prieto, 2008), and such psychiatric disorders as bipolar affective disorder (Yanik et al., 2004) and schizophrenia (Akyol et al., 2002; Herken et al., 2001).

Lipofuscin is an intralysosomal deposit of products of autophagocytosis and degradation of cytoplasmic components, including mitochondria, which cannot be degraded further or exocytosed. Oxidative stress is considered the factor contributing to lipid and protein damage and degradation, resulting in lipofuscin production and accumulation (Brunk et al., 1992; Sohal and Brunk, 1989). The presence of oxidatively modified proteins and lipids in lipofuscin supports the causative link between enhanced oxidative stress, autophagocytosis, and deposition of products of degradation in the lysosomal pathway and lipofuscin (Brunk and Terman, 2002a,b; Szweda et al., 2003; Terman and Brunk, 2004) and suggests that in autism, abnormal development is associated with early signs of oxidative stress and enhanced degradation and, possibly, turnover of cytoplasmic components.

1.5.3 β-Amyloid Precursor Protein and Intraneuronal Amyloid β in Autism

Sokol et al. (2006) detected signs of overexpression of APP in about 40% of autistic subjects. The levels of secreted APP in plasma in children with severe autistic behavior and aggression were two or more times the levels in children without autism, and up to fourfold more than in children with mild autism. The trend observed in autistic children, with higher levels of secreted β-APP and nonamyloidogenic secreted β-APP, and lower levels of Aβ 1–40 compared to controls, suggests an increased α-secretase pathway in autism (anabolic nonamyloidogenic APP processing). Enzyme-linked immunosorbent assay (ELISA) study of blood plasma from 25 autistic children 2–4 years of age and 25 age-matched control children revealed significantly increased level of secreted amyloid precursor protein alpha (sAPP-α) in 60% of autistic children (Bailey et al., 2008). Western blotting analysis confirmed higher levels of sAPP-α in autistic children.

Amino-terminally truncated intraneuronal amyloid (Aβ) is present in the neurons of control subjects, and the amount of intraneuronal Aβ increases with age (Wegiel et al., 2007). This study of 10 brains of autistic people revealed enhanced intraneuronal accumulation of amino-terminally truncated Aβ in 50% of autistic subjects, including in one 5-year-old child and four adults 20, 23, 52, and 62 years of age. A similar pattern was also found in four examined brains of people with autism and isodicentric chromosome 15 (idic15) (Brown et al., 2008). In idic15, excessive accumulation of intraneuronal Aβ might be related to an extra copy of one of the amyloid precursor protein-binding protein (APBA-2) genes localized on chromosome 15. In many brain regions, Aβ is accumulated in large cytoplasmic granules corresponding to deposits of lipofuscin. Numerous large lipofuscin deposits with very strong Aβ immunoreactivity in the neurons of several children and adults with autism appear to reflect severe metabolic stress affecting all of the neurons in the amygdala, all large neurons in the caudate/putamen, a majority of Purkinje cells, and the neurons in the dentate nucleus and nucleus olivaris, but only about 30%–40% of cortical pyramidal neurons. Accumulation of truncated Aβ appears to be a by-product of enhanced degradation of transmembrane APP. The aggregated intracellular Aβ induces the production of ROS and lipid peroxidation products and ultimately results in leakage of the lysosomal membrane (Glabe, 2001). This process appears to affect many neuronal populations, not only in young and old adults, but also in children diagnosed with autism. A metabolic shift with Aβ accumulation in neurons in these brain areas that are involved in the expression of emotions, stereotypic behaviors, and social deficits, such as the amygdala, hippocampus, some striatal subdivisions, and cerebellum, may contribute to cellular dysfunction and the clinical expression of autism.

1.6   CLINICOPATHOLOGICAL CORRELATIONS

Studies of clinicopathological correlations cover several domains of functional deficits in people with autism, including (a) speech, language, and verbal and nonverbal communication, (b) social deficits and face perception, (c) sensorimotor deficits, and (d) cognitive deficits.

1.6.1   SPEECH, LANGUAGE, AND VERBAL AND NONVERBAL COMMUNICATION

Expressive language function of individuals with autism ranges from complete mutism to verbal fluency. Verbal abilities are often accompanied by errors in word meaning (semantics) or language and communicative deficits in social context (social pragmatics) (Rapin, 1996; Stone et al., 1997; Wetherby et al., 1998). Studies of the language-related neocortex, including Wernicke's area (BA 22, speech recognition), Broca's area (BA 44, speech production) and the gyrus angularis (BA 39, reading) of 7- to 44-year-old autistic and 8- to 56-year-old control individuals, revealed reduced numerical density of neurons by 38% in area 22, and by 24% in area 39 in autistic subjects, as well as an increased numerical density of lipofuscin-containing neurons by 50% in BA 22, and 44% in BA 44. These neuronal changes were paralleled by an increase of numerical density of glial cells in all three examined regions. Lopez-Hurtado and Prieto (2008) hypothesized that structural alteration in one or more of these cortical areas may contribute to the communication impairment observed in autism.

1.6.2   FACE PERCEPTION

All subjects with ASDs have disturbance of social behavior, including abnormalities in social reciprocity and difficulties in use of eye contact, facial expression, and social motivation. Social functioning includes eye contact, processing of faces, identification of individuals, and monitoring of face expression (Baron-Cohen et al., 1994). Patients with autism reveal deficits in face-processing (Grelotti et al., 2001), perception (Schultz, 2005), and recognition (Joseph and Tanaka, 2003).

The face-processing network includes the visual cortex (BA17), which projects via the inferior occipital gyrus to the fusiform gyrus. Fibers from the fusiform gyrus project to the amygdala, and inferior frontal gyrus and orbital cortex (Fairhall and Ishai, 2007; van Kooten et al., 2008). Functional magnetic resonance imaging (fMRI) identified the fusiform gyrus and other cortical regions as supporting face-processing in control subjects, and hypoactivity of the fusiform gyrus in autistic patients (Bolte et al., 2006; Kanwisher et al., 1999; Pierce et al., 2004). Hypoactivation of the fusiform gyrus is believed to be associated with the failure to make direct eye contact in autism (Dalton et al., 2005). Results of imaging-based fusiform volume estimation are inconsistent. Increased (Waiter et al., 2004) and unchanged (Pierce et al., 2001) volume in both hemispheres and increased fusiform gyrus in the left hemisphere (Herbert et al., 2002) were reported. Morphometric studies of the brain of 7 autistic and 10 control subjects revealed a reduced number of neurons in layers III, V, and VI, and reduced volume of neuronal soma in layers V and VI in the fusiform gyrus. No alterations in Brodman area 17 in these autistic individuals suggest that the input from the visual cortex to the fusiform gyrus is intact. These results indicate the underdevelopment of connections in the fusiform gyrus that may contribute to abnormal face perception in autism (van Kooten et al., 2008).

Bailey et al. (1998) noted abnormalities in cytoarchitectonic organization and neuronal density in the superior frontal cortex and superior temporal gyrus in autism. Neurons in the superior temporal sulcus are sensitive to the angle of gaze (Perrett et al., 1985). Neurons that are attuned to particular facial expressions were found in the inferior and superior temporal lobes (Hasselmo et al., 1989). Cortical areas responsive to faces, facial expressions, and angle of gaze send direct projections to the amygdala (Stefanacci and Amaral, 2000). Pathological changes in the amygdala may play a central role in the dysfunction seen in autism, including disturbed components of social cognition such as attention to and interpretation of facial expressions. fMRI studies show that judging from the expression of another person's eyes what the other person might be thinking or feeling is associated with activation in the superior temporal gyrus, frontal cortex, and amygdala, whereas in subjects with autism, activation appears in the temporal and frontal cortex but not in the amygdala (Baron-Cohen et al., 1999).

1.6.3 SOCIAL ATTACHMENT—THE ROLE OF THE HYPOTHALAMUS IN BEHAVIORAL DEFICITS

Experimental studies revealed that the hypothalamic nucleus paraventricularis (NPV) and the nucleus supraopticus (NSO), producing oxytocin (OT) and vasopressin (VAS), regulate emotional responses, social attachment, cognitive functions, sleep, and appetite (Barden, 2004; Ehlert et al., 2001; Manaye et al., 2005). OT and VAS are relayed from the human brain into the bloodstream via the posterior pituitary. The presence of receptors for both peptides throughout the forebrain, limbic system, thalamus, brain stem, and spinal cord (Raggenbass, 2001) indicates that hypothalamic neuropeptides modulate the function of many brain regions. Developmental changes in the distribution and expression of receptors suggest that the hypothalamic peptides play a significant role both in brain development and function (Shapiro and Insel, 1989). OT is required for the development of social memory. In OT knockout mice, the loss of social memory could be rescued by OT treatment (Ferguson et al., 2000). VAS is necessary for the formation of social memory and OT for retention of newly formed social memories (Popik and Van Ree, 1992; Popik et al., 1992). OT facilitates the learning of social interactions and the formation of associations that are specifically related to the mother (Nelson and Panksepp, 1996).

The initial product of oxytocin mRNA is a polypeptide containing both nanopeptide OT and neurophysin I, separated by tripeptide glycine-lysine-arginine. The result of enzymatic cleavage are intermediate forms containing 10, 11, or 12 amino acids, collectively referred to as carboxy-extended forms of OT (OT-X), and oxytocin (Gabreels et al., 1998; Gainer et al., 1995; Mitchell et al., 1998; Rao et al., 1992). In 5.8- to 11.5-year-old autistic individuals, reduced plasma OT level, deficits in OT prohormone processing (increase in OT-X), and an increase in the ratio of C-terminal extended forms to OT were found. In control children, nearly all OT-X is metabolized to OT, whereas in autistic children, the immature OT forms serve as the primary circulating molecule in the absence of or in compensation for OT (Green et al., 2001). However, experimental studies show that OT-X is not an effective agonist at OT-sensitive sites (Mitchell et al., 1998). Deficient conversion of OT-X to OT in autism could be the result of alterations in the level of prohormone convertases associated with genetic defects (Cook, 1998; Szatmari et al., 1998). The identification of four single nucleotide polymorphisms located within the OT receptor gene of 195 Chinese autistic subjects indicates that abnormal modulation of the OT receptor results in autism (Wu et al., 2005). OT and VAS are known to play a role in repetitive behaviors. Patients with ASDs show a significant reduction in repetitive behaviors following OT infusion (Hollander et al., 2003). In about 60% of subjects with autism, abnormal sleep patterns are observed. VAS is involved in the control of circadian rhythmicity (Swaab, 1997). VAS enhances aggressiveness, anxiety, stress levels, and the consolidation of fear memory (Bielsky et al., 2004; Griebel et al., 2002; Landgraf and Neumann, 2004). OT decreases anxiety and stress; facilitates social encounters, maternal care, and the extinction of conditioned avoidance behavior (Bale et al., 2001; Champagne et al., 2001; Windle et al., 1997); reduces activation of the amygdala and modulates fear processing (Kirsch et al., 2005). The presence of abnormal levels of hypothalamic neuropeptides in patients with autism provides strong evidence that an abnormality in OT, VAS and other hypothalamic neuropeptides may have a significant contribution to the behavioral features of autism. However, the morphology and biochemistry of the hypothalamus of autistic subjects remains unknown. The only study of the hypothalamic mammillary body of a 26-year-old autistic man revealed that the cell-packing density was increased by 66% (Bauman and Kemper, 1985).

1.6.4 SENSORIMOTOR DEFICITS, AND REPETITIVE AND STEREOTYPED BEHAVIORS

In individuals with autism, impairments of gross and fine motor function recognized as hypotonia, limbic apraxia, and motor stereotypes are common findings and are more severe in subjects with lower IQ (Rogers et al., 1996). Hand mannerisms, body rocking, or unusual posturing are reported in 37% to 95% of individuals (Lord, 1995; Rapin, 1996; Rogers et al., 1996). In 42% to 88% of subjects with autism, aberrant sensory processing results in a preoccupation with sensory features of objects, over- or underresponsiveness to environmental stimuli or paradoxical responses to sensory stimuli (Kientz and Dunn, 1997). Sensorimotor deficits may by associated with pathological changes in both the nigrostriatal system (basal ganglia) and the cerebellum (Bailey et al., 1998; Kemper and Bauman, 1998; Ritvo et al., 1986; Saitoh and Courchesne, 1998; Sears et al., 1999). Cerebellar abnormality with a deficit/loss of Purkinje cells (Bailey et al., 1998; Kemper and Bauman, 1993, 1998; Ritvo et al., 1986) has been a common finding. Individuals with autism have been classified as affected by cerebellar hyper- or hypoplasia (Saitoh and Courchesne, 1998). A reduced number of Purkinje cells without significant glial activation and a reduced size of Purkinje cells were noticed in the majority of cerebellar reports (Bailey et al., 1998; Fehlow et al., 1993; Kemper and Bauman, 1993; Lee et al., 2002; Ritvo et al., 1986) in 21 of 29 examined cases (Palmen et al., 2004).

Results of evaluation of the size of the cerebellum using MRI are inconsistent. In several MRI studies, smaller cerebellar hemispheres (Gaffney et al., 1987; Murakami et al., 1989) and vermis (Ciesielski et al., 1997; Courchesne et al., 1988; Hashimoto et al., 1995) were reported. In a study by Piven et al. (1997a), the total cerebellar volume was found to be greater in subjects with autism than in the control group, and the increase was proportional to the increased total brain volume. In the cerebellum, boys with autism had less gray matter, a smaller ratio of gray to white matter, and smaller lobules VI and VII than did controls. Despite the inconsistency of reports characterizing topographic autism-associated vermian hypoplasia (Hashimoto et al., 1993; Kaufmann et al., 2003; Levitt et al., 1999; Piven et al., 1997a; Schaefer et al., 1996), several reports show associations between the size of the vermis and deficits in attention-orienting (Harris et al., 1999; Townsend et al., 1999), stereotypic behavior, and reduced exploration in autism (Pierce and Courchesne, 2001).

The reduced size of the pons, midbrain, and medulla in autism reported by Hashimoto et al. (1992, 1993, 1995) was not confirmed in other studies (Hsu et al., 1991; Piven et al., 1992).

Changes in neurons in the deep cerebellar nuclei were noticed by some authors (Kemper and Bauman, 1998) but not by others (Bailey et al., 1998). Structural MRI shows variable patterns of changes. Volumetry of the cerebellum may show no change, hypoplasia, or hyperplasia. Courchesne et al. (1988) reported selective hypertrophy of lobules VI and VII, but these results were not confirmed in other subjects. In part, the pattern may correspond to the functional status of subjects. In highly functioning subjects with autism, hypoplasia of the cerebellum has not been detected (Holttum et al., 1992).

A decrease in the number of GABAergic Purkinje cells is considered the most consistent neuropathological finding in autism, as it was detected in at least 50% of examined cases (Arin et al., 1991; Bailey et al., 1998). Recent studies indicate that preserved Purkinje cells reveal a 40% decrease in the expression of glutamic acid decarboxylase 67 (GAD67) mRNA in autistic subjects relative to control patients (Yip et al., 2007). Moreover, in autism, the basket cells likely provide increased GABAergic feed-forward inhibition to Purkinje cells. The result may include disruption in the timing of Purkinje cell firing and altered inhibition of the cerebellar nuclei, which could directly affect cerebellocortical output, leading to changes in motor behavior and cognition (Yip et al., 2008).

Repetitive and stereotyped behaviors defined as recurring, nonfunctional activities, or interests that occur regularly and interfere with daily functioning are a defining signs of autism. These behaviors include lower-order repetitive motor behavior, intense circumscribed patterns of interests, and higher-order rituals and compulsions (Gabriels et al., 2005). Several studies implicated the role of basal ganglia and frontostriatal circuitry in the pathophysiology of autism, especially in repetitive and stereotyped behaviors. Increased volume of the basal ganglia was reported in several MRI studies (Herbert et al., 2003; Hollander et al., 2005; Langen et al., 2007; Sears et al., 1999). Sears et al. (1999) and Hollander et al. (2005) observed a positive correlation between caudate volumes and repetitive behavior scores. A significant increase in caudate nucleus volume, disproportional to brain volume, was detected in MRI studies in two independent samples of medication-naive subjects with autism

(21 high-functioning children and adolescents, and 21 typically developing subjects; 21 high-functioning adolescents and young adults, and 21 healthy subjects) (Langen et al., 2007). Our studies showing a significantly smaller size of neurons in the caudate, putamen, and nucleus accumbens, especially in the brains of children 4–7 years of age suggest a developmental delay in the growth of neurons in the basal ganglia of autistic subjects, which may contribute to basal ganglia dysfunction (Wegiel et al., 2008). MRI and postmortem morphometric studies support the hypothesis that developmental abnormalities in frontostriatal circuitry contribute to repetitive and stereotyped behaviors, which are one of three defining symptoms of autism.

1.6.5 COGNITIVE DEFICITS

Many individuals with autism demonstrate a particular pattern on intellectual tests that is characteristic of autism. Performance IQ is usually higher than verbal IQ, and block design is the highest subtest, whereas comprehension is usually the lowest (Siegel et al., 1996). Individuals with autism have poorer adaptive function than would be predicted by IQ alone (Volkmar et al., 1993).

Cognitive deficits might be related in part to the memory system and limbic region abnormalities. Reduced volume of both the hippocampal formation and amygdala were noticed in subjects examined by Aylward et al. (1999), but not in populations examined by other researchers (Piven et al., 1998). Neurons in the hippocampus have reduced complexity of dendritic arbors. They are smaller and more densely packed in various portions of the hippocampal formation, entorhinal cortex, medial nuclei of the amygdala, medial septal nucleus, mammillary nuclei, and anterior cingulate gyrus (Bauman and Kemper, 1985; Kemper and Bauman, 1993). Haznedar et al. (1997) observed reduced volume of the anterior cingulate gyrus and decreased positron emission tomography (PET) activity in subjects with autism. Because the cerebellum is involved in a variety of cognitive and affective processes, abnormalities of both the limbic system and the cerebellum may be linked to the core social and communicative deficits in autism.

The caudate nucleus is an integral component of the frontostriatal network involved in cognitive functions (Chow and Cummings, 1999; Voelbel et al., 2006), including learning (Poldrack et al., 1999), short- and long-term memory (Fuh and Wang, 1995), and planning and problem-solving (Mendez et al., 1989; Schmidtke et al., 2002). The increased volume of the caudate observed in autistic children may be indicative of impaired neuronal pruning, contributing to a decrease in executive function (Voelbel et al., 2006).

1.6.6 EPILEPSY-ASSOCIATED PATHOLOGY

The 1% prevalence of epilepsy in the general population increases to 8% in DS, 10% in AD (Menendez, 2005; Risse et al., 1990; Velez and Selwa, 2003), and 33% in autism (Tuchman and Rapin, 2002). The interpretation of developmental changes in autism has been challenged by the need to differentiate among lesions that are not associated with epilepsy, that cause epilepsy, and that are produced by epilepsy (Sutula and Pitkanen, 2001). Recent studies support the hypothesis that epilepsy induces brain alterations that contribute to changes in circuitry, which potentiates the seizure-genic focus (Armstrong, 2005).

Studies of nonautistic subjects indicate that epilepsy-associated pathology includes patchy or laminar neuronal loss and gliosis in the cerebral cortex in one or both hemispheres. In temporal epilepsy, abnormalities were reported in 75% of the specimens examined, and hippocampal sclerosis was found in 50% (Bruton, 1988). Loss of hippocampal neurons correlates with the frequency of tonic-cloning seizures and the total duration of epilepsy (Dam, 1980; Tasch et al., 1999). Loss is accentuated in the CA4 sector and is observed in the granule cell layer in the dentate gyrus. Dispersion of dentate gyrus granular neurons might be a result of seizure-related, disturbed migration of neurons (Bengzon et al., 1997), or epilepsy-enhanced neurogenesis (Ericksson et al., 1998). Ammon horn sclerosis is a progressive lesion that can be induced and propagated by seizures (Armstrong, 2005).

In nearly all cases with hippocampal pathology, changes are also observed in other brain regions. In about 25%, the amygdala, thalamus and mammillary body are affected with neuronal loss. More severe neuronal loss and gliosis in the hippocampus is paralleled by severe neuronal loss and gliosis in the lateral nucleus in the amygdala (Bruton, 1988; Hudson et al., 1993; Thom et al., 1999). Ectopias with more than 8 neurons per 2 sq. mm of white matter occurred in 43% of epileptic patients but in none of the controls (Hardiman et al., 1988). In 45% of severely affected epileptics, significant neuronal loss and astrocytosis spreading out into the overlying molecular layer is observed in the cerebellar cortex. The severity of the cerebellar damage may range from gross atrophy of most or many folia to the restricted neuronal loss in some folia, especially at their basal portion (Gessaga and Urich, 1985).

Central apnea, asphyxia, and pulmonary edema occurring during a seizure (Nashef et al., 1996) as well as life-threatening cardiac arrhythmias during seizures (Earnest et al., 1992; Jallon, 1997; Nashef et al., 1996; Reeves et al., 1996; Saussu et al., 1998) have been suggested as possible causes of sudden unexpected death in epilepsy (Thom et al., 1999).

Enhanced electric activity of neurons and/or increased cell synaptic transmission with enhanced vesicle exocytosis, both in normal and in disease-affected brains are a common cause of modifications of APP processing and Aβ levels. Epilepsy is associated with an elevation of APP expression (Sheng et al., 1994) and occurs in 10 of 11 examined subjects with diffuse nonfibrillar Aβ plaque formation (mean age 47.9 ± 8.8 years of age) (Mackenzie and Miller, 1994; Mackenzie et al., 1996).

1.7 MECHANISMS AFFECTING BRAIN DEVELOPMENT

1.7.1 BDNF AND NEUROTROPHINS IN AUTISM

The neurotrophins, a related family of growth factors, including nerve growth factor (NGF), brain-derived neurotrophic factor (BDNF), and neurotrophins (NT) NT-3 and NT-4/5, have a major role in the survival, growth, and differentiation of neurons (Conner et al., 1997). During typical brain development, only neurons making the appropriate connections survive and form synapses, whereas neurons that fail to obtain adequate neurotrophins die (Oppenheim, 1991). BDNF is broadly distributed throughout the human central nervous system (CNS) and provides neurotrophic support for many neuronal populations in the cortex, amygdala, hippocampus, and striatum (Murer et al., 2001; Schmidt-Kastner et al., 1996; Tapia-Arancibia et al., 2004). The hypothalamus is the brain structure that contains the highest BDNF protein levels (Katoh-Semba et al., 1997; Nawa et al., 1995; Yan et al., 1997) and BDNF mRNA (Castren et al., 1995; Kawamoto et al., 1996; Yan et al., 1997). In the cerebellum, immunoreactivity was observed in Purkinje cells and the olivary complex of the nuclei (Kawamoto et al., 1996; Murer et al., 2001).

In the basal forebrain of autistic individuals, the level of BDNF was three times higher than in controls (Perry et al., 2001). Miyazaki et al. (2004) observed a higher level of BDNF in the blood samples of young children with autism than in adult control subjects. The mean BDNF levels in sera of children diagnosed with autism and childhood disintegrative disorder were about four times higher than in control children (Connolly et al., 2006). Children with autism and childhood disintegrative disorder have both elevated BDNF levels and levels of autoantibodies against BDNF. Serum BDNF has been shown to be increased after seizures (Binder et al., 2001; Chavko et al., 2002).

1.7.2 BRAIN STEM AND THE ROLE OF SEROTONIN IN BRAIN DEVELOPMENT AND CLINICAL FEATURES OF AUTISM

Because 5-hydroxytryptamine (5-HT; serotonin) serves as both a neurotransmitter and an important developmental signal in the brain, dysregulation of the 5-HT system during development may be responsible for many of the abnormalities seen in autism (Whitaker-Azmitia, 2005). In fact, all known chemical inducers of autism including cocaine, thalidomide, valproate, and alcohol modulate 5-HT levels in the brain (Harris et al., 1995; Kramer et al., 1994; Narita et al., 2002; Rathbun and Druse, 1985; Stromland et al., 1994; Williams et al., 2001). A high proportion of children with autism exhibit elevated blood 5-HT levels (hyperserotonemia) and specific alterations in 5-HT biosynthesis. The severity of hyperserotonemia is correlated with the severity of autistic behaviors (Chandana et al., 2005; Chugani et al., 1999; Kuperman et al., 1987). A causal role for serotonergic abnormalities in the etiology of autism is also suggested by studies indicating autism-specific genetic polymorphisms in 5-HT metabolizing enzyme, transporter, or receptor genes (Cohen et al., 2003; Sutcliffe et al., 2005). Also, gender-specific differences in serotonergic regulation during development (Chandana et al., 2005; Chugani et al., 1999), combined with a 52% higher rate of 5-HT biosynthesis in the male than female brain (Nishizawa et al., 1997), and the increased susceptibility of males to early insults imposed by elevated levels of 5-HT (Johns et al., 2002), may contribute to the fourfold higher propensity of males to develop autism compared to females.

As a result of the regulatory role of serotonin affecting the size of neurons, the size of dendritic tree and the number of synapses in innervated cortical and subcortical structures and cerebellum, developmental abnormalities in the serotonergic system may contribute to structural and functional changes in target brain regions and structures. Virtually all regions of the brain receive serotonergic afferents from raphe system neurons. The rostral raphe nuclei form ascending pathways of axons mainly to the forebrain. The caudal raphe system innervates the lower brain stem and the spinal cord (Aitken and Törk, 1988; Lidov and Molliver, 1982). The functions of serotonin are mediated by 14 subtypes of 5-HT receptors in the nervous system (Hoyer et al., 1994; Martin and Humphrey, 1994; Saudou and Hen, 1994a,b). The serotonin$_{2A}$ (5-HT$_{2A}$) receptor is known to be one of the major subtypes and is associated with psychological and mental events (Roth, 1994). The 5-HT$_{2A}$ receptor plays a role in facilitating the formation and maintenance of synapses (Niitsu et al., 1995). Staining for 5-HT$_{2A}$ shows the entire somata and dendritic tree of Purkinje cells in a rat cerebellum (Maeshima et al., 1998). In vitro studies have shown that that 5-HT inhibits the growth and arborization of Purkinje cell dendrites through 5-HT$_{2A}$ receptors and stimulates them through the 5-HT$_{1A}$ receptor (Kondoh et al., 2004). 5-HT promotes the formation of synapses in developing and mature brain and spinal cord (Chen et al., 1997; Niitsu et al., 1995; Okado et al., 1993), and this process is mediated by the 5-HT$_{2A}$ receptor in the spinal cord (Niitsu et al., 1995). Biochemical studies support the hypothesis that developmental defects of the raphe nuclei may make a major contribution to the structural and functional defects of cortical and subcortical structures. However, raphe nuclei have not yet been examined in autistic subjects.

1.8   CLOSING REMARKS

The detected brain structure–specific patterns of structural aberrations in a majority of examined anatomic subdivisions in autism brain may contribute to deficits in expression of emotions, processing of social stimuli, learning of social behaviors, verbal and nonverbal communication, and stereotypic behaviors. Pathological acceleration of brain growth and immaturity of neurons and neuronal networks in early childhood indicate that (a) a significant portion of structural/functional defects starts in early infancy and (b) causative factors dysregulate the mechanisms controlling brain/neuron development. The deceleration of brain growth in the second year of life and the increase of neuronal size in late childhood/adulthood suggests delayed activation of correcting mechanisms. However, the delayed correction of brain and neuronal size does not result in functional recovery. Analysis of the detected pattern of abnormal brain development in autism indicates that early diagnosis and early treatment may prevent or reduce developmental delay, reduce/eliminate secondary structural and functional changes, and improve clinical status throughout the life span.

ACKNOWLEDGMENTS

This study was supported in part by funds from the New York State Office of Mental Retardation and Developmental Disabilities and grants from Autism Speaks and the Department of Defense Autism Spectrum Disorders Research Program (AS073234).

REFERENCES

Aitken, A. R. and I. Tork (1988). Early development of serotonin-containing neurons and pathways as seen in wholemount preparations of the fetal rat brain. *J. Comp. Neurol.* 274:32–47.

Akyol, O., H. Herken, E. Uz, E. Fadillioglu, S. Unal, S. Sogut, H. Ozyurt, and H. A. Savas (2002). The indices of endogenous oxidative and antioxidative processes in plasma from schizophrenic patients: The possible role of oxidant/antioxidant imbalance. *Prog. Neuropsychopharmacol. Biol. Psychiatry* 26:995–1005.

American Psychiatric Association (2000). *Diagnostic and Statistical Manual of Mental Disorders DSM-IV-TR.* American Psychiatric Association, Washington, DC.

Arin, D. M., M. L. Bauman, and T. L. Kemper (1991). The distribution of Purkinje cell loss in the cerebellum in autism. *Neurology* 41 (suppl.): 307.

Armstrong, D. D. (2005). Epilepsy-induced microarchitectural changes in the brain. *Pediatr. Dev. Pathol.* 8:607–614.

Aylward, E. H., N. J. Minshew, K. Field, B. F. Sparks, and N. Singh (2002). Effects of age on brain volume and head circumference in autism. *Neurology* 59:175–183.

Aylward, E. H., N. J. Minshew, G. Goldstein, N. A. Honeycutt, A. M. Augustine, K. O. Yates, P. E. Barta, and G. D. Pearlson (1999). MRI volumes of amygdala and hippocampus in non-mentally retarded autistic adolescents and adults. *Neurology* 53:2145–2150.

Bailey, A., C. A. Le, I. Gottesman, P. Bolton, E. Simonoff, E. Yuzda, and M. Rutter (1995). Autism as a strongly genetic disorder: Evidence from a British twin study. *Psychol. Med.* 25:63–77.

Bailey, A., P. Luthert, P. Bolton, C. A. Le, M. Rutter, and B. Harding (1993). Autism and megalencephaly. *Lancet* 341:1225–1226.

Bailey, A., P. Luthert, A. Dean, B. Harding, I. Janota, M. Montgomery, M. Rutter, and P. Lantos (1998). A clinicopathological study of autism. *Brain* 121 (Pt 5):889–905.

Bailey, A. R., B. N. Giunta, D. Obregon, W. V. Nikolic, J. Tian, C. D. Sanberg, D. T. Sutton, and J. Tan (2008). Peripheral biomarkers in autism: Secreted amyloid precursor protein-alpha as a probable key player in early diagnosis. *Int. J Clin. Exp. Med.* 1:338–344.

Bale, T. L., A. M. Davis, A. P. Auger, D. M. Dorsa, and M. M. McCarthy (2001). CNS region-specific oxytocin receptor expression: Importance in regulation of anxiety and sex behavior. *J. Neurosci.* 21:2546–2552.

Barden, N. (2004). Implication of the hypothalamic-pituitary-adrenal axis in the physiopathology of depression. *J. Psychiatry Neurosci.* 29:185–193.

Barkovich, A. J., R. I. Kuzniecky, G. D. Jackson, R. Guerrini, and W. B. Dobyns (2005). A developmental and genetic classification for malformations of cortical development. *Neurology* 65:1873–1887.

Baron-Cohen, S. (2004). The cognitive neuroscience of autism. *J. Neurol. Neurosurg. Psychiatry* 75:945–948.

Baron-Cohen, S., H. Ring, J. Moriarty, B. Schmitz, D. Costa, and P. Ell (1994). Recognition of mental state terms. Clinical findings in children with autism and a functional neuroimaging study of normal adults. *Br. J. Psychiatry* 165:640–649.

Baron-Cohen, S., H. A. Ring, S. Wheelwright, E. T. Bullmore, M. J. Brammer, A. Simmons, and S. C. Williams (1999). Social intelligence in the normal and autistic brain: An fMRI study. *Eur. J. Neurosci.* 11:1891–1898.

Bauman, M. L., P. A. Filipek, and T. L. Kemper (1997). Early infantile autism. *Int. Rev. Neurobiol.* 41:367–386.

Bauman, M. L. and T. L. Kemper (1985). Histoanatomic observations of the brain in early infantile autism. *Neurology* 35:866–867.

Bauman, M. L. and T. L. Kemper (1996). Observation on the Purkinje cells in the cerebellar vermis in autism. *J. Neuropath. Exp. Neurol.* 55:613.

Bengzon, J., Z. Kokaia, E. Elmer, A. Nanobashvili, M. Kokaia, and O. Lindvall (1997). Apoptosis and proliferation of dentate gyrus neurons after single and intermittent limbic seizures. *Proc. Natl. Acad. Sci. USA* 94:10432–10437.

Bielsky, I. F., S. B. Hu, K. L. Szegda, H. Westphal, and L. J. Young (2004). Profound impairment in social recognition and reduction in anxiety-like behavior in vasopressin V1a receptor knockout mice. *Neuropsychopharmacology* 29:483–493.

Binder, D. K., S. D. Croll, C. M. Gall, and H. E. Scharfman (2001). BDNF and epilepsy: Too much of a good thing? *Trends Neurosci.* 24:47–53.

Boddaert, N., M. Zilbovicius, A. Philipe, L. Robel, M. Bourgeois, C. Barthelemy, D. Seidenwurm, I. Meresse, L. Laurier, I. Desguerre, N. Bahi-Buisson, F. Brunelle, A. Munnich, Y. Samson, M-C. Mouren, and N. Chabane (2009). MRI findings in 77 children with non-syndromic autism. *PLOS one* (www.plosone.com) 4:4415e.

Bolte, S., D. Hubl, S. Feineis-Matthews, D. Prvulovic, T. Dierks, and F. Poustka (2006). Facial affect recognition training in autism: Can we animate the fusiform gyrus? *Behav. Neurosci.* 120:211–216.

Bolton, P., J. Powell, M. Rutter, V. Buckle, J. R. Yates, Y. Ishikawa-Brush, and A. P. Monaco (1995). Autism, mental retardation, multiple exostoses and short stature in a female with 46,X,t(X;8)(p22.13;q22.1). *Psychiatr. Genet.* 5:51–55.

Brown, W. T., T. Wisniewski, I. L. Cohen, E. London, M. Flory, H. Imaki, I. Kuchna, J. Wegiel, S. Y. Ma, K. Nowicki, J. Wang, and J. Wegiel (2008). Neuropathologic changes in chromosome 15 duplication and autism. In 7th Annual International Meeting for Autism Research (IMFAR).

Brunk, U. T., C. B. Jones, and R. S. Sohal (1992). A novel hypothesis of lipofuscinogenesis and cellular aging based on interactions between oxidative stress and autophagocytosis. *Mutat. Res.* 275:395–403.

Brunk, U. T. and A. Terman (2002a). Lipofuscin: Mechanisms of age-related accumulation and influence on cell function. *Free Radic. Biol. Med.* 33:611–619.

Brunk, U. T. and A. Terman (2002b). The mitochondrial–lysosomal axis theory of aging: Accumulation of damaged mitochondria as a result of imperfect autophagocytosis. *Eur. J Biochem.* 269:1996–2002.

Bruton, C. J. (1988). *The Neuropathology of Temporal Lobe Epilepsy*. In Maudsley Monographs. Oxford University Press, New York.

Butler, M. G., M. J. Dasouki, X. P. Zhou, Z. Talebizadeh, M. Brown, T. N. Takahashi, J. H. Miles, C. H. Wang, R. Stratton, R. Pilarski, and C. Eng (2005). Subset of individuals with autism spectrum disorders and extreme macrocephaly associated with germline PTEN tumour suppressor gene mutations. *J. Med. Genet.* 42:318–321.

Buxhoeveden, D. P. and M. F. Casanova (2002). The minicolumn and evolution of the brain. *Brain Behav. Evol.* 60:125–151.

Carper, R. A. and E. Courchesne (2005). Localized enlargement of the frontal cortex in early autism. *Biol. Psychiatry* 57:126–133.

Carper, R. A., P. Moses, Z. D. Tigue, and E. Courchesne (2002). Cerebral lobes in autism: Early hyperplasia and abnormal age effects. *Neuroimage* 16:1038–1051.

Casanova, M. F., D. P. Buxhoeveden, A. E. Switala, and E. Roy (2002). Minicolumnar pathology in autism. *Neurology* 58:428–432.

Casanova, M. F., K. van, I, A. E. Switala, H. van Engeland, H. Heinsen, H. W. Steinbusch, P. R. Hof, J. Trippe, J. Stone, and C. Schmitz (2006). Minicolumnar abnormalities in autism. *Acta Neuropathol.* 112:287–303.

Castren, E., H. Thoenen, and D. Lindholm (1995). Brain-derived neurotrophic factor messenger RNA is expressed in the septum, hypothalamus and in adrenergic brain stem nuclei of adult rat brain and is increased by osmotic stimulation in the paraventricular nucleus. *Neuroscience* 64:71–80.

Champagne, F., J. Diorio, S. Sharma, and M. J. Meaney (2001). Naturally occurring variations in maternal behavior in the rat are associated with differences in estrogen-inducible central oxytocin receptors. *Proc. Natl. Acad. Sci. USA* 98:12736–12741.

Chandana, S. R., M. E. Behen, C. Juhasz, O. Muzik, R. D. Rothermel, T. J. Mangner, P. K. Chakraborty, H. T. Chugani, and D. C. Chugani (2005). Significance of abnormalities in developmental trajectory and asymmetry of cortical serotonin synthesis in autism. *Int. J. Dev. Neurosci.* 23:171–182.

Chauhan, A., V. Chauhan, W. T. Brown, and I. Cohen (2004). Oxidative stress in autism: Increased lipid peroxidation and reduced serum levels of ceruloplasmin and transferrin—the antioxidant proteins. *Life Sci.* 75:2539–2549.

Chauhan, A. and V. Chauhan (2006). Oxidative stress in autism. *Pathophysiology* 13:171–181.

Chauhan, A., B. Muthaiyah, M. M. Essa, T. W. Brown, J. Wegiel, and V. Chauhan (2009). Increased lipid peroxidation in cerebellum and temporal cortex in autism. International Meeting for Autism Research, Chicago, IL, May 8, 2009.

Chavko, M., N. S. Nadi, and D. O. Keyser (2002). Activation of BDNF mRNA and protein after seizures in hyperbaric oxygen: Implications for sensitization to seizures in re-exposures. *Neurochem. Res.* 27:1649–1653.

Chen, L., K. Hamaguchi, S. Hamada, and N. Okado (1997). Regional differences of serotonin-mediated synaptic plasticity in the chicken spinal cord with development and aging. *J. Neural Transplant. Plast.* 6:41–48.

Chow, T. W. and J. L. Cummings (1999). Frontal-subcortical circuits. In B. L. Miller and J. L. Cummings, (eds.), *The Human Frontal Lobes: Functions and Disorders*. Guilford Press, New York, pp. 3–26.

Chugani, D. C., O. Muzik, M. Behen, R. Rothermel, J. J. Janisse, J. Lee, and H. T. Chugani (1999). Developmental changes in brain serotonin synthesis capacity in autistic and nonautistic children. *Ann. Neurol.* 45:287–295.

Ciesielski, K. T., R. J. Harris, B. L. Hart, and H. F. Pabst (1997). Cerebellar hypoplasia and frontal lobe cognitive deficits in disorders of early childhood. *Neuropsychologia* 35:643–655.

Cohen, I. L. (2007). A neural network model of autism: Implications for theory and treatment. In D. Mareschal, S. Sirois, G. Westerman, and M. H. Johnson (eds.), *Neuroconstructivism*. Oxford University Press, Oxford.

Cohen, I. L., X. Liu, C. Schutz, B. N. White, E. C. Jenkins, W. T. Brown, and J. J. Holden (2003). Association of autism severity with a monoamine oxidase A functional polymorphism. *Clin. Genet.* 64:190–197.

Conner, J. M., J. C. Lauterborn, Q. Yan, C. M. Gall, and S. Varon (1997). Distribution of brain-derived neurotrophic factor (BDNF) protein and mRNA in the normal adult rat CNS: Evidence for anterograde axonal transport. *J. Neurosci.* 17:2295–2313.

Connolly, A. M., M. Chez, E. M. Streif, R. M. Keeling, P. T. Golumbek, J. M. Kwon, J. J. Riviello, R. G. Robinson, R. J. Neuman, and R. M. Deuel (2006). Brain-derived neurotrophic factor and autoantibodies to neural antigens in sera of children with autistic spectrum disorders, Landau-Kleffner syndrome, and epilepsy. *Biol. Psychiatry* 59:354–363.

Cook, E. H. Jr. (1998). Genetics of autism. *Mental Retardation Dev. Disabil. Res. Rev.* 4:113–120.

Coon, H., D. Dunn, J. Lainhart, J. Miller, C. Hamil, A. Battaglia, R. Tancredi, M. F. Leppert, R. Weiss, and W. McMahon (2005). Possible association between autism and variants in the brain-expressed tryptophan hydroxylase gene (TPH2). *Am. J. Med. Genet. B Neuropsychiatr. Genet.* 135B:42–46.

Courchesne, E., D. M. Karns, H. R. Davis, R. Ziccardi, R. A. Carper, Z. D. Tigue, H. J. Hisum, P. Moses, K. Pierce, C. Lord, A. J. Lincoln, S. Pizzo, L. Schreibman, R. H. Haas, N. A. Akshoomoff, R. Y. Courchesne (2001). Unusual brain growth patterns in early life in patients with autistic disorder: an MRI study. *Neurology* 57:245–254.

Courchesne, E., R. Carper, and N. Akshoomoff (2003). Evidence of brain overgrowth in the first year of life in autism. *JAMA* 290:337–344.

Courchesne, E., J. R. Hesselink, T. L. Jernigan, and R. Yeung-Courchesne (1987). Abnormal neuroanatomy in a nonretarded person with autism. Unusual findings with magnetic resonance imaging. *Arch. Neurol.* 44:335–341.

Courchesne, E., C. M. Karns, H. R. Davis, R. Ziccardi, R. A. Carper, Z. D. Tigue, H. J. Chisum, P. Moses, K. Pierce, C. Lord, A. J. Lincoln, S. Pizzo, L. Schreibman, R. H. Haas, N. A. Akshoomoff, and R. Y. Courchesne, E., R. Yeung-Courchesne, G. A. Press, J. R. Hesselink, and T. L. Jernigan (1988). Hypoplasia of cerebellar vermal lobules VI and VII in autism. *N. Engl. J. Med.* 318:1349–1354.

Courchesne, E. and K. Pierce (2005a). Why the frontal cortex in autism might be talking only to itself: Local over-connectivity but long-distance disconnection. *Curr. Opin. Neurobiol.* 15:225–230.

Courchesne, E. and K. Pierce (2005b). Brain overgrowth in autism during a critical time in development: Implications for frontal pyramidal neuron and interneuron development and connectivity. *Int. J. Dev. Neurosci.* 23:153–170.

Dalton, K. M., B. M. Nacewicz, T. Johnstone, H. S. Schaefer, M. A. Gernsbacher, H. H. Goldsmith, A. L. Alexander, and R. J. Davidson (2005). Gaze fixation and the neural circuitry of face processing in autism. *Nat. Neurosci.* 8:519–526.

Dam, A. M. (1980). Epilepsy and neuron loss in the hippocampus. *Epilepsia* 21:617–629.

Damasio, H., R. G. Maurer, A. R. Damasio, and H. C. Chui (1980). Computerized tomographic scan findings in patients with autistic behavior. *Arch. Neurol.* 37:504–510.

Davidovitch, M., B. Patterson, and P. Gartside (1996). Head circumference measurements in children with autism. *J. Child Neurol.* 11:389–393.

Dawson, G., J. Munson, S. J. Webb, T. Nalty, R. Abbott, and K. Toth (2007). Rate of head growth decelerates and symptoms worsen in the second year of life in autism. *Biol. Psychiatry* 61:458–464.

Dementieva, Y. A., D. D. Vance, S. L. Donnelly, L. A. Elston, C. M. Wolpert, S. A. Ravan, G. R. DeLong, R. K. Abramson, H. H. Wright, and M. L. Cuccaro (2005). Accelerated head growth in early development of individuals with autism. *Pediatr. Neurol.* 32:102–108.

Department of Health and Human Services, Centers for Disease Control and Prevention (2007). *Morbidity and Mortality Weekly Report* 56:1–28.

Dissanayake, C., Q. M. Bui, R. Huggins, and D. Z. Loesch (2006). Growth in stature and head circumference in high-functioning autism and Asperger disorder during the first 3 years of life. *Dev. Psychopathol.* 18:381–393.

Earnest, M. P., G. E. Thomas, R. A. Eden, and K. F. Hossack (1992). The sudden unexplained death syndrome in epilepsy: Demographic, clinical, and postmortem features. *Epilepsia* 33:310–316.

Ehlert, U., J. Gaab, and M. Heinrichs (2001). Psychoneuroendocrinological contributions to the etiology of depression, posttraumatic stress disorder, and stress-related bodily disorders: The role of the hypothalamus-pituitary-adrenal axis. *Biol. Psychol.* 57:141–152.

Erden-Inal, M., E. Sunal, and G. Kanbak (2002). Age-related changes in the glutathione redox system. *Cell Biochem. Funct.* 20:61–66.

Ericksson, P. S., E. Perfilieva, T. Bjork-Eriksson, A. M. Alborn, C. Nordborg, D. A. Peterson, and F. H. Gage (1998). Neurogenesis in the adult human hippocampus. *Nat. Med.* 4:1313–1317.

Evans, T., S. L. Siedlak, L. Lu, X. Fu, Z. Wang, W. R. McGinnis, E. Fakhoury, R. J. Castellani, S. L. Hazen, W. L. Walsh, A. T. Levis, R. G. Salomon, M. A. Smith, G. Perry, and X. Zhu (2008). The autistic phenotype exhibits a remarkably localized modification of brain protein by products of free radical-induced lipid oxidation. *Am J Biochem. Biotechnol., Special Issue on Autism Spectrum Disorders* 4:61–72.

Fairhall, S. L. and A. Ishai (2007). Effective connectivity within the distributed cortical network for face perception. *Cereb. Cortex* 17:2400–2406.

Fehlow, P., K. Bernstein, A. Tennstedt, and F. Walther (1993). Early infantile autism and excessive aerophagy with symptomatic megacolon and ileus in a case of Ehlers-Danlos syndrome. *Padiatr. Grenzgeb.* 31:259–267.

Ferguson, J. N., L. J. Young, E. F. Hearn, M. M. Matzuk, T. R. Insel, and J. T. Winslow (2000). Social amnesia in mice lacking the oxytocin gene. *Nat. Genet.* 25:284–288.

Fidler, D. J., J. N. Bailey, and S. L. Smalley (2000). Macrocephaly in autism and other pervasive developmental disorders. *Dev. Med. Child Neurol.* 42:737–740.

Filipek, P. A. (1996). Brief report: Neuroimaging in autism: The state of the science 1995. *J. Autism Dev. Disord.* 26:211–215.

Filipek, P. A., P. J. Accardo, G. T. Baranek, E. H. Cook Jr., G. Dawson, B. Gordon, J. S. Gravel, C. P. Johnson, R. J. Kallen, S. E. Levy, N. J. Minshew, S. Ozonoff, B. M. Prizant, I. Rapin, S. J. Rogers, W. L. Stone, S. Teplin, R. F. Tuchman, and F. R. Volkmar (1999). The screening and diagnosis of autistic spectrum disorders. *J. Autism Dev. Disord.* 29:439–484.

Folstein, S. E. and B. Rosen-Sheidley (2001). Genetics of autism: Complex aetiology for a heterogeneous disorder. *Nat. Rev. Genet.* 2:943–955.

Folstein, S. E. and M. L. Rutter (1988). Autism: Familial aggregation and genetic implications. *J. Autism Dev. Disord.* 18:3–30.

Fombonne E. (2003). Epidemiological surveys of autism and other pervasive developmental disorders. *J. Autism Dev. Disord.* 33:365–382.

Fombonne, E., B. Roge, J. Claverie, S. Courty, and J. Fremolle (1999). Microcephaly and macrocephaly in autism. *J. Autism Dev. Disord.* 29:113–119.

Friede, R. L. (1975). *Developmental Neuropathology.* Springer-Verlag, Berlin.

Fuh, J. L. and S. J. Wang (1995). Caudate hemorrhage: Clinical features, neuropsychological assessments and radiological findings. *Clin. Neurol. Neurosurg.* 97:296–299.

Gabreels, B. A., D. F. Swaab, D. P. de Kleijn, N. G. Seidah, J. W. Van de Loo, W. J. Van de Ven, G. J. Martens, and F. W. Van Leeuwen (1998). Attenuation of the polypeptide 7B2, prohormone convertase PC2, and vasopressin in the hypothalamus of some Prader-Willi patients: Indications for a processing defect. *J. Clin. Endocrinol. Metab.* 83:591–599.

Gabriels, R. L., M. L. Cuccaro, D. E. Hill, B. J. Ivers, and E. Goldson (2005). Repetitive behaviors in autism: Relationships with associated clinical features. *Res. Dev. Disabil.* 26:169–181.

Gaffney, G. R., L. Y. Tsai, S. Kuperman, and S. Minchin (1987). Cerebellar structure in autism. *Am. J. Dis. Child* 141:1330–1332.

Gainer, H., M. O. Lively, and M. Morris (1995). Immunological and related techniques for studying neurohypophyseal peptide-processing pathways. *Methods Neurosci.* 23:195–207.

Garber, H. J. and E. R. Ritvo (1992). Magnetic resonance imaging of the posterior fossa in autistic adults. *Am. J. Psychiatry* 149:245–247.

Gessaga, E. C. and H. Urich (1985). The cerebellum of epileptics. *Clin. Neuropathol.* 4:238–245.

Ghaziuddin, M., L. Y. Tsai, and N. Ghaziuddin (1992). Autism in Down's syndrome: Presentation and diagnosis. *J. Intellect. Disabil. Res.* 36 (Pt 5):449–456.

Gillberg, C. (1998). Chromosomal disorders and autism. *J. Autism Dev. Disord.* 28:415–425.

Gillberg C. and M. Coleman (1996). Autism and medical disorders: A review of the literature. *Dev. Med. Child. Neurol.* 38:191–202.

Gillberg, C. and L. de Souza (2002). Head circumference in autism, Asperger syndrome, and ADHD: A comparative study. *Dev. Med. Child Neurol.* 44:296–300.

Glabe, C. (2001). Intracellular mechanisms of amyloid accumulation and pathogenesis in Alzheimer's disease. *J. Mol. Neurosci.* 17:137–145.

Green, L. A., D. Fein, C. Modahl, C. Feinstein, L. Waterhouse, and M. Morris (2001). Oxytocin and autistic disorder: Alteration in peptide forms. *Biol. Psychiatry* 50:609–613.

Grelotti, D., I. Gauthier, and R. T. Shultz (2001). Social interest and the development of cortical face specialization: What autism teaches us about face processing. *Dev. Psychobiol.* 40:213–225.

Griebel, G., J. Simiand, G. C. Serradeil-Le, J. Wagnon, M. Pascal, B. Scatton, J. P. Maffrand, and P. Soubrie (2002). Anxiolytic- and antidepressant-like effects of the non-peptide vasopressin V1b receptor antagonist, SSR149415, suggest an innovative approach for the treatment of stress-related disorders. *Proc. Natl. Acad. Sci. USA* 99:6370–6375.

Guerrini, R. and C. Marini (2006). Genetic malformations of cortical development. *Exp. Brain Res.* 173:322–333.

Hagerman, R. J. (2002). The physical and behavioral phenotype. In R. J. Hagerman and P. J. Hagerman (eds.), *Fragile X Syndrome: Diagnosis, Treatment, and Research.* Johns Hopkins University Press, Baltimore, MD, pp. 206–248.

Happe, F. (1999). Autism: Cognitive deficit or cognitive style? *Trends Cogn. Sci.* 3:216–222.

Happe, F., A. Ronald, and R. Plomin (2006). Time to give up on a single explanation for autism. *Nat. Neurosci.* 9:1218–1220.

Hardan, A. Y., N. J. Minshew, M. Mallikarjuhn, and M. S. Keshavan (2001). Brain volume in autism. *J. Child Neurol.* 16:421–424.

Hardiman, O., T. Burke, J. Phillips, S. Murphy, B. O'Moore, H. Staunton, and M. A. Farrell (1988). Microdysgenesis in resected temporal neocortex: Incidence and clinical significance in focal epilepsy. *Neurology* 38:1041–1047.

Harris, N. S., E. Courchesne, J. Townsend, R. A. Carper, and C. Lord (1999). Neuroanatomic contributions to slowed orienting of attention in children with autism. *Brain Res. Cogn. Brain Res.* 8:61–71.

Harris, S. R., L. L. MacKay, and J. A. Osborn (1995). Autistic behaviors in offspring of mothers abusing alcohol and other drugs: A series of case reports. *Alcohol Clin. Exp. Res.* 19:660–665.

Hashimoto, T., M. Tayama, M. Miyazaki, K. Murakawa, and Y. Kuroda (1993). Brainstem and cerebellar vermis involvement in autistic children. *J. Child Neurol.* 8:149–153.

Hashimoto, T., M. Tayama, M. Miyazaki, N. Sakurama, T. Yoshimoto, K. Murakawa, and Y. Kuroda (1992). Reduced brainstem size in children with autism. *Brain Dev.* 14:94–97.

Hashimoto, T., M. Tayama, K. Mori, K. Fujino, M. Miyazaki, and Y. Kuroda (1989). Magnetic resonance imaging in autism: Preliminary report. *Neuropediatrics* 20:142–146.

Hashimoto, T., M. Tayama, K. Murakawa, T. Yoshimoto, M. Miyazaki, M. Harada, and Y. Kuroda (1995). Development of the brainstem and cerebellum in autistic patients. *J. Autism Dev. Disord.* 25:1–18.

Hasselmo, M. E., E. T. Rolls, and G. C. Baylis (1989). The role of expression and identity in the face-selective responses of neurons in the temporal visual cortex of the monkey. *Behav. Brain Res.* 32:203–218.

Hazlett, H. C., M. Poe, G. Gerig, R. G. Smith, J. Provenzale, A. Ross, J. Gilmore, and J. Piven (2005). Magnetic resonance imaging and head circumference study of brain size in autism: Birth through age 2 years. *Arch. Gen. Psychiatry* 62:1366–1376.

Haznedar, M. M., M. S. Buchsbaum, M. Metzger, A. Solimando, J. Spiegel-Cohen, and E. Hollander (1997). Anterior cingulate gyrus volume and glucose metabolism in autistic disorder. *Am. J. Psychiatry* 154:1047–1050.

Haznedar, M. M., M. S. Buchsbaum, T. C. Wei, P. R. Hof, C. Cartwright, C. A. Bienstock, and E. Hollander (2000). Limbic circuitry in patients with autism spectrum disorders studied with positron emission tomography and magnetic resonance imaging. *Am. J. Psychiatry* 157:1994–2001.

Herbert, M. R., G. J. Harris, K. T. Adrien, D. A. Ziegler, N. Makris, D. N. Kennedy, N. T. Lange, C. F. Chabris, A. Bakardjiev, J. Hodgson, M. Takeoka, H. Tager-Flusberg, and V. S. Caviness Jr. (2002). Abnormal asymmetry in language association cortex in autism. *Ann. Neurol.* 52:588–596.

Herbert, M. R., D. A. Ziegler, C. K. Deutsch, L. M. O'Brien, N. Lange, A. Bakardjiev, J. Hodgson, K. T. Adrien, S. Steele, N. Makris, D. Kennedy, G. J. Harris, and V. S. Caviness Jr. (2003). Dissociations of cerebral cortex, subcortical and cerebral white matter volumes in autistic boys. *Brain* 126:1182–1192.

Herbert, M. R., D. A. Ziegler, N. Makris, P. A. Filipek, T. L. Kemper, J. J. Normandin, H. A. Sanders, D. N. Kennedy, and V. S. Caviness Jr. (2004). Localization of white matter volume increase in autism and developmental language disorder. *Ann. Neurol.* 55:530–540.

Herken, H., E. Uz, H. Ozyurt, S. Sogut, O. Virit, and O. Akyol (2001). Evidence that the activities of erythrocyte free radical scavenging enzymes and the products of lipid peroxidation are increased in different forms of schizophrenia. *Mol. Psychiatry* 6:66–73.

Hevner, R. F. (2007). Layer-specific markers as probes for neuron type identity in human neocortex and malformations of cortical development. *J. Neuropathol. Exp. Neurol.* 66:101–109.

Hollander, E., E. Anagnostou, W. Chaplin, K. Esposito, M. M. Haznedar, E. Licalzi, S. Wasserman, L. Soorya, and M. Buchsbaum (2005). Striatal volume on magnetic resonance imaging and repetitive behaviors in autism. *Biol. Psychiatry* 58:226–232.

Hollander, E., S. Novotny, M. Hanratty, R. Yaffe, C. M. DeCaria, B. R. Aronowitz, and S. Mosovich (2003). Oxytocin infusion reduces repetitive behaviors in adults with autistic and Asperger's disorders. *Neuropsychopharmacology* 28:193–198.

Holttum, J. R., N. J. Minshew, R. S. Sanders, and N. E. Phillips (1992). Magnetic resonance imaging of the posterior fossa in autism. *Biol. Psychiatry* 32:1091–1101.

Howlin, P., L. Wing, and J. Gould. 1995. The recognition of autism in children with Down syndrome—Implications for intervention and some speculations about pathology. *Dev. Med. Child Neurol.* 37: 406–414.

Hoyer, D., D. E. Clarke, J. R. Fozard, P. R. Hartig, G. R. Martin, E. J. Mylecharane, P. R. Saxena, and P. P. Humphrey (1994). International Union of Pharmacology classification of receptors for 5-hydroxytryptamine (Serotonin). *Pharmacol. Rev.* 46:157–203.

Hsu, M., R. Yeung-Courchesne, E. Courchesne, and G. A. Press (1991). Absence of magnetic resonance imaging evidence of pontine abnormality in infantile autism. *Arch. Neurol.* 48:1160–1163.

Hudson, L. P., D. G. Munoz, L. Miller, R. S. McLachlan, J. P. Girvin, and W. T. Blume (1993). Amygdaloid sclerosis in temporal lobe epilepsy. *Ann. Neurol.* 33:622–631.

Jallon, P. (1997). Epilepsy and the heart. *Rev. Neurol.* 153:173–184.

Jellinger, K., D. Armstrong, H. Y. Zoghbi, and A. K. Percy (1988). Neuropathology of Rett syndrome. *Acta Neuropathol.* 76:142–158.

Johns, J. M., D. A. Lubin, J. A. Lieberman, and J. M. Lauder (2002). Developmental effects of prenatal cocaine exposure on 5-HT1A receptors in male and female rat offspring. *Dev. Neurosci.* 24:522–530.

Joseph, R. M. and J. Tanaka (2003). Holistic and part-based face recognition in children with autism. *J. Child Psychol. Psychiatry* 44:529–542.

Just, M. A., V. L. Cherkassky, T. A. Keller, and N. J. Minshew (2004). Cortical activation and synchronization during sentence comprehension in high-functioning autism: Evidence of underconnectivity. *Brain* 127:1811–1821.

Juurlink, B. H. and P. G. Paterson (1998). Review of oxidative stress in brain and spinal cord injury: Suggestions for pharmacological and nutritional management strategies. *J. Spinal Cord. Med.* 21:309–334.

Kanwisher, N., D. Stanley, and A. Harris (1999). The fusiform face area is selective for faces not animals. *Neuroreport* 10:183–187.

Katoh-Semba, R., I. K. Takeuchi, R. Semba, and K. Kato (1997). Distribution of brain-derived neurotrophic factor in rats and its changes with development in the brain. *J. Neurochem.* 69:34–42.

Kaufmann, W. E., K. L. Cooper, S. H. Mostofsky, G. T. Capone, W. R. Kates, C. J. Newschaffer, I. Bukelis, M. H. Stump, A. E. Jann, and D. C. Lanham (2003). Specificity of cerebellar vermian abnormalities in autism: A quantitative magnetic resonance imaging study. *J. Child Neurol.* 18:463–470.

Kawamoto, Y., S. Nakamura, S. Nakano, N. Oka, I. Akiguchi, and J. Kimura (1996). Immunohistochemical localization of brain-derived neurotrophic factor in adult rat brain. *Neuroscience* 74:1209–1226.

Kemper, T. L. and M. L. Bauman (1993). The contribution of neuropathologic studies to the understanding of autism. *Neurol. Clin.* 11:175–187.

Kent, L., J. Evans, M. Paul, and M. Sharp (1999). Comorbidity of autistic spectrum disorders in children with Down syndrome. *Dev. Med. Child Neurol.* 41:153–158.

Kientz, M. A. and W. Dunn (1997). A comparison of the performance of children with and without autism on the sensory profile. *Am. J. Occup. Ther.* 51:530–537.

Kirsch, P., C. Esslinger, Q. Chen, D. Mier, S. Lis, S. Siddhanti, H. Gruppe, V. S. Mattay, B. Gallhofer, and A. Meyer-Lindenberg (2005). Oxytocin modulates neural circuitry for social cognition and fear in humans. *J. Neurosci.* 25:11489–11493.

Kondoh, M., T. Shiga, and N. Okado (2004). Regulation of dendrite formation of Purkinje cells by serotonin through serotonin 1A and serotonin 2A receptors in culture. *Neurosci. Res.* 48:101–109.

Koshino, H., P. A. Carpenter, N. J. Minshew, V. L. Cherkassky, T. A. Keller, and M. A. Just (2005). Functional connectivity in an fMRI working memory task in high-functioning autism. *Neuroimage* 24:810–821.

Kramer, K., E. C. Azmitia, and P. M. Whitaker-Azmitia (1994). In vitro release of [^{3}H]5-hydroxytryptamine from fetal and maternal brain by drugs of abuse. *Brain Res. Dev. Brain Res.* 78:142–146.

Kuperman, S., J. Beeghly, T. Burns, and L. Tsai (1987). Association of serotonin concentration to behavior and IQ in autistic children. *J. Autism Dev. Disord.* 17:133–140.

Lainhart, J. E., J. Piven, M. Wzorek, R. Landa, S. L. Santangelo, H. Coon, and S. E. Folstein (1997). Macrocephaly in children and adults with autism. *J. Am. Acad. Child Adolesc. Psychiatry* 36:282–290.

Landgraf, R. and I. D. Neumann (2004). Vasopressin and oxytocin release within the brain: A dynamic concept of multiple and variable modes of neuropeptide communication. *Front. Neuroendocrinol.* 25:150–176.

Langen, M., S. Durston, W. G. Staal, S. J. Palmen, and H. van Engeland (2007). Caudate nucleus is enlarged in high-functioning medication-naive subjects with autism. *Biol. Psychiatry* 62:262–266.

Lee, M., C. Martin-Ruiz, A. Graham, J. Court, E. Jaros, R. Perry, P. Iversen, M. Bauman, and E. Perry (2002). Nicotinic receptor abnormalities in the cerebellar cortex in autism. *Brain* 125:1483–1495.

Levitt, J. G., R. Blanton, L. Capetillo-Cunliffe, D. Guthrie, A. Toga, and J. T. McCracken (1999). Cerebellar vermis lobules VIII-X in autism. *Prog. Neuropsychopharmacol. Biol. Psychiatry* 23:625–633.

Lidov, H. G. and M. E. Molliver (1982). Immunohistochemical study of the development of serotonergic neurons in the rat CNS. *Brain Res Bull.* 9:559–604.

Lopez-Hurtado, E. and J. J. Prieto (2008). A microscopic study of language-related cortex in autism. *Am. J. Biochem. Biotechnol. Special Issue on Autism Spectrum Disorders,* 4:130–145.

Lord, C., S. Risi, L. Lambrecht, E. H. Cook Jr., B. L. Leventhal, P. C. DiLavore, A. Pickles, and M. Rutter (2000). The autism diagnostic observation schedule-generic: A standard measure of social and communication deficits associated with the spectrum of autism. *J. Autism Dev. Disord.* 30:205–223.

Lord, C. and M. Rutter (1995). Autism and pervasive developmental disorders. In M. Rutter, E. Taylor, and L. Hersov (eds.), *Child and Adolescent Psychiatry, Modern Approaches.* Blackwell Science, Oxford, pp. 569–593.

Mackenzie, I. R., R. S. McLachlan, C. S. Kubu, and L. A. Miller (1996). Prospective neuropsychological assessment of nondemented patients with biopsy proven senile plaques. *Neurology* 46:425–429.

Mackenzie, I. R. and L. A. Miller (1994). Senile plaques in temporal lobe epilepsy. *Acta Neuropathol.* 87:504–510.

Maeshima, T., F. Shutoh, S. Hamada, K. Senzaki, K. Hamaguchi-Hamada, R. Ito, and N. Okado (1998). Serotonin2A receptor-like immunoreactivity in rat cerebellar Purkinje cells. *Neurosci. Lett.* 252:72–74.

Manaye, K. F., D. L. Lei, Y. Tizabi, M. I. vila-Garcia, P. R. Mouton, and P. H. Kelly (2005). Selective neuron loss in the paraventricular nucleus of hypothalamus in patients suffering from major depression and bipolar disorder. *J. Neuropathol. Exp. Neurol.* 64:224–229.

Martin, G. R. and P. P. Humphrey (1994). Receptors for 5-hydroxytryptamine: Current perspectives on classification and nomenclature. *Neuropharmacology* 33:261–273.

Mason-Brothers, A., E. R. Ritvo, C. Pingree, P. B. Petersen, W. R. Jenson, W. M. McMahon, B. J. Freeman, L. B. Jorde, M. J. Spencer, and A. Mo (1990). The UCLA-University of Utah epidemiologic survey of autism: Prenatal, perinatal, and postnatal factors. *Pediatrics* 86:514–519.

McClelland, J. L. (2000). The basis of hyperspecificity in autism: A preliminary suggestion based on properties of neural nets. *J. Autism Dev. Disord.* 30:497–502.

Mendez, M. F., N. L. Adams, and K. S. Lewandowski (1989). Neurobehavioral changes associated with caudate lesions. *Neurology* 39:349–354.

Menendez, M. (2005). Down syndrome, Alzheimer's disease and seizures. *Brain Dev* 27:246–252.

Miles, J. H., L. L. Hadden, T. N. Takahashi, and R. E. Hillman (2000). Head circumference is an independent clinical finding associated with autism. *Am. J. Med. Genet.* 95:339–350.

Miles, J. H., T. N. Takahashi, S. Bagby, P. K. Sahota, D. F. Vaslow, C. H. Wang, R. E. Hillman, and J. E. Farmer (2005). Essential versus complex autism: Definition of fundamental prognostic subtypes. *Am. J. Med. Genet. A* 135:171–180.

Ming, X., T. P. Stein, M. Brimacombe, W. G. Johnson, G. H. Lambert, and G. C. Wagner (2005). Increased excretion of a lipid peroxidation biomarker in autism. *Prostaglandins Leukot. Essent. Fatty Acids* 73:379–384.

Mitchell, B. F., X. Fang, and S. Wong (1998). Role of carboxy-extended forms of oxytocin in the rat uterus in the process of parturition. *Biol. Reprod.* 59:1321–1327.

Miyazaki, K., N. Narita, R. Sakuta, T. Miyahara, H. Naruse, N. Okado, and M. Narita (2004). Serum neurotrophin concentrations in autism and mental retardation: A pilot study. *Brain Dev.* 26:292–295.

Muhle, R., S. V. Trentacoste, and I. Rapin (2004). The genetics of autism. *Pediatrics* 113:e472–e486.

Muller, R. A. (2007). The study of autism as a distributed disorder. *Ment. Retard. Dev. Disabil. Res. Rev.* 13:85–95.

Murakami, J. W., E. Courchesne, G. A. Press, R. Yeung-Courchesne, and J. R. Hesselink (1989). Reduced cerebellar hemisphere size and its relationship to vermal hypoplasia in autism. *Arch. Neurol.* 46:689–694.

Murer, M. G., Q. Yan, and R. Raisman-Vozari (2001). Brain-derived neurotrophic factor in the control human brain, and in Alzheimer's disease and Parkinson's disease. *Prog. Neurobiol.* 63:71–124.

Narita, N., M. Kato, M. Tazoe, K. Miyazaki, M. Narita, and N. Okado (2002). Increased monoamine concentration in the brain and blood of fetal thalidomide- and valproic acid-exposed rat: Putative animal models for autism. *Pediatr. Res.* 52:576–579.

Nashef, L., F. Walker, P. Allen, J. W. Sander, S. D. Shorvon, and D. R. Fish (1996). Apnoea and bradycardia during epileptic seizures: Relation to sudden death in epilepsy. *J. Neurol. Neurosurg. Psychiatry* 60:297–300.

Nawa, H., J. Carnahan, and C. Gall (1995). BDNF protein measured by a novel enzyme immunoassay in normal brain and after seizure: Partial disagreement with mRNA levels. *Eur. J. Neurosci.* 7:1527–1535.

Nelson, E. and J. Panksepp (1996). Oxytocin mediates acquisition of maternally associated odor preferences in preweanling rat pups. *Behav. Neurosci.* 110:583–592.

Newschaffer, C. J., D. Fallin, and N. L. Lee (2002). Heritable and nonheritable risk factors for autism spectrum disorders. *Epidemiol. Rev.* 24:137–153.

Niitsu, Y., S. Hamada, K. Hamaguchi, M. Mikuni, and N. Okado (1995). Regulation of synapse density by 5-HT2A receptor agonist and antagonist in the spinal cord of chicken embryo. *Neurosci. Lett.* 195:159–162.

Nishizawa, S., C. Benkelfat, S. N. Young, M. Leyton, S. Mzengeza, M. C. de, P. Blier, and M. Diksic (1997). Differences between males and females in rates of serotonin synthesis in human brain. *Proc. Natl. Acad. Sci. USA.* 94:5308–5313.

Okado, N., L. Cheng, Y. Tanatsugu, S. Hamada, and K. Hamaguchi (1993). Synaptic loss following removal of serotoninergic fibers in newly hatched and adult chickens. *J. Neurobiol.* 24:687–698.

Ono, H., A. Sakamoto, and N. Sakura (2001). Plasma total glutathione concentrations in healthy pediatric and adult subjects. *Clin. Chim. Acta* 312:227–229.

Oppenheim, R. W. (1991). Cell death during development of the nervous system. *Annu. Rev. Neurosci.* 14:453–501.

Palmen, S. J., H. van Engeland, P. R. Hof, and C. Schmitz (2004). Neuropathological findings in autism. *Brain* 127:2572–2583.

Pennington, B. F., P. A. Filipek, D. Lefly, N. Chhabildas, D. N. Kennedy, J. H. Simon, C. M. Filley, A. Galaburda, and J. C. DeFries (2000). A twin MRI study of size variations in human brain. *J. Cogn. Neurosci.* 12:223–232.

Perrett, D. I., P. A. Smith, D. D. Potter, A. J. Mistlin, A. S. Head, A. D. Milner, and M. A. Jeeves (1985). Visual cells in the temporal cortex sensitive to face view and gaze direction. *Proc. R. Soc. Lond B Biol. Sci.* 223:293–317.

Perry, E. K., M. L. Lee, C. M. Martin-Ruiz, J. A. Court S. G. Volsen, J. Merrit, E. Folly, P. E. Iversen, M. L. Bauman, R. H. Perry, and G. L. Wenk (2001). Cholinergic activity in autism: Abnormalities in the cerebral cortex and basal forebrain. *Am. J. Psychiatry* 158:1058–1066.

Perry, S. W., J. P. Norman, A. Litzburg, and H. A. Gelbard (2004). Antioxidants are required during the early critical period, but not later, for neuronal survival. *J. Neurosci. Res.* 78:485–492.

Pfefferbaum, A., E. V. Sullivan, G. E. Swan, and D. Carmelli (2000). Brain structure in men remains highly heritable in the seventh and eighth decades of life. *Neurobiol. Aging* 21:63–74.

Pickett, J. and E. London (2005). The neuropathology of autism: A review. *J. Neuropathol. Exp. Neurol.* 64:925–935.

Pierce, K. and E. Courchesne (2001). Evidence for a cerebellar role in reduced exploration and stereotyped behavior in autism. *Biol. Psychiatry* 49:655–664.

Pierce, K., R. A. Muller, J. Ambrose, G. Allen, and E. Courchesne (2001). Face processing occurs outside the fusiform "face area" in autism: Evidence from functional MRI. *Brain* 124:2059–2073.

Pierce, K., F. Haist, F. Sedaghat, and E. Courchesne (2004). The brain response to personally familiar faces in autism: Findings of fusiform activity and beyond. *Brain* 127:2703–2716.

Piven, J., E. Nehme, J. Simon, P. Barta, G. Pearlson, and S. E. Folstein (1992). Magnetic resonance imaging in autism: Measurement of the cerebellum, pons, and fourth ventricle. *Biol. Psychiatry* 31:491–504.

Piven, J., S. Arndt, J. Bailey, S. Havercamp, N. C. Andreasen, and P. Palmer (1995). An MRI study of brain size in autism. *Am. J. Psychiatry* 152:1145–1149.

Piven, J., S. Arndt, J. Bailey, and N. Andreasen (1996). Regional brain enlargement in autism: A magnetic resonance imaging study. *J. Am. Acad. Child Adolesc. Psychiatry* 35:530–536.

Piven, J., K. Saliba, J. Bailey, and S. Arndt (1997a). An MRI study of autism: The cerebellum revisited. *Neurology* 49:546–551.

Piven, J., J. Bailey, B. J. Ranson, and S. Arndt (1997b). An MRI study of the corpus callosum in autism. *Am. J. Psychiatry* 154:1051–1056.

Piven, J., J. Bailey, B. J. Ranson, and S. Arndt (1998). No difference in hippocampus volume detected on magnetic resonance imaging in autistic individuals. *J. Autism Dev. Disord.* 28:105–110.

Poldrack, R. A., V. Prabhakaran, C. A. Seger, and J. D. Gabrieli (1999). Striatal activation during acquisition of a cognitive skill. *Neuropsychology* 13:564–574.

Popik, P. and J. M. Van Ree (1992). Long-term facilitation of social recognition in rats by vasopressin related peptides: A structure–activity study. *Life Sci.* 50:567–572.

Popik, P., J. Vetulani, and J. M. Van Ree (1992). Low doses of oxytocin facilitate social recognition in rats. *Psychopharmacology* 106:71–74.

Prasher, V. P. and D. J. Clarke (1996). Case report: Challenging behaviour in a young adult with Down's syndrome and autism. *Brit. J. Learning Disab.* 24:167–169.

Raggenbass, M. 2001. Vasopressin- and oxytocin-induced activity in the central nervous system: Electrophysiological studies using in-vitro systems. *Prog. Neurobiol.* 64:307–326.

Rao, V. V., C. Loffler, J. Battey, and I. Hansmann (1992). The human gene for oxytocin-neurophysin I (OXT) is physically mapped to chromosome 20p13 by in situ hybridization. *Cytogenet. Cell Genet.* 61:271–273.

Rapin, I. (1996). *Preschool Children with Inadequate Communication: Developmental Language Disorder, Autism, Low IQ*. MacKeith Press, London.

Rathbun, W. and M. J. Druse (1985). Dopamine, serotonin, and acid metabolites in brain regions from the developing offspring of ethanol-treated rats. *J. Neurochem.* 44:57–62.

Redcay, E. and E. Courchesne.(2005). When is the brain enlarged in autism? A meta-analysis of all brain size reports. *Biol. Psychiatry* 58:1–9.

Reeves, A. L., K. E. Nollet, D. W. Klass, F. W. Sharbrough, and E. L. So (1996). The ictal bradycardia syndrome. *Epilepsia* 37:983–987.

Risse, S. C., T. H. Lampe, T. D. Bird, D. Nochlin, S. M. Sumi, T. Keenan, L. Cubberley, E. Peskind, and M. A. Raskind (1990). Myoclonus, seizures, and paratonia in Alzheimer disease. *Alzheimer Dis. Assoc. Disord.* 4:217–225.

Ritvo, E. R., B. J. Freeman, A. B. Scheibel, T. Duong, H. Robinson, D. Guthrie, and A. Ritvo (1986). Lower Purkinje cell counts in the cerebella of four autistic subjects: Initial findings of the UCLA-NSAC Autopsy Research Report. *Am. J. Psychiatry* 143:862–866.

Rodier, P. M., J. L. Ingram, B. Tisdale, S. Nelson, and J. Romano (1996). Embryological origin for autism: Developmental anomalies of the cranial nerve motor nuclei. *J. Comp. Neurol.* 370:247–261.

Rogers, S. J., L. Bennetto, R. McEvoy, and B. F. Pennington (1996). Imitation and pantomime in high-functioning adolescents with autism spectrum disorders. *Child Dev.* 67:2060–2073.

Roth, B. L. (1994). Multiple serotonin receptors: Clinical and experimental aspects. *Ann. Clin. Psychiatry* 6:67–78.

Rutter, M., A. Bailey, P. Bolton, and C. A. Le (1994). Autism and known medical conditions: Myth and substance. *J. Child Psychol. Psychiatry* 35:311–322.

Saitoh, O. and E. Courchesne (1998). Magnetic resonance imaging study of the brain in autism. *Psychiatry Clin. Neurosci.* 52 Suppl:S219–S222.

Sajdel-Sulkowska, E. M., B. Lipinski, H. Windom, T. Audhya, and W. McGinnis (2008). Oxidative stress in autism: Cerebellar 3-nitrotyrosine levels. *Am. J. Biochem. Biotechnol.* (*Special Issue on Autism Spectrum Disorders*) 4:73–84.

Sarnat, H. B. and L. Flores-Sarnat (2004). Integrative classification of morphology and molecular genetics in central nervous system malformations. *Am. J. Med. Genet. A* 126A:386–392.

Saudou, F. and R. Hen (1994a). 5-Hydroxytryptamine receptor subtypes in vertebrates and invertebrates. *Neurochem. Int.* 25:503–532.

Saudou, F. and R. Hen (1994b). 5-Hydroxytryptamine receptor subtypes: Molecular and functional diversity. *Adv. Pharmacol.* 30:327–380.

Saussu, F., K. van Rijckevorsel, and T. de Barsy (1998). Bradycardia: An unrecognized complication of some epileptic crises. *Rev Neurol.* 154:250–252.

Schaefer, G. B., J. N. Thompson, J. B. Bodensteiner, J. M. McConnell, W. J. Kimberling, C. T. Gay, W. D. Dutton, D. C. Hutchings, and S. B. Gray (1996). Hypoplasia of the cerebellar vermis in neurogenetic syndromes. *Ann. Neurol.* 39:382–385.

Schmidt-Kastner, R., C. Wetmore, and L. Olson (1996). Comparative study of brain-derived neurotrophic factor messenger RNA and protein at the cellular level suggests multiple roles in hippocampus, striatum and cortex. *Neuroscience* 74:161–183.

Schmidtke, K., H. Manner, R. Kaufmann, and H. Schmolck (2002). Cognitive procedural learning in patients with fronto-striatal lesions. *Learn. Mem.* 9:419–429.

Schultz, R. T. (2005). Developmental deficits in social perception in autism: The role of the amygdala and fusiform face area. *Int. J. Dev. Neurosci.* 23:125–141.

Sears, L. L., C. Vest, S. Mohamed, J. Bailey, B. J. Ranson, and J. Piven (1999). An MRI study of the basal ganglia in autism. *Prog. Neuropsychopharmacol. Biol. Psychiatry* 23:613–624.

Shapiro, L. E. and T. R. Insel (1989). Ontogeny of oxytocin receptors in rat forebrain: A quantitative study. *Synapse* 4:259–266.

Sheng, J. G., F. A. Boop, R. E. Mrak, and W. S. Griffin (1994). Increased neuronal beta-amyloid precursor protein expression in human temporal lobe epilepsy: Association with interleukin-1 alpha immunoreactivity. *J. Neurochem.* 63:1872–1879.

Shulman, R. G., D. L. Rothman, K. L. Behar, and F. Hyder (2004). Energetic basis of brain activity: Implications for neuroimaging. *Trends Neurosci.* 27:489–495.

Siegel, D. J., N. J. Minshew, and G. Goldstein (1996). Wechsler IQ profiles in diagnosis of high-functioning autism. *J. Autism Dev. Disord.* 26:389–406.

Smalley, S. L., R. F. Asarnow, and M. A. Spence (1988). Autism and genetics. A decade of research. *Arch. Gen. Psychiatry* 45:953–961.

Sohal, R. S. and U. T. Brunk (1989). Lipofuscin as an indicator of oxidative stress and aging. *Adv. Exp. Med. Biol.* 266:17–26.

Sokol, D. K., D. Chen, M. R. Farlow, D. W. Dunn, B. Maloney, J. A. Zimmer, and D. K. Lahiri (2006). High levels of Alzheimer beta-amyloid precursor protein (APP) in children with severely autistic behavior and aggression. *J. Child Neurol.* 21:444–449.

Sparks, B. F., S. D. Friedman, D. W. Shaw, E. H. Aylward, D. Echelard, A. A. Artru, K. R. Maravilla, J. N. Giedd, J. Munson, G. Dawson, and S. R. Dager (2002). Brain structural abnormalities in young children with autism spectrum disorder. *Neurology* 59:184–192.

Stefanacci, L. and D. G. Amaral (2000). Topographic organization of cortical inputs to the lateral nucleus of the macaque monkey amygdala: A retrograde tracing study. *J. Comp. Neurol.* 421:52–79.

Steg, J. P. and J. L. Rapoport (1975). Minor physical anomalies in normal, neurotic, learning disabled, and severely disturbed children. *J. Autism Child Schizophr.* 5:299–307.

Stevenson, R. E., R. J. Schroer, C. Skinner, D. Fender, and R. J. Simensen (1997). Autism and macrocephaly. *Lancet* 349:1744–1745.

Stojanovic, A., A. E. Roher, and M. J. Ball (1994). Quantitative analysis of lipofuscin and neurofibrillary tangles in the hippocampal neurons of Alzheimer disease brains. *Dementia* 5:229–233.

Stone, W. L., O. Y. Ousley, P. J. Yoder, K. L. Hogan, and S. L. Hepburn (1997). Nonverbal communication in two- and three-year-old children with autism. *J. Autism Dev. Disord.* 27:677–696.

Stromland, K., V. Nordin, M. Miller, B. Akerstrom, and C. Gillberg (1994). Autism in thalidomide embryopathy: A population study. *Dev. Med. Child Neurol.* 36:351–356.

Sutcliffe, J. S., R. J. Delahanty, H. C. Prasad, J. L. McCauley, Q. Han, L. Jiang, C. Li, S. E. Folstein, and R. D. Blakely (2005). Allelic heterogeneity at the serotonin transporter locus (SLC6A4) confers susceptibility to autism and rigid-compulsive behaviors. *Am. J. Hum. Genet.* 77:265–279.

Sutula, T. P. and A. Pitkanen (2001). More evidence for seizure-induced neuron loss: Is hippocampal sclerosis both cause and effect of epilepsy? *Neurology* 57:169–170.

Swaab, D. F. (1997). Prader-Willi syndrome and the hypothalamus. *Acta Paediatr. Suppl.* 423:50–54.

Szatmari, P., M. B. Jones, L. Zwaigenbaum, and J. E. MacLean (1998). Genetics of autism: Overview and new directions. *J. Autism Dev. Disord.* 28:351–368.

Szweda, P. A., M. Camouse, K. C. Lundberg, T. D. Oberley, and L. I. Szweda (2003). Aging, lipofuscin formation, and free radical-mediated inhibition of cellular proteolytic systems. *Ageing Res. Rev.* 2:383–405.

Tapia-Arancibia, L., F. Rage, L. Givalois, and S. Arancibia (2004). Physiology of BDNF: Focus on hypothalamic function. *Front. Neuroendocrinol.* 25:77–107.

Tasch, E., F. Cendes, L. M. Li, F. Dubeau, F. Andermann, and D. L. Arnold (1999). Neuroimaging evidence of progressive neuronal loss and dysfunction in temporal lobe epilepsy. *Ann. Neurol.* 45:568–576.

Terman, A. and U. T. Brunk (2004). Lipofuscin. *Int. J. Biochem. Cell Biol.* 36:1400–1404.

Thom, M., B. Griffin, J. W. Sander, and F. Scaravilli (1999). Amygdala sclerosis in sudden and unexpected death in epilepsy. *Epilepsy Res.* 37:53–62.

Torsdottir, G., J. Kristinsson, S. Sveinbjornsdottir, J. Snaedal, and T. Johannesson (1999). Copper, ceruloplasmin, superoxide dismutase and iron parameters in Parkinson's disease. *Pharmacol. Toxicol.* 85:239–243.

Townsend, J., E. Courchesne, J. Covington, M. Westerfield, N. S. Harris, P. Lyden, T. P. Lowry, and G. A. Press (1999). Spatial attention deficits in patients with acquired or developmental cerebellar abnormality. *J. Neurosci.* 19:5632–5643.

Tuchman, R. F., I. Rapin, and S. Shinner (1991). Autistic and dysphasic children II: Epilepsy. *Pediatrics* 88:1219–1225.

Tuchman, R. F. and I. Rapin (2002). Epilepsy in autism. *Lancet Neurol.* 1:352–358.

van Kooten, I., S. J. Palmen, P. von Cappeln, H. W. Steinbusch, H. Korr, H. Heinsen, P. R. Hof, H. van Engeland, and C. Schmitz (2008). Neurons in the fusiform gyrus are fewer and smaller in autism. *Brain* 131:987–999.

Velez, L. and L. M. Selwa (2003). Seizure disorders in the elderly. *Am. Fam. Physician* 67:325–332.

Voelbel, G. T., M. E. Bates, J. F. Buckman, G. Pandina, and R. L. Hendren (2006). Caudate nucleus volume and cognitive performance: Are they related in childhood psychopathology? *Biol. Psychiatry* 60:942–950.

Volkmar, F. R., A. Carter, S. S. Sparrow, and D. V. Cicchetti (1993). Quantifying social development in autism. *J. Am. Acad. Child Adolesc. Psychiatry* 32:627–632.

Vorstman, J. A. S., W. G. Staal, E. van Daalen, H. van Engeland, P. F. R. Hochstenbach, and L. Franke (2006). Identification of novel autism candidate regions through analysis of reported cytogenetic abnormalities associated with autism. *Mol. Psych.* 11:18–28.

Waiter, G. D., J. H. Williams, A. D. Murray, A. Gilchrist, D. I. Perrett, and A. Whiten (2004). A voxel-based investigation of brain structure in male adolescents with autistic spectrum disorder. *Neuroimage* 22:619–625.

Wakabayashi, S. (1979). A case of infantile autism associated with Down's syndrome. *J. Autism Dev. Disord.* 9:31–36.

Wegiel, J., I. Kuchna, K. Nowicki, J. Frackowiak, B. Mazur-Kolecka, H. Imaki, J. Wegiel, P. D. Mehta, W. P. Silverman, B. Reisberg, M. Deleon, T. Wisniewski, T. Pirttilla, H. Frey, T. Lehtimaki, T. Kivimaki, F. E. Visser, W. Kamphorst, A. Potempska, D. Bolton, J. R. Currie, and D. L. Miller (2007). Intraneuronal Abeta immunoreactivity is not a predictor of brain amyloidosis-beta or neurofibrillary degeneration. *Acta Neuropathol.* 113:389–402.

Wegiel, J., E. London, I. L. Cohen, M. Flory, T. Wisniewski, H. Imaki, I. Kuchna, J. Wegiel, S. Y. Ma, K. Nowicki, J. Wang, and W. T. Brown (2008). Detection of leading developmental defects in brains of autistic subjects. In 7th Annual International Meeting for Autism Research (IMFAR) London, U.K.

Wetherby, A. M., B. M. Prizant, and T. Hutchinson (1998). Communicative, social-affective, and symbolic profiles of young children with autism and pervasive developmental disorder. *Am. J. Speech Language Pathol.* 7:79–91.

Whitaker-Azmitia, P. M. (2005). Behavioral and cellular consequences of increasing serotonergic activity during brain development: A role in autism? *Int. J. Dev. Neurosci.* 23:75–83.

Williams, J. H., A. Whiten, T. Suddendorf, and D. I. Perrett (2001). Imitation, mirror neurons and autism. *Neurosci. Biobehav. Rev.* 25:287–295.

Windle, R. J., N. Shanks, S. L. Lightman, and C. D. Ingram (1997). Central oxytocin administration reduces stress-induced corticosterone release and anxiety behavior in rats. *Endocrinology* 138:2829–2834.

Wu, S. P., M. X. Jia, Y. Ruan, Y. Q. Guo, M. Shuang, X. H. Gong, Y. B. Zhang, X. L. Yang, and D. Zhang (2005). Positive association of the oxytocine receptor gene (OXTR) with autism in the Chinese Han population. *Biol. Psychiatry* 58:74–77.

Yan, Q., R. D. Rosenfeld, C. R. Matheson, N. Hawkins, O. T. Lopez, L. Bennett, and A. A. Welcher (1997). Expression of brain-derived neurotrophic factor protein in the adult rat central nervous system. *Neuroscience* 78:431–448.

Yanik, M., H. Vural, H. Tutkun, S. S. Zoroglu, H. A. Savas, H. Herken, A. Kocyigit, H. Keles, and O. Akyol (2004). The role of the arginine-nitric oxide pathway in the pathogenesis of bipolar affective disorder. *Eur. Arch. Psychiatry Clin. Neurosci.* 254:43–47.

Yip, J., J. J. Soghomonian, and G. J. Blatt (2007). Decreased GAD67 mRNA levels in cerebellar Purkinje cells in autism: Pathophysiological implications. *Acta Neuropathol.* 113:559–568.

Yip, J., J. J. Soghomonian, and G. J. Blatt (2008). Increased GAD67 mRNA expression in cerebellar interneurons in autism: Implications for Purkinje cell dysfunction. *J. Neurosci. Res.* 86:525–530.

Yonan, A. L., M. Alarcon, R. Cheng, P. K. Magnusson, S. J. Spence, A. A. Palmer, A. Grunn, S. H. Juo, J. D. Terwilliger, J. Liu, R. M. Cantor, D. H. Geschwind, and T. C. Gilliam (2003). A genomewide screen of 345 families for autism-susceptibility loci. *Am. J. Hum. Genet.* 73:886–897.

Zilbovicius, M., B. Garreau, Y. Samson, P. Remy, C. Barthelemy, A. Syrota, and G. Lelord (1995). Delayed maturation of the frontal cortex in childhood autism. *Am. J. Psychiatry* 152:248–252.

Zoroglu, S. S., F. Armutcu, S. Ozen, A. Gurel, E. Sivasli, O. Yetkin, and I. Meram (2004). Increased oxidative stress and altered activities of erythrocyte free radical scavenging enzymes in autism. *Eur. Arch. Psychiatry Clin. Neurosci.* 254:143–147.

2 Evidence for Oxidative Damage in the Autistic Brain

Teresa A. Evans,[1] George Perry,[1,3] Mark A. Smith,[1] Robert G. Salomon,[2] Woody R. McGinnis,[4] Elizabeth M. Sajdel-Sulkowska,[5] and Xiongwei Zhu[1,]*

Departments of [1]Pathology and [2]Chemistry, Case Western Reserve University, Cleveland, OH 44106, USA

[3]College of Sciences, University of Texas at San Antonio, San Antonio, TX 78249, USA

[4]Autism House of Auckland, Autism New Zealand, Inc., Auckland, New Zealand

[5]Department of Psychiatry, Brigham and Women's Hospital, Boston, MA 02115, USA

CONTENTS

* Corresponding author: Tel.: +1-216-368-5903; fax: +1-216-368-8964; e-mail: xiongwei.zhu@case.edu

2.1 OXIDATIVE STRESS IS A COMMON FEATURE DURING NEURODEGENERATION IN THE BRAIN

The production of reactive oxygen species (ROS) takes place in all biological systems, however, under normal physiological conditions, redox homeostasis is maintained through antioxidant defense systems including antioxidants and antioxidant enzymes (Zhu et al., 2005). Oxidative stress entails breaching antioxidant defense to an extent that is sufficient to lead to damage to cellular components. Increased ROS and oxidative stress markers such as oxidative modifications to lipids, proteins, and nucleic acids are all considered evidence of oxidative stress and these changes are frequently accompanied by changes in antioxidants and antioxidant enzymes (Zhu et al., 2005). Neurons of the central nervous system are subject to a number of unique conditions that make them particularly vulnerable to oxidative stress, including a high energy and oxygen consumption rate, a high unsaturated lipid content of neuronal membranes, high levels of transition metals, a relative scarcity of antioxidant defense systems compared with other organs, and the postmitotic nature of neuronal populations. Not surprisingly, extensive evidence suggests that oxidative stress occurs in the brain of various neurodegenerative diseases including Alzheimer's disease, Parkinson's disease, amyotrophic lateral sclerosis, Huntington's disease, Prion disease, and stroke (Smith et al., 1994; Takeda et al., 2000). Although it is debatable whether oxidative stress is the cause or consequence of the disease, multiple lines of evidence suggest that oxidative stress is one of the earliest and most prominent changes suggesting a more causative role in disease pathogenesis (Nunomura et al., 2001, 2004). The pathology in these cases is often considered to be the result of cellular damage from ROS or cellular response to elevated ROS (Lee et al., 2005). Furthermore, oxidative stress is not always linked to the brain of age-related neurodegenerative disease patients in their later stages of life since it is also found in younger patients like those with Down syndrome where it is also believed to play an essential role in disease pathogenesis (Nunomura et al., 2001).

It is well known that autism patients suffer extensive neuronal loss in the cerebellum (Courchesne et al., 1994). Recently, unbiased stereological studies also demonstrated significant neuronal loss in the amygdala area, especially at the lateral nucleus subdivision (Schumann and Amaral, 2005). How these neurons become lost is of debate in the field. Although it is widely believed that the neuronal loss in these brain areas is due to the neurodevelopmental abnormalities, emerging evidence suggest that neurodegeneration may also be involved. For example, younger autistic patients have larger amygdala, which becomes normal later in life where neuronal loss is identified. One important piece of support for the neurodevelopmental hypothesis is the lack of gliosis in the autistic brain, but at least in a subset of autism patients, gliosis is identified suggesting neuronal insults later in life (Ahlsen et al., 1993; Bailey et al., 1998; Laurence and Fatemi, 2005). Given the prominent role of oxidative stress in neurodegeneration, we hypothesized that oxidative stress occurs in the autistic brain and results in neurodegeneration that in turn contributes to the autistic symptoms. Indeed, the evidence that oxidative stress is present in children with autism continues to accumulate and, given the sharp increased incidence of autism, defining the mechanisms that result in clinical symptoms is urgently needed.

2.2   PERIPHERAL OXIDATIVE STRESS IN AUTISM

A number of factors have been implicated in the pathogenesis of autism, including genetic, environmental, immunological, and neurological. Nonetheless, the precise molecular mechanisms involved in the pathogenesis of autism remain unknown. Some similarities in groups of children with autism have been recognized. Chromosomal abnormalities have been found in 5%–10% of those with an autism spectrum disorder (ASD) and genetic susceptibility loci have also been identified in even greater numbers of those with ASD (Grice and Buxbaum, 2006). High concordance rates are present in siblings of autistic probands as well as in monozygotic twins (Bailey et al., 1995). From this and other evidence, it is generally accepted that autism has both genetic and environmental influences.

The presence of oxidative stress in peripheral tissues in children with autism has been well established (Keller and Persico, 2003; Chauhan and Chauhan, 2006). Children with autism often present with abnormal immune and digestive systems. Digestive pathology such as inflammation of the bowel and changes in digestive enzymes are common, and children often suffer from bowel problems and constipation and, more occasionally, liver problems (Horvath and Perman, 2002). The cause of these systemic changes is not entirely known but may be related to an increase in ROS. Increased nitric oxide (NO) levels in red blood cells and higher antioxidant enzyme activity as well as zinc deficiency and copper excess in plasma (Sogut et al., 2003; Chauhan et al., 2004; Sweeten et al., 2004) and elevated urinary isoprostanes levels, a lipid peroxidation product, are all reported in autism patients (Ming et al., 2005; Yao et al., 2006). Additionally, mitochondrial abnormalities (Filipek et al., 2003), with elevated levels of lactate, pyruvate, and ammonia, and lower levels of carnitine are reported in autistic case studies (McGinnis, 2004). However, how these oxidative products in the body in children with autism are related to the changes seen in the brain and the symptoms of autism is not known. Treatment with vitamin C, carnosine, or vitamin B_6 leads to significant improvement in autistic children compared with placebo (Kleijnen and Knipschild, 1991; Dolske et al., 1993; Chez et al., 2002), and this may be a result of protection against oxidative injury, perhaps caused by mitochondrial dysfunction.

The cause of the increase in oxidative species in the periphery is not known, but could be brought about by exposure to a number of environmental toxins such as mercury or infection that leads to increased production of ROS or decreased activity of superoxide dismutase (SOD), catalase, or glutathione peroxidase enzymes responsible for removing the ROS that are produced during normal metabolism in the cell. SOD catalyzes the conversion of the superoxide anion into hydrogen peroxide, and catalase and glutathione peroxidase act to convert this hydrogen peroxide into water. SOD, through the Haber–Weiss reaction, is also capable of mediating the formation of a hydroxide radical, a potent ROS, when free copper is present and other conditions are met. Related to this, significantly higher levels of ZnCuSOD, which could lead to an increase in the formation of hydroxide radicals, have been found in erythrocytes and in platelets of autistic individuals compared with controls (Zoroglu et al., 2004). Low levels of enzymes responsible for the removal of oxidative species are also seen in autism. Plasma concentrations of reduced glutathione (GSH) are lower ($4.1 \pm 0.5 \mu mol/L$) for autistics compared with healthy controls ($7.6 \pm 1.4 \mu mol/L$), $p < 0.001$ (James et al., 2004, 2006). Glutathione peroxidase, an antioxidant enzyme, requires GSH as a cofactor to break down oxidative species and lower levels of glutathione peroxidase (−44.4%) are found in erythrocytes of autistic individuals compared with controls (Golse et al., 1978; Yorbik et al., 2002). These lower levels of glutathione peroxidase can lead to a decrease in the ability of the cells to remove H_2O_2 formed by the action of ZnCuSOD. In autistic patients, the combination of an increase in the formation of oxidative species by SOD and a reduction in the removal of these species by glutathione peroxidase might result in an overall increase in oxidative stress.

Along with apparent genetic connections and the presence of systemic oxidative stress indicators, families with a high rate of autoimmune diseases and immune abnormalities also have higher rates of autism, for example, autoantibodies IgG, IgM, IgE, and IgA against brain proteins are present in some ASD patients (Jyonouchi et al., 2001) and proinflammatory cytokines can be produced in excessive amounts by peripheral blood mononuclear cells from autistic children (Jyonouchi et al., 2001). Inflammation including autoimmune conditions can cause an increase in oxidative stress since macrophage activity increases during inflammation and causes an increase in the production of ROS by the macrophages. Autoantibodies can be used as a marker for an increase in immune responses, and these are found at higher levels in patients with autism. For example, serum IgG antibrain autoantibodies are present in 35% of children with ASD compared with 5% from healthy children and IgM autoantibodies are present in 50% of children with ASD compared with 10% of controls (Vojdani et al., 2002). In another similar study, sera from 40 healthy subjects and 40 autistic children was analyzed for the presence of IgG, IgM, and IgA antibodies against nine neuron-specific antigens and three encephalitogenic and cross-reactive proteins. For one of these antigens, namely neurofilament, only up to 10% of controls had IgA, IgG, or IgM antibodies against this antigen compared to up to 57.5% of subjects with autism (Gu et al., 2003).

Our previous studies demonstrated significantly elevated levels of carboxyethyl pyrrole (CEP) epitopes and the corresponding autoantibodies in the blood of age-related macular degeneration (AMD) patients compared with healthy age- and sex-matched controls (Miyagi et al., 2002). However, while we measured levels of CEP and iso[4]levuglandin E_2 [iso[4]LGE$_2$]–protein adducts and levels of CEP and iso[4]LGE$_2$–protein autoantibodies in plasma from patients with documented ASD with age-matched healthy controls, we found no significant difference (Evans et al., 2008).

2.3   OXIDATIVE STRESS IN THE AUTISTIC BRAIN

The autistic brain is much younger than is typically seen in neurodegenerative diseases and may be at an increased risk for oxidative damage because the young brain has immature antioxidant systems that may be unable to protect against any increase in ROS (Meagher and FitzGerald, 2000). Oxidative species mediate the formation of lipid peroxides and other products that contribute to loss of membrane function and cellular damage. Lipids are likely very important in the physiology and function of the brain, and a decrease in their function and integrity likely plays a role in the etiology of neurodegenerative disorders. Membrane damage due to lipid peroxidation could lead to a decrease in functional neurons or a decrease in the conductive ability of axons in the white matter and a decrease in conductivity between different portions of the brain.

Lipid hydroperoxides and peroxidation products of common cellular lipids are produced in tissue after death, are unstable and short lived, making analysis of the levels of these substances in autopsy tissue difficult (Gu et al., 2003). Therefore, to avoid problems with directly measuring oxidative species, it is possible to identify other substances that are modified by these oxidative processes. We have recently developed and characterized a method of detecting CEP adducts using a specific antibody (Evans et al., 2008). CEP adduct is derived exclusively from free radical–induced oxidative cleavage of docosahexaenoates, e.g., the docohexaenoic acid (DHA) ester of 2-lysophosphatidylcholine (DHA-PC), to afford 4-hydroxy-7-oxohept-5-enoic acid (HOHA) ester of 2-lysophosphatidylcholine (HOHA-PC) that then reacts with protein to generate CEP modifications of the ε-amino groups of lysyl residues (Figure 2.1) (Gu et al., 2003). DHA is the most oxidizable fatty acid in humans, and while a minor lipid in most tissues, it is rich in specific regions of the brain and retina (Smith et al., 1994; Takeda et al., 2000). Since DHA is present in the brain at such high levels, CEP adducts can be used as a reliable and sensitive dosimeter for local oxidative damage (Skinner et al., 1993; Alvarez et al., 1994) and it provides a reasonable way for detecting oxidative damage in brain tissue in autism. We also used antibodies against iso[4]LGE$_2$–protein adducts that arise exclusively through free radical–induced cyclooxygenation of arachidonates, e.g., the arachidonic acid (AA) ester AA-PC, and subsequent adduction of an intermediate iso[4]LGE$_2$-PC with protein (Figure 2.1). Iso[4]LGE$_2$–protein adducts identify cumulative damage to cells from oxidative injury, such as that associated with inflammation (Money et al., 1971; Comi et al., 1999; Poliakov et al., 2003; Sweeten et al., 2003). In addition to oxidative modification, oxidative stress in biological systems usually elicits an antioxidant response and therefore some antioxidant enzymes such as heme oxygenase-1 (HO-1) that are induced by oxidative stress are also widely used as an acceptable oxidative stress marker in neurodegeneration (Chung et al., 2004).

Using immunocytochemistry, CEP was found localized primarily in the white matter, often extending well into the gray matter of axons in every case of autism examined, and was not found in any age-matched or even older control cases that were analyzed (Evans et al., 2008). Clearly, this pattern of staining is a hallmark of the autistic brain. The white matter is composed mostly of axons, and staining in

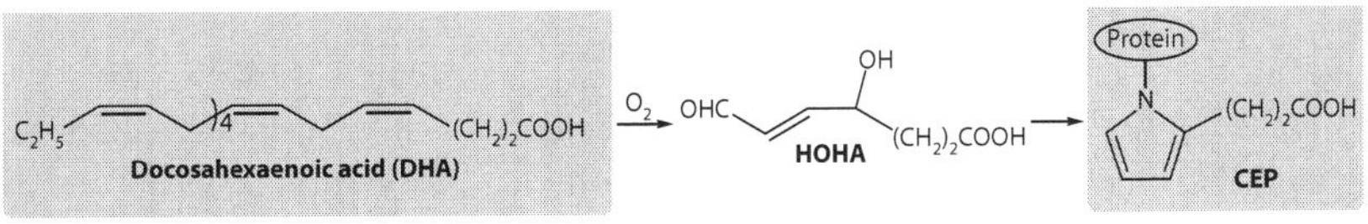

FIGURE 2.1   Generation of CEP.

this region may be indicative of a decreased functionality of the axons. Oxidative damage in the white matter in the autistic brain involves more than DHA-containing lipid since there are also elevated levels of iso[4]LGE$_2$–protein adducts, an oxidative protein modification derived from arachidonate-containing lipids. More importantly, the notion of elevated oxidative stress in autistic brain is further supported by the increased expression of HO-1, an inducible antioxidant enzyme. The induction of HO-1 is likely a response to elevated oxidative stress, which indicates that the elevated oxidative damage as evidenced by increased CEP and iso[4]LGE$_2$–protein adducts elicit functional consequences, e.g., by inducing an antioxidant response. The increase in HO-1 indicates that the antioxidant response is still intact and the body is attempting to retain homeostasis in the brain. In this regard, it is worthy of noting that brain-derived neurotrophic factor (BDNF), which can act as an antioxidant factor in brain development, is also increased in the autistic brain (Joosten and Houweling, 2004). However, given the presence of oxidative damage as evidenced by the CEP– and iso[4]LGE$_2$–protein adducts, it is likely that the total antioxidant response may be compromised and insufficient (Miyazaki et al., 2004; Connolly et al., 2006). Overall, our data represents the first direct experimental evidence of elevated oxidative stress in the autistic brain. The increase in ROS results in oxidative modifications, not limited to lipid, and recent studies also indicate an increased protein and DNA modification as evidenced by increased 3-nitrotyrosine (3-NT) levels (Sajdel-Sulkowska et al., 2008) and 8-OH-dG (Sajdel-Sulkowska et al., in press) in the autistic brain. The cause of the increased oxidative stress in the autistic brain is not known, but could be due to the exposure to environmental insults that lead to an increase in the production of oxidative species or a decrease in the ability of the body to process oxidative species that are normally produced in metabolism. It is now of great importance to understand the mechanisms underlying enhanced brain oxidative stress, whether they correlate with neuronal loss, and how they may lead to or compound the phenotype of autism patients.

2.4 AXON IS THE PRIMARY SITE FOR OXIDATIVE DAMAGE IN THE AUTISTIC BRAIN: POSSIBLE MECHANISMS UNDERLYING FUNCTIONAL UNDERCONNECTIVITY

One of the most astonishing aspects of our observation is that all three oxidative stress markers we used in our study demonstrated similar localizations within processes in the white matter in the autistic brain (Evans et al., 2008). The striking threadlike pattern in the white matter appears to be a hallmark of the autistic brain, suggesting that the axon may be the primary site of oxidative damage. Most of the axons connecting different sections of the brain are found in the white matter, and disruption of these connections may lead to a decrease in functional connectivity in the brain. This connection of parts of the brain has been shown to be responsible for many higher-order cognitive tasks such as reasoning, language, and social judgment (Halliwell et al., 1999). Likely not coincidentally, such tasks appear to be central in the symptoms seen in autism and it is suggested that underconnectivity in the brain may be responsible for the appearance of symptoms. Although more

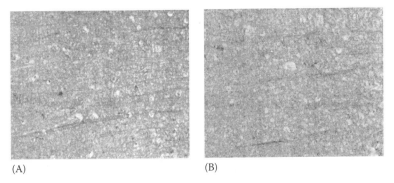

(A)   (B)

FIGURE 2.2 In autism, cellular processes contain choline acetyltransferase (A), in a pattern similar to that seen for CEP modifications (B).

research is warranted on the direct connection between white matter and connectivity in autism, our findings suggested a possible mechanism regarding how oxidative damage may be involved in underconnectivity and thereby contribute to the development of disease.

More recently, to characterize the identity of the neurons affected by oxidative modification, we have explored the association of CEP with various abnormal systems (i.e., GABAergic, glutamatergic, cholinergic, and serotoninergic systems) in autism and found that the immunostaining pattern of choline acetyltransferase, a marker of cholinergic neurons, was very similar to the pattern seen with the CEP antibody (Figure 2.2), suggesting that cholinergic neurons may be more vulnerable to CEP modifications in autism.

Consistent with the immunocytochemical detection of CEP primarily in axons, our further biochemical study suggested that neurofilament heavy (NFH) chain may be the primary target for CEP modification. Western blot analysis of CEP antibody revealed a band around 200 kDa, similar to the molecular size of NFH and, coimmunoprecipitation experiments using autism brain homogenates confirmed that NFH is modified by CEP. Indeed, NFH also demonstrated an immunostaining pattern very similar to that of CEP in autism tissues and a coimmunostaining assay confirmed the colocalization of CEP and NFH within the same processes (not shown). This is the first study implicating a specific protein in autism, which has the potential to advance our understanding of the mechanisms underlying functional underconnectivity.

2.5 FORMATION OF CEP–ADDUCT IS NOT A POSTMORTEM ARTIFACT

The most obvious concern of any immunocytochemical detection of oxidative modifications in postmortem human tissues is whether the positive signal is simply due to postmortem artifact. To test for the effect of postmortem interval (PMI) on the accumulation of these modifications within tissue structures, we examined CEP in a rat model of PMI. Initial experiments found no CEP immunoreactivity in the brain in any of the samples up to 24 h postmortem delay using WKY rat strain. However, use of an additional spontaneous hypertensive rat strain (SHR), proved to be very informative. Using

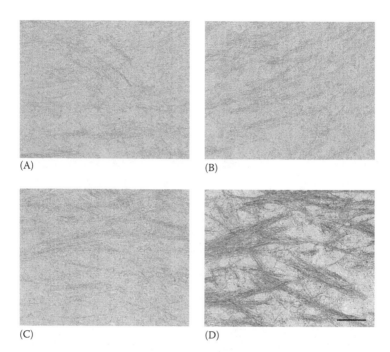

(A)   (B)

(C)   (D)

FIGURE 2.3 In a rat model, CEP is localized to cellular processes within the brain strikingly similar to the CEP localization in autism. To test for any postmortem changes in CEP modifications, rat pup brains were fixed following either 0 h (A), 4 h (B), or 8 h (C) postmortem delay. All rats displayed similar levels of CEP and following image analysis showed no significant differences (not shown). Paralleling the findings in human autism cases, CEP localization overlaps with neurofilament protein accumulation on adjacent sections (C, CEP and D, neurofilament protein). Scale bar = 50 μm.

this model, rat pups were kept at room temperature for different interval (0–8 h) prior to brain dissection to simulate increased PMI. All rat pups from all dams tested accumulated CEP in areas of the brain that overlapped significantly with neurofilaments accumulation as seen using monoclonal antibody SMI-31 (Covance) (Figure 2.3). Image analysis was performed to measure both the percent area stained and the intensity of labeling for both CEP and neurofilaments. No correlation was found between either the amount or intensity of CEP accumulation and PMI. These data strongly argue for neurofilament protein being a specific target for CEP modification (Evans et al., 2008).

To further correlate the rat model data with human disease, the levels of CEP modifications were compared in autism and control brain sections, which had varying and disparate PMI. There was no significant correlation between CEP and PMI, with times ranging from 13 to 39 h (Figure 2.4). Even in the control case with the longest PMI (36 h), there was no recognizable immunoreactivity to CEP (data not shown). Densitometric analysis of the staining in these autistic cases clearly did not show any significant correlation with differences in PMI (Figure 2.4).

Taken together, the human and rat models provide strong evidence that CEP modifications do not accumulate after death, and therefore may be a direct result

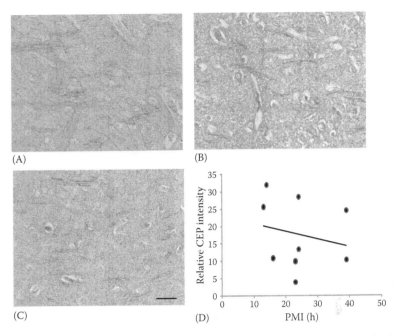

FIGURE 2.4 In autism, CEP is localized specifically to processes within the brain. Morphologically, no differences are apparent between cases collected following a relatively short PMI of 13 h (A), or 24 h (B), or even after a long PMI of 39 h (C). Computer-assisted image analysis of the intensity of CEP accumulation in nine cases of autism found no significant correlation when compared with PMI (D). Scale bar = 50 μm.

of oxidative damage in the living brain. Although this excludes a direct correlation between postmortem time and staining, this does not account for any differences in the presence of these substances in the rat brain.

2.6 CONCLUSION

There is ample evidence suggesting systemic oxidative stress in autism patients and evidence for brain oxidative stress is now beginning to accumulate. Our immunocytochemical and biochemical studies provide the first experimental evidence demonstrating lipid modification in autistic brain and suggests CEP– and iso[4]LGE$_2$–protein adducts, products of lipid peroxidation, as possible hallmark oxidative stress markers for the autistic brain. Supplementary animal experiments show that CEP formation is unlikely due to postmortem artifact, supporting CEP as a specific oxidative stress marker. From a structural perspective, our findings suggest that axons of cholinergic neurons in the white matter are the primary site of oxidative damage. At the molecular level, we have identified NFH to be the major target for CEP modification. Our findings not only support the notion that brain oxidative stress plays an important role in autism but now warrant future in-depth mechanistic studies, which have the potential to provide new targets for therapeutic efforts.

ACKNOWLEDGMENTS

This research was supported by Autism Research Institute. Human tissue was obtained from the NICHD Brain and Tissue Bank for Developmental Disorders at the University of Maryland under contracts N01-HD-4-3368 and N01-HD-4-3383.

REFERENCES

Ahlsen, G., Rosengren, L., Belfrage, M., Palm, A., Haglid, K., Hamberger, A., and Gillberg, C. (1993). Glial fibrillary acidic protein in the cerebrospinal fluid of children with autism and other neuropsychiatric disorders. *Biol. Psychiatry* 33:734–743.

Alvarez, R. A., Aguirre, G. D., Acland, G. M., and Anderson, R. E. (1994). Docosapentaenoic acid is converted to docosahexaenoic acid in the retinas of normal and *prcd*-affected miniature poodle dogs. *Invest. Ophthalmol. Vis. Sci.* 35:402–408.

Bailey, A., Le Couteur, A., Gottesman, I., Bolton, P., Simonoff, E., Yuzda, E., and Rutter, M. (1995). Autism as a strongly genetic disorder: Evidence from a British twin study. *Psychol. Med.* 25:63–77.

Bailey, A., Luthert, P., Dean, A., Harding, B., Janota, I., Montgomery, M., Rutter, M., and Lantos, P. (1998). A clinicopathological study of autism. *Brain* 121 (Pt 5):889–905.

Chauhan, A. and Chauhan, V. (2006). Oxidative stress in autism. *Pathophysiology* 13:171–181.

Chauhan, A., Chauhan, V., Brown, W. T., and Cohen, I. (2004). Oxidative stress in autism: Increased lipid peroxidation and reduced serum levels of ceruloplasmin and transferrin— the antioxidant proteins. *Life Sci.* 75:2539–2549.

Chez, M. G., Buchanan, C. P., Aimonovitch, M. C., Becker, M., Schaefer, K., Black, C., and Komen, J. (2002). Double-blind, placebo-controlled study of L-carnosine supplementation in children with autistic spectrum disorders. *J. Child Neurol.* 17:833–837.

Chung, M. K., Dalton, K. M., Alexander, A. L., and Davidson, R. J. (2004). Less white matter concentration in autism: 2D voxel-based morphometry. *Neuroimage* 23:242–251.

Comi, A. M., Zimmerman, A. W., Frye, V. H., Law, P. A., and Peeden, J. N. (1999). Familial clustering of autoimmune disorders and evaluation of medical risk factors in autism. *J. Child Neurol.* 14:388–394.

Connolly, A. M., Chez, M., Streif, E. M., Keeling, R. M., Golumbek, P. T., Kwon, J. M., Riviello, J. J., Robinson, R. G., Neuman, R. J., and Deuel, R. M. (2006). Brain-derived neurotrophic factor and autoantibodies to neural antigens in sera of children with autistic spectrum disorders, Landau–Kleffner syndrome, and epilepsy. *Biol. Psychiatry* 59:354–363.

Courchesne, E., Townsend, J., and Saitoh, O. (1994). The brain in infantile autism: Posterior fossa structures are abnormal. *Neurology* 44:214–223.

Dolske, M. C., Spollen, J., McKay, S., Lancashire, E., and Tolbert, L. (1993). A preliminary trial of ascorbic acid as supplemental therapy for autism. *Prog. Neuropsychopharmacol. Biol. Psychiatry* 17:765–774.

Evans, T., Siedlak, S. L., Lu, L., Fu, X., Wang, Z., McGinnis, W. R., Fakhoury, E., Castellani, R. J., Hazen, S. L., Walsh, W. L., Lewis, A. T., Salomon, R. G., Smith, M. A., Perry, G., and Zhu, X. (2008). The autistic phenotype exhibits a remarkably localized modification of brain protein by products of free radical-induced lipid oxidation. *Am. J. Biochem. Biotechnol. (Special Issue on Autism Spectrum Disorders)* 4:61–72.

Filipek, P. A., Juranek, J., Smith, M., Mays, L. Z., Ramos, E. R., Bocian, M., Masser-Frye, D., Laulhere, T. M., Modahl, C., Spence, M. A., and Gargus, J. J. (2003). Mitochondrial dysfunction in autistic patients with 15q inverted duplication. *Ann. Neurol.* 53:801–804.

Golse, B., Debray-Ritzen, P., Durosay, P., Puget, K., and Michelson, A. M. (1978). Alterations in two enzymes: Superoxide dismutase and glutathione peroxidase in developmental infantile psychosis (infantile autism). *Rev. Neurol.* 134:699–705.

Grice, D. E. and Buxbaum, J. D. (2006). The genetics of autism spectrum disorders. *Neuromol. Med.* 8:451–460.

Gu, X., Meer, S. G., Miyagi, M., Rayborn, M. E., Hollyfield, J. G., Crabb, J. W., and Salomon, R. G. (2003). Carboxyethylpyrrole protein adducts and autoantibodies, biomarkers for age-related macular degeneration. *J. Biol. Chem.* 278:42027–42035.

Halliwell, B., Zhao, K., and Whiteman, M. (1999). Nitric oxide and peroxynitrite. The ugly, the uglier and the not so good: A personal view of recent controversies. *Free Radic. Res.* 31:651–669.

Horvath, K. and Perman, J. A. (2002). Autism and gastrointestinal symptoms. *Curr. Gastroenterol. Rep.* 4:251–258.

James, S. J., Cutler, P., Melnyk, S., Jernigan, S., Janak, L., Gaylor, D. W., and Neubrander, J. A. (2004). Metabolic biomarkers of increased oxidative stress and impaired methylation capacity in children with autism. *Am. J. Clin. Nutr.* 80:1611–1617.

James, S. J., Melnyk, S., Jernigan, S., Cleves, M. A., Halsted, C. H., Wong, D. H., Cutler, P., Bock, K., Boris, M., Bradstreet, J. J., Baker, S. M., and Gaylor, D. W. (2006). Metabolic endophenotype and related genotypes are associated with oxidative stress in children with autism. *Am. J. Med. Genet. B Neuropsychiatr. Genet.* 141B:947–956.

Joosten, E. A. and Houweling, D. A. (2004). Local acute application of BDNF in the lesioned spinal cord anti-inflammatory and anti-oxidant effects. *Neuroreport* 15:1163–1166.

Jyonouchi, H., Sun, S., and Le, H. (2001). Proinflammatory and regulatory cytokine production associated with innate and adaptive immune responses in children with autism spectrum disorders and developmental regression. *J. Neuroimmunol.* 120:170–179.

Keller, F. and Persico, A. M. (2003). The neurobiological context of autism. *Mol. Neurobiol.* 28:1–22.

Kleijnen, J. and Knipschild, P. (1991). Niacin and vitamin B6 in mental functioning: A review of controlled trials in humans. *Biol. Psychiatry* 29:931–941.

Laurence, J. A. and Fatemi, S. H. (2005). Glial fibrillary acidic protein is elevated in superior frontal, parietal and cerebellar cortices of autistic subjects. *Cerebellum* 4:206–210.

Lee, H. G., Perry, G., Moreira, P. I., Garrett, M. R., Liu, Q., Zhu, X., Takeda, A., Nunomura, A., and Smith, M. A. (2005). Tau phosphorylation in Alzheimer's disease: Pathogen or protector? *Trends Mol. Med.* 11:164–169.

McGinnis, W. R. (2004). Oxidative stress in autism. *Altern. Ther. Health Med.* 10:22–36.

Meagher, E. A. and FitzGerald, G. A. (2000). Indices of lipid peroxidation in vivo: Strengths and limitations. *Free Radic. Biol. Med.* 28:1745–1750.

Ming, X., Stein, T. P., Brimacombe, M., Johnson, W. G., Lambert, G. H., and Wagner, G. C. (2005). Increased excretion of a lipid peroxidation biomarker in autism. *Prostaglandins Leukot. Essent. Fatty Acids* 73:379–384.

Miyagi, M., Sakaguchi, H., Darrow, R. M., Yan, L., West, K. A., Aulak, K. S., Stuehr, D. J., Hollyfield, J. G., Organisciak, D. T., and Crabb, J. W. (2002). Evidence that light modulates protein nitration in rat retina. *Mol. Cell Proteomics* 1:293–303.

Miyazaki, K., Narita, N., Sakuta, R., Miyahara, T., Naruse, H., Okado, N., and Narita, M. (2004). Serum neurotrophin concentrations in autism and mental retardation: A pilot study. *Brain Dev.* 26:292–295.

Money, J., Bobrow, N. A., and Clarke, F. C. (1971). Autism and autoimmune disease: A family study. *J. Autism Child Schizophr.* 1:146–160.

Nunomura, A., Perry, G., Aliev, G., Hirai, K., Takeda, A., Balraj, E. K., Jones, P. K., Ghanbari, H., Wataya, T., Shimohama, S., Chiba, S., Atwood, C. S., Petersen, R. B., and Smith, M. A. (2001). Oxidative damage is the earliest event in Alzheimer disease. *J. Neuropathol. Exp. Neurol.* 60:759–767.

Nunomura, A., Chiba, S., Lippa, C. F., Cras, P., Kalaria, R. N., Takeda, A., Honda, K., Smith, M. A., and Perry, G. (2004). Neuronal RNA oxidation is a prominent feature of familial Alzheimer's disease. *Neurobiol. Dis.* 17:108–113.

Poliakov, E., Brennan, M. L., Macpherson, J., Zhang, R., Sha, W., Narine, L., Salomon, R. G., and Hazen, S. L. (2003). Isolevuglandins, a novel class of isoprostenoid derivatives, function as integrated sensors of oxidant stress and are generated by myeloperoxidase in vivo. *FASEB J.* 17:2209–2220.

Sajdel-Sulkowska, E. M., Lipinski, B., Windom, H., Audhya, T., and McGinnis, W. (2008). Oxidative stress in autism: Cerebellar 3-nitrotyrosine levels. *Am. J. Biochem. Biotechnol. (Special Issue on Autism Spectrum Disorders)* 4:73–84.

Sajdel-Sulkowska, E. M., Ming, X., and Koibuchi, N. (2009). Increase in brain neurotrophin-3 and oxidative stress in autism. *Cerebellum* [Epub PMID 19357934].

Schumann, C. M. and Amaral, D. G. (2005). Stereological estimation of the number of neurons in the human amygdaloid complex. *J. Comp. Neurol.* 491:320–329.

Skinner, E. R., Watt, C., Besson, J. A., and Best, P. V. (1993). Differences in the fatty acid composition of the grey and white matter of different regions of the brains of patients with Alzheimer's disease and control subjects. *Brain* 116 (Pt 3):717–725.

Smith, M. A., Kutty, R. K., Richey, P. L., Yan, S. D., Stern, D., Chader, G. J., Wiggert, B., Petersen, R. B., and Perry, G. (1994). Heme oxygenase-1 is associated with the neurofibrillary pathology of Alzheimer's disease. *Am. J. Pathol.* 145:42–47.

Sogut, S., Zoroglu, S. S., Ozyurt, H., Yilmaz, H. R., Ozugurlu, F., Sivasli, E., Yetkin, O., Yanik, M., Tutkun, H., Savas, H. A., Tarakcioglu, M., and Akyol, O. (2003). Changes in nitric oxide levels and antioxidant enzyme activities may have a role in the pathophysiological mechanisms involved in autism. *Clin. Chim. Acta* 331:111–117.

Sweeten, T. L., Bowyer, S. L., Posey, D. J., Halberstadt, G. M., and McDougle, C. J. (2003). Increased prevalence of familial autoimmunity in probands with pervasive developmental disorders. *Pediatrics* 112:420–424.

Sweeten, T. L., Posey, D. J., Shankar, S., and McDougle, C. J. (2004). High nitric oxide production in autistic disorder: A possible role for interferon-gamma. *Biol. Psychiatry* 55:434–437.

Takeda, A., Smith, M. A., Avila, J., Nunomura, A., Siedlak, S. L., Zhu, X., Perry, G., and Sayre, L. M. (2000). In Alzheimer's disease, heme oxygenase is coincident with Alz50, an epitope of tau induced by 4-hydroxy-2-nonenal modification. *J. Neurochem.* 75:1234–1241.

Vojdani, A., Campbell, A. W., Anyanwu, E., Kashanian, A., Bock, K., and Vojdani, E. (2002). Antibodies to neuron-specific antigens in children with autism: Possible cross-reaction with encephalitogenic proteins from milk, *Chlamydia pneumoniae* and Streptococcus group A. *J. Neuroimmunol.* 129:168–177.

Yao, Y., Walsh, W. J., McGinnis, W. R., and Pratico, D. (2006). Altered vascular phenotype in autism: Correlation with oxidative stress. *Arch. Neurol.* 63:1161–1164.

Yorbik, O., Sayal, A., Akay, C., Akbiyik, D. I., and Sohmen, T. (2002). Investigation of antioxidant enzymes in children with autistic disorder. *Prostaglandins Leukot. Essent. Fatty Acids* 67:341–343.

Zhu, X., Lee, H. G., Casadesus, G., Avila, J., Drew, K., Perry, G., and Smith, M. A. (2005). Oxidative imbalance in Alzheimer's disease. *Mol. Neurobiol.* 31:205–217.

Zoroglu, S. S., Armutcu, F., Ozen, S., Gurel, A., Sivasli, E., Yetkin, O., and Meram, I. (2004). Increased oxidative stress and altered activities of erythrocyte free radical scavenging enzymes in autism. *Eur. Arch. Psychiatry Clin. Neurosci.* 254:143–147.

3 Oxidative Stress and Neurotrophin Signaling in Autism

Elizabeth M. Sajdel-Sulkowska[1,2,*]

[1]Department of Psychiatry, Harvard Medical School
and [2]Department of Psychiatry, Brigham and
Women's Hospital, Boston, MA 02115, USA

CONTENTS

Autism is a neurodevelopmental disorder characterized by social and language deficits, ritualistic-repetitive behaviors, and disturbance in motor functions. As concordance in monozygotic twins is less than 100% and the phenotypic expression is variable, both genetic predispositions and environmental triggers, many of which induce oxidative stress, are likely to be involved in the etiology of autism, but the cause(s) remain elusive. Data from brain imaging and head-circumference studies, as well as Purkinje cell analysis showing early brain overgrowth followed by slow brain growth and a decrease in Purkinje cell number in a subset of autistic cases suggest that regulatory mechanisms in brain growth and differentiation are abnormal

---

* Corresponding author: Tel.: +1-617-732-5859; fax: +1-617-713-3078; e-mail: esulkowska@rics.bwh.harvard.edu

in autism. Cell proliferation, differentiation, and the elimination of an excess number of neurons produced during the course of normal brain development are regulated by neurotrophins. We have recently reported an altered expression of brain neurotrophins, and specifically an increased level of neurotrophin 3 (NT-3) in the autistic cerebellum. Neurotrophin imbalance is likely to result in the initial overgrowth of brain tissue followed by an arrested growth resulting in abnormal brain connectivity. Here, we review the evidence for increased oxidative stress in autism, the role of neurotrophins in brain development, data supporting altered neurotrophin signaling in autism, as well as animal data suggesting both the dual role of neurotrophins in the developing brain and the possible association between oxidative stress and altered neurotrophin expression. We also address the therapeutic potential of neurotrophins in autism.

3.1 FURTHER EVIDENCE FOR INVOLVEMENT OF OXIDATIVE STRESS IN AUTISM

Autistic pathology results most likely from the interplay between genetic predisposition and the action of environmental triggers. Several environmental toxins, such as heavy metals (Bokara et al., 2008) including mercury (Palmer et al., 2009; Windham et al., 2006) and pesticides (D'Amelio et al., 2005), polychlorinated biphenyls (PCBs) (Kimura-Kuroda et al., 2007), as well as maternal infection (Brown et al., 2008) have been implicated in autism; these in turn share the ability to increase oxidative stress.

Oxidative stress occurs in the course of normal physiological processes. The damaging action of reactive oxygen species (ROS) targets key cellular macromolecules, including lipids, carbohydrates, proteins, DNA, and RNA. This action is kept in check by the body's natural antioxidant defense system that includes metal-binding metalloproteins and other antioxidants. In response to exposure to environmental toxins and in a number of disease conditions, this defense system appears to be overburdened, leading to unchecked oxidative stress damage. Specifically, oxidative damage to proteins is mediated by peroxynitrate formed by the reaction of superoxide with nitric oxide (NO), reacting with tyrosine residues (Beckman and Koppenol, 1996), and resulting in the formation of 3-nitrotyrosine (3-NT, a specific marker of oxidative damage to proteins). Modification of tyrosine residues in proteins can alter their conformation and function, which in turn has a profound effect on the developing brain.

There is growing evidence supporting the role of oxidative stress and specifically modification of proteins, as evidenced by increased 3-nitrotyrosine in over 50 pathologies including Alzheimer disease (AD), Parkinson disease (PD), and cancer (Beal, 2002; Neumann et al., 2008). Increased oxidative stress is also being implicated in autistic pathology. We have recently reported an increase in 3-nitrotyrosine in autistic cerebella (Sajdel-Sulkowska et al., 2008). Furthermore, it appears that tyrosine residues likely to be modified under increased oxidative stress are specifically related to the particular pathology and are genetically determined (Neumann et al., 2008). A proteonomic approach has identified specific target proteins of nitration in the Alzheimer's hippocampus (Sultana et al., 2006); others have shown that more than half of the modified proteins in AD and PD were related to the respective pathologies

(Sacksteder et al., 2006). It is possible that the genetic predisposition implicated in autism involves genes involved in oxidative defense systems that render the individuals more sensitive to oxidative stress triggers. Such a possibility is very intriguing since early screening could identify individuals "allergic" to environmental toxins. Once identified, the families may be able to implement dietary and other measures to reduce the risk of autism and/or control the extent of symptoms.

Indeed, there is evidence for the disruption of antioxidant defense mechanisms in autism manifested by lower than control levels of glutathione peroxidase (GSPHx) (Yorbik et al., 2002), by lower levels of plasma glutathione levels and higher ratios of oxidized glutathione to reduced glutathione (James et al., 2004, 2006) and by lower levels of two major serum antioxidant metalloproteins ceruloplasmin (copper-binding protein) and transferrin (iron-binding protein (Chauhan and Chauhan, 2006; Chauhan et al., 2004).

Concomitant with a decrease in the oxidative defense in autism, there is an increased oxidative stress in autism indicated by observations of increased lipid oxidation markers in blood (Chauhan et al., 2004; Zoroglu et al., 2004) and in urine (Ming et al., 2005; Yao et al., 2006), increased levels of NO in red blood cells (Sogut et al., 2003), and plasma levels of NO metabolites (Sweeten et al., 2004).

We have previously reported a 65% increase in cerebellar 3-nitrotyrosine (Figure 3.1; Sajdel-Sulkowska et al., 2008). More recently, we have observed an increase in the DNA oxidation marker, 8-OH-dG, in the autistic cerebellum (Sajdel-Sulkowska et al., 2009). Our study showed an overall 63.4% increase in the level of 8-OH-dG in the autistic cerebellum with four out of five autistic samples higher than mean control level. However, one of the autistic cases fell within the control values, suggesting that there may be a subset of autistic cases with little or no DNA damage. A similar conclusion was recently arrived at with respect to decrease in Purkinje cell number in a subset of autistic cases (Whitney et al., 2008); it would be of interest to compare directly Purkinje cell number and the levels of 8-OH-dG directly in the same cerebellar samples. A trend toward increased urinary 8-OH-dG levels in

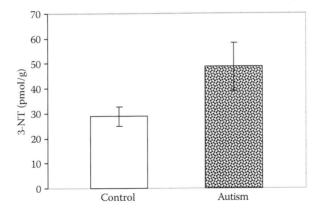

FIGURE 3.1 Increased 3-nitrotyrosine levels in autistic cerebella. 3-NT, 3-nitrotyrosine. (From Sajdel-Sulkowska, E. M. et al., *Am. J. Biochem. Biotechnol.* (*Special Issue on Autism Spectrum Disorders*), 4, 73, 2008. With permission.)

children has been reported in autism (Ming et al., 2005). Increased 8-OH-dG levels have been also observed in lymphocytes (Mecocci et al., 2002), the cerebrospinal fluid (CSF)-DNA (Lovell et al., 1999), and in the urine of patients with AD (Lee et al., 2007) and PD (Sato et al., 2005). The children with brain damage showed increased urinary 8-OH-dG levels (Fukuda et al., 2008). An immunohistochemical approach showed 10 times higher brain levels of 8-OH-dG in schizophrenia (Nishioka and Arnold, 2004).

The oxidative stress in autism could result from (1) the exposure to high levels of environmental pro-oxidants such as pesticides (Abdollahi et al., 2004; D'Amelio et al., 2005) and mercury (Hg) (Mutter et al., 2005a,b; Palmer et al., 2008; Windham et al., 2006); (2) inability to metabolize and clear the toxicant, such as heavy metals, from the system (Bradstreet et al., 2003; McGinnis 2004; Serajee et al., 2004); (3) the decreased internal antioxidant defense mechanisms (James et al., 2004; Yorbik et al., 2002, 2006; Zoroglu et al., 2004); or (4) increased sensitivity to oxidative stress (Buyske et al., 2006; Yang et al., 2008). It is possible that all four mechanisms may be involved in precipitating autistic pathology.

3.2 NEUROTROPHINS AND BRAIN DEVELOPMENT: COULD THE IMBALANCE IN BRAIN NEUROTROPHIN EXPRESSION LEAD TO THE ABNORMALITIES OBSERVED IN AUTISM?

Neurotrophins play a critical role in the regulation of growth, development, survival, differentiation, and function of neurons in both central and peripheral nervous system and synaptic development and maintenance, thus they are likely players in autistic pathology. Each of the four major mammalian neurotrophins, brain-derived neurotrophic factor (BDNF), nerve growth factor (NGF), neurotrophin 3 (NT-3), and NT-4, binds to its receptors, tropomysin-related kinase (TrkA, TrkB, TrkC), and neurotrophin receptor (75NTR), and activates signaling pathways affecting transcription. Neurotrophins are synthesized and secreted by the target organs, bind to the receptors, and act locally to regulate target innervations and nerve function. The neurotrophin–receptor complexes are also internalized and transported to cell bodies where they promote neuronal survival and differentiation (Reichardt, 2006). Thus the activity of neurotrophins can be regulated by factors involved in the transcriptional and posttranscriptional steps, receptor binding, and transport.

During development, neurotrophins are involved in the regulation of neuronal density. Developmental expression of neurotrophins has been examined in the rat hippocampus, neocortex, and cerebellum (Das et al., 2001). The results of this study indicate brain region–specific neurotrophin expression and independent regulation of neurotrophin mRNAs and proteins.

The involvement of neurotrophins in neuronal plasticity is suggested by the observations of altered brain levels of neurotrophins in response to social and physical stimulation in mice (Zhu et al., 2006) and learning in rats (Klinstova et al., 2004). Furthermore, exposure to environmental toxins such as lead (Bokara et al., 2008) or chlorpyrifos (Betancourt et al., 2007), resulting in increased oxidative stress, is associated with an increase in hippocampal BDNF (Chao et al., 2007), and maternal infection during pregnancy results in altered levels of brain NGF and BDNF (Marx et al., 1999).

3.2.1 EVIDENCE FOR ALTERED NEUROTROPHIN EXPRESSION IN AUTISM

Analysis of archived neonatal blood samples by recycling immunoaffinity chroma-tography showed an increase in BDNF and NT-4 in newborns that subsequently developed autism and mental retardation (Nelson et al., 2001). However, subsequent enzyme-linked immunosorbent assay (ELISA) analysis of these samples did not confirm the increase (Nelson et al., 2006). Yet serum BDNF levels were elevated severalfold in older children with autism (Connolly et al., 2006). Similarly, increased levels of plasma BDNF were observed in children with early-onset autism (Enstrom et al., 2008). In the archived neonatal samples, the NT-3 levels were significantly lower than in controls (Nelson et al., 2006). More recently, serum BDNF has been found to increase with age, while that of NT-3 and NT-4/5 decreased with age (Nelson et al., 2006). Serum BDNF levels were found to increase during the first several years, which then decreased slightly in adults. They were significantly lower in autism cases aged 0–9 years compared to age-matched controls (Katoh-Semba et al., 2007). In adult (25 years of age) autistic cases, serum levels of BDNF were lower than in controls (Hashimoto et al., 2006). An increase in serum BDNF and NT-4 levels in autism has been reported (Miyazaki et al., 2004). Serum levels of BDNF were lower in adult male patients with autism than controls (Hashimoto et al., 2006). BDNF hyperactivity may be associated with early brain overgrowth and increased prevalence of seizures in autism. These differences in the results of indi-vidual studies may reflect an expected spectrum of changes in neurotrophin expres-sion in autism. However, irrespective of the direction, altered brain neurotrophin levels are likely to be associated with impaired brain structure and function.

Despite evidence pointing to the role of neurotrophins in the pathophysiology of autism discussed above, data on the levels of brain neurotrophins in autism have been limited to two studies, and NT-3 between control and autistic cases have not been directly compared. The only direct assay of brain neurotrophin levels was reported by Perry et al. (2001). Using an ELISA, they reported a threefold higher level of BDNF in the basal forebrain in autism with no changes in NGF in teen-age cases. NT-3 levels were not measured in this particular study. They interpreted this increase as an intrinsic component of the autism disease process. The results of the only other study of human brain neurotrophins in control subjects using an immunohistochemical approach indicated that all four neurotrophins (NGF, BDNF, NT-3, and NT-4) are expressed in the human hippocampus at all ages, with the higher number of immunoreactive perikarya present in pre- and perinatal ages than in adults (Quartu et al., 1999).

Our recent report (Sajdel-Sulkowska et al., 2009) is the first to compare the levels of NT-3 between autistic and control brains. We examined the possible link between increased oxidative stress and brain neurotrophin levels in autism using cerebellar samples from the subset of autistic and control cases used in our previ-ous study on brain 3-nitrotyrosine levels (Sajdel-Sulkowska et al., 2008). We have selected the cerebellum because of its intimate involvement in autism indicated by increased cerebellar volume, decreased ratio of gray to white matter (Courchesne et al., 2001, 2003), and decrease in Purkinje cell number (Courchesne, 1991; Kemper and Bauman, 1993; Rivto et al., 1986; Whitney et al., 2008). NT-3 was

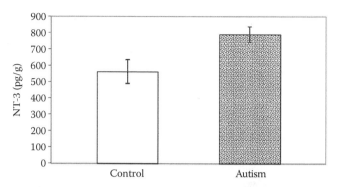

FIGURE 3.2 Increased NT-3 levels in autistic cerebella. (From Sajdel-Sulkowska, E.M., Ming, X., and Koibuchi, N. (2009), *Cerebellum* [Epub PMID 19357934] With permission.)

selected because of its high expression in the developing rat cerebellum (Das et al., 2001) and its critical role in migration and survival of cerebellar granule (Li et al., 2004) and Purkinje cells (Kawakami et al., 2000). The data presented in Figure 3.2 shows a statistically significant NT-3 increase (40.3%) in the autistic cerebellum and support a concept of altered brain neurotrophin expression in autism. As stated above, NT-3 levels in human brain have not been previously quantified; our data is thus the first on the brain levels of NT-3 in autism. It is intriguing that the expression of this particular neurotrophin expression appears to decrease with age in the rodent brain (Das et al., 2001). Consequently, if a similar developmental pattern is present in human cerebellum, then prolonged and persistent elevation of NT-3 in autism could upset the balance of neurotrophic factors and affect brain growth and development. Specifically, overexpression of NT-3 could contribute to the cerebellar overgrowth observed in some autistic cases (Courchesne et al., 2001). Furthermore, persistent elevation of NT-3, specifically involved in neuronal differentiation (Ghosh and Greenberg, 1995), neurite fasciculation (Segal et al., 1995), and axonal targeting, may have other profound effects such as on synapse formation.

We also observed a positive correlation between cerebellar NT-3 and cerebellar 3-nitrotyrosine, which suggests an association between increased oxidative stress and altered brain neurotrophin levels in autism. This association is not perfect ($r = .83$), suggesting the presence of a subset of autistic cases with normal neurotrophin levels. It is possible that subsets of autistic cases with unique clinical symptoms are related to specific molecular changes.

3.2.2 POSSIBLE MECHANISMS INVOLVED IN ALTERED NEUROTROPHIN SIGNALING IN AUTISM: AN ENVIRONMENTAL IMPACT

The discussion presented above thus seems to support the notion that abnormalities in neurotrophin signaling pathway are involved in autistic pathology. Evidence discussed below suggests that changes in neurotrophin expression could be brought about by the environmental triggers of oxidative stress as well as a genetic component.

Neonatal exposure to lead induces an increase in hippocampal BDNF (Chao et al., 2007), and the levels of NGF and BDNF are lower in women with evidence of infection during pregnancy (Marx et al., 1999). Our data revealing the correlation between NT-3 and oxidative stress seems to support environmental cause of neurotrophin imbalance in the autistic brain and increased oxidative stress as a causal factor in autism.

3.2.3 Neurotrophin Signaling in Autism: Genetic Component

It is quite likely that mutations affecting neurotrophin signaling pathway are also involved in autism. While the polymorphism in BDNF has been linked to impaired hippocampal function (Egan et al., 2003), a significant association has been reported between autism and SNP 16 in lymphocyte BDNF DNA (Nishimura et al., 2007). Such association is also found with obsessive compulsive disorder, attention deficit disorders, anxiety disorders, and anxiety-related personality traits (Nishimura et al., 2007). Abnormal, alternatively spliced forms of protein, Ca^{2+}-dependent activator protein (CAPS2/CADPS2), involved in release of neurotrophins, have been reported in some of the autistic cases (Sadakata et al., 2007). Because of the close association between BDNF and Trk-B, a polymorphism in the receptor could affect BDNF trafficking. Hyperactivity of BDNF-TrkB signaling, associated with epilepsy (Binder et al., 2001), has also been found in autism (Tsai, 2005). With respect to NT-3, one would expect to find mutations in Sp3/4 (Tabuchi, 2008). Finally, in the context of abnormal neurotrophin signaling in autism, one should not ignore possible mutations in the BDNF transcriptional repressor (MeCP2) in Rett syndrome (Chen et al., 2003). It is possible that polymorphic forms of proteins involved in the neurotrophin signaling cascade in autism express an increased number of tyrosine residues in the positions that render them more accessible to oxidative modification and formation of 3-nitrotyrosine. A model incorporating this concept is presented in Figure 3.3.

3.2.4 Dual Role of Neurotrophins

This discussion would be incomplete without pointing out the dual role of neurotrophins. In addition to the trophic function, NT-3 may also under certain conditions exacerbate oxidative stress (Bates et al., 2002) as part of a response to hypoxia (Pasarica et al., 2005). NT-3 is also known to reduce survival of Purkinje cells in vitro (Morrison and Mason, 1998).

In that respect, NT-3 behaves like NO that plays an important role in neuronal differentiation by nitrative modification of specific proteins (Cappelletti et al., 2003). However, overproduction of nitric oxide leads to peroxynitrite formation and is a source of neurotoxicity (Vargas et al., 2004). Increase in peroxynitrite results in 3-NT protein modification, which is observed in a number of human pathologies. It has been suggested that the negative action of NT-3 may be related to altered glutamate receptors (Behrens et al., 1999). In this respect, it is of interest that glutaminergic system abnormalities (Yip et al., 2007) have been implicated in a selective Purkinje cell decrease in autism (Rout and Dhossche, 2008).

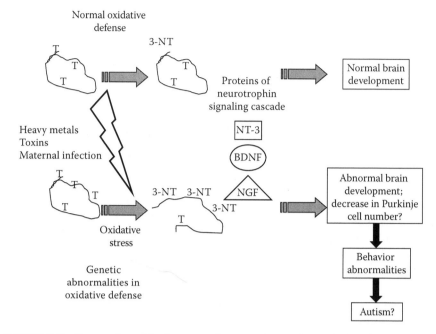

FIGURE 3.3 Proposed model of gene–environment interaction and altered neurotrophin signaling cascade in autism. 3-NT, 3-nitrotyrosine; NT-3, neurotrophin 3.

3.2.5 NEUROTROPHIN SIGNALING AND GENDER

Autism disproportionately affects boys more than girls, with a male-to-female ratio of 4:1 for autism (Baird et al., 2000; Scott et al., 2002). Thus, it is of interest that sexual dimorphism can be observed in response to environmental toxins, oxidative stress, neurotrophin expression, brain structure, and behavior.

A number of environmental or pharmacological toxins, whose action involves oxidative stress, have been observed to evoke different responses in males and in females. These include exposure to chlorpyrifos, organophosphate pesticides (Dam et al., 2000), ethanol (Rintala et al, 2001), methylazoxymethanol acetate (MAM) (Ferguson et al., 1996), glucocorticoids (Vicedomini et al., 1986), and naltrexone use in ethanol detoxification (de Cabo and Paz Viveros, 1997). Rats exposed prenatally to cocaine had impaired motor coordination, with males being more affected than females (Markowski et al., 1998).

Gender appears to affect the extent of hypertension-associated oxidative stress, lipid peroxidation, and protein damage in heart and brain tissue (Ren, 2007). In male rats, infection just before birth results in increase in protein carboxylation and reduced ratio of reduced/oxidized forms of glutathione in the hippocampus. The effect appears to be sex-dependent because it does not occur in the female offspring (Lante et al., 2007). Furthermore, other studies suggest that females are more efficient in dealing with oxidative stress (Ballerio et al., 2007).

Brain neurotrophins also exhibit a sexually dimorphic profile of expression (Gilmore et al., 2003), and gender differences in hippocampal BDNF expression have been suggested (Das et al., 2001) but not directly studied.

3.2.6 Possible Role of Neurotrophins as Targets of Future Therapies

Neurotrophin expression appears to be plastic; it can be affected by various disease states, but also by pharmacological means. Decreased BDNF activity is found in Rett syndrome (Chen et al., 2003), a severe neurodevelopmental disorder that is caused by mutations in the gene encoding methyl-CpG-binding protein 2 (MeCP2), which is thought to act as a transcriptional repressor of BDNF. MeCP2 null mice, which develop a Rett-like phenotype, exhibit progressive deficits in BDNF expression (Ogier et al., 2007). Ampakine (a regulator of glutamate receptors) treatment of MeCP2 null mice increases BDNF and results in functional improvement (Ogier et al., 2007). Rare mutations in MeCP2 as well as polymorphic markers have also been identified in autistic individuals (Loat et al., 2008). Semax, a heptapeptide analog of adrenocorticotropic hormone, stimulates memory and attention in rats and stimulates BDNF synthesis (Tsai, 2007). Further studies are needed to profile signaling cascades of other neurotrophins in autism. However, the studies discussed above suggest a potential for regulation of neurotrophin expression and possible therapeutic means of improving neurotrophin imbalance in autism.

3.3 CONCLUSIONS

The data discussed here support the key role of the following abnormalities in autism: (1) increased oxidative stress targeting both cerebellar protein and DNA; (2) genetic predisposition to oxidative stress triggers; (3) altered expression of brain neurotrophins; and (4) interaction between oxidative stress and neurotrophins. In particular, developmental elevation in cerebellar NT-3 expression could contribute to the initial cerebellar overgrowth and a subsequent reduction on cerebellar Purkinje cell number and/or result in abnormal brain connectivity in a subset of autistic cases. Chronic elevation in NT-3 in autism could further predispose the autistic individuals to oxidative damage.

ACKNOWLEDGMENTS

We thank Autism Research Institute for continuing support. We thank NICHD Brain and Tissue Bank for Developmental Disorders at the University of Maryland for providing us with human postmortem brain specimens.

REFERENCES

Abdollahi, M., Ranjbar, A., Shadnia S., Nikfar, S., and Rezaiee, A. (2004). Pesticides and oxidative stress: A review. *Med. Sci. Monit.* 10:141–147.

Baird, G., Charman, T., Baron-Cohen, S., Cox, A., Swettenham, J., Wheelwright, S., and Drew, A. (2000). A screening instrument for autism at 18 months of age: A 6-year follow-up study. *J. Am. Acad. Child Adolesc. Psychiatry* 39:694–702.

Ballerio, R., Ginazza, E., Mussoni, L., Miller, I., Gelosa, P., Guerrini, U., Eberini, I., Gemeiner, M., Belcredito, S., Tremoli, E., and Sironi, L. (2007). Gender differences in endothelial function and inflammatory markers align the occurrence of pathological events in stroke-prone rats. *Exp. Mol. Pathol.* 82:33–41.

Bates, B., Hirt, L., Thomas, S. S., Akbarian, S., Le, D., Amin-Hanjani, S., Whalen, M., Jaenisch, R., and Moskowitz, M. A. (2002). Neurotrophin-3 promotes cell death induced in cerebellar ischemia, oxygen-glucose deprivation, and oxidative stress: Possible involvement of oxygen free radicals. *Neurobiol. Dis.* 9:24–37.

Beal, M. F. (2002). Oxidatively modified proteins in aging and disease. *Free Radic. Biol. Med.* 32:797–803.

Beckman, J. S. and Koppenol, W. H. (1996). Nitric oxide, superoxide, and peroxynitrite the good, the bad and the ugly. *Am. J. Physiol.* 271:c1424–c1437.

Behrens, M. M., Strasser, U., Lobner, D., and Dugan, L. L. (1999). Neurotrophin-mediated potentiation of neuronal injury. *Microsc. Res. Tech.* 45:276–284.

Betancourt, A. M., Filipov, N. M., and Carr, L. R. (2007). Alteration of neurotrophins in the hippocampus and cerebral cortex of young rats exposed to chlorpyrifos and methyl parathion. *Toxicol. Sci.* 100:445–455.

Binder, D. K., Croll, S. D., Gall, C. M., and Scharfman, H. E. (2001). BDNF and epilepsy: Too much of a good thing? *Trends Neurosci.* 24:318–319.

Bokara, K. K., Brown, E., McCormick, R., Yallapragada, P. R., Rajanna, S., and Bettaiya, R. (2008). Lead-induced increase in antioxidant enzymes and lipid peroxidation products in developing rat brain. *Biometals* 21:9–16.

Bradstreet, J., Geier, D. A., Kartzinel, J. J., Adams, J. B., and Geier, M. R. (2003). A case–control study of mercury burden in children with autistic disorders. *J. Am. Phys. Surg.* 8:76–80.

Brown, G. E., Jones, S. D., MacKewn, A. S., and Plank, E. J. (2008). An exploration of possible pre- and postnatal correlates of autism: A pilot survey. *Psychol. Rep.* 102:273–282.

Buyske, S., Williams, T. A., Mars, A. E., Stenroos, E. S., Ming, S. X., Wang, R., Sreenath, M., Factura, M. F., Reddy, C., Lambert, G. H., and Johnson, W. G. (2006). Analysis of case–parent trios at a locus with a deletion allele: Association of GSTM1 with autism. *BMC Genet.* 7:8.

Cappelletti, G., Maggioni, M. G. Tedeschi, G., and Maci, R. (2003). Protein tyrosine nitration is triggered by nerve growth factor during neuronal differentiation of PC12 cells. *Exp. Cell. Res.* 288:9–20.

Chao, S. L., Moss, J. M., and Harry, G. J. (2007). Lead-induced alterations of apoptosis and neurotrophic factor mRNA in the developing rat cortex, hippocampus, and cerebellum. *J. Biochem. Mol. Toxicol.* 21:265–272.

Chauhan, A. and Chauhan, V. (2006). Oxidative stress in autism. *Pathophysiology* 13:171–181.

Chauhan, A., Chauhan, V., Brown, W. T., and Cohen, I. (2004). Oxidative stress in autism: Increased lipid peroxidation and reduced serum levels of ceruloplasmin and transferrin—the antioxidant proteins. *Life Sci.* 75:2539–2549.

Chen, W. G., Chang, Q., Lin, Y., Meissner, A., West, A. E., Griffith, E. C., Jaenisch, R., and Greeberg, M. E. (2003). Derepression of BDNF transcription involves calcium-dependent phosphorylation of MeCP2. *Science* 302:885–889.

Connolly, A. M., Chez, M., Streif, E. M., Keeling, R. M., Golumbek, P. T., Kwon, J. M., Riviello, J. J., Robinson, R. G., Neuman, R. J., and Deuel, R. M. K. (2006). Brain-derived neurotrophic factor and autoantibodies to neural antigens in sera of children with autistic spectrum disorders, Landau–Kleffner syndrome, and epilepsy. *Biol. Psychiatry* 59:354–363.

Courchesne, E. (1991). Neuroanatomic imaging in autism. *Pediatrics* 87:781–790.

Courchesne, E., Carper, R., and Akshoomoff, N. (2003). Evidence of brain overgrowth in the first year life in autism. *JAMA* 290:393–394.

Courchesne, E., Karns, C. M., Davis, H. R., Ziccardi, R., Carper, R. A., and Tigue, Z. D. (2001). Unusual brain growth patterns in early life in patients with autistic disorder: An MRI study. *Neurology* 57:245–254.

Dam, K., Seidler, F. J., and Slotkin, T. A. (2000). Chlorpyrifos exposure during a critical neonatal period elicits gender-selective deficits in the development of coordination skill and locomotor activity. *Brain Res. Dev. Brain Res.* 121:179–187.

D'Amelio, M., Ricci, I., Sacco, R., Liu, X., D'Agruma, L., Muscarella, L.A., Guarnieri, V., Militerni, R., Bravaccio, C., Elia, M., Schneider, C., Melmed, R., Trillo, S., Pascucci, T., Puglisi-Allegra, S., Reichelt, K. L., Macciardi, F., Holden, J.J., and Persico, A. M. (2005). Paraoxonase gene variants are associated with autism in North America, but not in Italy: Possible regional specificity in gene-environment interactions. *Mol. Psychiatry* 10:1006–1016.

Das, K. P., Chao, S. L., White, L. D., Haines, W. T., Harry, G. J., Tilson, H. A., and Barone, S. Jr. (2001). Differential patterns of nerve growth factor, brain-derived neurotrophic factor and neurotrophin-3 mRNA and protein levels in developing regions of rat brain. *Neuroscience* 103:739–761.

de Cabo, C. and Viveros, M. P. (1997). Effects of neonatal naltrexone on neurological and somatic development in rats of both genders. *Neurotoxicol. Teratol.* 19:499–509.

Egan, M. F., Kojima, M., Callicott, J. H., Goldberg, T. E., Kolachana, B. S., Bertolino, A., Zaitsev, E., Gold, B., Goldman, D., Dean. M., Lu, B., and Weinberger, D. R. (2003). The BDNF val66met polymorphism affects activity-dependent secretion of BDNF and human memory and hippocampal function. *Cell* 112:257–269.

Enstrom, A., Onore, C., Tarver, A., Hertz-Picciotto, I., Hansen, R., Croen, L., Van de Walter, J., and Ashwood, P. (2008). Peripheral blood leukocyte production of BDNF following mitogen stimulation in early onset and regressive autism. *Am. J. Biochem. Biotechnol. (Special Issue on Autism Spectrum Disorders)* 4:121–129.

Ferguson, S. A., Paule, M. G., and Holson, R. R. (1996). Functional effects of methylazoxymeth-anol-induced cerebellar hypoplasia in rats. *Neurotoxicol. Teratol.* 18:529–537.

Fukuda, M., Yamaguchi, H., Yamamoto, H., Aminaka, M., Murakami, H., Kamiyama, N., Miyamoto, Y., and Koitabashi, Y. (2008). The evaluation of oxidative damage in children with brain damage using 8-hydroxydeoxyguanosine levels. *Brain Dev.* 30:131–136.

Ghosh, A. and Greenberg, M. E. (1995). Distinct roles for bFGF and NT-3 in the regulation of cortical neurogenesis. *Neuron* 15:89–103.

Gilmore, J. H., Jarskog, L. F., and Vadlamudi, S. (2003). Maternal infection regulates BDNF and NGF expression in fetal and neonatal brain and maternal–fetal unit of rat. *J. Neuroimmunol.* 138:49–55.

Hashimoto, K., Iwata, Y., Nakamura, K., Tsuji, M., Tsuchiya, K. J., Sekine, Y., Suzuki, K., Minabe, Y., Takei, N., Iyo, M., and Mori, N. (2006). Reduced serum levels of brain-derived neurotrophic factor in adult male patients with autism. *Prog. Neuropsychopharmacol. Biol. Psychiatry* 30:1529–1531.

James, S. J., Cutler, P., Melnyk, S., Jernigan, S., Janak, L., Gaylor, D. W., and Neubrander, J. A. (2004). Metabolic biomarkers of increased oxidative stress and impaired methylation capacity in children with autism. *Am. J. Clin. Nutr.* 80:1611–1617.

James, S. J., Melny, S., Jernigan, S., Cleves, M. A., Halsted, C. H., Wong, D. H., Cutler, P., Bock, K., Boris, M., Bradstreet, J. J., Baker, S. M., and Gaylor, D. W. (2006). Metabolic endotype and related genotypes are associated with oxidative stress in children with autism. *Am. J. Genet. B. Neuropsychiat. Genet.* 141:947–956.

Katoh-Semba, R., Wakako, R., Komori, T., Shigemi, H., Miyazaki, N., Ito, H., Kumagai, T., Isuzuki, M., Shigemi, K., Yoshida, F., and Nakayama, A. (2007). Age-related changes in BDNF protein levels in human serum: Differences between autism cases and normal controls. *Int. J. Dev. Neurosci.* 25:367–372.

Kawakami, H., Nitta, A., Matsuyama, Y., Kamiya, M., Satake, K., Sato, K., Kondou, K., Iwata, H., and Furukawa, S. (2000). Increase in neurotrophin-3 expression followed by Purkinje cell degeneration in the adult rat cerebellum after spinal cord transaction. *J. Neurosci. Res.* 62:668–674.

Kemper, T. L. and Bauman, M. L. (1993). The contribution of neuropathologic studies to the understanding of autism. *Neurol. Clin.* 11:175–187.

Kimura-Kuroda, J., Nagata, I., and Kuroda, Y. (2007). Disrupting effect of hydroxyl-polychlorinated biphenyl (PCB) congeners on neuronal development of cerebellar Purkinje cells: A possible causal factor for the developmental brain disorders. *Chemosphere* 67:S412–S420.

Klinstova, A. Y., Dickson, E., Yoshida, R., and Greenough, W. T. (2004). Altered expression of BDNF and its high affinity receptor TrkB in response to complex motor learning and moderate exercise. *Brain Res.* 1028:92–104.

Lante, F., Meunier, J., Guiramand, J., Maurice, T., Cavalier, M., de Jesus Ferriera, M. C., Aimar, R., Cohen-Solal, C., Vignes, M., and Barbanel, G. (2007). Neurodevelopmental damage after prenatal infection: Role of oxidative stress in the fetal brain. *Free Radic. Biol. Med.* 42:1231–1245.

Lee, S. H., Kim, I., and Chung, B. C. (2007). Increased urinary level of oxidized nucleosides in patients with mild-to-moderate Alzheimer's disease. *Clin. Biochem.* 40:936–938.

Li, S., Qiu, F., Xu, A., Price, S. M., and Xiang, M. (2004). Barhl1 regulates migration and survival of cerebellar granule cells by controlling expression of neurotrophin-3 gene. *J. Neurosci.* 24:3104–3114.

Loat, C., Curran, S., Lewis, C., Abrahams, B., Duvall, J., Geschwind, D., Bolton, P., and Craig, I. (2008). Methyl-CpG-binding protein (MECP2) polymorphism and vulnerability to autism. *Genes Brain Behav.* 7:754–760.

Lovell, M. A., Gabbita, S. P., and Markesbery, W. R. (1999). Increased DNA oxidation and decreased levels of repair products in Alzheimer's disease ventricular CSF. *J. Neurochem.* 72:771–776.

Markowski, V. P., Cox, C., and Weiss, B. (1998). Prenatal cocaine exposure produces gender-specific motor effects in aged rats. *Neurotoxicol. Teratol.* 20: 43–53.

Marx, C. E., Vance, B. J., Jarskog, L. F., Chescheir, N. C., and Gilmore, J. H. (1999). Nerve growth factor, brain derived neurotrophic factor, and neurotrophin-3 levels in human amniotic fluid. *Am. J. Obstet. Gynecol.* 181:1225–1230.

McGinnis, W. R. (2004). Oxidative stress in autism. *Altern. Ther. Health Med.* 10:22–37.

Mecocci, P., Polidori, M. C., Cherubini, A., Ingegni, T., Mattioli, P., Catani, M., Rinaldi, P., Cechetti, R., Stahl, W., Senin, U., and Beal, M. F. (2002). Lymphocyte oxidative DNA damage and plasma antioxidants in Alzheimer disease. *Arch. Neurol.* 59:794–798.

Ming, X., Stein, T. P., Brimacombe, M., Johnson, W. G., Lambert, G. H., and Wagner, G. C. (2005). Increased excretion of lipid peroxidation biomarker in autism. *Prostaglandins Leukot. Essent. Fatty Acids* 73:379–384.

Miyazaki, K., Narita, N., Sakuta, R., Miyahara, T., Naruse, H., Okado, N., and Narita, M. (2004). Serum neurotrophin concentrations in autism and mental retardation: A pilot study. *Brain Dev.* 26:292–295.

Morrison, M. E. and Mason, C. A. (1998). Granule neuron regulation of Purkinje cell development: Striking a balance between neurotrophin and glutamate signaling. *J. Neurosci.* 18:3563–3573.

Mutter, J., Naumann, J., Schneider, R., Walach, H., and Haley, B. (2005a). Mercury and autism: Accelerating evidence? *Neuro. Endocrinol. Lett.* 26:439–446.

Mutter, J., Naumann, J., Walach, H., and Daschner, F. (2005b). Amalgam risk assessment with coverage of references up to 2005. *Gesundheitswesen* 67:204–216.

Nelson, K. B., Grether, J. K., Croen, L. A., Dambrosia, J. M., Dickens, B., Jelliffe, L. L., Hansen, R. L., and Philips, T. M. (2001). Neuropeptides and neurotrophins in neonatal blood of children with autism or mental retardation. *Ann. Neurol.* 49:597–606.

Nelson, P. G., Kuddo, T., Song, E. Y., Dambrosia, J. M., Kohler, S., Satyanarayana, G., Vandunk, C., Grether, J. K., and Nelson, K. B. (2006). Selected neuropeptides and cytokines: Developmental trajectory and concentrations in neonatal blood of children with autism or Down syndrome. *Int. J. Dev. Neurosci.* 241:73–80.

Neumann, H., Hazen, L., Weinstein, J., Mehl, R. A., and Chin, J. W. (2008). Genetically encoding protein oxidative damage. *J. Am. Chem. Soc.* 130:4028–4033.

Nishimura, K., Nakamura, K., Anitha, A., Yamada, K., Tsuji, M., and Iwayama, Y. (2007). Genetic analyses of the brain-derived neurotrophic factor (BDNF) gene in autism. *Biochem. Biophys. Res. Commun.* 356:200–206.

Nishioka, N. and Arnold, S. E. (2004). Evidence for oxidative DNA damage in the hippocampus of elderly patients with chronic schizophrenia. *Am. J. Geriatr. Psychiatry* 12:167–175.

Ogier, M., Wang, H., Hong, E., Wang, Q., Greenberg, M. E., and Katz, D. M. (2007). Brain-derived neurotrophic factor expression and respiratory function improve after ampakine treatment in a mouse model of Rett syndrome. *J. Neurosci.* 27:10912–10917.

Palmer, R. F., Blanchard, S., and Wood, R. (2009). Proximity to point sources of environmental mercury release as a predictor of autism prevalence. *Health Place* 15:18–24.

Pasarica, D., Gheorghiu, M., Toparceanu, F., Bleotu, C., Ichim, L., and Trandafir, T. (2005). Neurotrophin-3, TNF-alpha and IL-6 relations in serum and cerebrospinal fluid of ischemic stroke patients. *Roum. Arch. Microbiol. Immunol.* 64:27–33.

Perry, E. K., Lee, M. W., Martin-Ruiz, C. M., Court, J. A., Volsen, S. G., Merrit, J., Folly, E., Iversen, P. E., Bauman, M. L., Perry, R. H., and Wenk, G. L. (2001). Cholinergic activity in autism: Abnormalities in the cerebral cortex and basal forebrain. *Am. J. Psychiatry* 158:1058–1066.

Quartu, M., Lai, M. L., and Del Fiacco, M. (1999). Neurotrophin-like immunoreactivity in the human hippocampal formation. *Brain Res. Bull.* 48:375–382.

Reichardt, L. F. (2006). Neurotrophin-regulated signaling pathway. *Phil. Trans R. Soc. B* 361:1545–1564.

Ren, J. (2007). Influence of gender on oxidative stress, lipid peroxidation, protein damage and apoptosis in hearts and brains from spontaneously hypertensive rats. *Clin. Exp. Pharmacol. Physiol.* 34:432–438.

Rintala, J., Jaatinen, P., Kiianmaa, K., Iikonen, J., Kemppainen, O., Sarviharju, M., and Hervonen, A. (2001). Dose-dependent decrease in glial fibrillary acidic protein-immunoreactivity in rat cerebellum after lifelong ethanol consumption. *Alcohol* 23:1–8.

Rivto, E. R., Freeman, B. J., Scheibel, A. B., Duong, T., Robinson, H., Guthrie, D., and Ritvo, A. (1986). Lower Purkinje cell counts in the cerebella of four autistic subjects: Initial findings of the UCLA-NSac Autopsy Research Report. *Am. J. Psychiatry* 143:862–866.

Rout, U. K. and Dhossche, D. M. (2008). A pathogenetic model of autism involving Purkinje cell loss through anti GAD antibodies. *Med. Hypotheses* 71:218–221.

Sacksteder, C. A., Qian, W. J., Knyushko, T. V., Wang, H., Chin, M. H., Lacan, G., Melega, W. P., Camp, D. G. II, Smith, R. D., Smith, D. J., Squier, T. C., and Bigelow, D. J. (2006). Endogenously nitrated proteins in mouse brain: Links to neurodegenerative disease. *Biochemistry* 45:8009–8022.

Sadakata, T., Washida, M., Iwayama, Y., Shoji, S., Sato, Y., and Ohkura, T. (2007). Autistic-like phenotypes in Cadps2-knockout mice and aberrant CADPS2 splicing in autistic patients. *J. Clin. Invest.* 117:931–943.

Sajdel-Sulkowska, E. M., Lipinski, B., Windom, H., Audhya, T., and McGinnis, W. (2008). Oxidative stress in autism: Cerebellar 3-nitrotyrosine levels. *Am. J. Biochem. Biotechnol.* (*Special Issue on Autism Spectrum Disorders*) 4:73–84.

Sajdel-Sulkowska, E. M., Ming, X., and Koibuchi, N. (2009). Increase in brain neurotrophin-3 and oxidative stress in autism. *Cerebellum* [Epub PMID 19357934].

Sato, S., Mizuno, Y., and Hattori, N. (2005). Urinary 8-hydroxydeoxyguanosine levels as a biomarker for progression of Parkinson disease. *Neurology* 64:1081–1083.

Scott, F. J., Baron-Cohen, S., Bolton, P., and Brayne, C. (2002). Brief report: Prevalence of autism spectrum conditions in children aged 5–11 years in Cambridgeshire, UK. *Autism* 6:231–237.

Segal, R. A., Pomeroy, S. L., and Stiles, C. D. (1995). Axonal growth and fasciculation linked to differential expression of BDNF and NT-3 receptors in developing granule cells. *J. Neurosci.* 15:4970–4981.

Serajee, F. J., Nabi, R., Zhong, H., and Huq, M. (2004). Polymorphism in xenobiotic metabolism genes and autism. *J. Child Neurol.* 19:413–417.

Sogut, S., Zoroglu, S. S., Ozyurt, H., Yilmaz, H. R., Ozuğurlu, F., Sivasli, E., Yetkin, O., Yanik, M., Tutkun, H., Savaş, H. A., Tarakçioğlu, M., and Akyol, O. (2003). Changes in nitric oxide levels and antioxidant enzyme activities may have a role in the pathological mechanisms involved in autism. *Clin. Chim. Acta* 33:1111–1117.

Sultana, R., Perluigi, M., and Butterfield, D. A. (2006). Protein oxidation, lipid peroxidation in brain of subjects with Alzheimer's disease: Insights into mechanism of neurodegeneration from redox proteomics. *Antioxid. Redox. Signal.* 8:2021–2037.

Sweeten, T. L., Posey, D. J., Shankar, S., and McDougle, C. J. (2004). High nitric oxide production in autistic disorder: A possible role for interferon-gamma. *Biol. Psychiatry* 55:434–437.

Tabuchi, A. (2008). Synaptic plasticity-regulated gene expression: A key event in the long-lasting changes of neuronal function. *Biol. Pharm. Bull.* 31:327–335.

Tsai, S. J. (2005). Is autism caused by early hyperactivity of brain derived neurotrophic factor? *Med. Hypotheses* 65:79–82.

Tsai, S. J. (2007). Semax, an analogue of adrenocorticotropin (4–10), is a potential agent for the treatment of attention-deficit hyperactivity disorder and Rett syndrome. *Med. Hypotheses* 68:1144–1146.

Vargas, M. R., Pehar, M., Cassina, P., Estavez, A. G., Beckman, J. S., and Barbeito, L. (2004). Stimulation of nerve growth factor expression in astrocytes by peroxynitrite. *In Vivo* 18:269–274.

Vicedomini, J. P., Nonneman, A. J., DeKosky, S. T., and Scheff, S. W. (1986). Perinatal glucocorticoids disrupt learning: A sexually dimorphic response. *Physiol. Behav.* 36:145–149.

Whitney, E. R., Kemper, T. L., Bauman, M. L., Rosene, D. L., and Blatt, G. J. (2008). Cerebellar Purkinje cells are reduced in a subpopulation of autistic brains: A stereological experiment using calbindin-D28k. *Cerebellum* 7:406–416.

Windham, G. C., Zhang, L., Gunier, R., Croen, L. A., and Grether, J. K. (2006). Autism spectrum disorders in relation to distribution of hazardous air pollutants in the San Francisco bay area. *Environ. Health Perspect.* 114:1438–1444.

Yang, I. A., Fong, K. M., Zimmerman, P. V., Holgate, S. T., and Holloway, J. W. (2008). Genetic susceptibility to the respiratory effects of air pollution. *Thorax* 63:555–563.

Yao, Y., Walsh, W. J., McGinnis, W. R., and Pratico, D. (2006). Altered vascular phenotype in autism: Correlation with oxidative stress. *Arch. Neurol.* 63:1161–1164.

Yip, J., Soghomonian, J. J., and Blatt, G. J. (2007). Decreased GAD67 mRNA levels in cerebellar Purkinje cells in autism: Pathophysiological implications. *Acta Neuropathol.* 113:559–568.

Yorbik, O., Sayal, A., Akay, C., Akbiyik, D. I., and Sohmen, T. (2002). Investigation of antioxidant enzymes in children with autistic disorder. *Prostaglandins Leukot. Essent. Fatty Acids* 67:341–343.

Zhu, S.-W., Pham, T. M., Aberg, E., Brene, S., Winblad, B., Mohammed, A. H., and Baumans, V. (2006). Neurotrophin levels and behavior in BALB/c mice: Impact of intermittent exposure to individual housing and wheel running. *Behav. Brain Res.* 167:1–8.

Zoroglu, S. S., Armutcu, F., Ozen, S., Gurel, A., Sivasli, E., Yetkin, O., and Meram, I. (2004). Increased oxidative stress and altered activities of erythrocyte free radical scavenging enzymes in autism. *Eur. Arch. Psychiatr. Clin. Neurosci.* 254:143–147.

4 Genetics of Autism

*W. Ted Brown**

Department of Human Genetics, New York State Institute for Basic Research in Developmental Disabilities, Staten Island, NY 10314, USA

CONTENTS

4.1   INTRODUCTION

Autism has a strong genetic component. It is highly heritable. Heritability is a genetic term that provides an estimate of the proportion of phenotypic variation in a population that is due to genetic variation. Studies comparing the ratio of concordance of autism in monozygotic twin pairs (70%–90%) to dizygotic twin pairs (0%–10%) have provided heritability estimates for autism of >90% (Folstein and Rosen-Sheidley, 2001; Freitag, 2007). The autism heritability estimate of >90% suggests that the environmental component of autism is <10%, but not zero. The identical twin discordances may be due to epigenetic changes (Cheung et al., 2008; Kaminsky et al., 2009), somatic mutations (Bruder et al., 2008), and chorionic environmental influences (Bohm and Stewart, 2009). The inheritance of autism is not simple: it is rather complex (Abrahams and Geschwind, 2008). Autism is a heterogeneous condition of variable severity, ranging from severe cognitive impairment with seizures and lack of speech to the milder Asperger syndrome (AS) with social communication deficits but normal intelligence. It is now commonly regarded as an autism spectrum disorder (ASD), a classification that includes autism, pervasive developmental disability disorder—not otherwise specified (PDD-NOS), and AS (Freitag, 2007).

---

* Corresponding author: Tel.: +1-718-494-5117; fax: +1-718-494-0833; e-mail: Ted.Brown@omr.state.ny.us

It is likely that there are subtypes of ASDs. For example, regression is seen in a certain proportion of cases. One recent study reported that regression was seen in 41% of a sample of 333 subjects with autism; 26% lost either language or social skills, while 15% lost both (Hansen et al., 2008). Other domains in which subtypes are likely include the presence or absence of behavioral inflexibility, macrocephaly, seizures, and syndromic appearance.

4.2   EPIDEMIOLOGY OF AUTISM

A large epidemiological study overseen by the Centers for Disease Control and Prevention (CDC) concluded that in 14 large areas in the United States, among over 400,000 eight-year-old children, the mean prevalence of ASD was 6.6/1,000 (one of every 152 children). The male-to-female ratio overall was found to be approximately 4 to 1. With the altered sex ratio, approximately 1 in 81 boys and 1 in 325 girls were found to have an ASD. Among all sites, 42% of males and 58% of females with ASD had IQ scores of ≤70. Since the males in general had higher IQ scores, it would be expected that the sex ratio would be higher for those with IQ scores >70. Compared to findings of a CDC study done 2 years earlier, for the majority of sites, there was no variation in prevalence over 2 years (CDC, 2007). The prevalence figures of 6.6/1000 are similar to those in other recent epidemiological studies (Chakrabarti and Fombonne, 2001, 2005; Fombonne et al., 2006; Williams et al., 2008).

AS is a fairly new diagnosis and is a subcategory of ASD, representing a high-functioning subgroup of ASD. Whether it is a genetically separate subtype of ASD is an open question. It does occur within families in which there is also autism (Ghaziuddin, 2005). The main clinical features are markedly impaired social interactions and repetitive patterns of behavior, but no delay in language and cognitive development (American Psychiatric Association, 1994). Witwer and Lecavalier (2008) reviewed 22 studies on ASD subtypes and concluded that differences between autism and AS were largely unsupported on the basis of current criteria. Currently universal consensus for the essential clinical features does not exist, and several different sets of criteria are used. Kopra et al. (2008) compared four widely used criteria (ICD-10, DSM-IV, Gillberg and Gillberg, 1989; Szatmari et al., 1989), and found the highest agreement between the ICD-10 and the DSM-IV criteria. Mattila et al. (2007) reviewed the literature and conducted an epidemiological study of AS among 5484 eight-year-olds in Finland. These researchers reported that previous prevalence surveys for AS had widely ranged from 0.03 to 6 per 1000 due to varying criteria and age of diagnosis. Their study found prevalence rates per 1000 of 2.5, according to DSM-IV (American Psychiatric Association, 1994); 2.9 as per ICD-10 (World Health Organization, 1992); 2.7, to Gillberg and Gillberg (1989); and 1.6 as per Szatmari criteria (Szatmari et al., 1989), emphasizing the need to carefully reconsider the diagnostic criteria in epidemiological studies. When all children who meet any of the clinical criteria for AS were included, the male-to-female ratio was relatively low (1.7:1). Thus, the true prevalence and the actual sex ratio of AS, if different from those of ASD in general, are not known.

4.3   HERITABILITY OF AUTISM

In autism, as in many other complex genetic conditions, we are dealing with a lack of success in identifying the underlying genetic components. For example, the heritability of height is estimated to be 80%–90%. However, large genome-wide association studies (GWASs) have identified genetic variants that account for little more than 5% of the heritability of height (Maher, 2008). The same is true for large-scale studies of schizophrenia, attention-deficit hyperactivity disorder (ADHD), obesity, diabetes, and heart disease. A large-scale GWAS of general cognitive ability (IQ) recently reported only six potential genetic loci, with the strongest candidate having an effect size of only 0.4% (Butcher et al., 2008; Zimmer, 2008).

Where is the missing heritability? One possibility is that the assumptions about the underlying genetic basis of these conditions may be wrong. The most popular model employs the common disease common variant (CDCV) model, which assumes the existence of genetic variants that are common and confers relative risks on the order of 1.1–1.5. Most GWASs use genetic variants (single-nucleotide polymorphisms [SNPs]) when the polymorphisms under study are relatively common, with allele frequencies of 5%–50%. An alternative assumption is the common disease multiple rare variant (CDMRV) model, which postulates that complex genetic conditions result from many different mutations, each of which is relatively or exceedingly rare but has very strong effects when, for example, the relative risk conferred is greater than 10-fold (Psychiatric GWAS Consortium Steering Committee, 2009). If these conditions or disorders are caused by a large number of rare mutations, then larger sample sizes, and possibly the sequencing of each individual, may be required, which is not currently economically feasible, although it may be so in the near future. A second possibility is that due to the heterogeneous nature of ASD, it will be necessary to categorize families for linkage analysis by underlying phenotypes. An initial application of this approach, for the domains of social interaction and repetitive behaviors, produced modestly higher linkage scores for several loci (Liu et al., 2008).

4.4   INTEGRATIVE GENETICS

An alternative perspective to autism heritability is that it may be necessary to take an integrative genetics approach and identify multiple interacting networks that may be involved. With this approach, variations in hundreds of thousands of DNA markers are correlated to expression levels of many multiples of genes as measured by microarrays, which in turn are related to quantitative phenotypes or disease traits (Schadt et al., 2005). Data derived by this approach are used to develop models of how (1) DNA variations, (2) variations in gene expression, and (3) variations in disease trait are related, often by complex interacting networks. This approach has been applied with success to the study of gene expression related to human obesity (Emilsson et al., 2008) and to the study of human liver, a metabolically active tissue important in a number of common human diseases, such as diabetes and atherosclerosis (Schadt et al., 2008). Analysis of such multiple interacting networks requires intense computing power, but already has provided a number of new pharmaceutical compounds that are in various phases of clinical trials (Nelson, 2008; Zhu et al., 2008). Applications of this approach to neurodevelopmental disorders such as autism will be a challenge because of difficulties in measuring gene expression levels in the target tissue. Perhaps initially these difficulties will be addressed with mouse models. A similar approach has been proposed that employs a probabilistic framework to combine genetic linkage information with whole-genome molecular-interaction data to predict networks of interacting genes that contribute to common disorders (Feldman et al., 2008; Goh et al., 2007; Lossifov et al., 2008). This approach was applied to three disorders— autism, bipolar disorder, and schizophrenia—and it yielded a number of candidate genes and predicted gene targets that are likely to be shared among the disorders (Lossifov et al., 2008).

4.5   SINGLE-GENE MUTATIONS ASSOCIATED WITH AUTISM

A wide variety of chromosomal abnormalities, submicroscopic copy number variations (CNVs), single-gene disorders, and rare point mutations have been associated with ASDs (Abrahams and Geschwind, 2008). A list of some 25 ASD candidate genes can be compiled, each of which may be found in mutated form in various ASD subjects (Table 4.1). As a whole, the various identified abnormalities probably now account for up to 20% of ASDs (Abrahams and Geschwind, 2008; Marshall et al., 2008). Among single-gene disorders, fragile X syndrome was originally found in as many as 18% of autistic subjects (Brown et al., 1982). As the criteria for ASDs broadened to include more high-functioning individuals, and molecular testing for fragile X eliminated some subjects (originally considered to be cytogenetically positive for fragile X at low frequencies of <2%), the number of autism subjects with fragile X syndrome decreased, and now about 3% of males with ASD test positive for fragile X (Szatmari et al., 2007). Chromosome 15q11–13 duplications are found in 1%–2% of ASD subjects (Abrahams and Geschwind, 2008). Tuberous sclerosis (mutations of TSC1 or TSC2) is found in about 1% of ASD subjects. Down syndrome (DS) has been associated with ASD in 7%–10% of cases (Lowenthal et al., 2007), but because it is generally recognized at birth, it is probably not included in most studies of ASDs (alternatively, if 0.1% of the population has DS, then by chance 0.1% of ASD subjects would have DS). Other syndromes associated with ASD, each accounting for about 1%, include Chr16p11 del, 22q13 del (SHANK3 gene), and Rett syndrome (Abrahams and Geschwind, 2008).

The overlapping phenotypes of fragile X syndrome and autism have been of considerable interest for some time because approximately 30% of males with fragile X syndrome meet the full criteria for autism, and an additional 30% have PDD-NOS (Harris et al., 2008). Based on promising animal studies, trials of metabotropic glutamate receptor 5 antagonists as well as several other drugs are beginning with individuals with fragile X syndrome, with exciting preliminary results (Berry-Kravis et al., 2009; Bilousova et al., 2009; Hagerman et al., 2009). If fragile X and autism have some underlying pathophysiological genetic networks in common, as appears likely (Belmonte and Bourgeron, 2006), then these new drugs may have promising therapeutic roles for ASDs as well.

TABLE 4.1
ASA Gene Candidates

Gene Name	Gene Description
RELN	Reelin
UBE3A	Ubiquitin protein ligase E3A
MECP2	Methyl CpG binding protein 2
GABRB3	Gamma-aminobutyric acid (GABA) A receptor beta 3
TSC1	Tuberous sclerosis 1
TSC2	Tuberous sclerosis 2
PTEN	Phosphatase and tensin homolog
NLGN3	Neuroligin 3
NLGN4	Neuroligin 4
FMR1	Fragile X mental retardation 1
DHCR7	7-Dehydrocholesterol reductase
CADPS2	Ca^{2+}-dependent activator protein for secretion 2
SLC6A4	Solute carrier family 6 (tr-serotonin) member 4
SHANK3	SH3 and multiple ankyrin repeat domains 3
OXTR	Oxytocin receptor
MET	Met protooncogene
CNTNAP2	Contactin-associated protein-like 2
CACNA1C	Calcium channel voltage-dependent L type alpha 1C subunit
SLC25A12	Solute carrier family 25 (mitochondrial, Aralar) member 12
NRXN1	Neurexin 1
GRIK2	Glutamate receptor ionotropic kainate 2 precursor
EN2	Engrailed homeobox 2
AHI1	Abelson helper integration site 1
ITGB3	Integrin beta 3

Source: After Abrahams, B.S. and Geschwind, D.H., *Nat. Rev. Genet.*, 9, 341, 2008; for original references, see OMIM, *Online Mendelian Inheritance in Man.*

Note: These genes are found mutated or strongly associated in some families with autism.

4.6 COPY NUMBER VARIATIONS IN AUTISM

CNVs include insertion, deletions, and duplications of DNA and can range from less than a kilobase to several million bases. To determine the role of CNVs in ASDs, a number of studies using differing approaches (oligonucleotides, SNPs, and clones) have come to reasonably similar results (reviewed in Cook and Scherer, 2008). Resolution of the minimum size of the CNV is an important variable, because the frequency of detected CNVs should increase as the resolution increases. De novo or noninherited CNVs are found in 7%–10% of ASD samples from simplex families (having only one child affected, the majority), in 2%–3% from multiplex families, and in ~1% in non-ASD controls; ~10% of ASD subjects with de novo CNVs carry two or more (Christian et al., 2008; Marshall et al., 2008; Sebat et al., 2007; Szatmari et al., 2007). In these studies, a relatively increased frequency of CNVs involving neuronal synaptic complex genes, such as SHANK3, NLGN4, and NRXN1, has been found. In about 1% of ASD subjects, a duplication or deletion of a 600 kb region at chromosome 16p11.2 that contains some 25 genes has also been found (Weiss et al., 2008). In subjects with syndromic ASD (having an unusual or dysmorphic appearance), up to 27% may have de novo CNVs (Jacquemont et al., 2006).

Recent studies on CNVs in schizophrenia have reported similar findings to those on CNVs in ASDs (Walsh et al., 2008; Xu et al., 2008). For example, in the Xu study, de novo CNVs were found in 10% of sporadic cases and in 1.3% of unaffected controls (Xu et al., 2008). It is anticipated that further research will be forthcoming regarding the role of de novo CNVs in other neuropsychiatric conditions such as bipolar disorder, obsessive-compulsive disorder, Tourette's syndrome, and ADHD (Cook and Scherer, 2008).

Inherited CNVs reportedly are found in up to 50% of ASD subjects for whom one of the presumably normal parents also has the duplication/deletion. These familial CNVs could include candidate genes relevant to ASD if they are rare in the normal population, but further analysis of this possibility is needed. As regards to what is normal, a recent analysis of 2500 controls found that 5%–10% of individuals carry individual CNVs larger than 500 kb in size, and 1%–2% of controls carry CNVs greater than 1 Mb. Resolution of the minimum size of the CNV is an important variable, and when size was assayable down to 10 kb, it was found that an average of 3–7 CNVs were present per control subject, with a global average of 540 kb of CNV DNA per person (Itsara et al., 2009).

Zhao et al. (2007) have proposed a unified theory for the genetic basis of autism based on the observed high frequency of CNVs found in ASD. They propose that most families with ASD fall into two types. The large majority are families in which male offspring have a low risk of having a de novo mutation such as a CNV. A small minority of families includes those in which the risk of ASD in male offspring is close to 50%, essentially a dominant model with reduced penetrance in female offspring and carrier mothers. To explain the 4:1 male-to-female ratio, Zhao et al. hypothesize, that for unknown reasons that are yet to be determined, females have a greatly reduced risk of expressing the mutation, such as a CNV. This model nicely fits with the prevalence data for ASD, but the sex-dependent penetrance assumption is not satisfying: why should random CNVs be four times more penetrant in males?

4.7   PARENTAL AGE AND AUTISM

Advanced parental ages have been associated with increased risk of ASDs. A CDC-sponsored study of a 1994 birth cohort of ~250,000 study-site births, including 1250 ASD cases with complete parental age information, concluded that the odds ratio for maternal age ≥35 versus 25–29 years was 1.3, and the odds ratio for paternal age ≥40 versus 25–29 years was 1.4 (Durkin et al., 2008). This study came to essentially the same conclusions as an earlier study of 593 children with ASD, in which the risk of ASDs increased significantly with each 10 year increase in maternal age (RR of 1.31) and paternal age (RR of 1.28), and generally confirmed several earlier studies (Croen et al., 2007). The observed paternal age effect could suggest the role of accumulating new mutations because spermatogonia constantly divide in the male. The independent effect of maternal age could suggest environmental exposures during pregnancy, complications of pregnancy, or age-related chromosomal changes.

4.8 PRENATAL MATERNAL STRESS AND AUTISM

Do hurricanes cause autism? Kinney et al. (2008a) reviewed weather service data to identify hurricanes and severe weather storms in Louisiana from 1980 to 1995 and correlated these data with autism prevalences in the various localities. They found that the prevalence of autism increased in a dose–response fashion with severity of prenatal storm exposure. This effect was most significant near the middle and near the end of gestation. Children who had been exposed to storms during prenatal gestation months 5–6 or in the last month of pregnancy had a 3.8 times greater risk of having an ASD than did children exposed during other months of gestation ($p < 0.001$). Kinney et al. (2008b) suggest a number of potential mechanisms by which prenatal stress could disrupt normal brain development in the fetus, including neuroinflammatory effects; reduced fetal blood circulation; stimulated release of maternal stress hormones that could cross the placenta, causing altered development of the hypothalamic-pituitary-adrenal axis; complications of pregnancy; and epigenetic effects on expression of genes involved in the stress response. An interesting hypothesis is that prenatal stress could cause elevations of maternal stress hormones including testosterone (Cruess et al., 2000) and that risk for ASD may be increased by fetal exposure to high levels of testosterone during critical periods of pregnancy, which would support the "extreme male brain" theory of ASD (Baron-Cohen, 2002; Baron-Cohen et al., 2005; Knickmeyer and Baron-Cohen, 2006). The "extreme male brain" theory proposes that the behaviors seen in autism are an exaggeration of typical sex differences and that exposure to high levels of prenatal testosterone might be an added risk factor. This theory offers a potential explanation for the 4:1 male-to-female ratio for ASDs.

4.9 POTENTIAL ROLE OF NONCODING RNAs IN AUTISM

The human genome is more complex than was originally thought. Although only about 1.5% of the genome codes for proteins, about 5% is evolutionarily highly conserved, but even more than 5% may encode important functional information and, in fact, at least 70% of the human genome is transcribed (Pheasant and Mattick, 2007). A number of classes of functional nonprotein-coding RNAs (ncRNAs) are being identified, including microRNAs (miRNAs), small interfering RNAs (siRNAs), Piwi-interacting RNAs (piRNAs), and long noncoding RNAs (lincRNAs) (Ghildiyal and Zamore, 2009). There are over 1000 miRNAs, more than 1000 lincRNAs and possibly, 200,000 different piRNAs in the human genome (Betel et al., 2007; Guttman et al., 2009). The functions of these various ncRNAs are being intensively investigated. They very likely have important roles in regulating the expression of protein-coding RNAs. They may even be enriched in regions that are involved with CNVs in autism (Armengol et al., 2007).

A search for regions of the genome that are highly evolutionarily conserved among mammals but have rapidly diverged from our last common ancestor, chimpanzees, led to the discovery of human accelerated region 1 (HAR1) (Pollard et al., 2006). This 118 bp sequence had accumulated 18 base pair changes, when zero or one would have been expected to occur by chance. The expression of HAR1 in the brain overlaps nearly identically with that of the reelin gene, which is a protein that helps regulate processes of neuronal migration as well as neuronal positioning in the cortex and the hippocampus, and modulates synaptic plasticity (Niu et al., 2008). Thus, a rapidly evolving ncRNA gene appears to play an important role in human brain development. Further, other ncRNAs appear to play key roles in dendritic spine development (Schratt et al., 2006) and in long-term memory formation (Mercer et al., 2008). Further research in this exciting new area could help us to better understand the genetics of autism.

4.10   SUMMARY AND CONCLUSIONS

ASDs have a strong genetic component, but they have a complex pattern of inheritance and are highly heterogeneous. GWASs have not defined strong gene candidates, leading to the conclusion that multiple rare variants may be involved. Genetic network and integrative genetic approaches are leading to deeper insights into the underlying genetic problems. A number of single-gene disorders, such as fragile X, have been associated with ASDs and may lead the way for the development of new drug therapeutic approaches. The recent discovery of the significant role that CNVs play in ASD and other neurodevelopmental disorders also may help us understand and explain the underlying common genetic networks that are involved. Parental age effects in ASD suggest genetic mechanisms. Prenatal exposure to hurricanes has been associated with autism, pointing to the potential role of environmental stressors. Finally, the exciting role that the ncRNAs may play in regulating brain development and functioning are just beginning to help explain the complex genetics of autism.

REFERENCES

Abrahams, B.S. and D.H. Geschwind (2008). Advances in autism genetics: On the threshold of a new neurobiology. *Nat. Rev. Genet.* 9:341–355.
American Psychiatric Association (1994). *Diagnostic and Statistical Manual of Mental Disorders*, 4th ed. Washington, DC: American Psychiatric Association.
Armengol, L., M. Caceres, A. Brunet, and X. Estivill (2007). Enrichment and variability of PIWI-interacting RNAs (piRNAs) in segmental duplications and copy number variants (CNVs) suggest a functional role in the integrity of the genome. Abstract #153 presented at the Annual Meeting of the American Society of Human Genetics, San Diego, CA.
Baron-Cohen, S. (2002). The extreme male brain theory of autism. *Trends Cogn. Sci.* 6:248–254.
Baron-Cohen, S., R.C. Knickmeyer, and M.K. Belmonte (2005). Sex differences in the brain: Implications for explaining autism. *Science* 310:819–823.
Belmonte, M.K. and T. Bourgeron (2006). Fragile X syndrome and autism at the intersection of genetic and neural networks. *Nat. Neurosci.* 9:1221–1225.

Berry-Kravis, E.M., D. Hessl, S. Coffey, C. Hervey, A. Schneider, J. Yuhas, J. Hutchison, M. Snape, M. Tranfaglia, D.V. Nguyen, and R. Hagerman (2009). A pilot open-label single-dose trial of fenobam in adults with fragile X syndrome. *J. Med. Genet.* 46:266–271.

Betel, D., R. Sheridan, D.S. Marks, and C. Sander (2007). Computational analysis of mouse piRNA sequence and biogenesis. *PLoS Comput. Biol.* 3:e222.

Bilousova, T.V., L. Dansie, M. Ngo, J. Aye, J.R. Charles, D.W. Ethell, and I.M. Ethell (2009). Minocycline promotes dendritic spine maturation and improves behavioural performance in the fragile X mouse model. *J. Med. Genet.* 46:94–102.

Bohm, H.V. and M.G. Stewart (2009). Brief report: On the concordance percentages for autistic spectrum disorder of twins. *J. Autism Dev. Disord.* 39:806–808.

Brown, W.T., E.C. Jenkins, E. Friedman, J. Brooks, K. Wisniewski, S. Raguthu, and J. French (1982). Autism is associated with the fragile-X syndrome. *J. Autism Dev. Disord.* 12:303–308.

Bruder, C.E., A. Piotrowski, A.A. Gijsbers, R. Andersson, S. Erickson, T.D. de Ståhl, U. Menzel, J. Sandgren, D. von Tell, A. Poplawski, M. Crowley, C. Crasto, E.C. Partridge, H. Tiwari, D.B. Allison, J. Komorowski, G.J. van Ommen, D.I. Boomsma, N.L. Pedersen, J.T. den Dunnen, K. Wirdefeldt, and J.P. Dumanski (2008). Phenotypically concordant and discordant monozygotic twins display different DNA copy-number-variation profiles. *Am. J. Hum. Genet.* 82:763–771.

Butcher, L.M., O.S. Davis, I.W. Craig, and R. Plomin (2008). Genome-wide quantitative trait locus association scan of general cognitive ability using pooled DNA and 500K single nucleotide polymorphism microarrays. *Genes Brain Behav.* 7:435–446.

Centers for Disease Control and Prevention (2007). Prevalence of autism spectrum disorders—Autism and developmental disabilities monitoring network, 14 sites, United States, 2002. *MMWR Surveill. Summ.* 56:1–40.

Chakrabarti, S. and E. Fombonne (2001). Pervasive developmental disorders in preschool children. *JAMA* 285:3093–3099.

Chakrabarti, S. and E. Fombonne (2005). Pervasive developmental disorders in preschool children: Confirmation of high prevalence. *Am. J. Psychiatry* 162:1133–1141.

Cheung, V.G., A. Bruzel, J.T. Burdick, M. Morley, J.L. Devlin, and R.S. Spielman (2008). Monozygotic twins reveal germline contribution to allelic expression differences. *Am. J. Hum. Genet.* 82:1357–1360.

Christian, S.L., C.W. Brune, J. Sudi, R.A. Kumar, S. Liu, S. Karamohamed, J.A. Badner, S. Matsui, J. Conroy, D. McQuaid, J. Gergel, E. Hatchwell, T.C. Gilliam, E.S. Gershon, N.J. Nowak, W.B. Dobyns, and E.H. Cook Jr. (2008). Novel submicroscopic chromosomal abnormalities detected in autism spectrum disorder. *Biol. Psychiatry* 63:1111–1117.

Cook, E.H. Jr. and S.W. Scherer (2008). Copy-number variations associated with neuropsychiatric conditions. *Nature* 455:919–923.

Croen, L.A., D.V. Najjar, B. Fireman, and J.K. Grether (2007). Maternal and paternal age and risk of autism spectrum disorders. *Arch. Pediatr. Adolesc. Med.* 161:334–340.

Cruess, D.G., M.H. Antoni, M. Kumar, B. McGregor, S. Alferi, A.M. Boyers, C.S. Carver, and K. Kilbourn (2000). Effects of stress management on testosterone levels in women with early-stage breast cancer. *Int. J. Behav. Med.* 8:194–207.

Durkin, M.S., M.J. Maenner, C.J. Newschaffer, L.C. Lee, C.M. Cunniff, J.K. Daniels, R.S. Kirby, L. Leavitt, L. Miller, W. Zahorodny, and L.A. Schieve (2008). Advanced parental age and the risk of autism spectrum disorder. *Am. J. Epidemiol.* 168:1268–1276.

Emilsson, V., G. Thorleifsson, B. Zhang, A.S. Leonardson, F. Zink, J. Zhu, S. Carlson, A. Helgason, G.B. Walters, S. Gunnarsdottir, M. Mouy, V. Steinthorsdottir, G.H. Eiriksdottir, G. Bjornsdottir, I. Reynisdottir, D. Gudbjartsson, D. Helgadottir, A. Jonasdottir, A. Jonasdottir, U. Styrkarsdottir, S. Gretarsdottir, K.P. Magnusson, H. Stefansson, R. Fossdal, K. Kristjansson, H.G. Gislason, T. Stefansson, B.G. Leifsson, U. Thorsteinsdottir, J.R. Lamb, J.R. Gulcher, M.L. Reitman, A. Kong, E.E. Schadt, and

K. Stefansson (2008). Genetics of gene expression and its effect on disease. *Nature* 452:423–428.

Feldman, I., A. Rzhetsky, and D. Vitkup (2008). Network properties of genes harboring inherited disease mutations. *Proc. Natl. Acad. Sci. USA* 105:4323–4328.

Folstein, S.E. and B. Rosen-Sheidley (2001). Genetics of autism: Complex aetiology for a heterogeneous disorder. *Nat. Rev. Genet.* 2:943–955.

Fombonne, E., R. Zakarian, A. Bennett, L. Meng, and D. McLean-Heywood (2006). Pervasive developmental disorders in Montreal, Quebec, Canada: Prevalence and links with immunizations. *Pediatrics* 118:e139–e150.

Freitag, C.M. (2007). The genetics of autistic disorders and its clinical relevance: A review of the literature. *Mol. Psychiatry* 12:2–22.

Ghaziuddin, M. (2005). A family history study of Asperger syndrome. *J. Autism Dev. Disord.* 38:11735:177–182.

Ghildiyal, M. and P.D. Zamore (2009). Small silencing RNAs: An expanding universe. *Nat. Rev. Genet.* 10:94–108.

Gillberg, I.C. and C. Gillberg (1989). Asperger syndrome—Some epidemiological considerations: A research note. *J. Child Psychol. Psychiatry* 30:631–638.

Goh, K.I., M.E. Cusick, D. Valle, B. Childs, M. Vidal, and A.L. Barabási (2007). The human disease network. *Proc. Natl. Acad. Sci. USA* 104:8685–8690.

Guttman, M., I. Amit, M. Garber, C. French, M.F. Lin, D. Feldser, M. Huarte, O. Zuk, B.W. Carey, J.P. Cassady, M.N. Cabili, R. Jaenisch, T.S. Mikkelsen, T. Jacks, N. Hacohen, B.E. Bernstein, M. Kellis, A. Regev, J.L. Rinn, and E.S. Lander (2009). Chromatin signature reveals over a thousand highly conserved large non-coding RNAs in mammals. *Nature* 458:223–227.

Hagerman, R.J., E. Berry-Kravis, W.E. Kaufmann, M.Y. Ono, N. Tartaglia, A. Lachiewicz, R. Kronk, C. Delahunty, D. Hessl, J. Visootsak, J. Picker, L. Gane, and M. Tranfaglia (2009). Advances in the treatment of fragile X syndrome. *Pediatrics* 123:378–390.

Hansen, R.L., S. Ozonoff, P. Krakowiak, K. Angkustsiri, C. Jones, L.J. Deprey, D.N. Le, L.A. Croen, and I. Hertz-Picciotto (2008). Regression in autism: Prevalence and associated factors in the CHARGE Study. *Ambul. Pediatr.* 8:25–31.

Harris, S.W., D. Hessl, B. Goodlin-Jones, J. Ferranti, S. Bacalman, I. Barbato, F. Tassone, P.J. Hagerman, H. Herman, and R.J. Hagerman (2008). Autism profiles of males with fragile X syndrome. *Am. J. Ment. Retard.* 113:427–438.

Itsara, A., G.M. Cooper, C. Baker, S. Girirajan, J. Li, D. Absher, R.M. Krauss, R.M. Myers, P.M. Ridker, D.I. Chasman, H. Mefford, P. Ying, D.A. Nickerson, and E.E. Eichler (2009). Population analysis of large copy number variants and hotspots of human genetic disease. *Am. J. Hum. Genet.* 84:148–161.

Jacquemont, M.L., D. Sanlaville, R. Redon, O. Raoul, V. Cormier-Daire, S. Lyonnet, J. Amiel, M. Le Merrer, D. Heron, M.C. de Blois, M. Prieur, M. Vekemans, N.P. Carter, A. Munnich, L. Colleaux, and A. Philippe (2006). Array-based comparative genomic hybridisation identifies high frequency of cryptic chromosomal rearrangements in patients with syndromic autism spectrum disorders. *J. Med. Genet.* 43:843–849.

Kaminsky, K.A., T. Tang, S.C. Wang, C. Ptak, G.H. Oh, A.H. Wong, L.A. Feldcamp, C. Virtanen, J. Halfvarson, C. Tysk, A.F. McRae, P.M. Visscher, G.W. Montgomery, I.I. Gottesman, N.G. Martin, and A. Petronis (2009). DNA methylation profiles in monozygotic and dizygotic twins. *Nat. Genet.* 41:240–245.

Kinney, D.K., A.M. Miller, D.J. Crowley, E. Huang, and E. Gerber (2008a). Autism prevalence following prenatal exposure to hurricanes and tropical storms in Louisiana. *J. Autism Dev. Disord.* 38:481–488.

Kinney, D.K., K.M. Munir, D.J. Crowley, and A.M. Miller (2008b). Prenatal stress and risk for autism. *Neurosci. Biobehav. Rev.* 32:1519–1532.

Knickmeyer, R.C. and S. Baron-Cohen (2006). Fetal testosterone and sex differences in typical social development and in autism. *J. Child. Neurol.* 21:825–845.

Kopra, K., L. von Wendt, T. Nieminen-von Wendt, and E.J. Paavonen (2008). Comparison of diagnostic methods for Asperger syndrome. *J. Autism Dev. Disord.* 38:1567–1573.

Liu, X.Q., A.D. Paterson, and P. Szatmari; Autism Genome Project Consortium (2008). Genome-wide linkage analyses of quantitative and categorical autism subphenotypes. *Biol. Psychiatry* 64:561–570.

Lossifov, I., T. Zheng, M. Baron, T.C. Gilliam, and A. Rzhetsky (2008). Genetic-linkage mapping of complex hereditary disorders to a whole-genome molecular-interaction network. *Genome Res.* 18:1150–1162.

Lowenthal, R., C.S. Paula, J.S. Schwartzman, D. Brunoni, and M.T. Mercadante (2007). Prevalence of pervasive developmental disorder in Down's syndrome. *J. Autism Dev. Disord.* 37:1394–1395.

Maher, B. (2008). The case of the missing heritability. *Nature* 456:18–21.

Marshall, C.R., A. Noor, J.B. Vincent, A.C. Lionel, L. Feuk, J. Skaug, M. Shago, R. Moessner, D. Pinto, Y. Ren, B. Thiruvahindrapduram, A. Fiebig, S. Schreiber, J. Friedman, C.E. Ketelaars, Y.J. Vos, C. Ficicioglu, S. Kirkpatrick, R. Nicolson, L. Sloman, A. Summers, C. A. Gibbons, A. Teebi, D. Chitayat, R. Weksberg, A. Thompson, C. Vardy, V. Crosbie, S. Luscombe, R. Baatjes, L. Zwaigenbaum, W. Roberts, B. Fernandez, P. Szatmari, and S.W. Scherer (2008). Structural variation of chromosomes in autism spectrum disorder. *Am. J. Hum. Genet.* 82:477–488.

Mattila, M.-L., M. Kielinen, and K. Jussila (2007). An epidemiological and diagnostic study of Asperger syndrome according to four sets of diagnostic criteria. *J. Am. Acad. Child Adol. Psych.* 46:636–646.

Mercer, T.R., M.E. Dinger, J. Mariani, K.S. Kosik, M.F. Mehler, and J.S. Mattick (2008). Noncoding RNAs in long-term memory formation. *Neuroscientist* 14:434–445.

Nelson, B. (2008). A disruptive personality, disrupted. *Nature* 456:26–28.

Niu, S., O. Yabut, and G. D'Arcangelo (2008). The Reelin signaling pathway promotes dendritic spine development in hippocampal neurons. *J. Neurosci.* 28:10339–10348.

Pheasant, M. and J.S. Mattick (2007). Raising the estimate of functional human sequences. *Genome Res.* 17:1245–1253.

Pollard, K.S., S.R. Salama, N. Lambert, M.A. Lambot, S. Coppens, J.S. Pedersen, S. Katzman, B. King, C. Onodera, A. Siepel, A.D. Kern, C. Dehay, H. Igel, Ares, Jr., M.P. Vanderhaeghen, and D. Haussler (2006). An RNA gene expressed during cortical development evolved rapidly in humans. *Nature* 443:167–172.

Psychiatric GWAS Consortium Steering Committee (2009). A framework for interpreting genome-wide association studies of psychiatric disorders. *Mol. Psychiatry* 14:10–17.

Schadt, E.E., J. Lamb, X. Yang, J. Zhu, S. Edwards, D. Guhathakurta, S.K. Sieberts, S. Monks, M. Reitman, C. Zhang, P.Y. Lum, A. Leonardson, R. Thieringer, J.M. Metzger, L. Yang, J. Castle, H. Zhu, S.F. Kash, T.A. Drake, A. Sachs, and A.J. Lusis (2005). An integrative genomics approach to infer causal associations between gene expression and disease. *Nat. Genet.* 37:710–717.

Schadt, E.E., C. Molony, E. Chudin, K. Hao, X. Yang, P.Y. Lum, A. Kasarskis, B. Zhang, S. Wang, C Suver, J. Zhu, J. Millstein, S. Sieberts, J. Lamb, D. GuhaThakurta, J. Derry, J.D. Storey, I. Avila-Campillo, M.J. Kruger, J.M. Johnson, C.A. Rohl, A. van Nas, M. Mehrabian, T.A. Drake, A.J. Lusis, R.C. Smith, F.P. Guengerich, S.C. Strom, E. Schuetz, T.H. Rushmore, and R. Ulrich (2008). Mapping the genetic architecture of gene expression in human liver. *PLoS Biol.* 6:e107.

Schratt, G.M., F. Tuebing, E.A. Nigh, C.G. Kane, M.E. Sabatini, M. Kiebler, and M.E. Greenberg (2006). A brain-specific microRNA regulates dendritic spine development. *Nature* 439:283–289.

Sebat, J., B. Lakshmi, D. Malhotra, J. Troge, C. Lese-Martin, T. Walsh, B. Yamrom, S. Yoon, A. Krasnitz, J. Kendall, A. Leotta, D. Pai, R. Zhang, Y.H. Lee, J. Hicks, S.J. Spence, A.T. Lee, K. Puura, T. Lehtimäki, D. Ledbetter, P.K. Gregersen, J. Bregman, J.S. Sutcliffe, V. Jobanputra, W. Chung, D. Warburton, M.C. King, D. Skuse, D.H. Geschwind, T.C. Gilliam, K. Ye, and M. Wigler (2007). Strong association of de novo copy number mutations with autism. *Science* 316:445–449.

Szatmari, P., R. Bremner, and J. Nagy (1989). Asperger's syndrome: A review of clinical features. *Can. J. Psychiatry* 34:554–560.

Szatmari, P., et al. The Autism Genome Project Consortium (2007). Mapping autism risk loci using genetic linkage and chromosomal rearrangements. *Nat. Genet.* 39:319–328.

Walsh, T., J.M. McClellan, S.E. McCarthy, A.M. Addington, S.B. Pierce, G.M. Cooper, A.S. Nord, M. Kusenda, D. Malhotra, A. Bhandari, S.M. Stray, C.F. Rippey, P. Roccanova, V. Makarov, B. Lakshmi, R.L. Findling, L. Sikich, T. Stromberg, B. Merriman, N. Gogtay, P. Butler, K. Eckstrand, L. Noory, P. Gochman, R. Long, Z. Chen, S. Davis, C. Baker, E.E. Eichler, P.S. Meltzer, S.F. Nelson, A.B. Singleton, M.K. Lee, J.L. Rapoport, M.C. King, and J. Sebat (2008). Rare structural variants disrupt multiple genes in neurodevelopmental pathways in schizophrenia. *Science* 320:539–543.

Weiss, L.A., Y. Shen, J.M. Korn, D.E. Arking, D.T. Miller, R. Fossdal, E. Saemundsen, H. Stefansson, M.A. Ferreira, T. Green, O.S. Platt, D.M. Ruderfer, C.A. Walsh, D. Altshuler, A. Chakravarti, R.E. Tanzi, K. Stefansson, S.L. Santangelo, J.F. Gusella, P. Sklar, B.L. Wu, and M.J. Daly; Autism Consortium (2008). Association between microdeletion and microduplication at 16p11.2 and autism. *N. Engl. J. Med.* 358:667–675.

Williams, E., K. Thomas, H. Sidebotham, and A. Emond (2008). Prevalence and characteristics of autistic spectrum disorders in the ALSPAC cohort. *Dev. Med. Child Neurol.* 50:672–677.

Witwer, A.N. and L.J. Lecavalier (2008). Examining the validity of autism spectrum disorder subtypes. *J. Autism Dev. Disord.* 38:1611–1624.

World Health Organization (1992). *The ICD-10 Classification of Mental and Behavioral Disorders: Clinical Descriptions and Diagnostic Guidelines.* Geneva, Switzerland: WHO.

Xu, B., J.L. Roos, S. Levy, E.J. van Rensburg, J.A. Gogos, and M. Karayiorgou (2008). Strong association of de novo copy number mutations with sporadic schizophrenia. *Nat. Genet.* 40:880–885.

Zhao, X., A. Leotta, V. Kustanovich, C. Lajonchere, D.H. Geschwind, K. Law, P. Law, S. Qiu, C. Lord, J. Sebat, K. Ye, and M. Wigler (2007). A unified genetic theory for sporadic and inherited autism. *Proc. Natl. Acad. Sci. USA* 104:12831–12836.

Zhu, J., B. Zhang, and E.E. Schadt (2008). A systems biology approach to drug discovery. *Adv. Genet.* 60:603–635.

Zimmer, C. (2008). The search for intelligence. *Sci. Am.* 299 (4): 68–75.

5 Phenotypic Expression of Autism, Maternal Depression, and the Monoamine Oxidase-A Gene

Ira L. Cohen*

Department of Psychology, New York State
Institute for Basic Research in Developmental
Disabilities, Staten Island, NY 10314, USA

CONTENTS

5.1 INTRODUCTION

Autism and the other pervasive developmental disorders (PDD), including childhood disintegrative disorder, Rett's disorder, Asperger's disorder, and PDD—not otherwise specified, comprise a set of disorders which share a "triad" of impairments in socialization and communication along with repetitive and ritualistic behaviors (American Psychiatric Association, 2000). Etiologically, autism is a disorder with a strong genetic basis (Bailey et al., 1995) but research has yet to identify a single gene or even a set of genes that account for the vast majority of the identified cases

---

* Corresponding author: Tel.: +1-718-494-5181; fax: +1-718-494-4837; e-mail: ira.cohen@omr.state.ny.us

although progress is being made (Abrahams and Geschwind, 2008). Indeed, Happe and Ronald (2008) have noted that the triad of impairments characteristic of autism fractionate when examined in large-scale twin populations and are associated with nonoverlapping genes, suggesting that it may be fruitless to assume a single cause is responsible for the disorder. To complicate the matter further, there is strong heterogeneity not only across diagnostic classes in PDD but within autism itself. For example, Miles et al. (2005) have suggested two groupings: essential versus complex autism, with the latter categorized by evidence of significant dysmorphology or microcephaly. Such individuals were also more likely to have an identifiable syndrome. Yet the notion that autism is a syndrome with many different "organic" etiologies is not new (Coleman, 1976).

These observations suggest that when attempting to understand the puzzle of autism, it may be more beneficial to consider examining how behavioral components of the disorder (rather than the syndrome as a whole) are individually linked to specific, theoretically relevant, biobehavioral variables. The advantages of this approach include identifying possible etiologies for behaviors associated with autism as well with as other overlapping disorders, identifying targets for intervention, and for explaining the wide variation in the severity of autism. The latter factor impacts development over time, as well as stress within the family. This tactic has been the focus of our research on autism over the past 25 years, starting with our initial studies on behaviors that differ in children with autism who have fragile X syndrome relative to those who do not (Cohen, 1992, 1995, 1996; Cohen et al., 1989, 1991, 1996).

5.2   ASSESSMENT ISSUES AND THE PDD BEHAVIOR INVENTORY

Of course, in order for this approach to be efficacious, it is critical to have relevant measures of autism that are reliable, valid, and continuous or "dimensional" in nature. Categorical classifications of behaviors into "normal" or "abnormal" are often not very productive from a research perspective (e.g., statistical power), are difficult to interpret, and do not readily map onto the way behaviors occur in the natural environment, i.e., in a continuously varied manner. For example, impairments in social interaction can manifest themselves as varying degrees of shyness, aloofness, avoidance, aggressiveness, or a combination of these behaviors. This varying nature of behavior is often better captured by dimensional rating scales rather than by categorical diagnostic classification systems.

Tools for assessing autism, such as the Autism Diagnostic Interview-Revised (ADI-R; Lord et al., 1994), the Autism Screening Questionnaire (ASQ; Berument et al., 1999), now known as the Social Communication Questionnaire (SCQ), and the Autism Diagnostic Observation Schedule (ADOS; Lord et al., 1999), do yield dimensional measures of the severity of components of the disorder. However, these measures provide "raw scores" and not "standardized scores." That is, there is no reference against which the meaningfulness of the size of the scores can be interpreted. For example, IQ scores are easily understood because they are standardized against the "typical" population. Therefore, if two people receive IQ scores of 95 and 100, it tells us that they are actually quite similar to each other as well as to most people in the population (since most IQ tests are standardized with a mean of 100 and an SD of 15). However, raw scores do not provide this type of information. There is no way to know if raw scores of 10 and 15 in two different people on an autism measure such as the ADI-R represent "normal" variation or an actual meaningful difference in severity. Similar criticism applies to other autism scales such as the Childhood Autism Rating Scale (CARS) (Schopler et al., 1980). Related to this, such assessment tools are not age-standardized. This is a critical issue since children with autism at 2 years of age do not behaviorally look the same as children with autism at age 12.

Finally, most assessment tools for autism exclusively assess problem behaviors. They do not measure the person's abilities in socialization, communication, and play. There are several problems with this approach. First, there is no way to measure actual improvement or worsening in skills over time, only a change in problem behaviors can be assessed. Second, there is no way to differentiate subgroups within the autism spectrum that differ mainly in their relative assets (e.g., Asperger's cases that have intact language but poor social skills). Third, there is no way of identifying cases that differ on the basis of a relative lack of appropriate skills, and not the presence of deviant behaviors (e.g., language impaired children).

For the above reasons, we developed the PDD Behavior Inventory (PDDBI) (Cohen, 2003; Cohen et al., 2003b; Cohen and Sudhalter, 2005), a reliable and valid informant-based assessment tool standardized on a large, well-diagnosed sample of children, aged 2–12.5 years with PDD (autism in 86%; PDD-NOS in 12%, and other PDD 2%). Three hundred sixty-nine parents and 277 teachers comprised the informant sample. Filling out the PDDBI is relatively straightforward (items are between the fifth and eighth grade reading level) and can be completed by most informants in about 30–45 min.

The PDDBI provides age- and norm-referenced (T-scores: mean = 50; SD = 10) measures of behaviors typically seen in children with autism across two primary dimensions designated "Approach/Withdrawal Problems" and "Receptive/Expressive Social Communication Abilities." The Approach/Withdrawal Problems dimension is comprised of seven behavioral domains covering a variety of the problem behaviors seen in children with autism while the Receptive/Expressive Social Communication Abilities dimension is comprised of three domains capturing social, language, and memory skills that may be deficient in some children with autism. Domain T-scores are also used to compute an "Autism Composite" score designed to reflect overall severity. Each of these domain and composite T-scores are normally distributed within the reference sample. T-scores from the PDDBI have proven to be sensitive to relevant independent variables (Chauhan et al., 2004; Cohen et al., 2003a,b; Cohen and Tsiouris, 2006) and correlate well with diagnosis (Cohen, 2003; Cohen et al., 2003a,b; Cohen and Sudhalter, 2005).

In this chapter, I will summarize what we have learned, using the PDDBI, about two related factors influencing the severity of autism: maternal depression and a polymorphism in the monoamine oxidase A (MAOA) gene. Overall, our data indicate that maternal depression influences the behavioral profile of autism in a somewhat paradoxical manner and this effect is remarkably similar to what we see with this MAOA polymorphism, suggesting a link between mood disorders and autism.

5.3 MATERNAL DEPRESSION AND AUTISM SEVERITY

One of the most unusual factors influencing the severity of autism is a family history of anxiety and depression. Familial mood and anxiety disorders and autism have been shown to be associated in a number of studies (DeLong and Dwyer, 1988; Piven et al., 1991; DeLong, 1994; DeLong and Nohria, 1994; Smalley et al., 1995; Piven and Palmer, 1999). Smalley et al. (1995) reported a lifetime prevalence of DSM (*Diagnostic and Statistical Manual of Mental Disorders-III-Revised*) (American Psychiatric Association, 1987) defined major mood disorders in 40.3% of parents of children with autism, relative to 19.2% of parents of children with tuberous sclerosis, or of children with an unspecified seizure disorder. The majority of these parents (64%) had their first onset of depression prior to the birth of their child with autism. Further, 32.4% of siblings (mean age = 17 years) were found to have developed major mood disorders. Similar results were reported by Piven et al. (1999). Smalley et al. (1995) also reported that 20% of parents and 20.6% of siblings of children with autism had social phobia. Although depression occurs at higher rates in families with autism, the two disorders are not directly related. That is, in families, autism does not cause depression and depression does not cause autism (Bolton et al., 1998; Piven and Palmer, 1999).

Given the fact that one of the primary characteristics of depression is withdrawal from the environment and that social phobia is characterized by intense social withdrawal, one would expect that caregivers who suffer from these conditions would have children with autism whose outcome would be less than optimal. This expectation would be wrong. Smalley et al. (1995) found that a history of social phobia was more likely in families where the child with autism had an IQ greater than or equal to 70. Similar observations have been noted by DeLong (2004) with respect to a family history or mood disorders. We reported (Cohen and Tsiouris, 2006), based on a large sample of 122 families of young children (mean (SD) age = 5.4 (1.4) years) with an autism spectrum disorder, that a maternal lifetime history of recurrent major depression (there were no significant paternal effects or maternal anxiety disorder effects) is associated with significantly higher IQs (differences as great as 20 IQ points), higher adaptive skills and higher T-scores on the Receptive/Expressive Social Communication Abilities dimension of the PDDBI ($p < 0.025$) in these children.

Associations between recurrent major depression in the mothers and the Approach/ Withdrawal domain scores on the PDDBI were complicated but suggestive of increased anxiety and more social withdrawal in these young children. Specifically, teachers, but not parents, rated the children whose mothers had a history of recurrent depression as having more problems with sensory behaviors, rituals, and fears, and fewer problems with overarousal (i.e., relatively less hyperactivity), a more fearful and inhibited (internalizing) behavior style. These types of problems are suggestive of early-onset anxiety or internalizing problems. The fact that these effects were evident in the teacher but not the parent reports could reflect separation anxiety or social phobia problems in this young age group. In the non-PDD population, social phobia and major depression have been noted to be more common among young children (mean age of 6.7 years) whose parents have a history of major depression

(Biederman et al., 2001). Thus, the children of mothers with recurrent depression in our study resembled, to some extent, their non-PDD cohorts. Unlike these children, however, their internalizing problems manifested as an increased severity of certain "autistic" behaviors.

These observations are indeed puzzling. Why would high functioning autism be linked to a lifetime history of mood disorders in their families, especially their mothers? In our study, we could not attribute the relatively increased IQ association to psychosocial factors, selection bias, or other treatments such as applied behavior analysis (ABA). While it is conceivable that those mothers with a depression history may be more intelligent and, therefore, their children with autism would be more likely to be higher functioning, IQs of the children in our study were unrelated to maternal educational level, and type of maternal depression was unrelated to maternal educational level. Further, studies have concluded that IQs of children with autism do not correlate significantly with IQs of their parents (Szatmari and Jones, 1991; Fombonne et al., 1997).

Genetic factors could be a possible explanation. Smalley et al. (1995) speculated that the association of familial mood/anxiety disorders with high functioning autism is due to greater etiological heterogeneity in children with autism who also have intellectual disabilities. That is, in such children, genetic and/or environmental factors unrelated to mood disorder likely play a role in contributing to causation. DeLong (2004) has made a similar argument. However, there is no a priori reason for why genes associated with intellectual disability should not also be involved in depression or social phobia. Intellectual disability is a common feature in males with fragile X syndrome. Yet, social anxiety is prominent in these males at all levels of intelligence (Cohen et al., 1988) and major depression has been reported to be common in their mothers (Thompson et al., 1996).

In our paper (Cohen and Tsiouris, 2006), we hypothesized a "genetic modifier" model (cf. Slavotinek and Biesecker, 2003) as an explanation. In this model, "autism genes" and "depression genes" share common alleles, which interact with one another (epistatic interactions) to modify the expression of each disorder. In the case of autism, this would include a relatively "protective" effect of recurrent depression alleles on IQ in children with autism.

This modifier model is displayed in the Venn diagram (Figure 5.1). Here, the phenotypes of autism and depression are depicted as separate entities arising from gene sets that are largely independent. However, the two disorders share some risk alleles (denoted here as DEP/AUT alleles). When these DEP/AUT alleles are present, they interact with each other to modify the expression of each disorder (the shaded regions). Therefore, this model predicts that DEP/AUT alleles should result in individuals more likely to have a specific autism or depression phenotype, depending upon the number and type of these alleles, and that these DEP/AUT alleles have a protective effect on the deleterious effects on language and IQ caused by other autism genes, accounting for the increased cognitive ability in these affected children. If this hypothesis were true, it would have clear implications for prognosis and treatment. Is there any evidence that genes associated with mood and anxiety disorders have a protective effect on language and IQ in children with autism? The answer is yes.

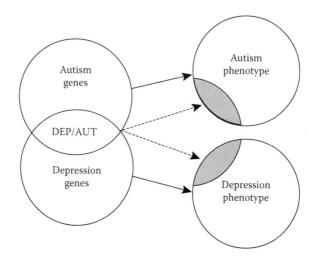

FIGURE 5.1 This figure presents a Venn diagram of the hypothesized overlap of risk alleles (DEP/AUT alleles) that are common to both autism and recurrent mood disorders. The dashed arrows emerging from the DEP/AUT overlap represent this modifier gene effect. The shaded regions represent DEP/AUT modified subgroups of autism and depression. (From Cohen, I.L. and Tsiouris, J.A., *J. Aut. Dev. Disord.*, 36, 1077, 2006. With permission.)

5.4   MONOAMINE OXIDASE-A GENE AS A DEP/AUT GENE

In searching for genes that would have an impact on both autism and depression, genes involved with the catecholamine and serotonin systems are reasonable candidates. There are two reasons for this. First, the catecholamines and serotonin, as neurotransmitters, are involved with mood, arousal, reward, and neural development (Azmitia, 2001). Second, drugs that affect these neurotransmitters improve some of the symptoms of autism, especially repetitive behaviors (Campbell et al., 1978, 1988; Cohen et al., 1980; Anderson et al., 1989; Hollander et al., 2005; McDougle et al., 2005) as well as depression.

Serotonin plays an important role in neurogenesis in utero, along with its well-characterized neurotransmitter role (Gillberg and Coleman, 2000; Azmitia, 2001). As such, it has theoretical relevance for autism, as well as for mood disorders. There is evidence that serotonin function is abnormal in autism. One of the earliest and most consistent findings is that serotonin blood concentration is elevated in a subset of cases with autism (Anderson, 1987). However, the meaning of these elevated blood serotonin levels is unclear. Elevated blood serotonin levels are not specific to autism (Gillberg and Coleman, 2000) and are not necessarily indicative of elevated brain serotonin levels. For example, Coleman et al. (1977) reported the case of a boy with infantile spasms who had consistently elevated levels of blood serotonin. This child died at 21 months of age and, on autopsy, gray matter levels of serotonin were lower than a control case. Nevertheless, elevated blood serotonin levels may indicate a dysfunction in the serotonin system that is indirectly related to the function of the central nervous system (CNS). For example, in some studies, blood serotonin levels have been found to correlate inversely with verbal IQ (Cook et al., 1990) and to correlate positively with severity of autism (Kuperman et al., 1987). Blood serotonin levels have also been found to be related to mood and anxiety disorders. Cook et al. (1994) reported that parents of children with autism who had elevated blood serotonin levels also had increased levels of symptoms of depression and obsessive–compulsive disorder, relative to parents of children with autism who had normal serotonin levels. More evidence for a serotonin dysfunction is found in the fact that increased binding of paroxetine to the serotonin transporter in blood platelets has been observed in autism (Marazziti et al., 2000), suggesting that a similar mechanism may be present centrally. Indeed, at the CNS level, Chugani et al. (1999) reported, in a positron emission tomography (PET) scan study, that brain serotonin synthesis declines with age in typically developing children; but in children with autism, brain serotonin synthesis fails to decrease with age.

Many factors affect overall CNS serotonin levels as well as the availability of serotonin in the synapse. Metabolically, serotonin is synthesized from 5-hydroxytryptophan (5-HTP) by L-amino acid decarboxylase (L-AADC). 5-HTP is synthesized from tryptophan by tryptophan hydroxylase (TPH), the rate-limiting enzyme in serotonin synthesis. When released into the synapse, serotonin interacts with a multitude of pre- and postsynaptic receptor sites. These postsynaptic receptors can induce gene expression by activating CREB1 (cAMP-responsive element-binding protein), a gene that has been implicated in recurrent depression in women (Zubenko et al., 2003). An inhibitory presynaptic autoreceptor (HTR1B/HTR1DB) modulates the release of serotonin into the synapse. The serotonin reuptake transporter (SERT/SLC6A4/5-HTT) brings serotonin back into the presynaptic neuron where it is eventually metabolized by MAO in the mitochondria. Thus, the extent to which serotonin can effect changes on the postsynaptic neuron is influenced by availability of precursors, enzyme activity, presynaptic receptor sensitivity and function, genes involved with the cAMP signaling pathway, and excitatory or inhibitory influences of other neuronal systems. The density of serotonergic synapses will also influence overall brain serotonin levels. Understanding how the serotonin system affects behavior in autism will ultimately require examining the contribution of many of these factors, both singly and in combination. For reasons enumerated below, the gene that codes for MAOA is a reasonable starting point.

Two forms of MAO exist (A and B). The genes that encode these isoenzymes map to Xp11.23~11.4. MAOA is of interest in this discussion because it preferentially deaminates serotonin and norepinephrine while MAOB acts on the phenethylamines and benzylamine (Sabol et al., 1998). Both MAOA and MAOB are present in various regions of the body including the brain and fibroblasts. Some tissues preferentially express only one of these isoenzymes. For example, platelets only express MAOB (Sabol et al., 1998).

A number of different studies indicate that MAOA levels and MAOA gene differences are associated with neurotransmitter and behavioral changes. For example, MAOA knockout mice show large increases in brain serotonin levels and disturbed CNS development (Cases et al., 1998). Thus, absence of MAOA has marked effects on brain development and serotonin function. Abnormal behaviors (aggression), borderline mental retardation, and marked decreases in MAOA activity have been reported in a family with a point mutation in the MAOA gene (Brunner et al., 1993). A blind male with Norrie disease, who also had a microdeletion in both MAOA and MAOB genes, had profound retardation and stereotypy habit disorder (Collins et al., 1992). Psychiatric problems were noted in his mother. This obligate carrier had been diagnosed with "chronic hypomania and schizotypal features," suggesting that MAO plays a role in mood and thought disorders. A recent PET scan study in fact has indicated that MAOA levels are uniformly increased in the brain during major depression (Meyer et al., 2006). A study of females with Turner syndrome has implicated the MAO gene (MAOB and, possibly, MAOA) in behaviors associated with autism (such as deficits in recognition of fear expression in faces) and in neuroanatomical regions associated with processing of emotion such as the amygdala and orbitofrontal cortex (Good et al., 2003).

An upstream variable number tandem repeat (uVNTR) polymorphism within the MAOA promoter region has been identified by Sabol et al. (1998). It consists of a 30-bp repeat sequence consisting of 3, 3.5, 4, or 5 copies. Expression studies indicate that the number of repeats is related to transcriptional efficiency of the gene. The 3-repeat allele (i.e., the one with 3 copies of the 30 bp repeat sequence) is associated with reduced transcription (Denney et al., 1999) relative to the other alleles (Sabol et al., 1998), leading to less MAOA activity. These same MAOA-uVNTR alleles have been shown to affect central serotonin functioning, as well as behavior. The low activity alleles have been found to be associated with increased serotonergic responsivity (prolactin response to fenfluramine challenge) (Manuck et al., 2000). Williams et al. (2003) reported that males ($N = 48$) carrying the 3.5 and 4 repeat alleles have higher 5-hydroxyindoleacetic acid (5-HIAA) levels in cerebrospinal fluid (CSF) than those with 3 or 5 repeats ($N = 36$). This effect was independent of racial background. These effects were, however, not present in women.

Behaviorally, Caspi et al. (2002) reported that the low activity 3-repeat MAOA allele was associated with antisocial behavior (an "externalizing" behavior) only in those males who had been subjected to abuse as children, suggesting a gene–environmental stress interaction effect. More germane to our model, alleles with more than 3 copies of the repeat sequence were found to be associated with recurrent major depression in females in at least two studies (Schulze et al., 2000; Yu et al., 2005). Thus, the 3-repeat allele seems to be involved with "externalizing"-type behaviors while the longer repeats may be associated with more "internalizing" (withdrawal) behaviors.

Given that (a) MAOA affects serotonin levels; (b) serotonin function may be abnormal in autism; (c) serotonin reuptake inhibitors are potent antidepressants; (d) MAOA polymorphisms associated with high activity of the gene are associated with depression; (e) MAOA polymorphisms associated with low transcriptional activity of the gene are associated with externalizing behavior (perhaps in reaction to stress); (e) MAOA plays an important role in brain development; and (f) MAO inhibitors are antidepressants, the MAOA gene is a reasonable DEP/AUT candidate gene for modulating the pattern of expression of autism.

5.5 ASSOCIATION OF AN MAOA-uVNTR POLYMORPHISM WITH BEHAVIOR IN AUTISM

We have reported (Cohen et al., 2003a,b), in a study of 41 males hemizygous for low or high activity MAOA alleles, that these alleles are associated with unique behavior patterns as measured by the PDDBI, IQ, and Adaptive Behavior assessments. In order to control for age-related effects and variability in assessment procedures, all of the males were less than 12.5 years of age and all received the same behavioral tests.

We found the high activity (4-repeat) allele in boys was associated with both higher IQ and lower Autism Composite scores (as measured by the parent and teacher forms of the PDDBI). There were no significant informant effects. That is, results were the same from both the parent and teacher PDDBIs. Analysis to determine which domains were specifically affected in the Approach/Withdrawal Problems dimension indicated that the SENSORY (a measure of repetitive interest in sensory-type behaviors such as hand flapping, staring at objects, repetitive play with objects, etc.) ($p < 0.002$) and AROUSAL (a measure of hyperactivity and lack of responsiveness) ($p < 0.02$) domains were highest in the 3-repeat group. These externalizing-type behavior effects replicate the above studies performed in other populations. Within the Receptive/Expressive Social Communication Abilities dimension, domains assessing social skills ($p < 0.005$), and measures of language and memory ($p < 0.02$) were highest in the 4-repeat group. These effects are shown in Figure 5.2. Thus, the 4-repeat behavior pattern resembled that of children having mothers with a history of recurrent depression.

The results of our study differed from that of Jones et al. (2004). They reported an effect of these MAOA alleles on Leiter performance IQ, but their data indicated that the effect was only seen when the mother's genotype was examined, i.e., a maternal effect. Mothers who were homozygous for the 3-repeat allele ($N = 9$) had children with much lower IQs (mean (SD)=51.1 (32.7)) than mothers who were heterozygous (i.e., with both the 3-repeat and 4-repeat alleles; $N=37$; mean (SD) = 78.5(25.5)) or homozygous for the 4-repeat allele ($N = 31$; mean (SD)=72.5 (26.8)). The explanation may relate, in part, to the nature of the two samples. Our sample consisted of boys less than 12.5 years of age whereas age was undefined in the study by Jones et al. (2004). Further, the MAOA allelic distribution of their affected males was atypical. The distribution of 3-repeat and 4-repeat alleles in affected males in the Jones et al. (2004) sample significantly differed from our study sample (Yates corrected χ^2 (1)=7.4, $p < 0.01$; numbers provided by M.B. Jones, personal communication), suggesting population stratification effects. Fifty-nine percent of their sample had the 3-repeat allele whereas only 36% of our sample had this same allele, a percentage identical to that of the general male population (Sabol et al., 1998). As well, effects may only be on verbal IQ and not performance IQ, although we did not see this in our study. More importantly, in order to disentangle maternal and child MAOA associations, boys should be stratified in groups according to their and their mothers' genotypes. An interaction between the alleles of the mothers and their sons, for example, could have wiped out any child effect. We have since examined this question in a larger sample. There is indeed a maternal effect for most behaviors.

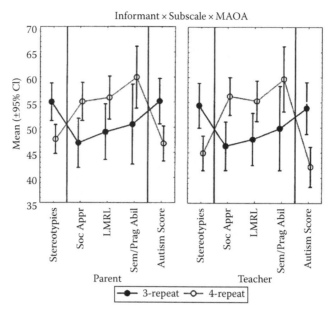

FIGURE 5.2 This figure shows the similarity in parent and teacher profiles for the significant PDDBI domain *T*-scores (mean ± 95% confidence interval) across 3-repeat and 4-repeat MAOA-uVNTR genotypes (see text). Note that the domain names differ slightly from the current version of the PDDBI (Cohen and Sudhalter, 2005) and these changes are noted below. Vertical lines separate the SENSORY (stereotypies) domain (higher scores indicate increased severity) from the Receptive-Expressive Social Communication Abilities domains (where higher scores indicate increased ability) and from the overall Autism Score (higher scores indicate increased severity). Soc Appr, Social Approach domain; LMRL, Learning, Memory and Receptive Language domain; Sem/Prag Abil is a component of the Expressive Language domain. (From Cohen, I.L. et al., *Clin. Genet.*, 64, 190, 2003. With permission.)

5.6   MAOA GENE AND BEHAVIOR PROFILES IN AUTISM, A MATERNAL EFFECT

Since our paper was published, my collaborators and I have recruited additional boys on whom we have both PDDBI and MAOA-uVNTR data. Some of this information has been reported elsewhere (Holden et al., 2006). We currently have data on 115 simplex and multiplex families who have sons who are positive for autism or autism spectrum disorder on the ADI-R or ADOS-G, have autism scores on the PDDBI greater than 36 (a cutoff that agrees well with the above measures as well as with clinical diagnosis of autism), have no other medical explanation for their disorder, who were born full-term, and who were in the correct age range for the PDDBI (18 months to 12.5 years of age). For multiplex families, only the earliest born affected male was selected for analysis. Of the 115 mothers, 4 were homozygous for the 3-repeat allele, 63 were heterozygous for the 3- and 4-repeat alleles (34 boys with the 3-repeat allele and 29 with the 4-repeat allele), and 48 were homozygous for the 4-repeat allele. Due to the small sample size of the homozygous

3-repeat mothers, their data were dropped from the rest of the analyses yielding three groups: (1) 3_34, i.e., 3-repeat boys from heterozygous mothers; (2) 4_34, or 4-repeat boys from heterozygous mothers; and (3) 4_44 or 4-repeat boys from homozygous 4-repeat mothers. If the associations with the MAO-A were maternal in nature, we would predict that groups 1 and 2 would be similar and both would differ from group 3. If the associations were strictly due to the alleles inherited by the boys, then group 1 would differ from groups 2 and 3, with the latter groups similar to one another. If the boys' and the mothers' alleles interacted, then all three groups would differ from one another.

Data were analyzed with multivariate analyses of variance (MANOVAs) with domains within each dimension of the PDDBI serving as the dependent variables. Analysis of variance (ANOVA) was used to analyze the overall Autism Composite score. Family status (simplex or multiplex) also served as a predictor to control for the effects of living with a sibling having autism. Post-hoc analyses were used to compare groups.

Within the Receptive/Expressive Social Communication Abilities dimension, higher levels of ability in association with the 4-repeat allele were predicted based on our previous data. This was confirmed for the Social Approach Behaviors domain (SOCAPP; a measure of nonvocal social skills such as eye contact, gesture, play, and empathy), Expressive Language domain (EXPRESS; a measure of phonological, semantic and pragmatic verbal ability), and the Learning, Memory and Receptive Language domain (LMRL; a measure of memory and receptive skills) except that these were indeed maternal in nature. The 3_34, 4_34, and 4_44 groups had mean SOCAPP (SE) T-scores of 44.9 (2.1), 47.2 (2.3), and 51.1 (1.6). Thus, there was about a 0.5 SD difference between the 4_44 group and the other two groups ($p < 0.022$) who did not differ from each other. Similar effects were present for the other two domains. Interestingly, the LMRL domain has the highest correlation with IQ (r (74) = 0.77; Cohen and Sudhalter, 2005) and the difference across groups for this domain was the largest: the 3_34, 4_34, and 4_44 groups had mean (SE) T-scores of 47.5 (2.2), 47.3 (2.4), and 54.6 (1.7). Thus, there was almost a 1 SD difference between the 4_44 group and the other two groups ($p < 0.014$). These results confirm our earlier findings but indicate that these differences are maternal in nature.

Within the Approach/Withdrawal Problems dimension of the PDDBI, significant differences ($p < 0.05$) were evident across the three groups for three domains: Sensory/Perceptual Approach Behaviors (SENSORY), replicating our original observation; Ritualisms/Resistance to Change (RITUAL; a measure of engaging in rituals or resisting changes in routines or in the environment); and Specific Fears (FEARS; a measure of overall anxiety, sensitivity to noises, separation problems, etc.). The SENSORY effect was not maternal with the 3_34 group showing higher T-scores (mean (SE)=52.7 (1.7)) than the 4_34 or 4_44 groups (mean = (SE) 48.1 (1.8) and 48.4 (1.4), respectively, $p < 0.05$). All of these scores were in the autism range but the means differed by about 0.5 SD. However, the RITUAL and FEARS effects were maternal in nature. The 3_34, 4_34, and 4_44 groups had mean (SE) RITUAL T-scores of 50.8 (1.5), 47.7 (1.7), and 53.6 (1.3) and mean (SE) FEARS T-scores of 50.2 (1.6), 48.0 (1.8), and 54.6 (1.4). Thus, again, there was about a 0.5 SD difference between the 4_44 group and the other two groups

($p<0.005$). Conceptually, both fears and ritualistic behaviors are related to one another as "internalizing" behaviors. Indeed, obsessive–compulsive disorder is characterized in the DSM as an anxiety disorder.

A nonmaternal effect was present, however. Boys with the 3-repeat allele had higher SENSORY scores, as noted, and higher Autism Composite Scores, a measure of overall severity, as predicted based on our previous data. The Autism Composite was worse in boys with the 3-repeat allele by about 0.5 SD ($p<0.028$). The 3_34, 4_34, and 4_44 groups had mean (SE) T-scores of 55.2 (1.6), 49.6 (1.7), and 50.9 (1.4).

5.7 SUMMARY AND CONCLUSIONS

These results are consistent with the maternal depression effects cited above. This particular MAOA polymorphism (or a closely linked site) is associated with anxiety-like behaviors in children with autism and with adaptive abilities in socialization and language, and these effects are maternal in nature. Recurrent major depression in the mothers of these children is also associated with the same behavior pattern. Thus, the "maternal environment" seems to play a role in modulating internalizing behaviors and social and language skills in these children. Mothers homozygous for the higher-activity 4-repeat MAOA allele have children on the autism spectrum who appear to be relatively better off compared to children with autism who have heterozygous mothers, irrespective of their MAO genotype in that they are "higher functioning," a good prognosticator for future development.

It should be noted that our results were specific to only certain behaviors; there was no "global" association of these alleles with the full spectrum of behaviors characteristic of autism. Thus, we did not find evidence for any associations of these MAOA alleles with PDDBI domains assessing social pragmatic problems and repetitive language (or aggression, at this age). The association with the global autism score was quantitative in nature and unlikely to be associated with an actual difference in diagnostic category. The 3-repeat cases were simply "more autistic," by 0.5 SD, than the other two groups whose scores were at the expected mean for children with autism. Therefore the notion that genes affect only certain behaviors linked to autism is supported by our data.

Recent data indicate that this MAOA-uVNTR polymorphism is also associated with brain size differences in autism. Davis et al. (2008) reported in an MRI study that cerebral gray and white matter volume was increased in children with autism having the low-activity 3-repeat allele ($n=12$) versus those with the high activity 4-repeat allele ($n=17$). Thus, there is an association of this polymorphism with brain growth in autism. These researchers did not determine if their effects were maternal in nature or not but they did note that MAOA is expressed early in development.

Taken together, these studies are consistent with the idea that alleles associated with depression are protective for cognitive functioning in children on the autism spectrum but enhance internalizing problems. These effects are maternal in nature, and, given the MRI data, likely prenatal in origin. Indeed, as noted, the primary substrate for MAO is serotonin and Cote et al. (2007) noted that this molecule plays a strong role in development prior to its role as a neurotransmitter. In mice, these researchers reported that this morphogen effect is maternal, i.e., that embryonic development is dependent on serotonin that is of maternal, and not fetal, origin. They also noted (Cote et al., 2007, p. 333), with respect to autism, that "it is conceivable that variations in maternal serotonin levels exert subtle effects on brain development during early ontogeny irrespective of the proper levels of peripheral serotonin in the affected child." Our data are consistent with this notion. Perhaps genes like MAOA that may affect maternal serotonin levels during early gestation mitigate some of the deleterious effect of other autism genes (or autism predisposing prenatal stress or epigenetic factors) on cognitive development but enhance the child's disposition to react with intense anxiety to the environment. This behavior pattern is typically seen in Asperger's type individuals. These findings suggest it may be beneficial to explore the use of maternal and child genotyping for these alleles in order to predict the therapeutic efficacy of medications affecting the serotonin system or MAOA activity.

It should also be noted that the notion that prenatal factors are involved in autism has been of increasing interest to the research community. Studies have noted increased risk for development of autism in association with a variety of birth complications (Kolevzon et al., 2007; Durkin et al., 2008; Kinney et al., 2008; Limperopoulos et al., 2008; Pinelli and Zwaigenbaum, 2008; Schendel, 2008; Schendel and Bhasin, 2008; Tsuchiya et al., 2008; Williams et al., 2008).

My colleagues and I (Karmel et al., 2008) have reported on factors associated with the later diagnosis of autism in neonatal intensive care unit (NICU) infants. Such infants were more likely than the rest of the cohort to be of low birth weight, to have shorter gestations, to show evidence for greater CNS involvement, to be male, and to have more educated mothers. We also noted that, by 4 months of age, the group that went on to develop autism had a greater preference for high frequency visual stimulation than a matched cohort, suggesting unique problems with the attention-arousal system in these infants. In fact, this preference was strongly correlated with a variety of domains on the PDDBI in a subgroup of these children ($n = 12$) who were seen at an average age of 4 years. When compared with other autistic children seen by me who were not in a NICU, the NICU children, at 4 years of age, showed higher RITUAL and AGGRESS (aggressiveness and irritability) domain scores, suggesting long-term influences of these birth complications on certain aspects of their behaviors. It would be interesting to analyze the MAOA genotypes of these children and their mothers to see if there is an association with the severity of their disorder, the specific type of birth complication or their interaction.

In summary, our data indicate that, by assuming that autism is a syndrome comprised of several different behavioral categories that can be independently influenced by many different factors, and by having appropriate assessment tools, it is possible to determine which variables modulate their severity and the magnitude of these effects. Further, to the extent that these variables yield similar effects, it may be possible to determine what they have in common. Our data indicate that a maternal lifetime history of recurrent depression and the high activity alleles of the MAOA-uVNTR polymorphism yield similar PDDBI profiles, and both may theoretically be linked through a common effect on prenatal serotonin levels.

REFERENCES

Abrahams, B. S. and D. H. Geschwind (2008). Advances in autism genetics: On the threshold of a new neurobiology. *Nat. Rev. Genet.* 9:341–355.

American Psychiatric Association (1987). *Diagnostic and Statistical Manual of Mental Disorders-III-R.* Washington, DC.

American Psychiatric Association (2000). *Diagnostic and Statistical Manual of Mental Disorders Fourth Edition Text Revision.* Washington, DC.

Anderson, G. M. (1987). Monoamines in autism: An update of neurochemical research on a pervasive developmental disorder. *Med. Biol.* 65:67–74.

Anderson, L. T., M. Campbell, P. Adams, A. M. Small, R. Perry, and J. Shell (1989). The effects of haloperidol on discrimination learning and behavioral symptoms in autistic children. *J. Autism Dev. Disord.* 19:227–239.

Azmitia, E. C. (2001). Neuronal instability: Implications for Rett's syndrome. *Brain Dev.* 23, Suppl 1:S1–S10.

Bailey, A., A. Le Couteur, I. Gottesman, P. Bolton, E. Simonoff, E. Yuzda, and M. Rutter (1995). Autism as a strongly genetic disorder: Evidence from a British twin study. *Psychol. Med.* 25:63–77.

Berument, S. K., M. Rutter, C. Lord, A. Pickles, and A. Bailey (1999). Autism screening questionnaire: Diagnostic validity. *Br. J. Psychiatry* 175:144–451.

Biederman, J., S. V. Faraone, D. R. Hirshfeld-Becker, D. Friedman, J. A. Robin, and J. F. Rosenbaum (2001). Patterns of psychopathology and dysfunction in high-risk children of parents with panic disorder and major depression. *Am. J. Psychiatry* 158:49–57.

Bolton, P. F., A. Pickles, M. Murphy, and M. Rutter (1998). Autism, affective and other psychiatric disorders: Patterns of familial aggregation. *Psychol. Med.* 28:385–395.

Brunner, H. G., M. Nelen, X. O. Breakefield, H. H. Ropers, and B. A. van Oost (1993). Abnormal behavior associated with a point mutation in the structural gene for monoamine oxidase A. *Science* 262:578–580.

Campbell, M., L. T. Anderson, M. Meier, I. L. Cohen, A.M. Small, C. Samit, and E. J. Sacher (1978). A comparison of haloperidol and behavior therapy and their interaction in autistic children. *J. Am. Acad. Child Adolesc. Psychiatry* 7:640–655.

Campbell, M., I. L. Cohen, R. Perry, A. M. Small, and M. Hersen (1988). Psychopharmacological treatment. In T. H. Ollendick (ed.), *Handbook of Child Psychopathology.* New York: Plenum Press.

Cases, O., C. Lebrand, B. Giros, T. Vitalis, E. De Maeyer, M. G. Caron, D. J. Price, P. Gaspar, and I. Seif (1998). Plasma membrane transporters of serotonin, dopamine, and norepinephrine mediate serotonin accumulation in atypical locations in the developing brain of monoamine oxidase A knock-outs. *J. Neurosci.* 18:6914–6927.

Caspi, A., J. McClay, T. E. Moffitt, J. Mill, J. Martin, I. W. Craig, A. Taylor, and R. Poulton (2002). Role of genotype in the cycle of violence in maltreated children. *Science* 297:851–854.

Chauhan, A., V. Chauhan, W. T. Brown, and I. L. Cohen (2004). Oxidative stress in autism: Increased lipid peroxidation and reduced serum levels of ceruloplasmin and transferrin— the antioxidant proteins. *Life Sci.* 75:2539–2549.

Chugani, D. C., O. Muzik, M. Behen, R. Rothermel, J. J. Janisse, J. Lee, and H. T. Chugani (1999). Developmental changes in brain serotonin synthesis capacity in autistic and nonautistic children. *Ann. Neurol.* 45:287–295.

Cohen, I. L., G. S. Fisch, E. G. Wolf Schein, V. Sudhalter, D. Hanson, R. Hagerman, E. C. Jenkins, and W. T. Brown (1988). Social gaze, social avoidance and repetitive behavior in fragile X males: A controlled study. *Am. J. Ment. Retard.* 92:436–446.

Cohen, I. L. (1992). The behavioral phenotype of Fragile X Syndrome and its association with autism. In R. J. Hagerman (ed.), *Third International Fragile X Conference.* Denver, CO: Spectra Publishing.

Cohen, I. L. (1995). Behavioral profiles of autistic and non-autistic fragile X males. *Dev. Brain Dysfunc.* 8:252–269.

Cohen, I. L. (1996). A theoretical analysis of the role of hyperarousal in the behavior and learning of fragile X males. *Mentl. Retard. Dev. Disabil. Res. Rev.* 1:286–291.

Cohen, I. L. (2003). Criterion-related validity of the PDD Behavior Inventory. *J. Autism Dev. Disord.* 33:47–53.

Cohen, I. L. and V. Sudhalter (2005). *The PDD Behavior Inventory.* Lutz, FL: Psychological Assessment Resources, Inc.

Cohen, I. L. and J. Tsiouris (2006). Maternal recurrent mood disorders and high-functioning autism. *J. Autism Dev. Disord.* 36:1077–1078.

Cohen, I. L., M. Campbell, D. Posner, A. M. Small, D. Triebel, and L. T. Anderson (1980). Behavioral effects of haloperidol in young autistic children. An objective analysis using a within-subjects reversal design. *J. Am. Acad. Child Psychiatry* 19:665–677.

Cohen, I. L., P. M. Vietze, V. Sudhalter, E. C. Jenkins, and W. T. Brown (1989). Parent–child dyadic gaze patterns in fragile X males and in non-fragile X males with autistic disorder. *J. Child Psychol. Psychiatry* 30:845–856.

Cohen, I. L., V. Sudhalter, A. Pfadt, E. C. Jenkins, W. T. Brown, and P. M. Vietze (1991). Why are autism and the fragile-X syndrome associated? Conceptual and methodological issues. *Am. J. Hum. Genet.* 48:195–202.

Cohen, I. L., S. L. Nolin, V. Sudhalter, X. H. Ding, C. S. Dobkin, and W. T. Brown (1996). Mosaicism for the FMR1 gene influences adaptive skills development in fragile X-affected males. *Am. J. Med. Genet.* 64:365–369.

Cohen, I. L., X. Liu, C. Schutz, B. N. White, E. C. Jenkins, W. T. Brown, and J. J. A. Holden (2003a). Association of autism severity with a monoamine oxidase A functional polymorphism. *Clin. Genet.* 64:190–197.

Cohen, I. L., S. Schmidt-Lackner, R. Romanczyk, and V. Sudhalter (2003b). The PDD Behavior Inventory: A rating scale for assessing response to intervention in children with PDD. *J. Autism Dev. Disord.* 33:31–45.

Coleman, M. (1976). *The Autistic Syndromes.* Amsterdam: North-Holland.

Coleman, M., P. N. Hart, J. Randall, J. Lee, D. Hijada, and C. G. Bratenahl (1977). Serotonin levels in the blood and central nervous system of a patient with sudanophilic leukodystrophy. *Neuropadiatrie* 8:459–466.

Collins, F. A., D. L. Murphy, A. L. Reiss, K. B. Sims, J. G. Lewis, L. Freund, F. Karoum, D. Zhu, I. H. Maumenee, and S. E. Antonarakis (1992). Clinical, biochemical, and neuropsychiatric evaluation of a patient with a contiguous gene syndrome due to a microdeletion Xp11.3 including the Norrie disease locus and monoamine oxidase (MAOA and MAOB) genes. *Am. J. Med. Genet.* 42:127–134.

Cook, E. H., B. L. Leventhal, W. Heller, J. Metz, M. Wainwright, and D. X. Freedman (1990). Autistic children and their first-degree relatives: Relationships between serotonin and norepinephrine levels and intelligence. *J. Neuropsychiatry Clin. Neurosci.* 2:268–274.

Cook, E. H., D. A. Charak, J. Arida, J. A. Spohn, N. J. Roizen, and B. L. Leventhal (1994). Depressive and obsessive-compulsive symptoms in hyperserotonemic parents of children with autistic disorder. *Psychiatry Res.* 52:25–33.

Cote, F., C. Fligny, E. Bayard, J. M. Launay, M. D. Gershon, J. Mallet, and G. Vodjani (2007). Maternal serotonin is crucial for murine embryonic development. *Proc. Natl. Acad. Sci. USA* 104:329–334.

Davis, L. K., H. C. Hazlett, A. L. Librant, P. Nopoulos, V. C. Sheffield, J. Piven, and T. H. Wassink (2008). Cortical enlargement in autism is associated with a functional VNTR in the monoamine oxidase A gene. *Am. J. Med. Genet. B Neuropsychiatr. Genet.* 5:1145–1151.

DeLong, R. (1994). Children with autistic spectrum disorder and a family history of affective disorder. *Dev. Med. Child Neurol.* 36:674–687.

DeLong, G. R. (2004). Autism and familial major mood disorder: Are they related? *J. Neuropsychiatry Clin. Neurosci.* 16:199–213.

DeLong, G. R. and J. T. Dwyer (1988). Correlation of family history with specific autistic subgroups: Asperger's syndrome and bipolar affective disease. *J. Autism Dev. Disord.* 18:593–600.

DeLong, R. and C. Nohria (1994). Psychiatric family history and neurological disease in autistic spectrum disorders. *Dev. Med. Child Neurol.* 36:441–448.

Denney, R. M., H. Koch, and I. W. Craig (1999). Association between monoamine oxidase A activity in human male skin fibroblasts and genotype of the MAOA promoter-associated variable number tandem repeat. *Hum. Genet.* 105:542–551.

Durkin, M. S., M. J. Maenner, C. J. Newschaffer, L. C. Lee, C. M. Cuniff, J. L. Daniels, R. S. Kirby, L. Leavitt, L. Miller, W. Zaharodny, and L. A. Schieve (2008). Advanced parental age and the risk of autism spectrum disorder. *Am. J. Epidemiol.* 168:1268–1276.

Fombonne, E., P. Bolton, J. Prior, H. Jordan, and M. Rutter (1997). A family study of autism: Cognitive patterns and levels in parents and siblings. *J. Child Psychol. Psychiat.* 38:667–683.

Gillberg, C. and M. Coleman (2000). *The Biology of the Autistic Syndromes.* London: Mac Keith Press.

Good, C. D., K. Lawrence, N. S. Thomas, C. J. Price, J. Ashburner, K. J. Friston, R. S. J. Frackowiak, L. Oreland, and D. H. Skuse (2003). Dosage-sensitive X-linked locus influences the development of amygdala and orbitofrontal cortex, and fear recognition in humans. *Brain* 126:1–6.

Happe, F. and A. Ronald (2008). The "Fractionable Autism Triad": A review of evidence from behavioural, genetic, cognitive and neural research. *Neuropsychol. Rev.* 18:287–304.

Holden, J. J. A., X. Liu, M. Floyd, E. C. Jenkins, W. T. Brown, S. Lewis, A. E. Chudley, ASD-CARC, M. Gonzalez, T. Rovito-Gomez, and I. L. Cohen (2006). Effects of maternal and child MAOA and serotonin transporter polymorphisms on the behavior patterns of children on the autism spectrum. Poster presented at the International Meeting for Autism Research, Montreal.

Hollander, E., A. Phillips, W. Chaplin, K. Zagursky, S. Novotny, S. Wasserman, and R. Iyengar (2005). A placebo controlled crossover trial of liquid fluoxetine on repetitive behaviors in childhood and adolescent autism. *Neuropsychopharmacology* 30:582–589.

Jones, M. B., R. M. Palmour, L. Zwaigenbaum, and P. Szatmari (2004). Modifier effects in autism at the MAO-A and DBH loci. *Am. J. Med. Genet. B Neuropsychiatr. Genet.* 126B:58–65.

Karmel, B. Z., J. M. Gardner, L. D. Swensen, I. L. Cohen, E. London, E. M. Lennon, and M. J. Flory (2008). Early medical and behavioral characteristics of NICU infants later diagnosed or suspected with autism spectrum disorder. Paper presented at the Pediatric Academic Societies and Asian Society for Pediatric Research, Honolulu, May 3–6.

Kinney, D. K., A. M. Miller, D. J. Crowley, E. Huang, and E. Gerber (2008). Autism prevalence following prenatal exposure to hurricanes and tropical storms in Louisiana. *J. Autism Dev. Disord.* 38:481–488.

Kolevzon, A., R. Gross, and A. Reichenberg (2007). Prenatal and perinatal risk factors for autism: A review and integration of findings. *Arch. Pediatr. Adolesc. Med.* 161:326–333.

Kuperman, S., J. Beeghly, T. Burns, and L. Tsai (1987). Association of serotonin concentration to behavior and IQ in autistic children. *J. Autism Dev. Disord.* 17:133–140.

Limperopoulos, C., H. Bassan, N. R. Sullivan, J. S. Soul, R. L. Robertson Jr., M. Moore, S. A. Ringer, J. J. Volpe, and A. J. du Plessis (2008). Positive screening for autism in ex-preterm infants: Prevalence and risk factors. *Pediatrics* 121:758–765.

Lord, C., M. Rutter, and A. Le Couteur (1994). Autism Diagnostic Interview-Revised: A revised version of a diagnostic interview for caregivers of individuals with possible pervasive developmental disorders. *J. Autism Dev. Disord.* 24:659–685.

Lord, C., M. Rutter, P. C. DiLavore, and S. Risi. (1999). *Autism Diagnostic Observation Schedule (ADOS)*. Los Angeles, CA: Western Psychological Services.

Manuck, S. B., J. D. Flory, R. E. Ferrell, J. J. Mann, and M. F. Muldoon (2000). A regulatory polymorphism of the monoamine oxidase-A gene may be associated with variability in aggression, impulsivity, and central nervous system serotonergic responsivity. *Psychiatry Res.* 95:9–23.

Marazziti, D., F. Muratori, A. Cesari, I. Masala, S. Baroni, G. Giannaccini, L. Dell'Osso, A. Cosenza, P. Pfanner, and G. B. Cassano (2000). Increased density of the platelet serotonin transporter in autism. *Pharmacopsychiatry* 33:165–168.

McDougle, C. J., L. Scahill, M. G. Aman, J. T. McCracken, E. Tierney, M. Davies, L. E. Arnold, D. J. Posey, A. Martin, J. K. Ghuman, B. Shah, S. Z. Chuang, N. B. Swiezy, N. M. Gonzalez, J. Hollway, K. Koenig, J. J. McGough, L. Ritz, and B. Vitiello (2005). Risperidone for the core symptom domains of autism: Results from the study by the autism network of the research units on pediatric psychopharmacology. *Am. J. Psychiatry* 162:1142–1148.

Meyer, J. H., N. Ginovart, A. Boovariwala, S. Sagrati, D. Hussey, A. Garcia, T. Young, N. Praschak-Rieder, A. A. Wilson, and S. Houle (2006). Elevated monoamine oxidase A levels in the brain: An explanation for the monoamine imbalance of major depression. *Arch. Gen. Psychiatry* 63:1209–1216.

Miles, J. H., T. N. Takahashi, S. Bagby, P. K. Sahota, D. F. Vaslow, C. H. Wang, R. E. Hillman, and J. E. Farmer (2005). Essential versus complex autism: Definition of fundamental prognostic subtypes. *Am. J. Med. Genet.* 135:171–180.

Pinelli, J. and L. Zwaigenbaum (2008). Chorioamnionitis, gestational age, male sex, birth weight, and illness severity predicted positive autism screening scores in very-low-birth-weight preterm infants. *Evid. Based Nurs.* 11:122.

Piven, J. and P. Palmer (1999). Psychiatric disorder and the broad autism phenotype: Evidence from a family study of multiple-incidence autism families. *Am. J. Psychiatry* 156:557–563.

Piven, J., G. A. Chase, R. Landa, M. Wzorek, J. Gayle, D. Cloud, and S. Folstein (1991). Psychiatric disorders in the parents of autistic individuals. *J. Am. Acad. Child Adol. Psychiat.* 30:471–478.

Sabol, S. Z., S. Hu, and D. Hamer (1998). A functional polymorphism in the monoamine oxidase A gene promoter. *Hum. Genet.* 103:273–279.

Schendel, D. E. (2008). Autism and prenatal exposure to storms. *Evid. Based Ment. Health* 11:32.

Schendel, D. and T. K. Bhasin (2008). Birth weight and gestational age characteristics of children with autism, including a comparison with other developmental disabilities. *Pediatrics* 121:1155–1164.

Schopler, E., R. J. Reichler, R. F. Devellis, and K. Daly (1980). Toward objective classification of childhood autism: Childhood Autism Rating Scale (CARS). *J. Autism Dev. Disord.* 10:91–103.

Schulze, T. G., D. J. Muller, H. Krauss, H. Scherk, S. Ohlraun, Y. V. Syagailo, C. Windemuth, H. Neidt, M. Grassle, A. Papassotiropoulos, R. Heun, M. M. Nothen, W. Maier, K. P. Lesch, and M. Rietschel (2000). Association between a functional polymorphism in the monoamine oxidase A gene promoter and major depressive disorder. *Am. J. Med. Genet.* 96:801–803.

Slavotinek, A. and L. G. Biesecker (2003). Genetic modifiers in human development and malformation syndromes, including chaperone proteins. *Hum. Mol. Genet.* 12:R45–R50.

Smalley, S. L., J. McCracken, and P. Tanguay (1995). Autism, affective disorders, and social phobia. *Am. J. Med. Genet.* 60:19–26.

Szatmari, P. and M. B. Jones (1991). IQ and the genetics of autism. *J. Child Psychol. Psychiat.* 32:897–908.

Thompson, N. M., G. A. Rogeness, E. McClure, R. Clayton, and C. Johnson (1996). Influence of depression on cognitive functioning in Fragile X females. *Psychiat. Res.* 64:97–104.

Tsuchiya, K. J., K. Matsumoto, T. Miyachi. M. Tsujii, K. Nakamura, S. Takagai, M. Kawai, A. Yagi, K. Iwaki, S. suda, G. Sugihara, Y. Iwata, H. Matsuzaki, Y. Sekine, K. Suzuki, T. Sugiyama, N. Mori, and N. Takei (2008). Paternal age at birth and high-functioning autistic-spectrum disorder in offspring. *Br. J. Psychiatry* 193:316–321.

Williams, R. B., D. A. Marchuk, K. M. Gadde, J. C. Barefoot, K. Grichnik, M. J. Helms, C. M. Kuhn, J. G. Lewis, S. M. Schanberg, M. Stafford-Smith, E. C. Suarez, G. L. Clary, I. K. Svenson, and I. C. Siegler (2003). A promoter polymorphism in the monoamine oxidase A gene and its relationships to monoamine metabolite concentrations in CSF of healthy volunteers. *Neuropsychopharmacology* 28:533–541.

Williams, K., M. Helmer, G. W. Duncan, J. K. Peat, and C. M. Mellis (2008). Perinatal and maternal risk factors for autism spectrum disorders in New South Wales, Australia. *Child Care Health Dev.* 34:249–256.

Yu, Y. W., S. J. Tsai, C. J. Hong, T. J. Chen, M. C. Chen, and C. W. Wang (2005). Association study of a monoamine oxidase a gene promoter polymorphism with major depressive disorder and antidepressant response. *Neuropsychopharmacology* 30:1719–1723.

Zubenko, G. S., B. Maher, H. B. Hughes III, W. N. Zubenko, J. S. Stiffler, B. B. Kaplan, and M. L. Marazita (2003). Genome-wide linkage survey for genetic loci that influence the development of depressive disorders in families with recurrent, early-onset, major depression. *Am. J. Med. Genet.* 123B:1–18.

6 Paraoxonase 1 Status, Environmental Exposures, and Oxidative Stress in Autism Spectrum Disorders

Maria Dronca[1],* and Sergiu P. Paşca[2]

[1]Department of Medical Biochemistry,
Iuliu Haţieganu University of Medicine
and Pharmacy, Cluj-Napoca, Romania

[2]Center for Cognitive and Neural
Studies, Cluj-Napoca, Romania

CONTENTS

6.1   INTRODUCTION

Autism spectrum disorders (ASDs) are a group of clinically and etiologically heterogeneous disorders, affecting the core domains of communication and social development and involving abnormal repetitive and restrictive behaviors (Rapin and Tuchman, 2008). To date, ASDs are considered to be genetically influenced disorders,

* Corresponding author: Tel.: +40-766-530-042; fax: +40-264-597-257 e-mail: m_dronca@yahoo.com

which are also subject to considerable environmental contributions (Abrahams and Geschwind, 2008; Herbert et al., 2006; Persico and Bourgeron, 2006). It is becoming increasingly recognized that no single explanation can account for all types of autism, and that multiple factors (genetic, epigenetic, and environmental) are involved in shaping the systemic phenotype. Exposures to environmentally toxic agents (e.g., pesticides), disturbances in the redox homeostasis (i.e., decrease in antioxidant defenses plus an increase in reactive oxygen species [ROS] production), as well as perturbed immune balance, have all been proposed, to a certain degree, as contributing factors to the pathophysiology of autism. Within this context, evidence has emerged in recent years to suggest the possible involvement in ASD of Paraoxonase 1 (PON1), an enzyme that travels in blood attached to high-density lipoprotein (HDL), which is involved in the degradation of neurotoxic pesticides, protects against oxidative stress, and is also a negative acute-phase protein. In this chapter, after briefly reviewing the basic structural and functional properties of PON1, we present the current evidence for an impaired PON1 status in ASD, as well as its relation to organophosphates (OP) exposure, oxidative stress, and immune/inflammatory modulation. In the end, we suggest future directions for research that could substantiate the knowledge on PON1's role in neurodevelopmental disorders.

6.2   HUMAN SERUM PARAOXONASE 1

Human paraoxonase 1 (PON1) is a member of a family of esterases/lactonases that also includes PON2 and PON3; the genes encoding for these enzymes are clustered in tandem on the long arm of chromosome 7 (7q21.3–q22.1), and appear to be approximately 27–28 kb long (Clendenning et al., 1996; Harel et al., 2004; Primo-Parmo et al., 1996). Their order was found to be PON1, PON3 and PON2, with PON1 being the most centromeric (Figure 6.1a) (Mochizuki et al., 1998). These genes share approximately 65% similarity at the amino acid level, and approximately 70% similarity at the nucleotide level, suggesting that they have arisen by gene duplication. Phylogenetic analysis demonstrated that PON2 is the oldest member of the family from which PON3 and afterwards PON1 arose (Draganov and La Du, 2004). In humans, PON1 and PON3 are expressed mainly in the liver and are then transferred from the hepatocyte membrane to HDL, while these HDL particle are transiently associated with the scavenger receptor SR-B1 (Deakin et al., 2002; Gaidukov and Tawfik, 2005; Reddy et al., 2001). PON1 can be competitively removed from HDL by phospholipids, thus being able to move between HDL and other phospholipid-rich areas, such as cell membranes and sites of lipid damage (Deakin et al., 2002; Sorenson et al., 1999). PON1 may also stimulate cellular cholesterol efflux, the first step in reverse cholesterol transport. In contrast, PON2 remains in the intracellular milieu, being expressed in a number of tissues, including the liver, kidney, heart, brain, and placenta, but also in the cells of the arterial wall (i.e., endothelial cells, smooth muscle cells, and macrophages) (Ng et al., 2001, 2005; Primo-Parmo et al., 1996).

Of the three PON enzymes, PON1 (paraoxonase activity, EC 3.1.8.1; arylesterase activity, EC 3.1.1.2) is the most studied and best understood, and has been repeatedly associated with cardiovascular diseases (Durrington, Mackness, and Mackness,

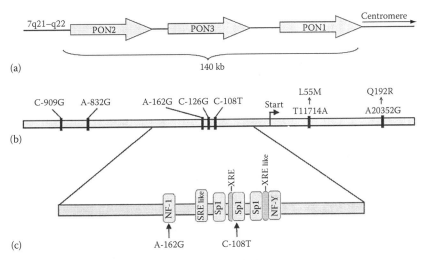

FIGURE 6.1 Structure of paraoxonases' genes. (a) PON gene family and location of PON1, PON2, and PON3 on human chromosome 7, bands q21–q22. (b) The locations of polymorphisms in the promoter and coding region of the PON1 gene; substitutions T11714A and A20352G in the exons 3 and 6 of the coding sequence correspond to L55M and Q192R variation in the protein sequence respectively. (c) The –162 and –108 polymorphisms and potential transcription factor binding sites in the 200 bp region of the promoter. SRE, sterol regulatory element; Sp1, transcription factor; XRE, xenobiotic responsive elements; NF-Y, nuclear factor-Y.

2001; Mackness, Arrol, and Durrington, 1991; Ng et al., 2005; Rozenberg, Shih, and Aviram, 2005). PON1 received its name because of the ability to hydrolyze paraoxon, the microsome-activated form of the insecticide parathion. Besides paraoxon, PON1 has the ability to hydrolyze other OP toxins, arylesters (e.g., phenylacetate), cyclic carbonates, and lactones (Draganov and La Du, 2004). Recent comprehensive structure–activity studies with PON1 and PON1 variants generated through directed evolution have demonstrated that PON1's native activity is that of a lactonase, while arylesterase and phosphotriesterase are promiscuous activities (Khersonsky and Tawfik, 2006).

From a structural perspective, PON1 consists of 354 amino acids residues (355 with N-terminal methionine) and has a molecular weight that can range from 38 to 45 kDa, depending on its glycosylation state (Clendenning et al., 1996; Gan et al., 1991). PON1 is unusual in retaining the N-terminal signal sequence, which provides a hydrophobic anchor for attachment to the HDL particle (Sorenson et al., 1999). Both activity and stability of PON1 are dramatically dependent on the HDL components (phospholipids and/or apolipoproteins) (Cabana et al., 2003; Rochu et al., 2007). At present, the exact structure and catalytic mechanism of the PON1 enzyme are still unknown, although a gene-shuffled bacterially expressed chimerical PON1 variant suggests that human PON1 is a six-bladed β-propeller (each blade consisting of four β-pleated sheets) with a "velcro" closure sealed by a disulfide bond between Cys_{42} and Cys_{353} (see Figure 6.2 for more details).

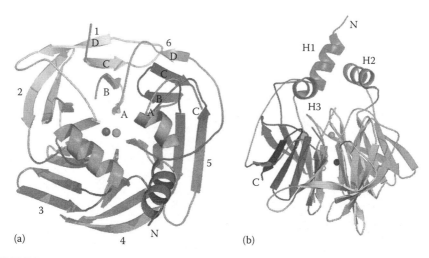

FIGURE 6.2   (See color insert following page 200.) Overall structure of PON1. (a) View of the six-bladed-propeller from above. Shown are the N- and C-termini, and the two calcium atoms in the central tunnel of the propeller (the "catalytic calcium" or Ca1, green (left); the "structural calcium" or Ca2, red (right)). (b) A side view of the propeller. At the top of the propeller, there are three helices H1–H3 which determine the PONs' cell distribution, translocation and secretion (H1), and protein–lipid and protein–protein interactions (H2 and H3). (Reproduced from Harel, M. et al., *Nat. Struct. Mol. Biol.*, 11, 412, 2004. With permission.)

From a functional perspective, PON1 displays several activities:

1. *Phosphotriesterase activity*: PON1 hydrolyzes the oxygen analogs of commonly used organophosphorus insecticides such as paraoxon, chlorpyrifos-oxon, diazinon, as well as nerve agents such as sarin, soman, tabun (Draganov and La Du, 2004).
2. *Arylesterase activity*: PON1 hydrolyzes phenylacetate and other aromatic arylesters, but it could also play a role in drug metabolism (i.e., the release of salicylate, the more active form of aspirin) (Santanam and Parthasarathy, 2007).
3. *Phopholipase A2-like activity*: PON1 has the ability to hydrolyze the platelet-activating factor (Rodrigo et al., 2001), and biologically active oxidized phospholipids (Ahmed et al., 2002).
4. *Peroxidase-like activity*: PON1 is implicated in the decomposition of lipid peroxides and H_2O_2 (Aviram et al., 2000; Ferretti et al., 2004), although there are some controversies in this regard (Kriska et al., 2007).
5. *Lactonase and lactonizing activities*: PON1 can alter the biological activity and/or distribution of endogenous (homocysteine thiolactone, δ-valerolactone derivatives) and exogenous lactones (e.g., antibacterial agents, glucocorticoid γ-lactones) (Draganov and Teiber, 2008; Draganov et al., 2005; Jakubowski, 2000).

At the moment, the physiological role of PON1 in vivo is uncertain. Experimental data support the hypothesis that PON1's antiatherosclerotic activity is due to its implication in HDL-mediated cholesterol efflux from macrophages (Rosenblat et al., 2005), protection of LDL and HDL against oxidation (Aviram et al., 1998; Mackness et al., 1993), and prevention of proteins' modification by homocysteine thiolactone (Jakubowski, 2000).

To a considerable degree, PON1 level and/or catalytic efficiency are determined by genetic variants (polymorphisms) in the coding and regulatory regions (Furlong et al., 2008; Roest et al., 2007). With respect to regulation of PON1 expression, it appears that only about 30% of the variability of PON1 plasma levels can be explained by known single-nucleotide polymorphisms (SNPs). Sequencing of promoter region of the PON1 gene led to the discovery of at least five SNPs with varying degrees of influence over gene expression: −909/907 (C or G), −832/824 (A or G), −162 (A or G), −126 (C or G), and −108/−107 (C or T) (Figure 6.1b). These SNPs are frequent in the population and, at least those at positions −108, −162, and −909, have an impact on promoter's activity of up to twofold difference in gene expression (Brophy et al., 2001). The −108 polymorphism, lying within a consensus binding site for transcription factors Sp1 and Sp3 (Figure 6.1c), has the greatest effect on PON1 levels in serum (23%–24% of the total variation), with −108C providing higher levels of plasma PON1 (Costa et al., 2003; Roest et al., 2007).

In the coding regions of PON1, two missense mutations were observed (T11714A and A20352G), resulting in a Leu(L)/Met(M) and Gln(Q)Arg(R) substitutions at codons 55 and 192, respectively (Humbert et al., 1993) (Figure 6.2b). Gene frequencies of $PON1_{L55M}$ range from 0.57 in Caucasians populations to 0.99 in Oji-Cree population, while the gene frequencies of $PON1_{Q192R}$ range from 0.75 in Caucasians of Northern European origin to 0.3 for some Asian populations (Brophy, Jarvik, and Furlong, 2002). The L55M substitution has not been found to affect catalytic efficiency (Adkins et al., 1993; Davies et al., 1996; Humbert et al., 1993), but the $PON1_{M55}$ alloenzyme has been associated with a lower plasma concentration (Mackness et al., 1998). In addition, due to the location in the N-terminal side of PON1, the L55M polymorphism influences the binding of PON1 to HDL (Humbert et al., 1993). Deakin et al. (2003) suggested that C-108T is the major genetic determinant of PON1 bioavailability while the effect of the L55M genotype on PON1 concentration may be the reflection of linkage between two loci. For a "nonpolymorphic" substrate such as phenylacetate, the amount of the enzyme is important, but for a "polymorphic" substrate such as paraoxon, both alleles present and the amount of protein are important. On the other hand, the Q192R polymorphism is responsible for a striking substrate specific difference in the hydrolytic activity of the enzyme (Davies et al., 1996; Humbert et al., 1993). The Gln/Arg polymorphism leads to two allozymes that clearly differ in paraoxon-hydrolyzing ability: the Arg allozyme has a relatively higher activity and shows a greater degree of stimulation by NaCl than does the Gln allozyme (Humbert et al., 1993). Further studies suggested that the effects of this polymorphism may be substrate-dependent, as the PON_{Q192} isoform hydrolyzes diazoxon, sarin and soman more rapidly than $PON1_{R192}$ with in vitro assays (Davies et al., 1996). It is noteworthy to mention that Q192R and L55M alleles are in strong linkage disequilibrium, which favors the simultaneous presence of those alleles associated with "high paraoxonase activity" (Garin et al., 1997).

In a given population, plasma PON1 activity can vary up to 40-fold (Davies et al., 1996; Richter and Furlong, 1999), and PON1 protein levels, within a given genotype class, can vary up to 13-fold (Jarvik et al., 2000). Although genetic determinants play an important role in determining the individual PON1 status, the contribution of other factors in modulating PON1 activity may also be important. Age, gender, ethnicity, diet (polyphenols, vitamin C and E, unsaturated fats), environmental chemicals (OP exposure, heavy metals), drugs (statins, fibrates), as well as certain disease conditions (e.g., liver disease, diabetes, inflammatory states), have been found to influence PON1 activity (Costa et al., 2005; Deakin and James, 2004; Rainwater et al., 2009).

6.3 PON1 IN AUTISM SPECTRUM DISORDERS

A relation between ASD and PON1 was first investigated by Serajee et al. (2004). These authors studied possible association between polymorphisms in xenobiotic metabolism genes (MTF1, ABCC1, SLC11A3, SLC11A2, PON1, and GSTP1) and autism. By genotyping the T/A polymorphism in exon 3 in the PON1 gene (L55M), they found that the marker showed deviation from Hardy–Weinberg equilibrium, while the transmission disequilibrium test did not demonstrate any association with autism in the 196 trios taken from the AGRE database ($p = 0.12$).

In 2005, D'Amelio et al. (2005) conducted a more extensive study by investigating three functional SNPs (C-108T, L55M, and Q192R) in the PON1 gene in 312 autistic patients and 676 first-degree relatives, belonging to 177 Italian families and 107 Caucasian-American families. Interestingly, they found that North American but not Italian families displayed a significant association between autism and a less active PON1 isoform on diazinon (L55/R192); patients also exhibited a nonsignificant trend toward increased allele frequencies and transmission rates of the −108T allele. Following these results, our group reported in a small cohort from Romania that the arylesterase activity of PON1 is reduced in children with ASD as compared to healthy control subjects, whereas PON1 paraoxonase activity was found to be similar (Paşca et al., 2006). The fact that the salt-stimulated paraoxonase activity was not found to be impaired in autistics could be explained by the higher variability in this catalytic activity or the modest sample of subjects in our study. More recently, we evaluated in 50 children with ASD and 30 age- and sex-matched controls from Romania whether the measurement of arylesterase and NaCl-stimulated paraoxonase enzymatic activities of PON1, together with the assessment of $PON1_{Q192R}$ and $PON1_{L55M}$ polymorphisms might yield more information than either genotype or activity alone in a cohort of patients with ASD (Paşca et al., 2009b). We found that both PON1 arylesterase (i.e., bioavailability) and PON1 paraoxonase (i.e., catalytic) activities were decreased in autistic patients ($p < 0.001$, $p < 0.05$, respectively), but no association with less active variants of the PON1 gene was found. Given that in a recent study investigating one-carbon metabolism, we found preliminary evidence for metabolic and genetic differences between clinical subtypes of ASD (Paşca et al., 2009a), we also checked for potential differences in the PON1 status between typical autism, pervasive developmental disorder—not otherwise specified (PDD-NOS), and Asperger syndrome, but we failed to locate any statistical dissimilarities (unpublished observations). The reduction in PON1 activities (arylesterase and diazoxonase) in children with autism has also been confirmed recently in a bigger sample size comprising children from Europe and North America (A.M. Persico et al., unpublished results).

Most studies investigating the association of PON1 with various diseases have examined only three SNPs: C-108T, L55M, Q192R. However, even if an individual was genotyped for all known PON1 polymorphisms, this analysis would not provide the level of plasma PON1 activity or the phase of polymorphisms (which polymorphisms are on each of an individual's two chromosomes). A functional genomic analysis provides a much more informative approach. This is accomplished through the use of a high-throughput enzyme assay involving two substrates: paraoxon and phenyl acetate (Eckerson et al., 1983), diazoxon and paraoxon (Richter and Furlong, 1999), and more recently the non-OP substrates: phenyl acetate and 4-(chloromethyl)-phenyl acetate (Richter et al., 2009). The two-dimensional enzyme analysis, referred to as the determination of "PON1 status," is much more useful and informative than PCR-based genotypes alone for epidemiological studies examining the role of PON1 in OP or lipid metabolism. Plotting rates of hydrolysis of one substrate against a second substrate provided a clear resolution of the individuals with low activities (phenotype AA) from individuals with intermediate and high activities (phenotype AB and BB, respectively). We examined the PON1 phenotype (using arylesterase and salt-stimulated paraoxonase activities) and found a similar distribution in the ASD group and the control group (Paşca et al., 2009b). The similar phenotypic distribution and the fact that there was no difference in the activities' ratio between groups suggest that the relationship between the two activities is generally maintained in autistics, regardless of a reduction in the hydrolytic protection. On the other hand, while in the ASD group, the PON1 catalytic activity/Q192R dependency was more pronounced than in controls, the dependency of the bioavailability of PON1 on the L55M polymorphism was absent in the ASD patients, whereas it reached a borderline small level in healthy participants. Interestingly, in children with ASD and first-degree relatives, the $PON1_{R192}$ allele has been previously associated with a reduction in PON1 arylesterase activity (Gaita and Persico, 2006). In a recent report, we also showed, although in a small sample, that the distribution of the PON1 C-108T genotypes was analogous in autistics and healthy controls (Kaucsár et al., 2009). Nevertheless, we observed in this study that the PON1 promoter polymorphism had a lower influence on the arylesterase activity's variance in autistic patients than controls, while the paraoxonase activity was not affected.

The intracellular status of PON2 still waits to be investigated in ASD, although there is circumstantial evidence for a disturbed gene expression in hypothalamic neurons in a rodent model for Rett syndrome (fold change in MeCP2-Tg versus WT was 0.327, $p = 0.0089$) (Chahrour et al., 2008). Although it is expected to find perturbations in PON2 in cells from autistic patients considering the previously reported alterations in intracellular redox status, the exact contribution of PON2 is worth exploring in future studies.

It is also worth mentioning that PON1 has a potentially imprinted expression in mouse placenta (Okita et al., 2003). If confirmed in humans, the imprinted status of PONs' genes could have implications for the imprinting hypothesis for the development of autism (Badcock and Crespi, 2006).

6.4   ENVIRONMENTAL EXPOSURES

In recent years, great concern has been raised about the negative impact of chronic OP (and other pesticides) exposure on the normal development of the nervous system (for a more comprehensive resource, see Eskenazi et al., 2008; Rosas and Eskenazi, 2008). Both animal studies and clinical reports of OP exposure in children have confirmed the deleterious effects of these agents on neurological functioning. Pesticides cross both the blood–brain barrier and placenta, and the fetus is generally more susceptible to neurotoxic agents intervening during development. As a matter of fact, significant decreases in birth weight and head circumference have been reported after OP exposure (Berkowitz et al., 2004; Whyatt et al., 2004). The CHAMACOS and Mt. Sinai studies revealed a dose-related number of impaired neonatal reflexes with higher in utero exposure to OP (Engel et al., 2007; Young et al., 2005). Noteworthy is that when an abnormal maternal PON1 status (i.e., lower first and second tertile) was taken into account, a higher risk for abnormal reflexes was detected (Engel et al., 2007). On the other hand, a study from Ecuador found only a decrease in the Stanford-Binet copying test with higher prenatal pesticide exposure in their cohort of older children (Grandjean et al., 2006).

Developmental disorders, including atypical autism, have been described among farming families who normally use OP (Worth, 2002). Currently, there are two studies reporting a statistical association between OP exposure during pregnancy and the risk for developing ASD. In a longitudinal birth cohort study in New York City, Rauh et al. (2006) reported that children exposed to higher levels of chlorpyrifos (i.e., levels of >6.17 pg/g cord plasma) were more likely to display mental and psychomotor developmental delays, attention problems, attention-deficit/hyperactivity disorder, and pervasive developmental disorder (PDD) at 36 months of age. Eskenazi et al. (2007) investigated the relationship between prenatal and postnatal biomarkers of OP exposure (as measured by six nonspecific dialkylphosphate [DAP] metabolites) and children's neurodevelopment in the CHAMACOS birth cohort living in an agricultural community in California. Children with higher prenatal and postnatal total DAPs were at significantly higher risk of being diagnosed with a PDD, displaying approximately twofold increase in the risk for each 10-fold increase in metabolites (prenatal DAPs: $OR = 2.3$; $CI_{95\%} = [1.0–5.2]$, $p = 0.05$; 24 month DAPs: $OR = 1.7$; $CI_{95\%} = [1.0–2.9]$, $p = 0.04$). Not only OP, but also other pesticides widely dispersed in human environment have been associated with a risk for neurological impairment or autism. For example, an association between residential proximity to organochlorine pesticide applications during gestation and ASD among children was reported ($OR = 6.1$, $CI_{95\%} = [2.4–15.3]$) (Roberts et al., 2007). In addition, noncoplanar polychlorinated biphenyls (PCBs) cause abnormal development of the auditory cortex in rats, including a perturbed balance of neuronal inhibition to excitation (Kenet et al., 2007), while use of household pesticides from pet shampoos (containing pyrethrins) were associated with an increased risk for autism (adjusted $OR = 2.0$, $CI_{95\%} = [1.2–3.6]$; strongest effect during the second trimester) (Hertz-Picciotto et al., 2008).

Chronic, occupational exposure to OP toxins has been shown to reduce PON1 activity (Costa et al., 2005), while temporary inhibition of PON1 activity has been reported after acute poisoning with OP pesticides (Sozmen et al., 2002). In smaller children, this effect could be enhanced due to a physiologically precarious PON1 status. Studies in humans have shown that serum PON1 activity in newborns is fourfold lower than the mothers' PON1 levels, and it increases over time to reach a plateau between 15 and 25 months of age (Cole et al., 2003; Furlong et al., 2005). Moreover, there is an increased influence of genetic variation on PON1 activity in neonates (Chen et al., 2003), while low PON1 activity was also reported to be associated with smaller neonatal head circumference (Berkowitz et al., 2004). Interestingly, birth outcomes (e.g., birth length, head circumference) have been connected with PON1 status in mothers (Wolff et al., 2007). In premature babies (33–36 weeks of gestation), PON1 activity measured using phenyl acetate as a substrate is 24% lower compared to full-term babies (Ecobichon and Stephens, 1973).

Therefore, the highly reactive intermediates of pesticides might account for the decreased paraoxonase activity of PON1 in ASD, as these compounds can inactivate the enzyme (Hernandez et al., 2004). An upregulation of PON1 following chronic OP exposure was described only in carriers of the $PON1_{192R}$ allele (Browne et al., 2006), but this allele has been associated with a reduction in PON1 arylesterase activity in children with ASD and first-degree relatives (Gaita and Persico, 2006). In addition, it was also reported that carriers of the $PON1_{192R}$ allele, as compared to individuals with the QQ genotype, exhibited lower acetylcholinesterase activity (Hernandez et al., 2004). Notably, neonatal exposure to parathion in rats (at doses straddling the threshold for cholinesterases inhibition) compromises the indices of acetylcholine synaptic function in adolescence and adulthood (Slotkin, Levin, and Seidler, 2009). Therefore, an altered PON1 status could also be related, at least conceptually for now, with the previously described alterations in the cholinergic system in autism (Perry et al., 2001). Differences in the regional expression (e.g., parietal cortex, cerebellum, and thalamus) of nicotinic acetylcholine receptors' subunits have been documented in postmortem brains from autistics and these results are suggestive of a potential enhanced susceptibility to OP exposure (Court et al., 2000; Lee et al., 2002). Consequently, an impaired catalytic efficacy of PON1 to degrade OP during an environmental exposure could have far more deleterious consequences in children displaying subtle alterations in the central cholinergic transmission (Pessah et al., 2008). This gene (PON1, AchR subunits) × environment (OP exposure, inhibitors of PON1 activity) interaction should be further explored in future prospective studies in relation to the autism risk.

The data indicating OP exposure as a risk factor for ASD (Eskenazi et al., 2007; Rauh et al., 2006) and the fact that overall these patients display lower PON1 activities (Paşca et al., 2006; Paşca et al., 2009b) are congruent with another recently proposed gene×environment interaction model, which includes PON1, a history of OP exposure, and a genetic or epigenetic based impairment in Reelin (Persico and Bourgeron, 2006) (Figure 6.3). Reelin is an extracellular serine protease that plays a pivotal role in the central nervous system by regulating the processes of neuronal migration and positioning in the developing brain and by modulating synaptic plasticity in the adult cerebral cortex. Reelin, secreted by Cajal–Retzius cells in the cortex and external granular layer and cerebellar nuclear neurons in the cerebellum, is crucial for the configuration of the mature cortical architecture, and exerts its functions by binding to a variety of receptors (Vldlr, ApoER2, a3b1 integrins) and

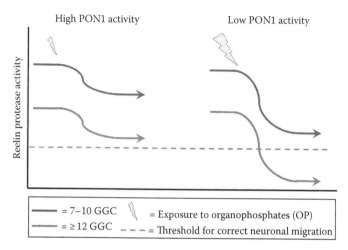

FIGURE 6.3   (See color insert following page 200.) The gene × environment model for autism. The model involves the Reelin (RELN) and Paraoxonase 1 (PON1) genes, and prenatal exposure to organophosphates (OP). RELN variants carrying either "normal" (7–10 repeats) or "long" (≥12 repeats) GGC alleles genetically determine whether levels of reelin are normal or reduced, respectively. In principle, both conditions are compatible with normal neurodevelopment. However, prenatal exposure to OP can transiently inhibit the proteolytic activity of reelin, which might then fall below the threshold required for correct neuronal migration, also depending on baseline levels of RELN gene expression determined genetically and epigenetically. In addition, exposure to identical doses of OP can affect reelin to a different extent depending on the amount and affinity spectrum of the OP- inactivating enzyme paraoxonase produced by the PON1 alleles of each individual. (Reproduced from Persico, A.M. and Bourgeron, T., *Trends Neurosci.*, 29, 349, 2006. With permission.)

by means of a proteolytic activity on extracellular proteins (Huang and D'Arcangelo, 2008). Several lines of evidence suggested that Reelin is associated to autism (Lintas and Persico, 2008). Case–control and family-based studies pointed out that longer triplet repeats (≥11 GGC) in the in 5′ untranslated region of the RELN gene confer vulnerability to autistic disorder (Persico et al., 2001), while in vivo and in vitro experiments suggested that the "long" RELN allele significantly reduces the expression of the gene. Moreover, postmortem studies have confirmed reductions in Reelin protein and mRNA in brains from ASD patients (Fatemi et al., 2005). Although a malfunctioning RELN gene variant may contribute to the pathogenesis of ASD, it is credible to say that the "long" allele is not sufficient to cause autism (Lintas and Persico, 2008). Following these observations, Persico and Bourgeron (2006) proposed that an autistic phenotype could arise in genetically or epigenetically vulnerable individuals producing lower amounts of RELN (i.e., carriers of the "long" allele) that are exposed to OP during critical pre/postnatal neurodevelopmental periods and in which neuronal migration, corticogenesis, and synaptogenesis would be affected to a different extent depending on the enzymatic efficacy of PON1. An interaction between prenatal chlorpyrifos exposure and *reeler* mutation has been uncovered, although these interactions were more complex than expected (Laviola et al., 2006). While the model was initially conceived as a gene × gene × environment interaction (i.e., less active PON1 variants × "long" allele of RELN × pre/postnatal OP exposure), results from our studies indicated that PON1 activities may be impaired in ASD patients in the absence of an association with less active PON1 gene variants (i.e., Q192R, L55M, C-108T) (Kaucsár et al., 2009; Paşca et al., 2009b). Future studies should better delineate the effects of RELN dosage in the context of a pesticides exposure and reduced PON1-mediated degradation of toxic agents.

Besides OP, exposure to several other environmental chemicals can have a substantial impact on serum PON1 activity, and could therefore, be relevant to autism. For instance, heavy metals cations (cadmium, iron, zinc, and mercury) have been shown to be, at least in vitro, potent inhibitors of $PON1_{R192}$ activity, while $PON1_{Q192}$ appear to be less sensitive to metal inhibition, excepting lead (Cole et al., 2002).

6.5   OXIDATIVE STRESS

The brain is highly vulnerable to oxidative stress, particularly during the early part of development, due to its naturally low levels of antioxidants, higher energy requirement, and higher content of fat and iron (Juurlink and Paterson, 1998). Due to a deficient glutathione-producing capacity, neurons are the first cells to be affected by an increase in ROS and/or a shortage in antioxidants (Perry et al., 2004). Especially in genetically susceptible individuals (e.g., carrying polymorphic oxidative genes), free radicals resulting from ingested or inhaled environmental toxins, food or food additives, inflammation or infection, may seriously disrupt neurodevelopmental milestones and lead to neuropsychiatric impairments.

Currently, it is generally recognized that autism is associated with a perturbed redox homeostasis (Chauhan and Chauhan, 2006). Increased oxidative stress in autism may be due to environmental pro-oxidants exposure, intensive production of endogenous pro-oxidants (i.e., nitric oxide [NO], xanthine oxidase, homocysteine), and/or decreased level/activity of antioxidants (i.e., ceruloplasmin, transferrin, superoxide dismutase [SOD]), glutathione peroxidase (GPx), catalase (CAT), PON1, and reduced glutathione (GSH). In fact, reduced levels of GPx (Yorbik et al., 2002), CAT (Zoroglu et al., 2004), and GSH (GPx cosubstrate) (James et al., 2004, 2006; Paşca et al., 2009a) are found in erythrocytes/whole blood of autistic individuals compared with controls. On the contrary, higher erythrocyte's SOD was observed in autism by Zoroglu et al. (2004). Oxidative stress in ASD is associated with increased plasma levels of malonyldialdehyde, a lipid peroxidation biomarker (Chauhan et al., 2004). Recently, carboxyethyl pyrrole and iso[4]levuglandin–protein adducts, markers of oxidative damage resulting from lipid peroxidation, were detected in postmortem brain tissue from autistic subjects (Evans et al., 2008).

ASDs have also been associated with one-carbon metabolism perturbations, as reported in studies investigating plasma metabolites (Adams et al., 2007; Geier and Geier, 2006; Geier et al., 2009; James et al., 2004, 2006; Paşca et al., 2006, 2009a) or immune cells (Suh et al., 2008). For instance, our group recently reported differences in the severity of the metabolite profiles across the spectrum of autistic disorders, with typical autistic patients exhibiting disturbances in both the methionine cycle and the transsulfuration pathway concomitant with a slightly more prevalent T allele frequency for the MTHFR C677T polymorphism, while patients with the less severe form of the disease (i.e., PDD-NOS) presented only with disturbances in the methionine cycle; in addition, since the levels of both folate and vitamin B_{12} were within the normal range, we excluded vitamin deficiencies as a cause for these impairments (Paşca et al., 2009a). A disturbed one-carbon metabolism, although (apparently) nonspecific to autism, could lead to a diminished capacity for methylation, with consequences on gene expression, neurotransmitter synthesis, and, potentially, on neuronal synchronization. It remains to be further investigated how much the metabolic profiles in plasma echo the actual intracellular metabolic dynamics, and whether corrections of these impairments will lead to genuine clinical improvements.

PON1 was found to efficiently hydrolyze not only lipoprotein-associated peroxides (including cholesteryl linoleate hydroperoxides), but also hydrogen peroxide (H_2O_2), and may thus play an important role in eliminating potent oxidants involved in atherogenesis (Aviram et al., 1998). Conversely, PON1 also serves as a target for lipid peroxidation products, resulting in an inhibition of PON1 activities (arylesterase and lactonase) and a reduction in PON1 gene expression (Aviram et al., 1999; Van Lenten et al., 2001). PON1 induces the lysophosphatidylcholine (LPC) formation, which might act in both direction as pro-oxidant (based on the upregulated effects on adhesive molecules) and antioxidant (by increasing the expression of extracellular SOD in monocyte-macrophages) (Rosenblat, Oren, and Aviram, 2006). Moreover, PON1 can be inactivated by S-glutathionylation, resulting from a reaction between its free sulfhydryl group at Cys_{284} and oxidized glutathione (GSSG) (Rozenberg and Aviram, 2006). Considering these facts, one may assume that in ASD, an altered PON1 could contribute to the perturbed redox homeostasis, while an enhanced oxidative stress could easily disturb the PON1 status.

6.6   INFLAMMATION

Experimental and clinical evidence accumulated in the last decades have led to the idea that, at least in a subgroup of patients with autism, immune imbalance or even autoimmune processes may play a considerable role in the pathophysiology of the autistic disorder (Ashwood, Wills, and Van de Water, 2006; Pardo, Vargas, and Zimmerman, 2005). Previous studies have already reported a wide plethora of immune abnormalities, including T-cell, B-cell, and NK-cell dysfunction; autoantibody production; and increased proinflammatory cytokines.

Studies published more than a decade ago indicated that HDL protects against bacterial lipopolysaccharide (LPS), the endotoxin found in the outer membrane of Gram-negative bacteria (Levine et al., 1993). Animal experiments have later showed that purified PON1 (type Q) is able to protect cells from LPS and prevent or greatly reduce the release of cytokines (La Du et al., 1999), suggesting a potential role for PON1 in modulating immune responses. Interestingly, Jyonouchi and coworkers showed that peripheral blood mononuclear cells (PBMCs) from ASD patients exposed to LPS produced excessive amounts of tumor necrosis factor-α (TNF-α), interleukin 1 (IL-1), and/or interleukin 6 (IL-6) compared to controls, indicative of an aberrant innate immune response in a considerable percentage of children with ASD (Jyonouchi, Sun, and Le, 2001). Moreover, Sweeten, Posey, and McDougle, (2003) showed that the mean absolute monocyte count was significantly higher in the autistic children, which was accompanied by increased levels of neopterin; these findings were interpreted as heightened cell-mediated immunity in ASD. In the context of the maternal immune activation (MIA) model for developmental disorders, it is worth mentioning that maternal injections of LPS in rodents result in increased anxiety, deficits in social interaction in the adult offspring; this suggests that short systemic maternal inflammation has long-lasting consequences on the adult mouse stress and social behavior (Hava et al., 2006). On the other hand, the cytokine IL-6 was already identified as a key intermediary contributing to MIA in rodents (Smith et al., 2007). Vargas et al. (2005) demonstrated in postmortem autistic brain, excessive significantly higher level of subsets of cytokines (IL-6, IL-10, MCP-3, etc.) in brain regions that have been previously associated with autism (i.e., anterior cingulated gyrus). In a small sample of patients with autism displaying regressive features, Chez et al. (2007) reported elevated levels of TNF-α in cerebrospinal fluid. These and other studies suggest that at least some autistic children display a subclinical inflammatory state.

During inflammation, particularly during the acute-phase response, there is a reduction in several proteins important in reverse cholesterol transport and inhibiting oxidation. These include cholesterol ester transfer protein, lecithin cholesterol acyltransferase, hepatic lipase, apoA-I, and PON1. It is thought that reduction in these proteins, accompanied by an increase in proteins such as apoJ and serum amyloid A (SAA), changes HDL from an anti-inflammatory to a proinflammatory particle (Van Lenten et al., 2006). Several studies provide evidence that hepatic PON1 mRNA is downregulated in response to inflammatory cytokines (Deakin and James, 2008). Treatment with LPS and oxidized LDL, known to induce an immune response, reduced PON1 mRNA in human hepatocyte cells line (Feingold et al., 1998). A similar effect was observed with administration of TNF-α, IL-1, and IL-6 (Feingold et al., 1998; Kumon et al., 2002). Therefore, HDL loses its anti-inflammatory properties during acute infection, and PON1 activity and concentration are regulated by inflammatory cytokines and endotoxin administration. In this context, it could be concluded that PON1 is a negative acute-phase protein whose mRNA is rapidly downregulated (Feingold et al., 1998). In an ongoing study, we did not identify any statistical correlation between arylesterase or paraoxonase activities of PON1 and plasma C-reactive protein (CRP) levels in a population of children with typical autism (unpublished observation).

NO is a unique biological messenger molecule involved in neurodevelopment, but also a versatile player in the immune system. Recent studies have shown that NO may also play a role in the pathophysiology of autism. Apparently, autistic children display increased NO levels in red blood cells (Sogut et al., 2003) and increased levels of plasma NO metabolites (Sweeten et al., 2004; Zoroglu et al., 2003). A recent article reported a nitrite-mediated inactivation of PON1, in a dose- and time-dependent manner; this inactivation is probably generated through nitration of enzyme phenyl residues, while tryptophan could be of important value in minimizing this effect (Abd-Allah and Mariee, 2008). Future research should elucidate in more details the role of PON1 in modulation of immune responses and, consequently, how is the altered PON1 status in autism contributing to the aberrant inflammatory responses in autism.

6.7 CONCLUSIONS

The biochemical and genetics studies indicate that the PON1 status is impaired in children with ASD. The current evidence points toward differences in the frequency of PON1 gene variants in autistic patients between North America and Europe. Currently, the reasons behind the PON1 status alteration in autism are not known, nor are all its consequences. Besides the SNPs investigated (i.e., C192R, L55M, C-108T) to date, other SNPs in the PON1 gene or at distant loci could be associated with ASD. Chronic OP exposure, increased and prolonged oxidative stress, an altered hepatic status, environmental heavy metals, or a silent subclinical inflammatory state are all factors that could contribute to lessening the PON1 bioavailability and/ or catalytic activity. Whatever are the causes, an altered PON1 status would increase the susceptibility to neurotoxic pesticides (especially in Reelin-deficient subjects during critical periods) and lead to deficiencies in corticogenesis and cholinergic neurotransmission, as well as contribute to the perturbation in the redox homeostasis and immune dysfunctions; and all these despite the relative nonspecificity of the PON1 alterations in autism.

We suggest that future studies should be performed on bigger, prospective cohorts of ASD patients, and that they should address the following issues: (a) investigate for a possible relationship between PON1 and the severity of the clinical phenotype; (b) elucidate the effect of HDL, inflammation, and oxidative biomarkers on PON1 in autism; (c) replicate and verify for causality the association between OP exposure and autism; (d) measure the putative physiological activity of PON1, i.e., lactonase activity; and (e) investigate the effect of other SNPs or distant genetic loci.

ACKNOWLEDGMENTS

The authors would like to thank Drs. Anca M. Paşca, Raul C. Muresan, and Carmen Gherasim for fruitful discussions and pertinent comments on previous versions of this manuscript.

REFERENCES

Abd-Allah, G. M. and A. D. Mariee (2008). Nitrite-mediated inactivation of human plasma paraoxonase-1: Possible beneficial effect of aromatic amino acids. *Appl. Biochem. Biotechnol.* 150:281–288.

Abrahams, B. S. and D. H. Geschwind (2008). Advances in autism genetics: On the threshold of a new neurobiology. *Nat. Rev. Genet.* 9:341–355.

Adams, M., M. Lucock, J. Stuart, S. Fardell, K. Baker, and X. Ng (2007). Preliminary evidence for involvement of the folate gene polymorphism 19 bp deletion-DHFR in occurrence of autism. *Neurosci. Lett.* 422:24–29.

Adkins, S., K. N. Gan, M. Mody, and B. N. La Du (1993). Molecular basis for the polymorphic forms of human serum paraoxonase/arylesterase: glutamine or arginine at position 191, for the respective A or B allozymes. *Am. J. Hum. Genet.* 52:598–608.

Ahmed, Z., A. Ravandi, G. F. Maguire, A. Emili, D. Draganov, B. N. La Du, A. Kuksis, and P. W. Connelly (2002). Multiple substrates for paraoxonase-1 during oxidation of phosphatidylcholine by peroxynitrite. *Biochem. Biophys. Res. Commun.* 290:391–396.

Ashwood, P., S. Wills, and J. Van de Water (2006). The immune response in autism: A new frontier for autism research. *J. Leukoc. Biol.* 80:1–15.

Aviram, M., E. Hardak, J. Vaya, S. Mahmood, S. Milo, A. Hoffman, S. Billicke, D. Draganov, and M. Rosenblat (2000). Human serum paraoxonases (PON1) Q and R selectively decrease lipid peroxides in human coronary and carotid atherosclerotic lesions: PON1 esterase and peroxidase-like activities. *Circulation* 101:2510–2517.

Aviram, M., M. Rosenblat, S. Billecke, J. Erogul, R. Sorenson, C. L. Bisgaier, R. S. Newton, and B. La Du (1999). Human serum paraoxonase (PON 1) is inactivated by oxidized low density lipoprotein and preserved by antioxidants. *Free Radic. Biol. Med.* 26:892–904.

Aviram, M., M. Rosenblat, C. L. Bisgaier, R. S. Newton, S. L. Primo-Parmo, and B. N. La Du (1998). Paraoxonase inhibits high-density lipoprotein oxidation and preserves its functions. A possible peroxidative role for paraoxonase. *J. Clin. Invest.* 101:1581–1590.

Badcock, C. and B. Crespi (2006). Imbalanced genomic imprinting in brain development: An evolutionary basis for the aetiology of autism. *J. Evol. Biol.* 19:1007–1032.

Berkowitz, G. S., J. G. Wetmur, E. Birman-Deych, J. Obel, R. H. Lapinski, J. H. Godbold, I. R. Holzman, and M. S. Wolff (2004). In utero pesticide exposure, maternal paraoxonase activity, and head circumference. *Environ. Health Perspect.* 112:388–391.

Brophy, V. H., M. D. Hastings, J. B. Clendenning, R. J. Richter, G. P. Jarvik, and C. E. Furlong (2001). Polymorphisms in the human paraoxonase (PON1) promoter. *Pharmacogenetics* 11:77–84.

Brophy, V. H., G. P. Jarvik, and C. E. Furlong (2002). PON1 polymorphisms. In L. Costa and C. Furlong (eds.), *Paraoxonase (PON1) in Health and Disease: Basic and Clinical Aspects*. Boston, MA: Kluwer Academic Press.

Browne, R. O., L. B. Moyal-Segal, D. Zumsteg, Y. David, O. Kofman, A. Berger, H. Soreq, and A. Friedman (2006). Coding region paraoxonase polymorphisms dictate accentuated neuronal reactions in chronic, sub-threshold pesticide exposure. *FASEB J.* 20:1733–1735.

Cabana, V. G., C. A. Reardon, N. Feng, S. Neath, J. Lukens, and G. S. Getz (2003). Serum paraoxonase: Effect of the apolipoprotein composition of HDL and the acute phase response. *J. Lipid Res.* 44:780–792.

Chahrour, M., S. Y. Jung, C. Shaw, X. Zhou, S. T. Wong, J. Qin, and H. Y. Zoghbi (2008). MeCP2, a key contributor to neurological disease, activates and represses transcription. *Science* 320:1224–1229.

Chauhan, A. and V. Chauhan (2006). Oxidative stress in autism. *Pathophysiology* 13:171–181.

Chauhan, A., V. Chauhan, W. T. Brown, and I. Cohen (2004). Oxidative stress in autism: Increased lipid peroxidation and reduced serum levels of ceruloplasmin and transferrin—the antioxidant proteins. *Life Sci.* 75:2539–2549.

Chen, J., M. Kumar, W. Chan, G. Berkowitz, and J. G. Wetmur (2003). Increased influence of genetic variation on PON1 activity in neonates. *Environ. Health Perspect.* 111:1403–1409.

Chez, M. G., T. Dowling, P. B. Patel, P. Khanna, and M. Kominsky (2007). Elevation of tumor necrosis factor-alpha in cerebrospinal fluid of autistic children. *Pediatr. Neurol.* 36:361–365.

Clendenning, J. B., R. Humbert, E. D. Green, C. Wood, D. Traver, and C. E. Furlong (1996). Structural organization of the human PON1 gene. *Genomics* 35:586–589.

Cole, T. B., R. L. Jampsa, B. J. Walter, T. L. Arndt, R. J. Richter, D. M. Shih, A. Tward, A. J. Lusis, R. M. Jack, L. G. Costa, and C. E. Furlong (2003). Expression of human paraoxonase (PON1) during development. *Pharmacogenetics* 13:357–364.

Cole, T. B., W. F. Li, R. J. Richter, C. E. Furlong, and L. G. Costa (2002). Inhibition of Paraoxonase (PON1) by heavy metals. *Toxicol. Sci.* 66:312.

Costa, L. G., T. B. Cole, G. P. Jarvik, and C. E. Furlong (2003). Functional genomic of the paraoxonase (PON1) polymorphisms: Effects on pesticide sensitivity, cardiovascular disease, and drug metabolism. *Annu. Rev. Med.* 54:371–392.

Costa, L. G., A. Vitalone, T. B. Cole, and C. E. Furlong (2005). Modulation of paraoxonase (PON1) activity. *Biochem. Pharmacol.* 69:541–550.

Court, J. A., C. Martin-Ruiz, A. Graham, and E. Perry (2000). Nicotinic receptors in human brain: Topography and pathology. *J. Chem. Neuroanat.* 20:281–298.

D'Amelio, M., I. Ricci, R. Sacco, X. Liu, L. D'Agruma, L. A. Muscarella, V. Guarnieri, R. Militerni, C. Bravaccio, M. Elia, C. Schneider, R. Melmed, S. Trillo, T. Pascucci, S. Puglisi-Allegra, K. L. Reichelt, F. Macciardi, J. J. Holden, and A. M. Persico (2005). Paraoxonase gene variants are associated with autism in North America, but not in Italy: Possible regional specificity in gene-environment interactions. *Mol. Psychiatry* 10:1006–1016.

Davies, H. G., R. J. Richter, M. Keifer, C. A. Broomfield, J. Sowalla, and C. E. Furlong (1996). The effect of the human serum paraoxonase polymorphism is reversed with diazoxon, soman and sarin. *Nat. Genet.* 14:334–336.

Deakin, S., I. Leviev, M. C. Brulhart-Meynet, and R. W. James (2003). Paraoxonase-1 promoter haplotypes and serum paraoxonase: A predominant role for polymorphic position-107, implicating the Sp1 transcription factor. *Biochem. J.* 372:643–649.

Deakin, S., I. Leviev, M. Gomaraschi, L. Calabresi, G. Franceschini, and R. W. James (2002). Enzymatically active paraoxonase-1 is located at the external membrane of producing cells and released by a high affinity, saturable, desorption mechanism. *J. Biol. Chem.* 277:4301–4308.

Deakin, S. P. and R. W. James (2004). Genetic and environmental factors modulating serum concentrations and activities of the antioxidant enzyme paraoxonase-1. *Clin. Sci.* 107:435–447.

Deakin, S. P. and R. W. James (2008). Transcriptional regulation of the paraoxonase genes. In B. Mackness, M. Mackness, M. Aviram, and G. Paragh (eds.), *The Paraoxonase: Their Role in Disease Development and Xenobiotic Metabolism.* Dordrecht, the Netherlands: Springer.

Draganov, D. I. and B. N. La Du (2004). Pharmacogenetics of paraoxonases: A brief review. *Naunyn Schmiedebergs Arch. Pharmacol.* 369:78–88.

Draganov, D. I. and J. F. Teiber (2008). PON's natural substrates—The key for their physiological roles. In B. Mackness, M. Mackness, M. Aviram, and G. Paragh (eds.), *The Paraoxonase: Their Role in Disease Development and Xenobiotic Metabolism.* Dordrecht, the Netherlands: Springer.

Draganov, D. I., J. F. Teiber, A. Speelman, Y. Osawa, R. Sunahara, and B. N. La Du (2005). Human paraoxonases (PON1, PON2, and PON3) are lactonases with overlapping and distinct substrate specificities. *J. Lipid Res.* 46:1239–1247.

Durrington, P. N., B. Mackness, and M. I. Mackness (2001). Paraoxonase and atherosclerosis. *Arterioscler. Thromb. Vasc. Biol.* 21:473–480.

Eckerson, H. W., J. Romson, C. Wyte, and B. N. La Du (1983). The human serum paraoxonase polymorphism: Identification of phenotypes by their response to salts. *Am. J. Hum. Genet.* 35:214–227.

Ecobichon, D. J. and D. S. Stephens (1973). Perinatal development of human blood esterases. *Clin. Pharmacol. Ther.* 14:41–47.

Engel, S. M., G. S. Berkowitz, D. B. Barr, S. L. Teitelbaum, J. Siskind, S. J. Meisel, J. G. Wetmur, and M. S. Wolff (2007). Prenatal organophosphate metabolite and organochlorine levels and performance on the Brazelton Neonatal Behavioral Assessment Scale in a multiethnic pregnancy cohort. *Am. J. Epidemiol.* 165:1397–1404.

Eskenazi, B., A. R. Marks, A. Bradman, K. Harley, D. B. Barr, C. Johnson, N. Morga, and N. P. Jewell (2007). Organophosphate pesticide exposure and neurodevelopment in young Mexican-American children. *Environ. Health Perspect.* 115:792–798.

Eskenazi, B., L. G. Rosas, A. R. Marks, A. Bradman, K. Harley, N. Holland, C. Johnson, L. Fenster, and D. B. Barr (2008). Pesticide toxicity and the developing brain. *Basic Clin. Pharmacol. Toxicol.* 102:228–236.

Evans, T. A., S. L. Siedlak, L. Lu, X. Fu, Z. Wang, W. R. McGinnis, E. Fakhoury, R. J. Castellani, S. L. Hazen, W. J. Walsh, R. G. Salomon, M. A. Smith, G. Perry, and X. Zhu (2008). The autistic phenotype exhibits a remarkably localized modification of brain protein by products of free radical-induced lipid oxidation. *Am. J. Biochem. Biotechnol. Special issue on Autism Spectrum Disorders* 4:61–72.

Fatemi, S. H., A. V. Snow, J. M. Stary, M. Araghi-Niknam, T. J. Reutiman, S. Lee, A. I. Brooks, and D. A. Pearce (2005). Reelin signaling is impaired in autism. *Biol. Psychiatry* 57:777–787.

Feingold, K. R., R. A. Memon, A. H. Moser, and C. Grunfeld (1998). Paraoxonase activity in the serum and hepatic mRNA levels decrease during the acute phase response. *Atherosclerosis* 139:307–315.

Ferretti, G., T. Bacchetti, D. Busni, R. A. Rabini, and G. Curatola (2004). Protective effect of paraoxonase activity in high-density lipoproteins against erythrocyte membranes peroxidation: A comparison between healthy subjects and type 1 diabetic patients. *J. Clin. Endocrinol. Metab.* 89:2957–2962.

Furlong, C. E., T. B. Cole, G. P. Jarvik, C. Pettan-Brewer, G. K. Geiss, R. J. Richter, D. M. Shih, A. D. Tward, A. J. Lusis, and L. G. Costa (2005). Role of paraoxonase (PON1) status in pesticide sensitivity: Genetic and temporal determinants. *Neurotoxicology* 26:651–659.

Furlong, C. E., R. J. Richter, W. F. Li, V. H. Brophy, C. Carlson, M. Rieder, D. Nickerson, L. G. Costa, J. Ranchalis, A. J. Lusis, D. M. Shih, A. Tward, and G. P. Jarvik (2008). The functional consequences of polymorphisms in the PON1 gene. In B. Mackness, M. Mackness, M. Aviram, and G. Paragh (eds.), *The Paraoxonase: Their Role in Disease Development and Xenobiotic Metabolism.* Dordrecht, the Netherlands: Springer.

Gaidukov, L. and D. S. Tawfik (2005). High affinity, stability, and lactonase activity of serum paraoxonase PON1 anchored on HDL with ApoA-I. *Biochemistry* 44:11843–11854.

Gaita, L. and A. M. Persico (2006). The R192 allele of the PON1 gene is associated with reduced serum arylesterase activity in autistic patients and in their first degree relatives. In The 56th Annual Meeting of the American Society of Human Genetics, New Orleans, LA.

Gan, K. N., A. Smolen, H. W. Eckerson, and B. N. La Du (1991). Purification of human serum paraoxonase/arylesterase. Evidence for one esterase catalyzing both activities. *Drug Metab. Dispos.* 19:100–106.

Garin, M. C., R. W. James, P. Dussoix, H. Blanche, P. Passa, P. Froguel, and J. Ruiz (1997). Paraoxonase polymorphism Met-Leu54 is associated with modified serum concentrations of the enzyme. A possible link between the paraoxonase gene and increased risk of cardiovascular disease in diabetes. *J. Clin. Invest.* 99:62–66.

Geier, D. A. and M. R. Geier (2006). A clinical and laboratory evaluation of methionine cycle-transsulfuration and androgen pathway markers in children with autistic disorders. *Horm. Res.* 66:182–188.

Geier, D. A., J. K. Kern, C. R. Garver, J. B. Adams, T. Audhya, and M. R. Geier (2009). A prospective study of transsulfuration biomarkers in autistic disorders. *Neurochem. Res.* 34:386–393.

Grandjean, P., R. Harari, D. B. Barr, and F. Debes (2006). Pesticide exposure and stunting as independent predictors of neurobehavioral deficits in Ecuadorian school children. *Pediatrics* 117:e546–556.

Harel, M., A. Aharoni, L. Gaidukov, B. Brumshtein, O. Khersonsky, R. Meged, H. Dvir, R. B. Ravelli, A. McCarthy, L. Toker, I. Silman, J. L. Sussman, and D. S. Tawfik (2004). Structure and evolution of the serum paraoxonase family of detoxifying and anti-atherosclerotic enzymes. *Nat. Struct. Mol. Biol.* 11:412–419.

Hava, G., L. Vered, M. Yael, H. Mordechai, and H. Mahoud (2006). Alterations in behavior in adult offspring mice following maternal inflammation during pregnancy. *Dev. Psychobiol.* 48:162–168.

Herbert, M. R., J. P. Russo, S. Yang, J. Roohi, M. Blaxill, S. G. Kahler, L. Cremer, and E. Hatchwell (2006). Autism and environmental genomics. *Neurotoxicology* 27:671–684.

Hernandez, A., M. A. Gomez, G. Pena, F. Gil, L. Rodrigo, E. Villanueva, and A. Pla (2004). Effect of long-term exposure to pesticides on plasma esterases from plastic greenhouse workers. *J. Toxicol. Environ. Health A* 67:1095–1108.

Hertz-Picciotto, I., I. N. Pessah, R. Hansen, and P. Krakowiak (2008). Household pesticides use in relation to autism. In International Meeting for Autism Research, London, UK.

Huang, C-C. and G. D'Arcangelo (2008). The Reelin gene and its functions in brain development In S. H. Fatemi (ed.), *Reelin Glycoprotein: Structure, Biology and Roles in Health and Disease*. New York: Springer.

Humbert, R., D. A. Adler, C. M. Disteche, C. Hassett, C. J. Omiecinski, and C. E. Furlong (1993). The molecular basis of the human serum paraoxonase activity polymorphism. *Nat. Genet.* 3:73–76.

Jakubowski, H. (2000). Calcium-dependent human serum homocysteine thiolactone hydrolase. A protective mechanism against protein N-homocysteinylation. *J. Biol. Chem.* 275:3957–3962.

James, S. J., P. Cutler, S. Melnyk, S. Jernigan, L. Janak, D. W. Gaylor, and J. A. Neubrander (2004). Metabolic biomarkers of increased oxidative stress and impaired methylation capacity in children with autism. *Am. J. Clin. Nutr.* 80:1611–1617.

James, S. J., S. Melnyk, S. Jernigan, M. A. Cleves, C. H. Halsted, D. H. Wong, P. Cutler, K. Bock, M. Boris, J. J. Bradstreet, S. M. Baker, and D. W. Gaylor (2006). Metabolic endophenotype and related genotypes are associated with oxidative stress in children with autism. *Am. J. Med. Genet. B Neuropsychiatr. Genet.* 141B:947–956.

Jarvik, G. P., L. S. Rozek, V. H. Brophy, T. S. Hatsukami, R. J. Richter, G. D. Schellenberg, and C. E. Furlong (2000). Paraoxonase (PON1) phenotype is a better predictor of vascular disease than is PON1(192) or PON1(55) genotype. *Arterioscler. Thromb. Vasc. Biol.* 20:2441–2447.

Juurlink, B. H. and P. G. Paterson (1998). Review of oxidative stress in brain and spinal cord injury: Suggestions for pharmacological and nutritional management strategies. *J. Spinal Cord Med.* 21:309–334.

Jyonouchi, H., S. Sun, and H. Le (2001). Proinflammatory and regulatory cytokine production associated with innate and adaptive immune responses in children with autism spectrum disorders and developmental regression. *J. Neuroimmunol.* 120:170–179.

Kaucsár, T., S. P. Paşca, B. K. Ferencz, S. Chira, I. Lupan, E. Dronca, N. Nemeş, F. Iftene, and M. Dronca (2009). Investigation of the Paraoxonase 1 (PON1) promoter polymorphism C(–108)T and activities in autism spectrum disorders. *Romanian J. Biochem.* 46:13–23.

Kenet, T., R. C. Froemke, C. E. Schreiner, I. N. Pessah, and M. M. Merzenich (2007). Perinatal exposure to a noncoplanar polychlorinated biphenyl alters tonotopy, receptive fields, and plasticity in rat primary auditory cortex. *Proc. Natl. Acad. Sci. USA* 104:7646–7651.

Khersonsky, O. and D. S. Tawfik (2006). The histidine 115-histidine 134 dyad mediates the lactonase activity of mammalian serum paraoxonases. *J. Biol. Chem.* 281:7649–7656.

Kriska, T., G. K. Marathe, J. C. Schmidt, T. M. McIntyre, and A. W. Girotti (2007). Phospholipase action of platelet-activating factor acetylhydrolase, but not paraoxonase-1, on long fatty acyl chain phospholipid hydroperoxides. *J. Biol. Chem.* 282:100–108.

Kumon, Y., Y. Nakauchi, T. Suehiro, T. Shiinoki, N. Tanimoto, M. Inoue, T. Nakamura, K. Hashimoto, and J. D. Sipe (2002). Proinflammatory cytokines but not acute phase serum amyloid A or C-reactive protein, downregulate paraoxonase 1 (PON1) expression by HepG2 cells. *Amyloid* 9:160–164.

La Du, B. N., M. Aviram, S. Billecke, M. Navab, S. Primo-Parmo, R. C. Sorenson, and T. J. Standiford (1999). On the physiological role(s) of the paraoxonases. *Chem. Biol. Interact.* 119–120:379–388.

Laviola, G., W. Adriani, C. Gaudino, R. Marino, and F. Keller (2006). Paradoxical effects of prenatal acetylcholinesterase blockade on neuro-behavioral development and drug-induced stereotypies in reeler mutant mice. *Psychopharmacology* 187:331–344.

Lee, M., C. Martin-Ruiz, A. Graham, J. Court, E. Jaros, R. Perry, P. Iversen, M. Bauman, and E. Perry (2002). Nicotinic receptor abnormalities in the cerebellar cortex in autism. *Brain* 125:1483–1495.

Levine, D. M., T. S. Parker, T. M. Donnelly, A. Walsh, and A. L. Rubin (1993). In vivo protection against endotoxin by plasma high density lipoprotein. *Proc. Natl. Acad. Sci. USA* 90:12040–12044.

Lintas, C. and A. M. Persico. (2008). Reelin gene polymorphisms in autistic disorder. In S. H. Fatemi (ed.), *Reelin Glycoprotein: Structure, Biology and Roles in Health and Disease.* New York: Springer.

Mackness, B., M. I. Mackness, S. Arrol, W. Turkie, and P. N. Durrington (1998). Effect of the human serum paraoxonase 55 and 192 genetic polymorphisms on the protection by high density lipoprotein against low density lipoprotein oxidative modification. *FEBS Lett.* 423:57–60.

Mackness, M. I., S. Arrol, C. Abbott, and P. N. Durrington (1993). Protection of low-density lipoprotein against oxidative modification by high-density lipoprotein associated paraoxonase. *Atherosclerosis* 104:129–135.

Mackness, M. I., S. Arrol, and P. N. Durrington (1991). Paraoxonase prevents accumulation of lipoperoxides in low-density lipoprotein. *FEBS Lett.* 286:152–154.

Mochizuki, H., S. W. Scherer, T. Xi, D. C. Nickle, M. Majer, J. J. Huizenga, L. C. Tsui, and M. Prochazka (1998). Human PON2 gene at 7q21.3: Cloning, multiple mRNA forms, and missense polymorphisms in the coding sequence. *Gene* 213:149–157.

Ng, C. J., D. M. Shih, S. Y. Hama, N. Villa, M. Navab, and S. T. Reddy (2005). The paraoxonase gene family and atherosclerosis. *Free Radic. Biol. Med.* 38:153–163.

Ng, C. J., D. J. Wadleigh, A. Gangopadhyay, S. Hama, V. R. Grijalva, M. Navab, A. M. Fogelman, and S. T. Reddy (2001). Paraoxonase-2 is a ubiquitously expressed protein with antioxidant properties and is capable of preventing cell-mediated oxidative modification of low density lipoprotein. *J. Biol. Chem.* 276:44444–44449.

Okita, C., M. Meguro, H. Hoshiya, M. Haruta, Y. K. Sakamoto, and M. Oshimura (2003). A new imprinted cluster on the human chromosome 7q21-q31, identified by human–mouse monochromosomal hybrids. *Genomics* 81:556–559.

Pardo, C. A., D. L. Vargas, and A. W. Zimmerman (2005). Immunity, neuroglia and neuroinflammation in autism. *Int. Rev. Psychiatry* 17:485–495.

Paşca, S. P., E. Dronca, T. Kaucsár, E. C. Craciun, E. Endreffy, B. Ferenz, F. Iftene, I. Benga, R. Cornean, R. Banerjee, and M. Dronca (2009a). One carbon metabolism disturbances and the C677T MTHFR gene polymorphism in children with autism spectrum disorders. *J. Cell. Mol. Med.* (in press).

Paşca, S. P., E. Dronca, B. Nemeş, T. Kaucsár, E. Endreffy, F. Iftene, I. Benga, R. Cornean, and M. Dronca (2009b). Paraoxonase 1 activities and polymorphisms in autism spectrum disorders. *J. Cell. Mol. Med.* (in press).

Paşca, S. P., B. Nemes, L. Vlase, C. E. Gagyi, E. Dronca, A. C. Miu, and M. Dronca (2006). High levels of homocysteine and low serum paraoxonase 1 arylesterase activity in children with autism. *Life Sci.* 78:2244–2248.

Perry, E. K., M. L. Lee, C. M. Martin-Ruiz, J. A. Court, S. G. Volsen, J. Merrit, E. Folly, P. E. Iversen, M. L. Bauman, R. H. Perry, and G. L. Wenk (2001). Cholinergic activity in autism: abnormalities in the cerebral cortex and basal forebrain. *Am. J. Psychiatry* 158:1058–1066.

Perry, S. W., J. P. Norman, A. Litzburg, and H. A. Gelbard (2004). Antioxidants are required during the early critical period, but not later, for neuronal survival. *J. Neurosci. Res.* 78:485–492.

Persico, A. M. and T. Bourgeron (2006). Searching for ways out of the autism maze: Genetic, epigenetic and environmental clues. *Trends Neurosci.* 29:349–358.

Persico, A. M., L. D'Agruma, N. Maiorano, A. Totaro, R. Militerni, C. Bravaccio, T. H. Wassink, C. Schneider, R. Melmed, S. Trillo, F. Montecchi, M. Palermo, T. Pascucci, S. Puglisi-Allegra, K. L. Reichelt, M. Conciatori, R. Marino, C. C. Quattrocchi, A. Baldi, L. Zelante, P. Gasparini, and F. Keller (2001). Reelin gene alleles and haplotypes as a factor predisposing to autistic disorder. *Mol. Psychiatry* 6:150–159.

Pessah, I. N., R. F. Seegal, P. J. Lein, J. LaSalle, B. K. Yee, J. Van De Water, and R. F. Berman (2008). Immunologic and neurodevelopmental susceptibilities of autism. *Neurotoxicology* 29:532–545.

Primo-Parmo, S. L., R. C. Sorenson, J. Teiber, and B. N. La Du (1996). The human serum paraoxonase/arylesterase gene (PON1) is one member of a multigene family. *Genomics* 33:498–507.

Rainwater, D. L., S. Rutherford, T. D. Dyer, E. D. Rainwater, S. A. Cole, J. L. Vandeberg, L. Almasy, J. Blangero, J. W. Maccluer, and M. C. Mahaney (2009). Determinants of variation in human serum paraoxonase activity. *Heredity* 102:147–154.

Rapin, I. and R. F. Tuchman (2008). Autism: Definition, neurobiology, screening, diagnosis. *Pediatr. Clin. North Am.* 55:1129–1146.

Rauh, V. A., R. Garfinkel, F. P. Perera, H. F. Andrews, L. Hoepner, D. B. Barr, R. Whitehead, D. Tang, and R. W. Whyatt (2006). Impact of prenatal chlorpyrifos exposure on neurodevelopment in the first 3 years of life among inner-city children. *Pediatrics* 118:e1845–1859.

Reddy, S. T., D. J. Wadleigh, V. Grijalva, C. Ng, S. Hama, A. Gangopadhyay, D. M. Shih, A. J. Lusis, M. Navab, and A. M. Fogelman (2001). Human paraoxonase-3 is an HDL-associated enzyme with biological activity similar to paraoxonase-1 protein but is not regulated by oxidized lipids. *Arterioscler. Thromb. Vasc. Biol.* 21:542–547.

Richter, R. J. and C. E. Furlong (1999). Determination of paraoxonase (PON1) status requires more than genotyping. *Pharmacogenetics* 9:745–753.

Richter, R. J., G. P. Jarvik, and C. E. Furlong (2009). Paraoxonase 1 (PON1) status and substrate hydrolysis. *Toxicol. Appl. Pharmacol.* 235:1–9.

Roberts, E. M., P. B. English, J. K. Grether, G. C. Windham, L. Somberg, and C. Wolff (2007). Maternal residence near agricultural pesticide applications and autism spectrum disorders among children in the California Central Valley. *Environ. Health Perspect.* 115:1482–1489.

Rochu, D., E. Chabriere, F. Renault, M. Elias, C. Clery-Barraud, and P. Masson (2007). Stabilization of the active form(s) of human paraoxonase by human phosphate-binding protein. *Biochem. Soc. Trans.* 35:1616–1620.

Rodrigo, L., B. Mackness, P. N. Durrington, A. Hernandez, and M. I. Mackness (2001). Hydrolysis of platelet-activating factor by human serum paraoxonase. *Biochem. J.* 354:1–7.

Roest, M., T. M. van Himbergen, A. B. Barendrecht, P. H. Peeters, Y. T. van der Schouw, and H. A. Voorbij (2007). Genetic and environmental determinants of the PON-1 phenotype. *Eur. J. Clin. Invest.* 37:187–196.

Rosas, L. G. and B. Eskenazi (2008). Pesticides and child neurodevelopment. *Curr. Opin. Pediatr.* 20:191–197.

Rosenblat, M., R. Oren, and M. Aviram (2006). Lysophosphatidylcholine (LPC) attenuates macrophage-mediated oxidation of LDL. *Biochem. Biophys. Res. Commun.* 344:1271–1277.

Rosenblat, M., J. Vaya, D. Shih, and M. Aviram (2005). Paraoxonase 1 (PON1) enhances HDL-mediated macrophage cholesterol efflux via the ABCA1 transporter in association with increased HDL binding to the cells: a possible role for lysophosphatidylcholine. *Atherosclerosis* 179:69–77.

Rozenberg, O. and M. Aviram (2006). S-Glutathionylation regulates HDL-associated paraoxonase 1 (PON1) activity. *Biochem. Biophys. Res. Commun.* 351:492–498.

Rozenberg, O., D. M. Shih, and M. Aviram (2005). Paraoxonase 1 (PON1) attenuates macrophage oxidative status: Studies in PON1 transfected cells and in PON1 transgenic mice. *Atherosclerosis* 181:9–18.

Santanam, N. and S. Parthasarathy (2007). Aspirin is a substrate for paraoxonase-like activity: Implications in atherosclerosis. *Atherosclerosis* 191:272–275.

Serajee, F. J., R. Nabi, H. Zhong, and M. Huq (2004). Polymorphisms in xenobiotic metabolism genes and autism. *J. Child Neurol.* 19:413–417.

Slotkin, T. A., E. D. Levin, and F. J. Seidler (2009). Developmental neurotoxicity of parathion: Progressive effects on serotonergic systems in adolescence and adulthood. *Neurotoxicol. Teratol.* 31:11–17.

Smith, S. E., J. Li, K. Garbett, K. Mirnics, and P. H. Patterson (2007). Maternal immune activation alters fetal brain development through interleukin-6. *J. Neurosci.* 27:10695–10702.

Sogut, S., S. S. Zoroglu, H. Ozyurt, H. R. Yilmaz, F. Ozugurlu, E. Sivasli, O. Yetkin, M. Yanik, H. Tutkun, H. A. Savas, M. Tarakcioglu, and O. Akyol (2003). Changes in nitric oxide levels and antioxidant enzyme activities may have a role in the pathophysiological mechanisms involved in autism. *Clin. Chim. Acta* 331:111–117.

Sorenson, R. C., M. Aviram, C. L. Bisgaier, S. Billecke, C. Hsu, and B. N. La Du (1999). Properties of the retained N-terminal hydrophobic leader sequence in human serum paraoxonase/arylesterase. *Chem. Biol. Interact.* 119–120:243–249.

Sozmen, E. Y., B. Mackness, B. Sozmen, P. Durrington, F. K. Girgin, L. Aslan, and M. Mackness (2002). Effect of organophosphate intoxication on human serum paraoxonase. *Hum. Exp. Toxicol.* 21:247–252.

Suh, J. H., W. J. Walsh, W. R. McGinnis, A. Lewis, and B. N. Ames (2008). Altered sulfur amino acid metabolism in immune cells of children diagnosed with autism. *Am. J. Biochem. Biotechnol. (Special Issue on Autism Spectrum Disorders)* 4:105–113.

Sweeten, T. L., D. J. Posey, and C. J. McDougle (2003). High blood monocyte counts and neopterin levels in children with autistic disorder. *Am. J. Psychiatry* 160:1691–1693.

Sweeten, T. L., D. J. Posey, S. Shankar, and C. J. McDougle (2004). High nitric oxide production in autistic disorder: A possible role for interferon-gamma. *Biol. Psychiatry* 55:434–437.

Van Lenten, B. J., S. T. Reddy, M. Navab, and A. M. Fogelman (2006). Understanding changes in high density lipoproteins during the acute phase response. *Arterioscler. Thromb. Vasc. Biol.* 26:1687–1688.

Van Lenten, B. J., A. C. Wagner, M. Navab, and A. M. Fogelman (2001). Oxidized phospholipids induce changes in hepatic paraoxonase and ApoJ but not monocyte chemoattractant protein-1 via interleukin-6. *J. Biol. Chem.* 276:1923–1929.

Vargas, D. L., C. Nascimbene, C. Krishnan, A. W. Zimmerman, and C. A. Pardo (2005). Neuroglial activation and neuroinflammation in the brain of patients with autism. *Ann. Neurol.* 57:67–81.

Whyatt, R. M., V. Rauh, D. B. Barr, D. E. Camann, H. F. Andrews, R. Garfinkel, L. A. Hoepner, D. Diaz, J. Dietrich, A. Reyes, D. Tang, P. L. Kinney, and F. P. Perera (2004). Prenatal insecticide exposures and birth weight and length among an urban minority cohort. *Environ. Health Perspect.* 112:1125–1132.

Wolff, M. S., S. Engel, G. Berkowitz, S. Teitelbaum, J. Siskind, D. B. Barr, and J. Wetmur (2007). Prenatal pesticide and PCB exposures and birth outcomes. *Pediatr. Res.* 61:243–250.

Worth, J. 2002. Paraoxonase polymorphisms and organophosphates. *Lancet* 360:802–803.

Yorbik, O., A. Sayal, C. Akay, D. I. Akbiyik, and T. Sohmen (2002). Investigation of antioxidant enzymes in children with autistic disorder. *Prostaglandins Leukot. Essent. Fatty Acids* 67:341–343.

Young, J. G., B. Eskenazi, E. A. Gladstone, A. Bradman, L. Pedersen, C. Johnson, D. B. Barr, C. E. Furlong, and N. T. Holland (2005). Association between in utero organophosphate pesticide exposure and abnormal reflexes in neonates. *Neurotoxicology* 26:199–209.

Zoroglu, S. S., F. Armutcu, S. Ozen, A. Gurel, E. Sivasli, O. Yetkin, and I. Meram (2004). Increased oxidative stress and altered activities of erythrocyte free radical scavenging enzymes in autism. *Eur. Arch. Psychiatry Clin. Neurosci.* 254:143–147.

Zoroglu, S. S., M. Yurekli, I. Meram, S. Sogut, H. Tutkun, O. Yetkin, E. Sivasli, H. A. Savas, M. Yanik, H. Herken, and O. Akyol (2003). Pathophysiological role of nitric oxide and adrenomedullin in autism. *Cell Biochem. Funct.* 21:55–60.

7 The Redox/Methylation Hypothesis of Autism: A Molecular Mechanism for Heavy Metal-Induced Neurotoxicity

Richard C. Deth* and Christina R. Muratore

Department of Pharmaceutical Sciences,
Northeastern University, Boston, MA 02115, USA

CONTENTS

7.1   INTRODUCTION

The rapid rise of autism rates over the past 25 years suggests a potential toxic effect from one or more environmentally encountered substances on the normal trajectory of neurological development, although increased diagnosis may also contribute. Two major autism categories can be identified, based upon whether or not individuals did or did not initially exhibit normal cognitive function and language acquisition.

* Corresponding author: Tel.: +1-617-373-4064; fax: +1-617-373-8886; e-mail: r.deth@neu.edu

(1) Classical autism, described prior to 1980, corresponds to the latter pattern where infants fail to achieve standard developmental milestones from birth. (2) Regressive autism, which is more typical of the contemporary condition, reflects a loss of previously acquired abilities that can occur over a short period of time (i.e., days to weeks). Anecdotal reports from some parents link regression to the time period after vaccination, raising the possibility that vaccine components, including mercury and/ or aluminum and the accompanying inflammatory activation they promote, might contribute to autism. While this proposal is both frightening and controversial, it requires serious consideration and investigation. Autistic children exhibit signs of oxidative stress and neuroinflammation, which may be attributed in part to heavy metal toxicity. This chapter reviews clinical observations and relevant molecular mechanisms, which bear on this critical public health question.

7.2   REDOX: AN EVOLUTIONARY PERSPECTIVE

Many biochemical reactions involve reduction or oxidation, the gain or loss of electrons, respectively. This is especially true in aerobic organisms, such as humans, which utilize oxygen as a primary source of energy, creating a constant source of oxidative risk that must be counterbalanced by an effective antioxidant redox-buffering system (Benzie, 2000). Since the origin of life, molecules containing reduced sulfur (e.g., thiols) have served as primary antioxidants, based upon the ease with which they release their hydrogen atom, making them excellent reducing agents. Indeed, the simplest thiol, hydrogen sulfide, a gas released from underwater volcanic vents, may have been essential for earliest life forms (Clark et al., 1998). Thiols within proteins (e.g., enzymes) can be modified by reactive oxygen or nitrogen species, and by formation of mixed disulfides, resulting in a change of protein function. Via these mechanisms, a vast number of cellular processes come under the influence of cellular redox status. Under oxidative stress conditions, these thiol-based changes in protein function can serve to restore redox balance, representing a major example of homeostatic control.

It has been proposed that metabolic adaptation to increasing levels of oxygen has been an important driving force during the 2–3 billions of years over which life on earth has evolved (Falkowski, 2006; Raymond and Segrè, 2006). At the ocean depths where geothermal conditions allowed synthesis of biomolecules (e.g., amino acids) and primitive life forms, oxygen exists almost exclusively in its fully reduced state, i.e., water (H_2O). Accordingly, early organisms depended upon anaerobic metabolism, including the abstraction of reducing equivalents (hydrogen atoms) from hydrogen sulfide (H_2S). Photosynthesis by algae and plants began converting H_2O to O_2, a reaction that liberates both electrons and reducing equivalents, which can react with carbon dioxide (CO_2) to form organic materials (e.g., carbohydrates). Based upon the utility of these reactions, plants emerged from the ocean and became a dominant species, accelerating oxygenation of the atmosphere. As damage from accumulating oxygen became more problematic, organisms with novel antioxidant metabolic strategies emerged and evolved, illustrating the power of negative selection pressure. Along this evolutionary path, the selective advantage of combining cell types with different metabolic networks was realized, resulting in complex plant and animal organisms. As we reflect on the extreme complexity of humans, with multiple organ systems and a resident population of microorganisms in our intestine, we must appreciate that the primitive elements of our metabolic origins are still operative and the ability to sustain redox balance is the heart of metabolism for every cell type.

7.3   REDOX METABOLISM IN HUMAN BRAIN

Autism is primarily a neurodevelopmental disorder, and systemic oxidative stress has been documented in autistic children (Chauhan and Chauhan, 2006; James et al., 2004, 2006). This strongly suggests that the brain and neuronal function are more sensitive to disturbances involving redox metabolism than other tissue and cell types. This conclusion is consistent with the notion that the brain, indeed the human brain, reflects the highest degree of evolution with unique metabolic features that are necessary for its normal function. Reciprocally, this perspective implies that the human brain function is uniquely vulnerable to the toxic effects of agents such as heavy metals, which interfere with redox metabolism.

The tripeptide glutathione, in its reduced (GSH) and oxidized (GSSG) forms, is the primary determinant of redox status in all human cells, reflected by its high intracellular concentration (~10 mM) and the multiplicity of redox reactions in which it participates (Schafer and Buettner, 2001). The cysteine residue of GSH, flanked by glutamate and glycine, is the basis of its redox activity, reflecting its hydrogen sulfide origins. Prevailing levels of GSH depend upon its de novo synthesis, for which the concentration of cysteine is rate-limiting, as well as its dynamic utilization in multiple reactions, many of which are reversible, allowing regeneration of GSH. Most important among the latter is reduction of oxidized GSSG to GSH, which can be directly accomplished by glutathione reductase or indirectly via involvement of protein thiols in conjunction with the thioredoxin system. In both cases, reducing equivalents are provided by NADPH, whose level is maintained by glucose metabolism through the successive actions of hexokinase and glucose-6-phosphate dehydrogenase.

De novo synthesis of GSH is supported by cysteine made available from the breakdown of proteins, through cellular uptake, or via transsulfuration of homocysteine, which is elaborated during the methionine cycle of methylation (Figure 7.1). Various cell surface amino acid transporters bring either cysteine or oxidized cystine into cells. Cell type–specific differences in transporter expression can lead to variations in redox regulation and can also influence local glutamate levels. Astrocytes, for example, express a transporter which exchanges cystine for glutamate, EAAT1 (Excitatory Amino Acid Transporter 1), and within the cell cystine is reduced to provide cysteine for GSH synthesis (Banner et al., 2002). Under normal circumstances, astrocytes synthesize excess GSH, and the excess is released to the extracellular space where it is converted to cysteine by the action of two proteases. Neurons take up astrocyte-derived cysteine via EAAT3, which can alternatively transport glutamate or aspartate, the predominant transporter in mature neurons (Aoyama et al., 2006; Gegelashvili and Schousboe, 1998). EAAT3 activity is regulated by protein kinase C and phosphatidylinositol 3 kinase (Do et al., 2002; Huang and Zuo, 2005),

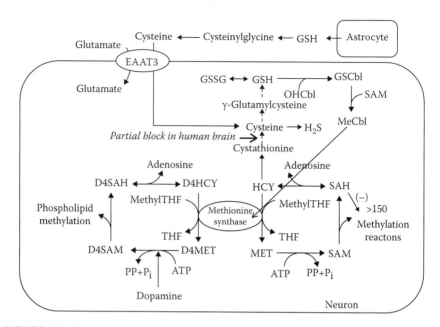

FIGURE 7.1 Pathways of thiol metabolism in human neuronal cells. In human neurons, transsulfuration is impaired and cysteine for synthesis of GSH is provided primarily by uptake via EAAT3, which is dependent upon GSH released from astrocytes. GSH is required for synthesis of methylcobalamin (MeCbl) and for activity of methionine synthase. During oxidative stress, low levels of GSH and MeCbl cause a decrease in a large number of SAM-dependent methylation reactions, and a decrease in dopamine-stimulated, D4 dopamine receptor-mediated phospholipid methylation.

linking it to receptor signaling pathways, and implying that neurotransmitters and neurotrophic factors may regulate redox status in neurons.

Transsulfuration of homocysteine (HCY) provides a major source of cysteine in most cells. However, in the brain, activity of cystathionine-gamma-lyase is low, resulting in accumulation of cystathionine and decreased cysteine availability (Finkelstein, 1990). Early studies concluded that transsulfuration did not function in brain, but more recent studies confirm partial activity, since inhibition of cystathionine-gamma-lyase leads to a significant decrease in GSH (Vitvitsky et al., 2006). Interestingly, levels of cystathionine are 40-fold higher in human brain versus rat or mouse, with intermediate levels in nonhuman primates, although levels in other human tissues are low (Tallan et al., 1958). This pattern reflects a progressive decrease in transsulfuration with evolution among these mammals, accompanied by a progressive increase in the risk of oxidative stress. It is also of interest that the transsulfuration pathway operates in the opposite direction in plants, allowing synthesis of HCY (and methionine) from cysteine, reflecting a lower requirement for GSH in association with the release of oxygen (Giovanelli and Mudd, 1967).

Restricted transsulfuration in human brain has several implications: (1) Capacity for GSH synthesis is limited. (2) EAAT3-dependent uptake of cysteine is more critical for maintaining cellular redox status. (3) Agents affecting EAAT3 activity will exert a more powerful influence on redox status. (4) The limited available pool of GSH may be more dynamically utilized. (5) Human brain function is more vulnerable to toxic substances, which impair redox metabolism.

7.4   REDOX AND METHYLATION

Methylation involves the addition of a carbon atom to a molecule, usually causing a change in the function of the methylated molecule. S-adenosylmethionine (SAM), the ATP-activated form of the essential amino acid methionine, is the methyl donor for more than 150 methyltransferase-dependent methylation reactions, which regulate a large number of cellular functions (Katz et al., 2003). Donation of a methyl group by SAM results in formation of S-adenosylhomocysteine (SAH), which inhibits methyltransferase activity by competing with SAM, and is reversibly converted to HCY (Figure 7.1). Ongoing activity of the methionine cycle of methylation is sustained by the cobalamin (vitamin B12)-dependent enzyme methionine synthase, which utilizes 5-methyltetrahydrofolate (methylfolate) as the methyl donor for conversion of HCY to methionine. Since HCY formation from SAH is reversible, any decrease in methionine synthase activity will be reflected as an increase in both HCY and SAH, resulting in inhibition of SAM-dependent methylation reactions. Clearly methionine synthase exerts a powerful influence over cell function via its control over methylation.

As illustrated in Figure 7.1, methionine synthase is positioned at the intersection between transsulfuration and methylation pathways. As a consequence, its level of activity exerts control over cellular redox status, since it determines the proportion of HCY that will be diverted toward cysteine and GSH synthesis. Methionine synthase activity is exceptionally sensitive to inhibition during oxidative stress, primarily because its cobalamin cofactor is easily oxidized (Liptak and Brunold, 2006). This allows methionine synthase to serve as a redox sensor, lowering its activity whenever the level of oxidation increases, until increased GSH synthesis brings the system back into balance. Electrophilic compounds, such as oxygen-containing xenobiotic metabolites, also react with cobalamin, inactivating the enzyme and increasing diversion of HCY toward GSH synthesis (Watson et al., 2004). Thus methionine synthase is a sensor of both redox and xenobiotic status.

One of the most important roles of methylation is epigenetic regulation of gene expression through DNA methylation. Cytidine residues preceding guanine residues (i.e., CpG sites) frequently occur in promoter regions and their methylation facilitates binding of a series of proteins that favor histone binding and inhibits transcription of adjacent genes (Miranda and Jones, 2007). Significant changes in patterns of DNA methylation occur during development, as genes are differentially turned off or on, and disruption of methylation by oxidative stress and impaired methionine synthase activity will therefore adversely affect development. Indeed, several neurodevelopmental disorders including Rett, Prader-Willi, and Angelman syndromes, as well as fragile X syndrome, have been linked to genetic defects involving DNA methylation (McConkie-Rosell et al., 1993; Thatcher et al., 2005; Wan et al., 1999). Oxidative stress associated with environmental exposure to xenotoxins may therefore mimic certain aspects of these disorders. Moreover, xenotoxin exposure can amplify the impact of methylation-related genetic risk factors, increasing the likelihood of developmental disorders.

7.5 HEAVY METALS AND REDOX STATUS

It is widely recognized that heavy metals exert many of their toxic effects via binding to thiols. Moreover, thiol-containing compounds, especially GSH, are critical for heavy metal detoxification and elimination. This is particularly true for mercury, and the term mercaptan is a synonym for thiol-containing compounds, which "capture mercury." Since thiols play a central role in maintaining cellular redox status, it is not surprising that mercury and other heavy metals would disrupt redox status. Moreover, cell type-specific differences in thiol metabolism, as described above, can lead to differences in vulnerability to heavy metals.

Mercury exists in elemental (Hg•), inorganic (Hg^{2+}), or organic (e.g., methyl-mercury or ethylmercury) states. Hg• is liquid at room temperature and has a high vapor pressure, which allows it to readily enter the gas phase. These unique physical properties increase the spread of mercury throughout the earth and its atmosphere and also facilitate its use in industrial products such as liquid electrical switches and light bulbs. Methylmercury from maternal seafood ingestion and dental amalgams is the primary source of in utero exposure for infants, while ethylmercury from the vaccine preservative thimerosal can be a postnatal source of exposure. Vaccination-associated mercury exposure significantly increased starting in the late 1980s, but was dramatically reduced following a 1999 FDA report (Centers for Disease Control and Prevention, 1999), which led to the availability of nominally thimerosal-free infant vaccines starting in 2001. Removal of thimerosal was not, however, associated with a decrease in rising autism rates (Schechter and Grether, 2008), casting doubt on a causative role for thimerosal (Fonbonne, 2008). Nonetheless, since epigenetic effects of toxic exposures can be transmitted across generations, significant concerns remain about the impact of mercury exposure during the two previous decades. In addition, aluminum, which shares many of the effects of mercury on thiol metabolism and redox status (Sharma and Mishra, 2006; Verstraeten et al., 2008), remains as an adjuvant additive in a number of vaccines at levels much higher than previous levels of mercury. Lead exposure, from paint, dust, contaminated soil, or other sources is an additional, potentially important contributor to neurotoxicity and autism via its effects on redox status (Quig, 1998; Verstraeten et al., 2008).

Organomercurials have greater access to the brain than inorganic mercury, since methyl and ethyl groups increase hydrophobic character and facilitate diffusion across the blood–brain barrier. However, the methyl and ethyl groups dissociate from mercury, leaving inorganic mercury trapped within the brain compartment, where it can remain for years. Studies in nonhuman primates showed that a greater proportion of inorganic mercury remained in the brain from thimerosal than from methylmercury, consistent with the weaker chemical bond of mercury to the ethyl group (Burbacher et al., 2005). Lacking methyl or ethyl groups, aluminum has an intrinsically lower ability to cross the blood–brain barrier than organomercurials, but significant levels in brain can be detected after vaccination (Flarend et al., 1997).

Within the brain compartment, mercury and other metals affect thiol metabolism in different cell types, including pluripotent stem cells, neurons, astrocytes, microglia, and oligodendrocytes. Under mild oxidative stress conditions, an increased proportion of pluripotent stem cells become astrocytes, whereas mild reducing conditions increase the proportion of neuronal cells (Prozorovski et al., 2008). Since astrocytes serve as reservoirs of GSH and provide cysteine for neurons (Figure 7.1), this mode of regulation appears to adjust cell fate in response to prevailing redox conditions, and heavy metal-induced oxidative stress would reduce neuronal development. Neuronal stem cells are particularly sensitive to mercury, and low nanomolar concentrations of methylmercury activate caspase-dependent apoptosis (Tamm et al., 2006). Heavy metal-induced oxidative stress in oligodendrocytes can lead to impaired myelination (Crang and Jacobson, 1982), while it can lead to activation and the release of proinflammatory cytokines in microglia (Kim and de Vellis, 2005). Importantly, each of these conditions has been observed in the brain of children with autism.

In 2004, our group first described the potent inhibitory effects of mercury, thimerosal, aluminum, and lead on methylation and methionine synthase activity in SH-SY5Y human neuronal cells (Waly et al., 2004). Subsequently, we determined that inhibition reflected the ability of these heavy metals to lower GSH levels (M. Waly et al., unpublished observation), resulting in decreased synthesis of methylcobalamin (methylB12), which is required for methionine synthase activity in these neuronal cells, as illustrated in Figure 7.1. These heavy metals potently inhibit EAAT3-mediated uptake of cysteine, which accounts for their ability to decrease GSH, methylB12, and methionine synthase activity. Together, these studies illustrate the critical role of EAAT3 in regulating redox status and methylation activity in human neuronal cells, as well as their vulnerability to heavy metals.

An important breakthrough in understanding the molecular mechanism of mercury toxicity was provided from studies carried out by Holmgren and colleagues at the Karolinska Institute in Sweden (Carvalho et al., 2008). They compared the potency of inorganic mercury and methylmercury to inhibit several enzymes, each of which promote a reduced intracellular redox state, including thioredoxin, thioredoxin reductase, glutathione reductase, and glutaredoxin. Among these, thioredoxin and thioredoxin reductase showed exceptionally high sensitivity to both mercury compounds, strongly suggesting that they are primary targets for mercury-induced neurotoxicity. Thioredoxin has multiple activities, including the ability to release GSH from glutathionylated proteins (i.e., proteins with a thiol-bound GSH), while thioredoxin reductase, a selenoprotein, serves to reactivate thioredoxin after it has carried out deglutathionylation (Figure 7.2). The extent of protein glutathionylation reflects the level of cellular oxidative stress, and mercury inhibition of the thioredoxin system will promote the accumulation of glutathionylated proteins, producing and sustaining a state of high oxidative stress. The ultrahigh affinity of mercury for selenoproteins has long been recognized, and selenium supplementation has been suggested as a treatment for mercury toxicity.

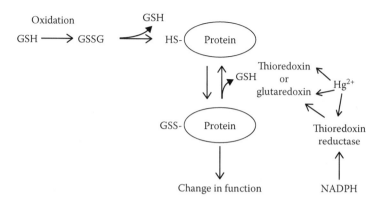

FIGURE 7.2   Mercury inhibits deglutathionylation of proteins. Mixed disulfide exchange allows glutathionylation of proteins by oxidized glutathione (GSSG), which can result in an alteration of protein function associated with oxidative stress. Thioredoxin and glutaredoxin remove glutathione utilizing NADPH-derived reducing equivalents provided by thioredoxin reductase. Mercury potently inhibits all three proteins involved in deglutathionylation.

7.6   OXIDATIVE STRESS AND NEUROINFLAMMATION IN AUTISM

As detailed in this book, a substantial and growing body of evidence indicates that oxidative stress and neuroinflammation are closely associated with autism and are likely to be critical factors in causing the disorder (for reviews see: Chauhan and Chauhan, 2006; Deth et al., 2008; Kern and Jones, 2006; McGinnis, 2004). Plasma levels of glutathione, as well as methionine cycle and transsulfuration metabolites are abnormal in autistic individuals (Geier and Geier, 2006; James et al., 2004, 2006). Adenosine and SAH levels are increased while HCY, methionine and SAM levels are low, consistent with decreased methionine synthase activity and increased cystathionine-beta-synthase (CBS) activity, while the SAM/SAH ratio is significantly reduced, indicating impaired methylation capacity. Cystathionine, cysteine, and GSH levels are decreased, along with the GSH/GSSG ratio, reflecting increased oxidative stress. Elevated HCY levels have also been reported in autism (Pasca et al., 2006). Supplementation with a combination of betaine (trimethylglycine) and folinic acid (5-formylTHF) normalized methionine cycle metabolites, but transsulfuration metabolites remained abnormal (James et al., 2004). Upon further addition of methylcobalamin, levels of all metabolites, as well as SAM/SAH and GSH/GSSG ratios returned to normal. If these abnormal metabolic profiles are confirmed by others, they will represent a critically important clue to the origins of autism.

Oxidative stress in autism is associated with increased plasma levels of malonyldialdehyde, urinary levels of fatty acid and lipid peroxidation biomarkers (Chauhan et al., 2004; Ming et al., 2005; Yao et al., 2006; Zoroglu et al., 2004). Elevated levels of inflammatory cytokines and evidence of microglial activation are observed in postmortem brain sections, indicating the presence of neuroinflammation (Vargas et al., 2005). Microglial cells monitor the local environment and provide a macrophage-like function in the brain, releasing proinflammatory substances upon activation. In addition, microglia take up organic mercury and convert it to the more toxic inorganic mercury (Charleston et al., 1995), and in primate cortex, chronic methylmercury exposure leads to a large increase in activated microglia (Charleston et al., 1994). Heavy metals can therefore cause oxidative stress in neurons not only by their direct influence on sulfur metabolism, but also by promoting microglia-based neuroinflammation.

Oxidation of cobalamin during oxidative insults provides a short-term mechanism to augment transsulfuration and GSH synthesis, but chronic neuroinflammation and prolonged oxidative stress can activate additional, longer-term adaptive responses to restrict methionine synthase activity. These could include decreased transcription of the methionine synthase gene, decreased translation of its mRNA, increased degradation of the protein, and/or decreased cellular uptake of cobalamin or folic acid cofactors. To evaluate brain methionine synthase status in autism, we carried out quantitative reverse transcriptase polymerase chain reaction (RT-PCR) using cortex RNA samples from autistic subjects and age-matched neurotypical control subjects. The tissues from which these RNA samples were derived included those in which Vargas et al. (2005) described the presence of neuroinflammation. We utilized primers directed against both cobalamin-binding and cap domains of methionine synthase and in both cases, the level of mRNA was significantly lower in autism samples, amounting to a decrease of two- to threefold (Figure 7.3; unpublished observation). As outlined above, lower activity of methionine synthase increases HCY diversion to transsulfuration and GSH synthesis, thus we interpret the reduction in methionine synthase mRNA as an adaptive response to oxidative stress and neuroinflammation. This finding confirms impaired methylation in the brain during autism, and in particular, it indicates that the supply of methyl groups for dopamine-stimulated phospholipid methylation (PLM) activity will be reduced.

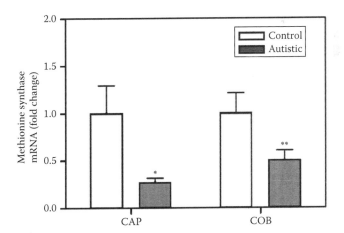

FIGURE 7.3 Methionine synthase mRNA levels in human cortex are reduced in autism. RNA samples from autistic and nonautistic subjects were probed using qRT-PCR with specific primers to the CAP and COB domains of methionine synthase. $n = 11$ for each group ($* = p < 0.05$ compared to control for the CAP primer set; $** = p < 0.05$ compared to control for the COB primer set).

Genes play a major role in autism, as reflected by high concordance rates between monozygotic twins (Smalley et al., 1988), but this does not necessarily imply that genetic defects are the cause of autism. A study of single-nucleotide polymorphisms (SNPs) in genes affecting redox and methylation found that autistic subjects had a significantly higher prevalence of risk-inducing SNPs (James et al., 2006). These genes included transcobalamin II and the reduced folate carrier, which transport cobalamin and folate into cells, as well as methionine synthase reductase, which is responsible for reduction of oxidized cobalamin, and catecholamine-O-methyltransferase (COMT), which inactivates dopamine and norepinephrine. Importantly, these SNPs are normal features of human genes, contributing to individual variability in the metabolic processes they control. When combinations of SNPs were evaluated, an odds ratio up to sevenfold was found, providing a clear example of how genetic risk factors might contribute to autism, but at the same time not necessarily represent the critical causative factor.

7.7   A MOLECULAR MECHANISM FOR HEAVY METAL-INDUCED AUTISM

The above-described observations provide a framework for specifying a molecular hypothesis of how exposure to heavy metals may cause autism in genetically vulnerable individuals. The hypothesis presented here uses organic mercury provided by thimerosal as a prototypical example, but other sources of exposure and other heavy metals can be expected to substantially act via the same mechanism. The possible involvement of thimerosal-derived mercury in autism is a highly controversial subject, which requires further research and investigation. The aim of providing a specific molecular mechanism is to bring clarity to the proposed link between mercury exposure and autism, and to guide further studies, which will ultimately refute or sustain the hypothesis. If sustained, the hypothesis should lead to measures that will reduce heavy metal exposure of infants in the future with the expectation that autism rates will cease to increase and may even decrease. In addition, a useful hypothesis should also lead to effective treatments for those who are already affected, a goal which is partially realized by current biomedical treatments. The hypothesis is directed toward "contemporary autism," whose rising prevalence suggests a critical role for environmental factors. It does not apply to "classical autism," which is more reflective of profound genetic abnormalities. If the prevalence of contemporary autism is taken as 10-fold higher than that for classical autism, this hypothesis is directed toward 90% of current cases.

7.7.1   PREEXISTING GENETIC RISK FACTORS

Risk of heavy metal-induced autism can arise from normally occurring genetic variants, which directly or indirectly affect the capacity for glutathione synthesis, the activity of methionine synthase, CBS, the methylation of DNA or histones, or the level of catecholamines and/or their receptor signaling activity. Additional genetic risk arises from variants affecting the formation of neural networks (e.g., neurogenesis, neural differentiation, synapse formation), particularly those networks supporting gamma frequency synchronized oscillations during aware-ness, attention, and cognition. Notably, these genetic risk factors would be latent in the absence of environmental exposures, giving rise to differences in neurological and cognitive function that would be considered to be normal individual variations within the population.

7.7.2 HEAVY METAL EXPOSURE

The opportunities for infants to be exposed to heavy metals are limited. Moreover, there are very few opportunities for exposure of sufficiently large number of infants in the United States to cause rates of autism to increase across the entire country. Prenatal exposure from maternal fish consumption is one possible source of heavy metal exposure with sufficiently broad influence to potentially contribute to the current "autism epidemic." Vaccine-associated ethylmercury and aluminum represent another potential source of society-wide heavy metal exposure.

Prenatal heavy metal exposure can occur through, for example, maternal consumption of fish containing significant quantities of methylmercury. Since fish provide an important source of ω-3 fatty acids and other nutrients important for brain development, contamination of this vital food category represents a major threat to human well-being. The Environmental Protection Agency (EPA) established a benchmark range for methylmercury in cord blood of 46–79 μg/L (213–367 nM), based upon neurocognitive testing of exposed populations, which they consider as a threshold value for significant "developmental neuropsychological impairment" (U.S. EPA, 2001). However, methylmercury levels above 6 μg/L (27 nM) are associated with lower IQ (Kjellstrom et al., 1986, 1989; Lederman et al., 2008), suggesting that neuronal function is impaired at low nanomolar concentrations of mercury. Neurological assessment of neonates revealed a correlation between blood mercury levels and developmental status, with a 10-fold higher mercury level being equivalent to a loss of 3 weeks in gestational development (Steuerwald et al., 2000). Since development substantially reflects epigenetic influences over gene expression, decreased methylation of DNA and histones is likely to be an important aspect of this mercury-induced developmental delay.

Vaccination with the ethylmercury-containing preservative thimerosal represented a significant source of mercury exposure for infants in the United States prior to its voluntary removal from mandated childhood vaccines starting in 2001. The preservative action of thimerosal reflects the ability of mercury to potently interfere with thiol metabolism in all organisms so as to limit their replication and survival. After administration of a thimerosal-containing vaccine, peak blood mercury levels reach 5.0, 3.6, and 2.8 μg/L in newborn, 2-month-old, and 6-month-old infants, respectively, and blood levels decrease with a $t_{1/2}$ of 3.7 days (Pichichero et al., 2008). However, for autism, the relevant issue is the level of mercury in brain tissue, particularly the level of inorganic mercury, which is retained for long periods of time. A study in nonhuman primate infants showed that total brain mercury reached approximately 40 ng/g immediately following four thimerosal-containing vaccinations, which were timed to replicate the schedule for human infants, and the level of inorganic mercury reached 16 ng/g of brain tissue (Burbacher et al., 2005). This tissue level of inorganic mercury would be equivalent to a concentration of 80 nM if the mercury was in solution, but the vast majority of mercury is undoubtedly bound to thiols and thiol- or selenium-containing proteins, where it exerts its neurotoxic effects (Ralston et al., 2007). Consistent with high-affinity and essentially irreversible binding, the level of inorganic mercury in brain failed to show any significant decline during 28 days of washout, although organic mercury decreased with a $t_{1/2}$ of 14 days.

The above studies indicate that vaccination with thimerosal-containing vaccines creates a steady-state level of inorganic mercury in the brain that can bind to thiol and selenium-containing proteins in the nanomolar concentration range. At the same time, dose–response studies in cultured human neuronal cells show that both thimerosal and inorganic mercury significantly lower GSH levels, inhibit methionine synthase, and reduce methylation activity at subnanomolar concentrations (Waly et al., 2004; M. Waly et al., unpublished observation). Thus vaccine-derived mercury exposure can produce brain levels of mercury sufficient to interfere with methylation of DNA and histone in a manner, which would lead to developmental disorders.

Aluminum is added to many vaccines, at concentrations 10-fold or higher than mercury, as an adjuvant to boost immunity by promoting Th2 cell-mediated antibody response (Lindblad, 2004), reflecting its ability to promote inflammation and induce oxidative stress (Oteiza et al., 2004). Aluminum lowers brain levels of GSH and disrupts neurodevelopment in rats (Domingo, 1995; Sharma and Mishra, 2006), and has been implicated as a factor in neurodegenerative disorders such as Alzheimer's disease (Campbell, 2006). In studies with cultured human neuronal cells, we found that aluminum inhibits methylation activity and lowers GSH in human neuronal cells at nanomolar concentrations, similar to mercury (Waly et al., 2004; M. Waly et al., unpublished observation). Thus although it has received less attention than mercury, vaccine-derived aluminum is a significant source of heavy metal exposure for infants, and may contribute to causing autism.

7.7.3 Molecular Targets

As outlined above, mercury binds strongly to thiols, even stronger to selenocysteine, and this binding forms the basis for its neurodevelopmental and neurotoxic effects. Organic mercury binds to lower molecular weight thiols (e.g., GSH, cysteine, HCY), which are present in the extracellular fluids at micromolar concentrations, via one bond, while inorganic mercury can bind two thiols. When thiol-bound mercury is excreted, this binding represents a mode of detoxification. Specialized proteins containing multiple cysteines (e.g., metallothionein) or selenocysteines (e.g., selenoprotein P) provide addition protection. When the mercury-thiol bond does break, mercury is free to redistribute to other partners, and over time, it migrates to sites of higher affinity. High-affinity binding of inorganic mercury binding is provided by proteins, in which it is able to simultaneously bind to two cysteine or selenocysteine residues. In such dual binding locations, the occasional breakage of one bond does not release mercury, resulting in ultrahigh-affinity binding, which can last for the lifetime of the protein. Accordingly, the activity of such proteins can be inhibited in an essentially irreversible manner.

Intramolecular disulfide bonds provide potential binding sites for mercury, particularly if they undergo cycles of oxidation and reduction. Vicinal (i.e., consecutive) cysteine residues provide a special case, and the oxidized and reduced proteins have significantly different conformations and activities. In such cases, the disulfide bond serves as a redox sensor, and the binding of mercury stabilizes a conformation, which mimics the oxidized condition. Another structural motif with high mercury binding affinity is the thioredoxin fold, named after the ubiquitous protein in which it was first characterized. In the thioredoxin fold, two cysteines are separated by two residues (e.g., glycine and proline), which allow the formation of a redox-sensitive disulfide bond that binds inorganic mercury with high affinity. Since thioredoxin catalyzes removal of thiols such as GSH or cysteine from proteins, mercury inhibition results in the accumulation of these thiol-modified proteins. Under normal circumstances, thiolation of proteins is increased when GSSG and cystine levels are high, so the net effect of mercury is to shift cells to an oxidative stress condition.

Mercury binds potently to thiols in their unprotonated thiolate state, but the prevalence of this state is much higher for selenocysteine, resulting in a millionfold higher affinity for mercury, as compared to cysteine, with a binding constant of 10^{45} (Dyrssen and Wedborg, 1991). This property is the basis for the unique redox capabilities of selenoproteins, but also makes them highly vulnerable to mercury inhibition. Moreover, redistribution of mercury away from thiols of lower affinity results in its increasing association with selenoproteins. Thus the targets of mercury, which are most likely to contribute to autism are selenoproteins, which include thioredoxin reductases, glutathione peroxidases, thyroid hormone deiodinases, selenoprotein P, and other proteins whose function remains to be established. Selenoproteins are particularly important in brain, and under deficiency conditions, other tissues release their selenium, which is taken up by the brain (Behne and Kyriakopoulos, 2001).

Since both thioredoxin and thioredoxin reductase possess molecular features, which render them highly sensitive to inorganic mercury, their combined inhibition will result in a highly amplified accumulation of thiol-modified proteins (Figure 7.2). When combined with the unique pattern of sulfur metabolism in human neuronal cells (Figure 7.1), these actions may account for the extremely potent reduction in GSH levels caused by mercury. Importantly, autistic subjects have a significantly lower level of selenium, which may increase their sensitivity to mercury (Jory and McGinnis, 2008).

7.7.4 CELLULAR CONSEQUENCES

A reduction in cellular GSH levels causes a decrease in the synthesis of methylcobalamin, which is absolutely required for the activity of methionine synthase in human neuronal cells (M. Waly et al., unpublished observation). Lower methionine synthase activity leads to a decrease in the SAM to SAH ratio, resulting in impaired methylation of DNA and histones, with adverse consequences for the highly orchestrated expression of genes during development. Differentiation of neuronal stem cells is particularly sensitive to mercury (Tamm et al., 2006). Lower methionine synthase activity interferes with D4 dopamine receptor-mediated PLM, which has been proposed to play a central role in gamma frequency synchronization of neural networks during attention (Kuznetsova and Deth, 2008).

Mitochondrial dysfunction is a recognized risk factor for autism (Oliveira et al., 2005; Poling et al., 2006). Complex I of the mitochondrial electron transport chain is subject to glutathionylation at several cysteine residues during oxidative stress, which is correlated with impaired activity (Hurd et al., 2008). Mercury-induced inhibition of thioredoxin activity will increase complex I glutathionylation, thereby providing a molecular link to the occurrence of mitochondrial dysfunction.

7.8 SUMMARY

The ability to counteract oxidation is a critical role for sulfur metabolism in all cells, but human neuronal cells are particularly vulnerable to oxidative stress. As illustrated in Figure 7.4, mercury and other heavy metals impair GSH synthesis and inhibit methylation activity by binding with high affinity to thiols and selenoproteins. Studies indicate that the concentration of inorganic mercury delivered to the brain following vaccination is sufficient to inhibit the activity of selenoproteins such as thioredoxin reductase. This inhibition creates a state of oxidative stress, which disrupts methylation activities including epigenetic regulation of gene expression and dopamine-stimulated PLM. Together, these observations provide a coherent and compelling molecular mechanism by which mercury and other heavy metals can contribute to the etiology of autism. Additional studies are needed to confirm specific aspects of this molecular hypothesis.

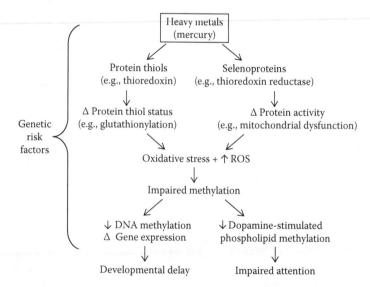

FIGURE 7.4 Molecular hypothesis for heavy metal-induced autism. Heavy metals such as mercury bind with high affinity to protein thiols and to selenoproteins, disrupting their role in redox regulation. The resulting oxidative stress inhibits methionine synthase activity, causing a decrease in DNA methylation and a decrease in D4 dopamine receptor-mediated phospholipid methylation. In a genetically vulnerable subpopulation, these neurotoxic effects are significant factors in the etiology of autism.

REFERENCES

Aoyama, K., Suh, S.W., Hamby, A.M., Liu, J., Chan, W.Y., Chen, Y., and Swanson, R.A. (2006). Neuronal glutathione deficiency and age-dependent neurodegeneration in the EAAC1 deficient mouse. *Nat. Neurosci.* 9:119–126.

Banner, S.J., Fray, A.E., Ince, P.G., Steward, M., Cookson, M.R., and Shaw, P.J. (2002). The expression of the glutamate re-uptake transporter excitatory amino acid transporter 1 (EAAT1) in the normal human CNS and in motor neurone disease: An immunohistochemical study. *Neuroscience* 109:27–44.

Behne, D. and Kyriakopoulos, A. (2001). Mammalian selenium-containing proteins. *Annu. Rev. Nutr.* 21:453–473.

Benzie, I.F. (2000). Evolution of antioxidant defence mechanisms. *Eur. J. Nutr.* 39:53–61.

Burbacher, T.M., Shen, D.D., Liberato, N., Grant, K.S., Cernichiari, E., and Clarkson, T. (2005). Comparison of blood and brain mercury levels in infant monkeys exposed to methylmercury or vaccines containing thimerosal. *Environ. Health Perspect.* 113:1015–1021.

Campbell, A. (2006). The role of aluminum and copper on neuroinflammation and Alzheimer's disease. *J. Alzheimers Dis.* 10:165–172.

Carvalho, C.M., Chew, E.H., Hashemy, S.I., Lu, J., and Holmgren, A. (2008). Inhibition of the human thioredoxin system. A molecular mechanism of mercury toxicity. *J. Biol. Chem.* 283:11913–11923.

Centers for Disease Control and Prevention (1999). Notice to Readers: Thimerosal in Vaccines: A Joint Statement of the American Academy of Pediatrics and the Public Health Service. *Morb. Mort. Wkly. Rep.* 48:563–565.

Charleston, J.S., Bolender, R.P., Mottet, N.K., Body, R.L., Vahter, M.E., and Burbacher, T.M. (1994). Increases in the number of reactive glia in the visual cortex of *Macaca fascicularis* following subclinical long-term methyl mercury exposure. *Toxicol. Appl. Pharmacol.* 129:196–206.

Charleston, J.S., Body, R.L., Mottet, N.K., Vahter, M.E., and Burbacher, T.M. (1995). Autometallographic determination of inorganic mercury distribution in the cortex of the calcarine sulcus of the monkey Macaca fascicularis following long-term subclinical exposure to methylmercury and mercuric chloride. *Toxicol. Appl. Pharmacol.* 132:325–333.

Chauhan, A. and Chauhan, V. (2006). Oxidative stress in autism. *Pathophysiology* 13:171–181.

Chauhan, A., Chauhan, V., Brown, W.T., and Cohen, I. (2004). Oxidative stress in autism: Increased lipid peroxidation and reduced serum levels of ceruloplasmin and transferrin—The antioxidant proteins. *Life Sci.* 75:2539–2549.

Clark, P.D., Dowling, N.I., and Huang, M. (1998). Comments on the role of H_2S in the chemistry of Earth's early atmosphere and in prebiotic synthesis. *J. Mol. Evol.* 47:127–132.

Crang, A.J. and Jacobson, W. (1982). The relationship of myelin basic protein (arginine) methyltransferase to myelination in mouse spinal cord. *J. Neurochem.* 39:244–247.

Deth, R., Muratore, C., Benzecry, J., Power-Charnitsky, V.A., and Waly, M. (2008). How environmental and genetic factors combine to cause autism: A redox/methylation hypothesis. *Neurotoxicology* 29:190–201.

Do, S.H., Fang, H.Y., Ham, B.M., and Zuo, Z. (2002). The effects of lidocaine on the activity of glutamate transporter EAAT3: The role of protein kinase C and phosphatidylinositol 3-kinase. *Anesth. Analg.* 95:1263–1268.

Domingo, J.L. (1995). Reproductive and developmental toxicity of aluminum: A review. *Neurotoxicol. Teratol.* 17:515–521.

Dyrssen, D. and Wedborg, M. (1991). The sulfur–mercury(II) system in natural waters. *Water Air Soil Pollut.* 56:507–519.

Falkowski, P.G. (2006). Evolution. Tracing oxygen's imprint on earth's metabolic evolution. *Science* 311:1724–1725.

Finkelstein, J.D. (1990). Methionine metabolism in mammals. *J. Nutr. Biochem.* 1:228–237.

Flarend, R.E., Hem, S.L., White, J.L., Elmore, D., Suckow, M.A., Rudy, A.C., and Dandashli, E.A. (1997). In vivo absorption of aluminium-containing vaccine adjuvants using 26Al. *Vaccine* 15:1314–1318.

Fonbonne, E. (2008). Thimerosal disappears but autism remains. *Arch. Gen. Psychiatry* 65:15–16.

Gegelashvili, G. and Schousboe, A. (1998). Cellular distribution and kinetic properties of high-affinity glutamate transporters. *Brain Res. Bull.* 45:233–238.

Geier, D.A. and Geier, M.R. (2006). A clinical and laboratory evaluation of methionine cycle-transsulfuration and androgen pathway markers in children with autistic disorders. *Horm. Res.* 66:182–188.

Giovanelli, J. and Mudd, S.H. (1967). Synthesis of homocysteine and cysteine by enzyme extracts of spinach. *Biochem. Biophys. Res. Commun.* 27:150–156.

Huang, Y. and Zuo, Z. (2005). Isoflurane induces a protein kinase C alpha-dependent increase in cell-surface protein level and activity of glutamate transporter type 3. *Mol. Pharmacol.* 67:1522–1533.

Hurd, T.R., Requejo, R., Filipovska, A., Brown, S., Prime, T.A., Robinson, A.J., Fearnley, I.M., and Murphy, M.P. (2008). Complex I within oxidatively stressed bovine heart mitochondria is glutathionylated on Cys-531 and Cys-704 of the 75-kDa subunit: Potential role of CYS residues in decreasing oxidative damage. *J. Biol. Chem.* 283:24801–24815.

James, S.J., Cutler, P., Melnyk, S., Jernigan, S., Janak, L., Gaylor, D.W., and Neubrander, J.A. (2004). Metabolic biomarkers of increased oxidative stress and impaired methylation capacity in children with autism. *Am. J. Clin. Nutr.* 80:1611–1617.

James, S.J., Melnyk, S., Jernigan, S., Cleves, M.A., Halsted, C.H., Wong, D.H., Cutler, P., Bock, K., Boris, M., Bradstreet, J.J., Baker, S.M., and Gaylor, D.W. (2006). Metabolic endophenotype and related genotypes are associated with oxidative stress in children with autism. *Am. J. Med. Genet. B Neuropsychiatr. Genet.* 141:947–956.

Jory, J. and McGinnis, W.R. (2008). Red-cell trace minerals in children with autism. *Am. J. Biochem. Biotechnol. (Special Issue on Autism Spectrum Disorders)* 4:101–104.

Katz, J.E., Dlakić, M., and Clarke, S. (2003). Automated identification of putative methyltransferases from genomic open reading frames. *Mol. Cell. Proteomics* 2:525–540.

Kern, J.K. and Jones, A.M. (2006). Evidence of toxicity, oxidative stress, and neuronal insult in autism. *J. Toxicol. Environ. Health B Crit. Rev.* 9:485–499.

Kim, S.U. and de Vellis, J. (2005). Microglia in health and disease. *J. Neurosci. Res.* 81:302–313.

Kjellstrom, T., Kennedy, P., Wallis, S., and Mantell, C. (1986). Physical and Mental Development of Children with Prenatal Exposure to Mercury from Fish. Stage I: Preliminary Tests at Age 4. Report 3080. Solna, Sweden: National Swedish Environmental Protection Board.

Kjellstrom, T., Kennedy, P., Wallis, S., Stewart, A., Friberg, L., Lind, B., and Mantell, C. (1989). Physical and Mental Development of Children with Prenatal Exposure to Mercury from Fish. Stage II: Interviews and Psychological Tests at Age 6. Report 3642. Solna, Sweden: National Swedish Environmental Protection Board.

Kuznetsova, A.Y. and Deth, R.C. (2008). A model for modulation of neuronal synchronization by D4 dopamine receptor-mediated phospholipid methylation. *J. Comput. Neurosci.* 24:314–329.

Lederman, S.A., Jones, R.L., Caldwell, K.L., Rauh, V., Sheets, S.E., Tang, D., Viswanathan, S., Becker, M., Stein, J.L., Wang, R.Y., and Perera, F.P. (2008). Relation between cord blood mercury levels and early child development in a World Trade Center cohort. *Environ. Health Perspect.* 116:1085–1091.

Lindblad, E.B. (2004). Aluminium adjuvants—In retrospect and prospect. *Vaccine* 22:3658–3668.

Liptak, M.D. and Brunold, T.C. (2006). Spectroscopic and computational studies of Co1 + cobalamin: Spectral and electronic properties of the "superreduced" B12 cofactor. *J. Am. Chem. Soc.* 128:9144–9156.

McConkie-Rosell, A., Lachiewicz, A.M., Spiridigliozzi, G.A., Tarleton, J., Schoenwald, S., Phelan, M.C., Goonewardena, P., Ding, X., and Brown, W.T. (1993). Evidence that methylation of the FMR-I locus is responsible for variable phenotypic expression of the fragile X syndrome. *Am. J. Hum. Genet.* 53:800–809.

McGinnis, W.R. (2004). Oxidative stress in autism. *Altern. Ther. Health Med.* 10:22–36.

Ming, X., Stein, T.P., Brimacombe, M., Johnson, W.G., Lambert, G.H., and Wagner, G.C. (2005). Increased excretion of a lipid peroxidation biomarker in autism. *Prostaglandins Leukot. Essent. Fatty Acids* 73:379–384.

Miranda, T.B. and Jones, P.A. (2007). DNA methylation: The nuts and bolts of repression. *J. Cell. Physiol.* 213:384–390.

NRC (National Research Council) (2000). *Toxicological Effects of Methylmercury.* Washington, DC: National Academy Press.

Oliveira, G., Diogo, L., Grazina, M., Garcia, P., Ataíde, A., Marques, C., Miguel, T., Borges, L., Vicente, A.M., and Oliveira, C.R. (2005). Mitochondrial dysfunction in autism spectrum disorders: A population-based study. *Dev. Med. Child. Neurol.* 47:185–189.

Oteiza, P.I., Mackenzie, G.G., and Verstraeten, S.V. (2004). Metals in neurodegeneration: Involvement of oxidants and oxidant-sensitive transcription factors. *Mol. Aspects Med.* 25:103–115.

Paşca, S.P., Nemes, B., Vlase, L., Gagyi, C.E., Dronca, E., Miu, A.C., and Dronca, M. (2006). High levels of homocysteine and low serum paraoxonase 1 arylesterase activity in children with autism. *Life Sci.* 78:2244–2248.

Pichichero, M.E., Gentile, A., Giglio, N., Umido, V, Clarkson, T., Cernichiari, E., Zareba, G., Gotelli, C., Gotelli, M., Yan, L., and Treanor, J. (2008). Mercury levels in newborns and infants after receipt of thimerosal-containing vaccines. *Pediatrics* 121:e208–e214.

Poling, J.S., Frye, R.E., Shoffner, J., and Zimmerman, A.W. (2006). Developmental regression and mitochondrial dysfunction in a child with autism. *J. Child Neurol.* 21:170–172.

Prozorovski, T., Schulze-Topphoff, U., Glumm, R., Baumgart, J., Schröter, F., Ninnemann, O., Siegert, E., Bendix, I., Brüstle,O., Nitsch, R., Zipp, F., and Aktas, O. (2008). Sirt1 contributes critically to the redox-dependent fate of neural progenitors. *Nat. Cell Biol.* 10:385–394.

Quig, D. (1998). Cysteine metabolism and metal toxicity. *Altern. Med. Rev.* 3:262–270.

Ralston, N.V., Blackwell, J.L. III, and Raymond, L.J. (2007). Importance of molar ratios in selenium-dependent protection against methylmercury toxicity. *Biol. Trace Elem. Res.* 119:255–268.

Raymond, J. and Segrè, D. (2006). The effect of oxygen on biochemical networks and the evolution of complex life. *Science* 311:1764–1767.

Schafer, F.Q. and Buettner, G.R. (2001). Redox environment of the cell as viewed through the redox state of the glutathione disulfide/glutathione couple. *Free Radic. Biol. Med.* 30:1191–1212.

Schechter, R. and Grether, G.K. (2008). Continuing increases in autism reported to California's developmental services system: Mercury in retrograde. *Arch. Gen. Psychiatry* 65:19–24.

Sharma, P. and Mishra, K.P. (2006). Aluminum-induced maternal and developmental toxicity and oxidative stress in rat brain: Response to combined administration of tiron and glutathione. *Reprod. Toxicol.* 21:313–321.

Smalley, S.L., Asarnow, R.F., and Spence, M.A. (1988). Autism and genetics. A decade of research. *Arch. Gen. Psychiatry* 45:953–961.

Steuerwald, U., Weihe, P., Jørgensen, P.J., Bjerve, K., Brock, J., Heinzow, B., Budtz-Jørgensen, E., and Grandjean, P. (2000). Maternal seafood diet, methylmercury exposure, and neonatal neurologic function. *J. Pediatr.* 136:599–605.

Tallan, H.H., Moore, S., and Stein, W.H. (1958). L-Cystathionine in human brain. *J. Biol. Chem.* 230:707–716.

Tamm, C., Duckworth, J., Hermanson, O., and Ceccatelli, S. (2006). High susceptibility of neural stem cells to methylmercury toxicity: Effects on cell survival and neuronal differentiation. *J. Neurochem.* 97:69–78.

Thatcher, K.N., Peddada, S., Yasui, D.H., and Lasalle, J.M. (2005). Homologous pairing of 15q11–13 imprinted domains in brain is developmentally regulated but deficient in Rett and autism samples. *Hum. Mol. Genet.* 14:785–797.

U.S. EPA. (2001). *Methylmercury Reference Dose for Chronic Oral Exposure.* U.S. Environmental Protection Agency, Integrated Risk Information System (IRIS). Washington, DC: U.S. Environmental Protection Agency: http://www.epa.gov/NCEA/iris/subst/0073.htm

Vargas, D.L., Nascimbene, C., Krishnan, C., Zimmerman, A.W., and Pardo, C.A. (2005). Neuroglial activation and neuroinflammation in the brain of patients with autism. *Ann. Neurol.* 57:67–81.

Verstraeten, S.V., Aimo, L., and Oteiza, P.I. (2008). Aluminium and lead: Molecular mechanisms of brain toxicity. *Arch. Toxicol.* 82:789–802.

Vitvitsky, V., Thomas, M., Ghorpade, A., Gendelman, H.E., and Banerjee, R. (2006). A functional transsulfuration pathway in the brain links to glutathione homeostasis. *J. Biol. Chem.* 281:35785–35793.

Waly, M., Olteanu, H., Banerjee, R., Choi, S.W., Mason, J.B., Parker, B.S., Sukumar, S., Shim, S., Sharma, A., Benzecry, J.M., Power-Charnitsky, V.A., and Deth, R.C. (2004). Activation of methionine synthase by insulin-like growth factor-1 and dopamine: A target for neurodevelopmental toxins and thimerosal. *Mol. Psychiatry* 9:358–370.

Wan, M., Lee, S.S., Zhang, X., Houwink-Manville, I., Song, H.R., Amir, R.E., Budden, S., Naidu, S., Pereira, J.L., Lo, I.F., Zoghbi, H.Y., Schanen, N.C., and Francke, U. (1999). Rett syndrome and beyond: Recurrent spontaneous and familial MECP2 mutations at CpG hotspots. *Am. J. Hum. Genet.* 65:1520–1529.

Watson, W.P., Munter, T., and Golding, B.T. (2004). A new role for glutathione: Protection of vitamin B12 from depletion by xenobiotics. *Chem. Res. Toxicol.* 17:1562–1567.

Yao, Y., Walsh, W.J., McGinnis, W.R., and Pratico, D. (2006). Altered vascular phenotype in autism: Correlation with oxidative stress. *Arch. Neurol.* 63:1161–1164.

Zoroglu, S.S., Armutcu, F., Ozen, S., Gurel, A., Sivasli, E., Yetkin, O., and Meram, I. (2004). Increased oxidative stress and altered activities of erythrocyte free radical scavenging enzymes in autism. *Eur. Arch. Psychiatry Clin. Neurosci.* 254:143–147.

8 Autism and Oxidative Stress: Evidence from an Animal Model

Michelle A. Cheh,[1] Alycia K. Halladay,[2,3] Carrie L. Yochum,[2] Kenneth R. Reuhl,[3] Marianne Polunas,[3] Xue Ming,[4] and George C. Wagner[2,]*

Departments of [1]Neuroscience, [2]Psychology, and [3]Pharmacology and Toxicology, Rutgers University, New Brunswick, NJ 08854, USA

[4]Department of Neuroscience, University of Medicine and Dentistry of New Jersey, Newark, NJ 07103, USA

CONTENTS

* Corresponding author: Tel.: +1-732-445-4660; fax: +1-732-445-2263; e-mail: gcwagner@rci.rutgers.edu

8.1   INTRODUCTION: AN OVERVIEW OF AUTISM

Autism is a neurodevelopmental disorder with core symptoms of impaired social interactions, deficits in verbal and nonverbal communication, and the appearance of stereotypic and sometimes self-injurious behaviors. These symptoms appear early and persist throughout the life of the individual (Rapin, 1997). The intensity of symptom manifestation varies along a continuum with mild but pervasive developmental disturbances at one end of the spectrum to severely retarded and compromised individuals at the other end. Patients with Asperger syndrome are higher functioning autistic individuals with impaired social skills but less severe language deficits. Some autistic individuals manifest exceptional skills for restricted topics, but these savant skills are embedded in an otherwise restricted behavioral repertoire that only serves to heighten their occurrence by contrast.

That autism is a neurobiological disorder has been apparent since its earliest description. In an editorial comment accompanying his initial report, Kanner (1943a) characterized autism as an "...innate inability to form affective contact with people in the ordinary way to which the human species is biologically disposed." He then provided 11 case histories of children; for each, the hallmark feature was a failure of the child to engage in proper social interactions. Of interest, of the 10 cases for whom the case history were reasonably complete, Kanner (1943b) noted that five had an unusually large head circumference. In addition, Kanner (1943b) also noted that six of these 10 cases had difficulty feeding, showing sensitivity to different diets, and five showed frequent illness during development. Most important, in one case (case 3), the child exhibited an adverse reaction to smallpox vaccination administered at the age of 12 months. Two years later, the mother reported: "It seems that he has gone backwards mentally gradually for the last two years." Kanner's case 3 appears to be the first association of autistic regression following an adverse reaction to a vaccination.

Several of the important biological features of autism include: (1) a male:female ratio of about 4:1 in the prevalence of autism (Rapin, 1997; Fombonne et al., 1999); (2) approximately 75% of those diagnosed with autism are also mentally retarded (Rutter, 1979); (3) about 30% of all individuals with autism exhibit an increase in plasma serotonin (Schain and Freedman, 1961); (4) about 40% of all autistic individuals have a seizure disorder (Volkmar and Nelson, 1990; Ballaban-Gil and Tuchman, 2000); (5) approximately 70% of those with autism engage in self-injurious behavior sometime during their life (Bartak and Rutter, 1976); and (6) there is a strong heritability of autism with about a 60% concordance rate between monozygotic twins as compared to about a 1% concordance rate for dizygotic twins (Bailey et al., 1996). Finally, one of the more dramatic features of autism is that about 35%–40% of those destined to be diagnosed with the disorder have apparent normal cognitive-social development through about the age of 18–30 months but then experience a "regression" where acquired skills are lost (Tuchman and Rapin, 1997). The lost skills are sometimes regained, at least partially, but only after considerable developmental delay. Collectively, these features reveal autism to have a neurobiological basis with early onset.

Although it is clear that autism has a neurobiological basis, its neuropathology has not been well characterized. Following histopathological analysis, Bauman and Kemper (1985) reported limbic system and cerebellar abnormalities in the brain of a 29-year-old mentally retarded individual with autism who had regressed at the age of 30 months and exhibited a seizure disorder thereafter. This individual engaged in stereotypic and self-injurious behavior and was medicated and institutionalized until the time of his death. The major drawback to the conclusion that the described brain pathology was attributable to autism was that there were no control cases for mental retardation, protracted institutionalization with medication, or seizure activity, in the absence of autism. In a later review summarizing histopathological observations of the brains of nine autistic individuals, Kemper and Bauman (1998) reported a consistent reduction in cerebellar Purkinje cells. Comparing these nine brains to the controls, the authors noted variability in cerebellar lobe size. They also note that two other cerebella from individuals with autism but normal intelligence both were similar to the control. Since Soto-Ares et al. (2003) observed cerebella atrophy in 27 of 30 individuals with mental retardation, evidence suggests that the cerebellar pathology is not specific to autism but better reflects the more common mental retardation.

Ritvo et al. (1986) also reported a reduction in cerebellar Purkinje cells in the brains of four individuals with autism. Once again, three of their subjects were severely retarded while the fourth (subject 2) had a normal IQ. The Purkinje cell counts of this individual were nearly identical to those of the controls. Collectively, these data led to the conclusion that cerebellar and limbic damage is associated with mental retardation, protracted institutionalization with medication, seizure disorders, and/or autism.

In well-controlled magnetic resonance imaging studies, an increase in cerebral gray and white matter was observed in autistic children as compared to normally developing children (Courchesne et al., 2001; Aylward et al., 2002; Sparks et al., 2002; Hazlett et al., 2005). These differences, which appear very early in life, slowly disappear between the ages of 5 and 12 (Courchesne et al., 2001; Aylward et al., 2002). Unfortunately, when individual regions are compared, such as the amygdala and the hippocampus, the results are less conclusive. Howard et al. (2000) reported increases in the volume of the amygdala while Aylward et al. (2002) reported decreases. Likewise, Saitoh et al. (1995) and Piven et al. (1995) reported no differences in the volume of the hippocampus but Aylward et al. (2002) noted decreases in the volume of this structure. Thus, one must use caution in concluding that neuropathological changes in limbic structures and the cerebellum are associated specifically with autism.

8.2 ETIOLOGY OF AUTISM

In an important paper, Wakefield et al. (1998) revealed an apparent link between gastrointestinal (GI) distress (including food intolerance, diarrhea, and/or abdominal pain) in children (12 case reports) and an autistic-like regression with loss of acquired skills (notably social and communication) and, less frequently, the appearance of stereotypic and self-injurious behaviors. This autistic regression followed the GI distress either immediately or gradually over a period of a few weeks.

Unfortunately, the Wakefield et al. (1998) paper became a source of controversy. In eight of the 12 cases, the authors noted that the GI distress and subsequent autistic regression followed delivery of the measles-mumps-rubella (MMR) vaccination. Specifically, in these eight cases, the GI distress along with other symptoms including fever, delirium, and/or convulsions were part of an adverse reaction to the MMR vaccination. The autistic regression appeared an average of 6.3 days after the onset of the reaction. The authors clearly state "We did not prove an association between measles, mumps, and rubella vaccine and the syndrome described" but despite this caution, the report triggered a debate about the possible link between MMR and autism. This debate soon expanded to include a possible association between one of the constituents of the MMR vaccine, organic mercury, and autism.

The observations of Wakefield et al. (1998) are of interest because they replicate aspects of Kanner's (1943b) original case descriptions of autism associated with frequent illness, food intolerance, and adverse reactions to a vaccination. There have been attempts to refute the basic observations of Wakefield et al. (1998), whose report focused on autistic regression and not the overall prevalence of autism. For example, Dales et al. (2001) compared the percentage of children immunized with MMR on a year-by-year basis in California over the years 1980 to 2000 with the number of diagnosed cases of autism. They observed that the percentage of children being immunized remained very stable while, during these same years, the absolute number of cases of autism increased dramatically. Although no correlation coefficient or any other statistical analysis was provided, they concluded that there was no relationship between the two and that the MMR vaccination was not associated with autism. Interestingly, there was an increase in the population of California over that 20-year period and, therefore, a comparable increase in the absolute number of MMR vaccinations delivered. This seems to indicate that the Dales et al. (2001) data reflect that the increased numbers of autism cases were associated with increased administration of MMR. However, the simplest conclusion is that the increase in the number of cases of autism was associated with an increase in the population of California. In any case, the link between the MMR vaccination and autistic regression was not addressed by Dales et al. (2001).

Taylor et al. (1999) reviewed autism cases in the United Kingdom born between 1979 and 1998, comparing the incidence before and after October 1988, when the MMR vaccine was introduced. They report that there was a dramatic increase in the incidence in autism in their population starting 3 years after the introduction of the MMR vaccination but concluded that there was no association between autism and the MMR vaccination because, by 1992, the vaccine coverage had already stabilized (while the autism rate was still climbing).

Madsen et al. (2002) assessed a large population of children born in Denmark between 1991 and 1998. They divided their population into those children who received the MMR vaccination and those who did not. They then looked for a diagnosis of autism or autism spectrum disorder in these two groups and concluded that there was strong evidence against the hypothesis that the MMR vaccination causes autism. Of interest, however, is that there were about 27% more cases of autism diagnosed over the age of 3 in the vaccinated group as compared to the unvaccinated group. More important, they failed to specifically examine autistic regression, preferring instead to combine all cases of autism. This controversy continues with most recent reports continuing to emphasize the safety of the MMR vaccine (Demicheli et al., 2005; Honig et al., 2008). Nonetheless, one consequence of the MMR controversy is that there has been increased awareness that early exposure to environmental toxicants may place certain individuals at risk for autism.

As noted, about one-third of those diagnosed with autism experience autistic regression, having apparently normal development interrupted at some point by a dramatic setback with a loss of acquired skills. Yet even in these cases, as well as for the remaining two-thirds of the cases where autism appears to be the result of a neurodevelopmental defect present at birth (Kanner, 1943b), it remains true that the etiology of autism remains unknown. Evidence for a genetic contribution for the disorder is clear, but no single gene has been identified; rather, a constellation of gene polymorphisms appears to increase the risk for individuals. The controversy surrounding the link between autism and the MMR vaccination suggested the involvement of an environmental toxicant exposure as a second factor, at least for autistic regression. Other studies have linked autism to prenatal exposure to toxicants such as thalidomide or valproic acid (VPA) (Rodier et al., 1997). Based upon these observations, together with the fact that autism fails to reach 100% concordance rates in monozygotic twins, a hypothesis has been developed that the etiology of autism may arise as the result of a gene by environment interaction with a gene polymorphism(s) enhancing the sensitivity of individuals to the deleterious effects of environmental toxicants (London and Etzel, 2000). Based upon our observations in humans (Ming et al., 2005, 2008a) and mice (Wagner et al., 2006; Ming et al., 2008b), we have advanced this hypothesis with the proposal that autism is the result of a gene by environment interaction where the environmental toxicant triggers oxidative stress while the genetic deficiency affects the ability of the individual to respond effectively to the deleterious effects of oxidative stress (Ming et al., 2008b). Toward this end, we have developed an animal model of autism and have used this model to assess the effects of gene alterations (Cheh et al., 2006) as well as early exposure to toxicants such as VPA (Wagner et al., 2006; Yochum et al., 2008) and mercury (Wagner et al., 2007) on neurobehavioral development.

8.3 ANIMAL MODEL OF AUTISM

The symptoms of autism have proven difficult to model in other species, though there has been some success, especially with respect to the stereotypic and self-injurious behaviors (e.g., Wagner et al., 2004). We have initiated work on a novel strategy to model the behavioral phenotype of autism in mice. In this model, the normal development of key behaviors is carefully monitored from birth through adolescence. Once the maturation of these key behaviors is understood (i.e., in terms of the postnatal day(s) of life in which subjects are able to successfully perform the task or engage in the behavior), the performance of mice with early toxicant exposure and/or genetic modification can be assessed. The model does not claim to produce autistic mice; rather, developmental deficits can be identified against the vehicle-treated, wild-type controls. Likewise, the model does not claim to be exclusive for autism. Rather, it provides a new strategy for classifying alterations in the normal maturation of individual mice consequent to toxicant exposure, genetic manipulation, or the interaction of the two.

The model strategy begins by characterizing behavioral manifestations of developmental disorders as retardations (i.e., a behavior fails to develop during a critical period), regressions (i.e., a behavior develops at about the right time but then is lost with later development, especially following toxicant exposure), or intrusions (i.e., the appearance of behaviors aberrant in form or frequency which mask normal development). Most developmental disorders (e.g., autism, attention deficit disorder, mental retardation) include some combination of these conditions. In this framework, the hypothesis that environmental toxicants are causally involved in developmental disorders can be readily tested. That is, acute or repeated exposure to a toxicant should disrupt neurobehavioral development, causing behavioral retardation, regression, or intrusions. These conditions can be identified only if normal developmental patterns are thoroughly understood.

For each of these three classes of developmental deficits (i.e., retardations, regressions, and intrusions), neurodevelopmental tests may be employed to target the cognitive, motor, emotional, and/or social maturation of the subject. Genetic manipulation or toxicant exposure may, for example, impact the social maturation of the subjects, causing a retardation or regression in its development or by obscuring its manifestation by inducing intrusive stereotypic or self-injurious behaviors.

Further refinement of this model enhances its relevance for autism. This may be accomplished by making genetic alterations known to be relevant to autism (e.g., Cheh et al., 2006) and by using toxicants that have been associated with autism (e.g., Wagner et al., 2006, 2007; Yochum et al., 2008). Likewise, the neurodevelopmental tasks that are employed may assess the maturation of the cerebellum or hippocampus, brain areas thought to be involved in autism and, likewise, known to be targets of the selected toxicants. Most recently, we have used this model strategy to further assess the hypothesis that oxidative stress may be a critical factor in the etiology of autism.

8.4   OXIDATIVE STRESS AND AUTISM

The involvement of enhanced oxidative stress in autism has been derived from several lines of evidence (reviewed in Chauhan and Chauhan, 2006). First, an increased excretion of oxidative stress biomarkers has been reported. Specifically, nitric oxide, a free radical that can block energy production, was increased in erythrocytes of patients with autism as compared to age- and sex-matched controls (Sogut et al., 2003). In addition, elevated nitrite concentrations along with thiobarbituric acid–reactive substances and xanthine oxidase activity were reported in the plasma and red blood cells of autistic individuals (Zoroglu et al., 2003, 2004; Chauhan et al., 2004). The elevation of these substances indicates excess generation of free radicals in individuals with autism compared to controls. Consistent with the increased oxidative stress biomarkers, children with autism were found to have increased body burdens of environmental toxicants that may generate oxidative stress (Edelson and Cantor, 1998, 2000).

A second line of evidence that oxidative stress may play a role in autism is suggested by a reduced endogenous antioxidant capacity. Specifically, altered glutathione peroxidase (Yorbik et al., 2002; Sogut et al., 2003), superoxide oxidase (Yorbik et al., 2002), and catalase (Zoroglu et al., 2004) activities as well as total glutathione, and GSH/GSSG and cysteine levels (James et al., 2004) were found in autistic individuals compared to controls. Likewise, levels of exogenous antioxidants were also found to be reduced in autism, including vitamin C, vitamin E, and vitamin A in plasma, and zinc and selenium in erythrocytes (James et al., 2004).

Finally, evidence of altered oxidative stress in autism is derived from evidence of impaired energy metabolism. Magnetic resonance spectroscopic study of the brains of individuals with autism showed reduced synthesis of ATP (Minshew et al., 1993). In addition, higher lactate (Coleman and Blass, 1985; Chugani et al., 1999) and pyruvate (Moreno et al., 1992) levels in autism may suggest mitochondrial dysfunction in autism (Filipek et al., 2003); one major cause of mitochondria dysfunction is a result of oxidative injury (Packer, 1984). Taken together, these lines of evidence support the hypothesis that at least some children with autism exhibit enhanced oxidative stress. As noted, we have used our animal model to examine the role of oxidative stress in causing the neurobehavioral deficits following early exposure to VPA (Ming et al., 2008b) and mercury.

8.5   VALPROIC ACID, AUTISM, AND OXIDATIVE STRESS

Following its administration, VPA elicits an oxidative stress response when it is metabolized by a cytochrome P450-dependent hydroxylation, leading to a decrease in cellular glutathione and suppressing the activities of hepatic glutathione reductase, glutathione peroxidase, and glucose-6 phosphate dehydrogenase (Simon et al., 1994; Jurima-Romet et al., 1996). Thus, it appears that the metabolism-dependent VPA-induced cytotoxicity is the result of generation of hydrogen peroxide and subsequent interaction with iron to produce the highly reactive hydroxyl free radicals. In this regard, a series of antioxidants and iron chelators protected against metabolism-dependent VPA-induced in vitro cytotoxicity (Jurima-Romet et al., 1996; Tabatabaei and Abbott, 1999).

In adults, VPA is used as an anticonvulsant with few side effects. However, prenatal exposure to VPA causes behavioral and neuroanatomical abnormalities in children that are strikingly similar to those found in autism. This fetal valproate syndrome is characterized by deficits in language and communication, stereotypic behavior, and hyperexcitability (Ardinger et al., 1988; Williams et al., 2001). In rodents, early VPA exposure results in a reduction in Purkinje cell number and cerebellar cell volume similar to what is observed in patients with autism (Rodier and Hyman, 1998; Ingram et al., 2000; Sobaniec-Lotowweska, 2001). Schneider and Przewlocki (2005) found that prenatally. VPA administration to rats resulted in the appearance of repetitive behaviors together with decreased social interaction.

In our previous study, we demonstrated that mice injected with sodium valproate at crucial developmental time points displayed a retardation and/or regression of certain critical behaviors such as surface righting, midair righting, and negative geotaxis (Wagner et al., 2006). In addition, we showed that similarly treated mice showed deficits in their later cognitive performance and social interactions (Wagner et al., 2006; Yochum et al., 2008) and a 30-fold increase in the number of cells staining for apoptosis in the cerebellum together with a 10-fold increase in cells staining for apoptosis in the hippocampus (Yochum et al., 2008).

In the context of our present chapter, we sought to determine if antioxidant pretreatment could protect against the behavioral deficits caused by VPA. Accordingly, male BALB/c mice were treated with vitamin E or its vehicle on day P14. Pups then received a second injection of either saline or 400 mg/kg of VPA for a total of four groups. As in our initial studies, the ability to right in midair was evaluated on P13–19 by holding the pups upside-down, 45 cm above a padded surface and dropped for three trials each test day. Their ability to right in midair was determined if the pup landed with all four paws on the surface.

Consistent with our previous studies, we found that midair righting first appears about postnatal day 14 of life. The VPA treatment caused a pronounced regression in this response; pups that could perform the task on P14 completely lost the ability to midair right after receiving the VPA. This regression-like loss of a motor skill did gradually return over about a 1-week period. Of importance, pretreatment with the antioxidant, vitamin E, completely protected the pups against the VPA-induced loss of midair righting (Ming et al., 2008b). As noted, VPA has been associated with human autism and its mechanism of action is thought to involve oxidative stress. Therefore, this first set of data suggests that antioxidants administered at the time of toxicant exposure might afford some protection against an autistic-like regression. We then sought to extend these observations to a second toxicant that has also, at least indirectly, been linked to autism.

8.6 MERCURY EXPOSURE AND AUTISM

It is well established that exposure to methylmercury (MeHg) can induce detrimental effects in humans (for review, see Chang and Annau, 1984; Mendola et al., 2002). The effects are most severe when exposure to high doses of MeHg occurs during neural development and are manifest as severe developmental disabilities often associated with brain malformations. MeHg is an environmental toxicant that bioaccumulates in large predatory fish and, thus, human exposure comes almost exclusively through fish consumption (Clarkson et al., 2003). A number of studies have examined the effects of low-level MeHg exposure in fish-eating populations. Unfortunately, the results of these studies are conflicting (reviewed in Davidson et al., 2004) with some reporting that increased blood concentrations of MeHg correlate with poor developmental outcomes while others observing no adverse effects. Nonetheless, it has been postulated that an increase in low-level exposure to MeHg could be involved in some neurodevelopmental disorders (Davidson et al., 2004).

The brain is the primary target for MeHg (Nagashima, 1997; Costa et al., 2004). Following exposure, MeHg initiates an increase in the generation of reactive oxygen species (ROS) and, simultaneously, decreases endogenous antioxidant activity (Andersen and Andersen, 1993; Yee and Choi, 1994, 1996; Shanker and Aschner, 2003; Vicente et al., 2004). Neurons are particularly vulnerable to MeHg toxicity because their endogenous antioxidant capacity is low compared to other cell types. Therefore, the brain is particularly sensitivity to oxidative stress-induced injury consequent to MeHg exposure (Usuki et al., 2001; Costa et al., 2004). The cerebellum is one of the principle brain regions disrupted by MeHg exposure, with cerebellar granule cells being a primary target in the adult human (Castoldi et al., 2000).

MeHg exposure during neural development leads to more severe toxicity than comparable exposure in adults. Specifically, early exposure results in a more diffuse neuropathology and can affect the organization of the cerebellum, cerebral cortex, and striatum (Chang et al., 1977; Chang and Annau, 1984; Sager et al., 1984; Sakamoto et al., 2002). Commonly reported neurobehavioral deficits in rodents following early MeHg exposure include deficits in reflex development and locomotor activity and coordination as well as cognitive deficits in learning and memory (Olson and Boush, 1975; Chang and Annau, 1984; Vorhees, 1985; Doré et al., 2001; Sakamoto et al., 2002; Stringari et al., 2006). In general, the severity of the behavioral deficits following MeHg increases with dose and earlier exposure times.

Antioxidants have been shown to confer significant protection against MeHg toxicity in vitro and in vivo, reducing the levels of ROS thereby attenuating the neuropathological damage (Chang et al., 1978; Andersen and Andersen, 1993; Yee and Choi, 1994; Usuki et al., 2001; Shanker and Aschner, 2003; Beyrouty and Chan, 2006). One recent study reported that pretreatment with vitamin E attenuated MeHg-induced behavioral deficits in the acoustic startle response of rats (Beyrouty and Chan, 2006). However, the protective effect of antioxidants on persistent MeHg-induced neurobehavioral disruption is not well studied. Using our animal model of autism, we have previously shown that early exposure to MeHg sensitizes the developing mouse to the later appearance of stereotypic and self-injurious intrusive behavior (Wagner et al., 2007).

8.7 TROLOX PROTECTS MICE AGAINST EARLY EXPOSURE TO MeHg

We now report that, as with VPA, antioxidant pretreatment protects mice against the neurobehavioral deficits induced by early exposure to MeHg. Mice were exposed to MeHg in the presence or absence of antioxidants during the first 2 weeks of postnatal life (see Wagner et al., 2007 for details). The developmental period selected for MeHg exposure corresponds to the third trimester in human gestation, a time, of rapid brain growth (Costa et al., 2004). Trolox (6-hydroxy-2,5,7,8-tetramethyl-chroman-2-carboxylic acid), a water-soluble vitamin E derivative, was used as the antioxidant pretreatment. Trolox has been reported to provide significant protection against MeHg toxicity both in cell culture and in neuropathological studies (Usuki et al., 2001; Shanker and Aschner, 2003).

Pregnant BALB/c mice (Taconic, Germantown, New York) were housed in plastic cages in a temperature- and humidity-regulated colony room with a 12 h light/12 h dark cycle, and given free access to food and water. Day of birth was recorded as postnatal day (PND) 0; litters were culled to all male pups prior to treatment and were weaned at PND 20.

Mice were treated with 4.0 mg/kg MeHg Cl (ICN, Costa Mesa) or phosphate-buffered saline (PBS) vehicle subcutaneously on alternate days between PND 3–15. Additional groups of pups were dosed with the same MeHg regimen, but given high-dose (2.5 mg/kg) or low-dose (1.0 mg/kg) Trolox subcutaneously 1 hour prior to each MeHg injection. We evaluated body weight during postnatal development and reflexes including midair righting, negative geotaxis, and hanging wire strength. Adolescent mice were then evaluated in the water maze. Finally, pairs of similarly treated adult mice were tested in a resident-intruder paradigm. Details of the behavioral test procedures may be found in Wagner et al. (2006, 2007).

We observed that MeHg-induced deficits in reflex development and spatial learning and memory as well as in adult social interactions, and that Trolox pretreatment protected the mice against these MeHg-induced neurodevelopmental deficits. Specific observations were as follows.

8.7.1 BODY WEIGHT

Body weight was monitored daily from PND 3–15. Across postnatal development, mice of all treatment groups gained weight ($F(6,450)=1099.1$, $p<0.0001$). There was a significant effect of treatment on body weight gain ($F(4,75)=4.5$, $p=0.003$) as well as a significant treatment by day interaction ($F(24,450)=2.5$, $p<0.0001$). Specifically, MeHg produced a significant decrease in body weight gain compared to controls from PND 5–15. In addition, pretreatment with both high-dose and low-dose Trolox attenuated the MeHg-induced reduction in weight gain, with high-dose Trolox reaching significance on PND 7–15 and low-dose Trolox reaching significance on PND 5–11.

8.7.2 REFLEX DEVELOPMENT

8.7.2.1 Midair Righting

Mice were assessed on three daily trials for their ability to successfully right in midair on PND 13–19. Control mice displayed significantly better performance in midair righting than MeHg-exposed mice. As shown in Figure 8.1a, significant impairment was observed in MeHg-exposed mice on PND 14–18 (day 14, $H=11.1$, $p=0.01$; day 15, $H=9.8$, $p=0.2$; day 16, $H=19.7$, $p<0.001$; day 17, $H=10.2$, $p<0.001$; day 18, $H=17.8$, $p<0.001$). Complete protection against this behavioral disruption was observed following pretreatment with high-dose Trolox on all test days, while pretreatment with low-dose Trolox resulted in a significant attenuation of this deficit on PND 17–18.

8.7.2.2 Negative Geotaxis

Mice were monitored for their performance of the negative geotaxis response on days 13–19. All mice showed an improvement in performance of this reflexive response across testing ($F(6,192)=7.3$, $p<0.001$). As shown in Figure 8.1b, MeHg-treated animals showed the longest latencies to perform the geotactic response, although this difference did not reach statistical significance.

8.7.2.3 Hanging Wire

Mice were evaluated for their latency to fall when suspended from a wire on days 13–19. All mice showed an improvement in their ability to hang from the wire across testing ($F(6,156)=30.4$, $p<0.001$). There was no significant effect of treatment on hanging wire performance (data not shown).

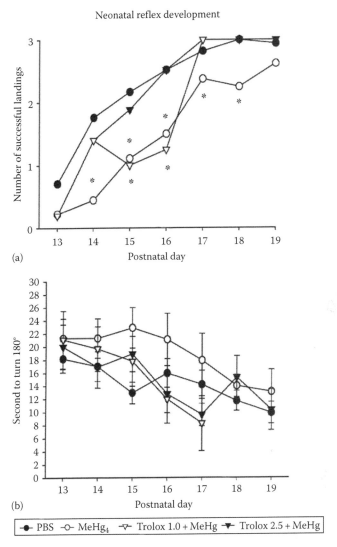

Neonatal reflex development

FIGURE 8.1   (a) The number of times out of three that mice were successful at midair righting across postnatal development is illustrated. * Indicates significantly different from control using a distribution free nonparametric post-hoc test. (b) Latency to perform the negative geotaxis response across postnatal development is depicted. Error bars indicate SEM.

8.7.3   Cognitive Development

8.7.3.1   Hidden Platform Water Maze

Mice were tested in the hidden-platform water maze for 16 trials across two days (8 trials a day for two consecutive days). All treatment groups showed a significant reduction in escape latency across the 16 trials of water maze testing ($F(15,630)=2.5$, $p<0.001$). As shown in Figure 8.2a and b, MeHg-exposed mice showed poorer hidden-platform water maze performance than controls ($F(4,42) = 5.9$, $p = 0.001$). Post-hoc analysis revealed that the escape latency for MeHg-exposed mice was significantly greater than controls for the average escape latency on day 1, as well as on trials 9, 10, 13, 14, 15 on day 2. This deficit was attenuated by high-dose of Trolox on day 2 of testing, but not by the lower dose. As an additional measure, escape latency was converted to the proportion of time spent in the quadrant where the platform was located. This

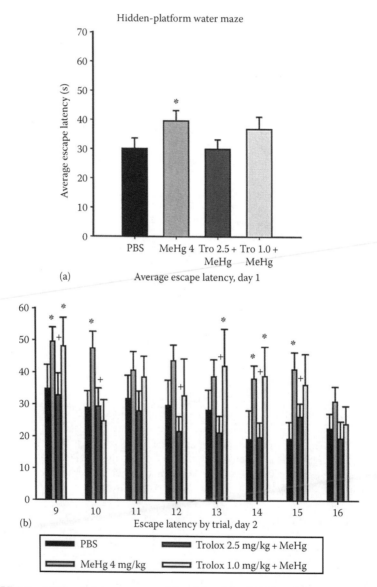

FIGURE 8.2 (a) Escape latency averaged for eight trials of hidden-platform water maze testing on day one and (b) escape latency across eight trials of hidden-platform water maze testing on day two is shown.

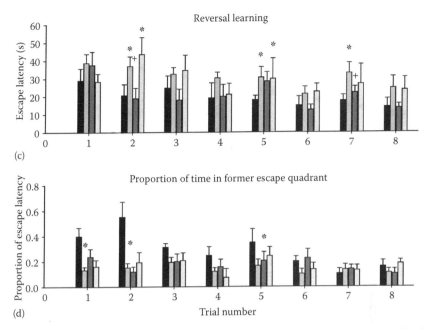

FIGURE 8.2 (continued) (c) Latency to escape to the hidden-platform when moved to the opposite quadrant across eight trials, and (d) the proportion of time spent in the quadrant where the platform was previously located across eight trials is depicted. * Indicates MeHg significantly different from control. + Indicates significantly different than MeHg-treated. Error bars indicate SEM.

proportion of time spent in the escape quadrant increased across trials for all mice ($F(15,630)=2$, $p=0.013$). MeHg-treated mice showed a smaller proportion of time in the escape quadrant compared to controls ($F(4,42)=3.5$, $p=0.015$), further indicating that they did not learn as well. Trolox pretreatment partially improved this measure, with both doses showing similar efficacy during the later trials (data not shown). Finally, in separate group of mice, high-dose Trolox was administered in the absence of MeHg and no effect on escape latency was observed (data not shown), indicating that Trolox itself does not affect spatial learning, but is effective at attenuating the MeHg-induced deficit in hidden-platform water maze performance.

8.7.3.2 Reversal Learning

One week after the initial spatial learning trials, the position of the hidden platform was changed to the opposite quadrant of the maze. For this reversal learning task, mice showed a significant reduction in escape latency across trials, demonstrating that they were able to find the position of the platform in its new location ($F(7,252)=4.3$, $p<0.0001$). There was also a significant effect of treatment on performance in this reversal learning task ($F(4,36)=3.1$, $p=0.026$). As shown in Figure 8.2c, MeHg-exposed mice did not learn the task as well as controls, displaying longer escape latencies across testing. Post-hoc analysis revealed significant differences on trials 2, 5, and 7. Pretreatment with high-dose Trolox significantly attenuated the MeHg-induced impairment in reversal learning performance, which reached significance on trials 2 and 7. However, pretreatment with low-dose Trolox did not significantly improve the MeHg-induced impairment. Again, high-dose Trolox by itself did not alter performance in this task (data not shown). This indicates that Trolox alone does not alter reversal learning, but is able to attenuate the MeHg-induced deficit in reversal learning.

During the reversal learning task, the time spent in the quadrant where the platform was previously located was also assessed. Control mice spent a larger proportion of time in this quadrant during early trials, which significantly decreased across repeated testing $(F(7,252)=3.9, p=0.001)$. This same pattern was not observed in MeHg- or Trolox-pretreated mice. Correspondingly, there was a treatment effect on the proportion of time spent in the previous platform location $(F(4,36)=4.2, p=0.006)$ and a significant interaction between trial and treatment $(F(28,252)=1.5, p=0.04)$. As shown in Figure 8.2d, MeHg-treated mice spent significantly less time in the former escape quadrant on trials 1, 2, and 5. This suggests that control mice developed a spatial memory for the former escape location and were able to adapt their strategy when they did not find the escape platform. Pretreatment with high-dose Trolox did not shorten the proportion of time MeHg-exposed mice spent in the previous platform location, even though it reduced the deficit in escape latency in both the hidden-platform and reversal learning paradigms. This suggests that Trolox confers partial protection against the MeHg-induced impairment in learning and memory.

8.7.3.3   Visible Platform

To determine whether motor skills may have influenced results of the water maze tasks, another group of treatment and age-matched mice were tested using a cued-version of the task. No significant difference was observed between groups in the latency to escape to a visible platform. This demonstrated that mice of all treatment groups were equally able to swim and escape to the visible platform. Therefore, a motor deficit likely did not contribute to the poorer performance observed by MeHg-exposed mice.

8.7.4   Social Development

The social behavior of adult mice treated as neonates was examined using the resident–intruder paradigm. The number of resident-to-intruder sniffing episodes and the number of attacks were recorded for two sessions run on consecutive days in treatment-matched pairs. Only mice pretreated with high-dose Trolox were assessed in this task.

8.7.4.1   Sniffing

There was a significant effect of day on the number of times resident mice sniffed an intruder $(F(1,26)=5.9, p<0.001)$. In addition, a significant effect of treatment $(F(1,26)=6.68, p<0.004)$ and a significant treatment-by-day interaction were found $(F(2,26)=9.0, p<0.001)$. As shown in Figure 8.3a, MeHg-exposed resident mice made significantly fewer sniffs of the intruder on day 1 compared to control mice. Pretreatment with Trolox resulted in complete reversal of the deficit in sniffing observed in MeHg-treated mice. Furthermore, both control and Trolox-pretreated mice engaged in a greater number of sniffing episodes on day one than on day 2. MeHg-exposed mice

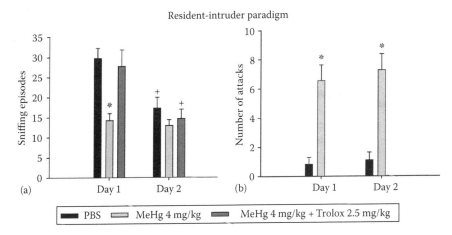

FIGURE 8.3 (a) The number of times a pair of mice sniffed one another and (b) the number of attacks resident mice made to the intruder in the resident–intruder paradigm on two consecutive days is illustrated. * Indicates significantly different than control. + Indicates significantly different than on day one of testing. Error bars indicate SEM.

engaged in a similar level of sniffing on both test days that was reduced compared to the control and Trolox-pretreated mice.

8.7.4.2 Attacks

A significant effect of treatment on the number of attacks was also observed in the resident–intruder paradigm ($F(1,26)=6.68$, $p<0.004$). MeHg-exposed resident mice made many more attacks than controls. This increased aggression was completely absent in Trolox-pretreated mice, such that none of the resident mice pretreated with Trolox attacked the intruder (see Figure 8.3b). All three groups maintained a similar level of attack behavior on the first and second day of testing. Results of the resident–intruder paradigm indicate that less social investigation and greatly enhanced aggressive behavior occur in adult mice that were exposed to MeHg during postnatal development. This behavioral pattern was completely protected by high-dose Trolox pretreatment.

8.8 CONCLUSIONS

Methylmercury is a developmental neurotoxicant that causes damage, in part, through the generation of ROS. A number of studies have reported that MeHg exposure during development leads to impaired cognitive and motor behavior. The postnatal MeHg exposure regimen used here resulted in behavioral impairments consistent with those reported by others including impaired reflex development and deficits in a spatial learning task. In addition, the present study also revealed that early MeHg exposure results in abnormal social and aggressive interactions behavior much later in life. Pretreatment with Trolox, a water-soluble vitamin E derivative, resulted in a robust protective effect against these MeHg-induced behavioral deficits. Trolox was particularly effective at abolishing the MeHg-induced deficits in midair righting and the increased aggressive behaviors of the adults. These data suggest that free-radical scavenging antioxidants might be an effective means of reducing the potential health risks of early MeHg exposure.

Dramatically increased aggressive behavior together with reduced social investigation was observed in MeHg-treated mice compared to controls. When control mice are paired in a small chamber with a target intruder mouse for the first time, they quickly develop a "social" memory (File and Seth, 2003). That is, they frequently approach and investigate the intruder on the first test day but this approach behavior decreases when they are exposed to the same intruder on subsequent days. MeHg-treated mice, however, approached the intruder significantly fewer times on the first test day, but maintained a similar level of investigation upon the second exposure to the same intruder. Moreover, MeHg-exposed mice attacked the intruder much more frequently than controls on both test days. This indicates that developmental MeHg exposure altered the social behavior expressed in adulthood, leading to increased aggression with reduced social investigation. We recently reported that mice treated with the same MeHg regimen exhibited significant increases in amphetamine-induced self-injurious behaviors as adults (Wagner et al., 2007). In the present study, Trolox pretreatment protected mice against the MeHg-induced alterations in social behavior observed in the resident–intruder paradigm, completely preventing increase in intrusive attack behavior.

Learning and memory deficits were observed in MeHg-treated mice tested in the water maze during adolescence. We found an increase in their escape latency in the hidden platform water maze, as well as in the reversal-learning task. Sensorimotor problems did not appear to contribute significantly to the MeHg-induced deficits, since no difference in escape latency was observed between groups in the visible platform version of the task. Trolox elicited a partial, dose-related protective effect on hidden-platform and reversal-learning performance.

The proportion of time that mice spent in the previous escape quadrant was recorded during the reversal-learning task. This measure functioned as a probe trial to assess memory for the former escape quadrant. The control mice spent more time in the former escape location on early trials. This decreased after just a few trials and the controls were able to quickly adapt their strategy to learn the new platform location. In contrast, mice exposed to MeHg showed a decreased proportion of time spent in the former escape location, reflecting their overall poor performance at finding the hidden-platform. However, Trolox pretreatment did not improve this measure. The lack of protection on this measure suggests that subtle abnormalities of MeHg exposure may still be present. Future studies determining the effect of Trolox in other learning and memory tasks may lead to a clearer understanding of the degree of protection conferred on MeHg-induced learning deficits.

Finally, the maturation of the mid-air righting reflex over the first 3 weeks of postnatal life is mediated, in part, by continuing cerebellar maturation. MeHg exposure resulted in a significant disruption in the maturation of the midair righting reflex and, as above, Trolox pretreatment effectively attenuated this deficit.

It appears likely that pretreatment with the free radical scavenging antioxidant, Trolox, protected mice against the behavioral deficits by decreasing the amount of oxidative damage to neurons induced by the MeHg. Gutierrez et al. (2006) recently reported that rats exposed to mercuric chloride displayed reduced levels of total radical trapping antioxidant potential following MeHg, suggesting that oxidative stress may be induced as intracellular stores of glutathione and other antioxidants become depleted. Shanker et al. (2005) showed that intracellular glutathione and antioxidants play an important role in protecting against MeHg-induced oxidative stress in the brain. Usuki et al. (2001) reported that high-dose Trolox resulted in significant protection against MeHg-induced toxicity in adult rats, reducing the number of apoptotic cells in the cerebellum as well as the degree of hind-limb crossing (a behavioral manifestation of MeHg toxicity in the adult). Likewise, Shanker and Aschner (2003) reported that Trolox was able to completely block the increase in ROS following MeHg exposure in isolated PND1 cerebral astrocytes. Thus, it is concluded that early exposure to MeHg leads to motor, cognitive, and social deficiencies that resemble human developmental disorders such as autism and that pretreatment with the antioxidant, Trolox, affords protection against the neurobehavioral deficits.

In summary, it appears that autism may be the result of early toxicant exposure acting upon individuals sensitive to their damaging effects because of a constellation of gene polymorphisms. While no single toxicant has been identified, a number of compounds have been associated indirectly with autism and these appear to share a common mechanism of generating ROS. Likewise, no single gene has been identified but a number of the polymorphisms that have been associated with autism directly or indirectly affect the response to ROS. We (and others) have previously linked the occurrence of autism to the proximity of toxic landfills (Ming et al., 2008a) and have demonstrated increased excretion of biomarkers of ROS in a cohort of autism cases compared to age-matched controls (Ming et al., 2005). Finally, using our animal model, we have shown that deletion of genes in mice that have been associated with human autism polymorphisms results in neurobehavioral deficits during development (Cheh et al., 2006), that early administration of toxicants that have been linked to human autism produces a spectrum of behavioral deficits quite similar to the gene deletions (Wagner et al., 2006, 2007; Yochum et al., 2008), and most recently, that pretreatment with antioxidants protects mice against the deleterious effects of these toxicants (Ming et al., 2008b; present chapter). The protective effects afforded by antioxidant pretreatment against the neurobehavioral deficits induced by VPA and MeHg are consistent with the interpretation that these compounds exert their damaging effects, at least in part, through the generation of ROS. The clinical ramifications of these observations await further study.

ACKNOWLEDGMENTS

Supported by: NIEHS grants ES05022, ES07148, ES11256, as well as the NJ Governor's Council on Autism (GCW) and Autism Speaks (GCW).

REFERENCES

Ardinger, H.H., Atkin, J.F., Blackston, R.D., Elsas, L.J, Clarren, S.K., Livingstone, S., Flannery, D.B., Pellock, J.M., Harrod, M.J., and Lammer, E.J. (1988). Verification of the fetal valproate syndrome phenotype. *Am. J. Med. Genet.* 29:171–185.
Andersen, H.R. and Andersen, O. (1993). Effects of dietary alpha-tocopherol and beta-carotene on lipid peroxidation induced by methyl mercuric chloride in mice. *Pharmacol. Toxicol.* 4:192–201.

Aylward, E.H., Minshew, N.J., Field, K., Sparks, B.F., and Singh, N. (2002). Effects of age on brain volume and head circumference in autism. *Neurology* 59:175–183.

Bailey, A., Phillips, W., and Rutter, M. (1996). Autism: Towards an integration of clinical, genetic, neuropsychological, and neurobiological perspectives. *J. Child Psychol. Psychiatry* 37:89–126.

Ballaban-Gil, K. and Tuchman, R. (2000). Epilepsy and epileptiform EEF: Association with autism and language disorders. *Ment. Retard. Dev. Disabil. Res. Rev.* 6:300–308.

Bartak, L. and Rutter, M. (1976). Differences between mentally retarded and normally intelligent autistic children. *J. Autism Child Schizophr.* 6:109–120.

Bauman, M. and Kemper, T.L. (1985). Histoanatomic observations of the brain in early infantile autism. *Neurology* 35:866–874.

Beyrouty, P. and Chan, H.M. (2006). Co-consumption of selenium and vitamin E altered the reproductive and developmental toxicity of methylmercury in rats. *Neurotox. Teratol.* 28:49–58.

Castoldi, A.F., Barni, S., Turin, I., Gandini, C., and Manzo, L. (2000). Early acute necrosis, delayed apoptosis and cytoskeletal breakdown in cultured cerebellar granule neurons exposed to methylmercury. *J. Neurosci. Res.* 59:775–787.

Chang, L.W. and Annau, Z. (1984). Developmental neuropathology and behavioral teratology of methylmercury. *Neurobehav. Teratol.* 18:405–432.

Chang, L.W., Gilbert, M., and Sprecher, J. (1978). Modification of methylmercury neurotoxicity by vitamin E. *Environ. Res.* 17:356–366.

Chang, L.W., Reuhl, K.R., and Lee, G.W. (1977). Degenerative changes in the developing nervous system as a result of in utero exposure to methylmercury. *Environ. Res.* 14:414–423.

Chauhan, A. and Chauhan, V. (2006). Oxidative stress in autism. *Pathophysiology* 13:171–181.

Chauhan, A., Chauham, V., Brown, W.T., and Cohen, I. (2004). Oxidative stress in autism: Increased lipid peroxidation and reduced serum levels of ceruloplasmin and transferring the antioxidant proteins. *Life Sci.* 75:2539–2549.

Cheh, M.A., Millonig, J.H., Roselli, L.M., Ming, X., Jacobsen, E., Kamdar, S., and Wagner, G.C. (2006). En2 mutant mice display neurobehavioral and neurochemical alterations relevant to disorder. *Brain Res.* 1116:166–176.

Chugani, D.C., Sundram, B.S., Behen, M., Lee, M.L., and Moore, G.J. (1999). Evidence of altered energy metabolism in autistic children. *Prog. Neuropsychopharmacol. Biol. Psychiatry* 23:635–641.

Clarkson, T.W., Magos, L., and Myers, G.J. (2003). The toxicology of mercury—Current exposures and clinical manifestations. *N. Engl. J. Med.* 349:1731–1737.

Coleman, M. and Blass, J.P. (1985). Autism and lactic acidosis. *J. Autism Dev. Disord.* 15:1–8.

Costa, L.G., Aschner, M., Vitalone, A., Syversen, T., and Soldin, O.P. (2004). Developmental neuropathology of environmental agents. *Annu. Rev. Pharmacol. Toxicol.* 44:87–110.

Courchesne, E., Karns, C.M., Davis, H.R., Ziccardi, R., Carper, R.A., Tigue, Z.D., Chisum, H.J., Moses, P., Pierce, K., Lord, C., Lincoln, A.J., Pizzo, S., Schreibman, L., Haas, R.H., Akshoofoff, N.A., and Courchesne, R.Y. (2001). Unusual brain growth patterns in early life in patients with autistic disorder: An MRI study. *Neurology* 57:245–254.

Dales, L., Hammer, S.J., and Smith, N.J. (2001). Time trends in autism and in MMR immunization coverage in California. *JAMA* 285:1183–1185.

Davidson, P.W., Myers, G.J., and Weiss, B. (2004). Mercury exposure and child development outcomes. *Pediatrics* 113:1023–1029.

Demicheli, V., Jefferson, T., Rivetti, A., and Price, D. (2005). Vaccines for measles, mumps and rubella in children. *The Cochrane Library* 4:CD004407.

Doré, F.Y., Goulet, S., Gallagher, A., Harvey, P.O., Cantin, J.F., Aigle, T.D., and Mirault, M.E. (2001). Neurobehavioral changes in mice treated with methylmercury at two different stages of fetal development. *Neurotoxicol. Teratol.* 23:463–472.

Edelson, S.B. and Cantor, D.S. (1998). Autism: Xenobiotic influences. *Toxicol. Ind. Health* 14:799–811.

Edelson, S.B. and Cantor, D.S. (2000). The neurotoxic etiology of the autistic spectrum disorder: A replicative study. *Toxicol. Ind. Health* 16:239–247.

File, S.E. and Seth, P. (2003). A review of 25 years of the social interaction test. *Eur. J. Pharmacol.* 463:35–53.

Filipek, P.A., Juranek,J., Smith, M., Mays, L.Z., Ramos, E.R., Bocian, M., Masser-Frye, D., Laulhere, T.M., Modahl, C., Spence, M.A., and Gargus, J.J. (2003). Mitochondrial dysfunction in autistic patients with 15q inverted duplication. *Ann. Neurol.* 53:801–804.

Fombonne, E., Roge, B., Claverie, J., Courty, S., and Fremolle, J. (1999). Microcephaly and macrocephaly in autism. *J. Autism Dev. Disord.* 29:113–119.

Gutierrez, L.L., Mazzotti, N.G., Araujo, A.S., Klipel, R.B., Fernandes, T.R., Llesuy, S.F., and Bello-Klein, A. (2006). Peripheral markers of oxidative stress in chronic mercuric chloride intoxication. *Braz. J. Med. Biol. Res.* 39:767–772.

Hazlett, H.C., Poe, M., Gerig, G., Smith, R.G., Provenzale, J., Ross, A., Gilmore, J., and Piven, J. (2005). Magnetic resonance imaging and head circumference study of brain size in autism: Birth through age 2 years. *Arch. Gen. Psychiatry* 62:1366–1376.

Honig, M., Briese, T., Buie, T., Bauman, M.L., Lauwers, G., Siemetzki, U., Hummel, K., Rota, P.A., Bellini, W.J., O'Leary, J.J., Sheils, O., Alden, E., Pickering, L., and Lipkin, W.I. (2008). Lack of association between measles virus vaccine and autism with enteropathy: A case–control study. *PLoS One* 3:3140.

Howard, M.A., Cowell, P.E., Boucher, J., Broks, P., Mayes, A., Farrant, A., and Roberts, N. (2000). Convergent neuroanatomical and behavioural evidence of an amygdala hypothesis of autism. *Neuroreport* 11:2931–2935.

Ingram, J.L., Peckharm, S.M., Tisdale, B., and Rodier, P. (2000). Prenatal exposure of rats to valproic acid reproduces the cerebellar anomalies associated with autism. *Neurotoxicol. Teratol.* 22:319–324.

James, S.J., Cutler, P., Melnyk, S., Jernigan, S., Janak, L., Gaylor, D.W., and Neubrander, J.A. (2004). Metabolic biomarkers of increased oxidative stress and impaired methylation capacity in children with autism. *Am. J. Clin. Nutr.* 80:1611–1617.

Jurima-Romet, M., Abbott, F.S., Tang, W., Huang, H.S., and Whitehouse, L.W. (1996). Cytotoxicity of unsaturated metabolites of valproic acid and protection by vitamins C and E in glutathione-depleted rat hepatocytes. *Toxicology* 112:69–85.

Kanner, L. (1943a). Co-editor's introduction. *Nervous Child* 2:216.

Kanner, L. (1943b). Autistic disturbances of affective contact. *Nervous Child* 2:217–250.

Kemper, T.L. and Bauman, M.L. (1998). Neuropathology of infantile autism. *J. Neuropath. Exp. Neurology* 57:645–652.

London, E. and Etzel, R.A. (2000). The environment as an etiologic factor in autism: A new direction for research. *Environ. Health Perspect.* 108:401–404.

Madsen, K.M., Hviid, A., Vestergaard, M.., Schendel, D., Wohlfahrt, J., Thorsen, P., Olsen, J., and Melbye, M. (2002). A population-based study of measles, mumps, and rubella vaccination and autism. *N. Eng. J. Med.* 347:1477–1482.

Mendola, P., Selevan, S.G., Gutter, S., and Rice, D. (2002). Environmental factors associated with a spectrum of neurodevelopmental deficits. *Ment. Retard. Dev. Disabil. Res. Rev.* 8:188–197.

Ming, X., Brimacombe, M., Malek, J.H., Jani, N., and Wagner, G.C. (2008a). Autism spectrum disorders and identified toxic land fills: Co-occurrence across States. *Environ. Health Insights* 2:55–59.

Ming, X., Cheh, M.A., Yochum, C.L., Halladay, A.K., and Wagner, G.C. (2008b). Evidence of oxidative stress in autism derived from animal models. *Am. J. Biochem. Biotechnol.* (*Special Issue on Autism Spectrum Disorders*) 4:218–225.

Ming, X., Stein, T.P., Johnson, W.G., Lambert, G.H., and Wagner, G.C. (2005). Increased excretion of a lipid peroxidation biomarker in autism. *Prostaglandins Leukot. Essent. Fatty Acids* 73:379–384.

Minshew, N.J., Goldstein, G., and Dombrowski, S.M. (1993). A preliminary ^{31}P MRS study of autism: Evidence for undersynthesis and increased degradation of brain membranes. *Biol. Psychiatry* 33:762–773.

Moreno, H., Borjas, L., Arrieta, A., Sáez, L., Prassad, A., Estévez, J., and Bonilla, E. (1992). Clinical heterogeneity of the autistic syndrome: A study of 60 families. *Invest. Clin.* 33:13–31.

Nagashima, K. (1997). A review of experimental methylmercury toxicity in rats: Neuropathology and evidence for apoptosis. *Toxicol. Pathol.* 25:624–631.

Olson, K. and Boush, M. (1975). Decreased learning capacity in rats exposed prenatally and postnatally to low doses of mercury. *Bull Environ. Contam. Toxicol.* 13:73–79.

Piven, J., Arndt, S., Bailey, J., Havercamp, S., Andreasen, N.C., and Palmer, P. (1995). An MRI study of brain size in autism. *Am. J. Psychiatry* 152:1145–1149.

Packer, L. (1984). Oxygen radicals in biological systems. In L. Packer (ed.), *Methods in Enzymology 105*. New York: Academic Press.

Rapin, I. (1997). Autism. *N. Eng. J. Med.* 337:97–104.

Ritvo, E.R., Freeman, B.J., Scheibel, A.B., Duong, T., Robinson, H., Guthrie, D., and Ritvo, A. (1986). Lower Purkinje cell counts in the cerebella of four autistic subjects: Initial findings of the UCLA-NSAC autopsy research report. *Am. J. Psychiatry* 143:862–866.

Rodier, P.M., Ingram, J.L., Tisdale, B., and Croog, V.J. (1997). Linking etiologies in humans and animal models: Studies of Autism. *Repro. Toxicol.* 11:417–422.

Rodier, P.M. and Hyman, S.L. (1998). Early environmental factors in autism. *Ment. Retard. Dev. Dis. Res. Rev.* 4:121–128.

Rutter, M. (1979). Language, cognition and autism. In R. Katzman (ed.), *Congenital and Acquired Cognitive Disorders*, New York, Raven Press, pp. 247–264.

Sager, P.R., Aschner, M., and Rodier, P.M. (1984). Persistent, differential alterations in developing cerebellar cortex of male and female mice after methylmercury exposure. *Brain Res.* 314:1–11.

Saitoh, O., Courchesne, E., Egaas, B., Lincoln, A.J., and Schreibman, L. (1995). Cross-sectional area of the posterior hippocampus in autistic patients with cerebellar and corpus callosum abnormalities. *Neurology* 45:317–324.

Sakamoto, M., Kakita, A., Wakabayashi, K., Takahashi, H., Nakano, A., and Akagi, H. (2002). Evaluation of changes in methylmercury accumulation in the developing rat brain and its effects: A study with consecutive and moderate dose exposure throughout gestation and lactation periods. *Brain Res.* 949:51–59.

Schain, R.J. and Freedman, D.X. (1961). Studies on 5-hydroxyindole metabolism in autistic and mentally retarded children. *J. Pediatrics* 58:315–320.

Schneider, T. and Przewlocki, R. (2005). Behavioral alterations in rats prenatally exposed to valproic acid: Animal model of autism. *Neuropsychopharmacology* 30:80–89.

Shanker, G. and Aschner, M. (2003). Methylmercury-induced reactive oxygen species formation in neonatal cerebral astrocytic cultures is attenuated by antioxidants. *Mol. Brain Res.* 110:85–91.

Shanker, G., Syversen, T., Aschner, J.L., and Aschner, M. (2005). Modulatory effect of glutathione status and antioxidants on methylmercury-induced free radical formation in primary cultures of cerebral astrocytes. *Mol. Brain Res.* 137:11–22.

Simon, G., Moog, C., and Obert, G. (1994). Valproic acid reduces the intracellular level of glutathione and stimulates human immunodeficiency virus. *Chem. Biol. Interact.* 91:111–21.

Sobaniec-Lotowweska, M.E. (2001). Ultrastructure of Purkinje cell perikarya and their dendritic processes in the rat cerebellar cortex in experimental encephalopathy induced by chronic application of valproate. *Int. J. Exp. Pathol.* 82:337–348.

Sögüt, S., Zoroglu, S.S., Ozyurt, H., Yilmaz, H.R., Ozugurlu, F., Sivasli, E., Yetkin, O., Yanik, M., Tutkun, H., Savas, H.A., Tarakçioglu. M., and Akyol, O. (2003). Changes in nitric oxide levels and antioxidant enzyme activities may have a role in the pathophysiological mechanisms involved in autism. *Clin. Chim. Acta* 331:111–117.

Soto-Ares, G., Joyes, B., Lemaitire, M.P., Vallee, L., and Pruvo, J.P. (2003). MRI in children with mental retardation. *Pediatr. Radiol.* 33:334–345.

Sparks, B.F., Friedman, S.D., Shaw, D.W., Aylward, E.H., Echelard, D., Artru, A.A., Maravilla, K.R., Giedd, J.N., Munson, J., Dawson, G., and Dager, S.R. (2002). Brain structural abnormalities in young children with autism spectrum disorder. *Neurology* 59:184–192.

Stringari, J., Meotti, F.C., Souza, D.O., Santos, A.R.S., and Farina, M. (2006). Postnatal methylmercury exposure induces hyperlocomotor activity and cerebellar oxidative stress in mice: Dependence on the neurodevelopmental period. *Neurochem. Res.* 31:563–569.

Tabatabaei, A.R. and Abbott, F.S. (1999). Assessing the mechanism of metabolism-dependent valproic acid-induced in vitro cytotoxicity. *Chem. Res. Toxicol.* 12:323–330.

Taylor, B., Miller, E., Farrington, C.P., Petropoulous, M-C., Favot-Mayaud, I., Li, J., and Waight, P.A. (1999). Autism and measles, mumps, and rubella vaccine: No epidemiological evidence for a causal association. *Lancet* 353:2026–2029.

Tuchman, R.F. and Rapin, I. (1997). Regression in pervasive developmental disorders: Seizures and epileptiform electroencephalogram correlates. *Pediatrics* 99:560–566.

Usuki, F., Yasutake, A., Umehara, F., Tokunaga, H., Matsumoto, M., Eto, K., Ishiura, S., and Higuchi, I. (2001). In vivo protection of a water-soluble derivative of vitamin E, Trolox, against methylmercury-intoxication in the rat. *Neurosci. Lett.* 304:199–203.

Vicente, É., Boer, M., Netto, C., Fochesatto, C., Dalmaz, C., Siqueira, I.R., and Gonçalves, C.A. (2004). Hippocampal antioxidant system in neonates from methylmercury-intoxicated rats. *Neurotoxicol. Teratol.* 26:817–823.

Volkmar, F.R. and Nelson, D.S. (1990). Seizure disorders in autism. *J. Am. Acad. Child Adolesc. Psychiatry* 29:127–129.

Vorhees, C.V. (1985). Behavioral effects of prenatal methylmercury in rats: A parallel trial to the collaborative behavioral teratology study. *Neurobehav. Toxicol. Teratol.* 7:717–725.

Wagner, G.C., Avena, N., Kita T., Nakashima T., Fisher H., and Halladay, A.K. (2004). Risperidone attenuation of amphetamine-induced self-injurious behavior in mice. *Neuropharmacology* 46:700–708.

Wagner, G.C., Reuhl, K.R., Cheh, M., McRae, P., and Halladay, A.K. (2006). A new neurobehavioral model of autism in mice: Pre- and postnatal exposure to sodium valproate. *J. Autism Dev. Disord.* 36:779–793.

Wagner, G.C., Reuhl, K.R., Ming, X., and Halladay, A.K. (2007). Behavioral and neurochemical sensitization to amphetamine following early postnatal administration of methylmercury. *NeuroToxicology* 28:59–66.

Wakefield, A.J., Murch, S.H., Anthony, A., Linnell, J., Casson, D.M., Maiik, M., Berelowitz, M., Dhillon, A.P., Thompson, M.A., Harvey, P., Valentine, A., Davies, S.E., and Walker-Smith, J.A. (1998). Ileal-lymphoid-nodular hyperplasia, non-specific colitis, and pervasive developmental disorder in children. *Lancet* 351:637–641.

Williams, G., King, J., Cunningham, M., Stephan, M., Kerr, B., and Hersh, J.H. (2001). Fetal valproate syndrome and autism: Additional evidence of an association. *Dev. Med. Child Neurol.* 43:202–206.

Yee, S. and Choi, B.H. (1994). Methylmercury poisoning induces oxidative stress in the mouse brain. *Exp. Mol. Pathol.* 60:188–196.

Yee, S. and Choi, B.H. (1996). Oxidative stress in neurotoxic effects of methylmercury poisoning. *NeuroToxicology* 17:17–26.

Yochum, C.L., Dowling, P., Reuhl, K.R., Wagner, G.C., and Ming, X. (2008). VPA-induced apoptosis and behavioral deficits in neonatal mice. *Brain Res.* 1203:126–132.

Yorbik, O., Sayalm A., Akay, C., Akbiyik, D.I., and Sohmen, T. (2002). Investigation of antioxidant enzymes in children with autistic disorder. *Prostaglandins Leukot. Essent. Fatty Acids* 67:341–343.

Zoroglu, S.S., Armutcu, F., Ozen, S., Gurel, A., Sivasli, E., Yetkin, O., and Meram, I. (2004). Increased oxidative stress and altered activities of erythrocyte free radical scavenging enzymes in autism. *Eur. Arch. Psychiatry Clin. Neurosci.* 254:143–147.

Zoroglu, S.S., Yürekli, M., Meram, I., Sögüt, S., Tutkun, H., Yetkin, O., Sivasli, E., Savas, H.A., Yanik, M., Herken, H., and Akyol, O. (2003). Pathophysiological role of nitric oxide and adrenomedullin in autism. *Cell. Biochem. Function* 21:55–60.

9 Neurotoxic Brainstem Impairment as Proposed Threshold Event in Autistic Regression

Woody R. McGinnis,[1,] Veronica M. Miller,[2]*
Tapan Audhya,[3,4] and Stephen M. Edelson[5]

[1]Autism House of Auckland, Autism New Zealand, Inc.,
Auckland, New Zealand

[2]Wadsworth Center for Laboratories and Research,
New York State Department of Health, Albany,
NY 12201, USA

[3]Vitamin Diagnostics Laboratory,
Cliffwood Beach, NJ 07735, USA

[4]Division of Endocrinology, Department of Medicine,
New York University School of Medicine,
New York, NY 10016, USA

[5]Autism Research Institute, San Diego, CA 92116, USA

CONTENTS

* Corresponding author: Tel.: +64-9-476-3605; fax: +64-9-846-0913; e-mail: woody.mcginnis@gmail.com

9.1 INTRODUCTION

In this chapter, we propose a model for autistic regression resulting from passage of toxicants into regions of brain unprotected by blood–brain barrier (BBB). These portals surround the primitive brainstem, a reportedly abnormal brain region in autistic subjects. We propose that toxicant-induced impairment of a specific structure, the dorsal vagal complex (DVC) of the medulla, sufficiently accounts for the primary neurophysiological changes of autistic regression. Toxicant effects on other unprotected sites may explain associated abnormalities in autism, including altered melatonin and oxytocin production. In autistic regression, it is possible that brainstem is primary target for toxicant-induced inflammation, which ramifies to higher structures in a pattern resembling the known stages of Parkinson disease (PD).

9.2 SOMATOBEHAVIORAL REGRESSION IN AUTISM

The earliest accounts of autism included descriptions of regression (Kanner, 1943), an intriguing phenomenon, which has been well documented as a true loss of acquired function in children later diagnosed with autism (Goldberg et al., 2003; Hansen et al., 2008; Lord et al., 2004; Werner and Dawson, 2005). The reported incidence of regression varies with methodology and approaches 50% in some studies (Goldberg et al., 2003). As reviewed by Goldberg, regression is well documented as a second-year phenomenon, usually occurring at 18–24 months (Goldberg et al., 2003). Behavioral changes are well-characterized in regression, and fall broadly into two domains which are congruent with classical diagnostic criteria for autism: (1) lost vocalization—acquired words, or babbling in preverbal children and (2) lost social skills.

In a study distinguished by a relatively brief period between regression and parental interview, Lord found that 29% of children with the diagnosis of autism lost meaningful words and another 9% lost nonword vocalizations (Lord et al., 2004). Word loss was found in 62% of autistic children with regression, and occurred over days or weeks (Goldberg et al., 2003). Loss of spoken words nearly always associates with loss in social behavior (Lord et al., 2004), but some children appear to suffer isolated social loss (Goldberg et al., 2003). Concomitant motor losses are very rare (Davidovitch et al., 2000; Tuchman and Rapin, 1997).

While regression commonly is viewed by parents as the first sign of abnormality in children who eventuate the diagnosis of autism, studies suggest that some children with discernible regression in the second year displayed prior developmental delay (Torrente et al., 2002), or difficulties in regulatory behavior (Werner and Dawson, 2005). Multiple distinct regressions are documented in some cases (Weissman et al., 2008). On the basis of parental questionnaires collected by the Autism Research Institute (ARI) over five decades, Rimland proposed a proportionate increase in regressive autism (Rimland and McGinnis, 2002).

Over the past decade, it has become clear that a variety of gastrointestinal problems—constipation, diarrhea, abdominal pain, and distension—commonly associate with autistic behavior. Over half of a mixed cohort of autistic children had radiographic fecal loading or megacolon (Afzal et al., 2003), as did 100% of a regressive cohort, with or without history of intercurrent diarrhea (Torrente et al., 2002). Endoscopy of regressed cohorts demonstrated very high incidence of enterocolitis (Wakefield et al., 1998, 2002) and reflux esophagitis (Horvath et al., 1999).

Case reports suggest that gastrointestinal symptoms and behavioral regression occur at about the same time (Madsen and Vestergaard, 2004). On the basis of hundreds of clinical interviews oriented to somatic as well as behavioral changes, we (McGinnis, Audhya, and Edelson) concur with Goldberg's published observation: "Parents often report their children as having gastrointestinal symptoms that started about the same time autistic symptoms appeared" (Goldberg, 2004). Refined data for onset of gastrointestinal symptoms are not sufficiently evolved, but the collective clinical knowledge strongly suggests a triad of changes in autistic regression: (1) lost vocalization, (2) lost social skills, AND (3) gastrointestinal impairment.

9.3 TOXICANTS AS POTENTIAL TRIGGERS FOR REGRESSION IN AUTISM

It has been postulated that regression results from brain damage after birth by environmental toxicants, particularly in light of evolving evidence of gliosis and neuronal loss in autism (Kern and Jones, 2006). The increasing incidence of autism parallels progressive contamination of the environment (Grandjean and Landrigan, 2006; Lathe, 2008), and autism rates correlate with presence of toxic landfill sites (Ming et al., 2008). A preliminary epidemiological study linked the incidence of autism most strongly to the estimated environmental concentrations of cadmium and mercury (Windham et al., 2006), and another suggested that proximity to point sources of environmental mercury associates with autism (Palmer et al., 2009). Greater cumulative exposure to mercury in autism is suggested by elevated dental concentrations of mercury (Adams et al., 2007), and urinary porphyrin abnormality, which correlates with autistic symptoms (Geier et al., 2008). A possible etiological role for mercury in autism (Bernard et al., 2001) is unproven (Institute of Medicine, 2004; Nelson and Bauman, 2003).

The very timing of regression in the second year is potentially significant, because the BBB, which shields brain from blood-born toxicants, is mature in humans by about 1 year of age. Select regions of brain known as the circumventricular organs (CVO) fail to develop BBB, so they are potential portals for toxicants otherwise impeded by BBB after 1 year. The CVO are located conspicuously within or around the subcortical brainstem, defined here broadly to include medulla, pons, midbrain, and diencephalon (Figure 9.1). An extensive neural network interconnects multiple CVO and receives input from the viscera.

A CVO of particular interest, the area postrema (AP), is the so-called "emesis center" of the medulla. AP is one of the most highly vascularized regions of brain (Wislocki and Putnam, 1920), and blood flowing through its capillaries has very long residence time in comparison to other regions of brain (Gross et al., 1990). The AP is

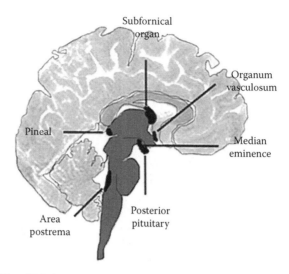

FIGURE 9.1   The CVO, in proximity to primitive brainstem (shaded), remain unprotected by BBB after its maturation in humans by about 12 months of age.

a central site of action for circulating angiotensin II (Kim et al., 2008). A rich network of axons emerges from the AP, including serotonergic connections to the pons.

AP-lesioned animals consume remarkable amounts of water (Curtis et al., 1996) or concentrated salt water (Johnson and Edwards, 1991)—an interesting observation in light of published reports of increased water consumption in autistic children (Terai et al., 1999) and an 8% (2,090/25,637) incidence of salt-craving in autistic children surveyed by ARI. Food aversions and cravings for carbohydrates and bland diets result from ablation of AP (Edwards et al., 1997), and although inadequately quantified in autism, are commonly reported by parents. Flavor aversion after cadmium exposure is reversed by dimercaptosuccinic acid (Peele et al., 1988), a chelating agent which does not cross the BBB, but which reportedly improved behavior in a number of children with autism (Geier and Geier, 2006).

AP is proximate to the dorsal motor nucleus of the vagus (DMV) and the nucleus tractus solitarius (NTS). The three structures comprise the DVC, which mediates autonomic function of the cervical, thoracic, and abdominal viscera (Figure 9.2). Ablation of the DMV blocks viscerosecretory as well as visceromotor function. The NTS receives abundant viscerosensory input via cranial nerves VII, IX, and X, integrates peripheral and central signals, and sends both sympathetic and parasympathetic efferents to the viscera. Conceivably, reported rapid improvement in children with autism after secretin infusion (Horvath et al., 1998) relates to NTS, where binding of intravenous secretin is most prominent (Yang et al., 2004).

DMV is the consistent site of initial pathology in PD, which ascends in stages to outlying brainstem and distal structures including neocortex (Figure 9.3). Not surprisingly, digestive symptoms are frequent in PD and occasionally dominate the clinical picture (Spellman and Warner, 1977). Disorders of gastrointestinal motility are prominent in PD (Cersosimo and Benarroch, 2008). The gastroesophageal sphincter is lax, and 61% of patients with PD complained of esophageal

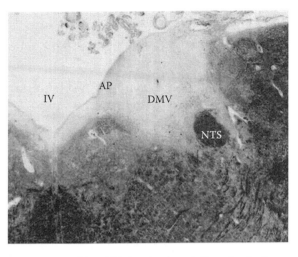

FIGURE 9.2   Cross section of luxol-blue stained medulla at level of area postrema (AP), which adjoins the dorsal motor nucleus of the vagus (DMV) and the NTS in the floor of the fourth ventricle (IV). AP lacks tight BBB and tight CSF barrier and is envisioned as key portal for neurotoxicants in autistic regression.

symptoms (Bassotti et al., 1998). Many environmental risk factors have been identified for PD (Onyango, 2008).

Years after autistic regression, reported physical changes in brain are evident in widespread areas not limited to brainstem. Plausible mechanisms exist within our model for ramifying changes after initial brainstem injury. Brainstem injury itself may disturb development of higher structures (Geva and Feldman, 2008; Tanguay and Edwards, 1982). The spread of pathology from brainstem CVO conceivably involves diffusion of toxicants or reactive inflammatory cytokines. Elevated cytokine levels in cerebrospinal fluid (CSF) of subjects with autism (Vargas et al., 2005) plausibly result from toxicant-induced production in CVO, two of which—AP and median eminence (ME)—lack tight junctions with CSF (Broadwell et al., 1983).

Experimentally, inflammatory cytokine diffuses from lateral ventricle along white matter nerve bundles of the corpus callosum, external capsule, and striatum all the way to amygdala (Vitkovic et al., 2000). Cytokine injected in striatum exacerbates excitoxicity in cortex (Lawrence et al., 1998). The pattern of inflammatory cytokine diffusion along nerve bundles suggests an anisotropic diffusion pathway in small channels located outside myelinated axons (Agnati et al., 1995).

9.4   TOXICANT ACCUMULATION AND INJURY IN CVO

As will be shown, cadmium, monosodium glutamate (MSG), and paraquat exemplify a class of neurotoxicants, which do not readily cross the BBB and which preferentially accumulate in areas of brain unprotected by BBB. The data we will discuss shows that mercury in its inorganic form poorly crosses BBB and therefore

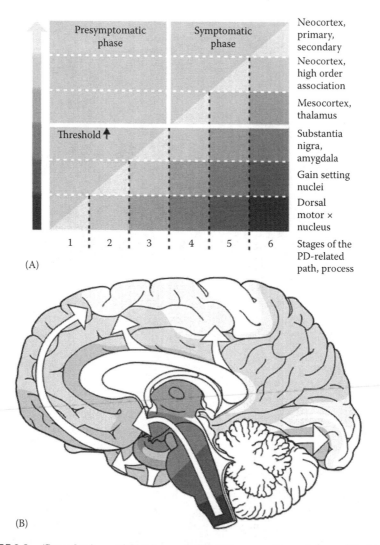

(A)

(B)

FIGURE 9.3   (See color insert following page 200.) The ascending pathology of Parkinson's disease occurs in six recognizable stages, beginning in the DMV of the medulla. Progressive shading in table (A) corresponds to the like-shaded anatomic regions represented in diagram (B). (From Braak, H. et al., *Cell. Tissue Res.*, 31, 121, 2004. With permission.)

concentrates in CVO, and also that administration of mercury in the organic form—which is commonly understood to traverse the BBB—results in accumulation of inorganic mercury in CVO, with long-term residence after remote conversion and redistribution via blood. A review of the literature will make it clear that oxidative mechanisms of cytotoxicity are prominent for each of the aforementioned toxicants.

Cadmium injected intravenously into adult rats accumulated only in regions outside the BBB, including AP and pineal, but did not appear elsewhere in the brain (Arvidson, 1986; Arvidson and Tjalve, 1986). Cadmium induces oxidative stress, histopathological damage, and increased lipid peroxidation in brain tissue (Mendez-Armenta et al., 2003; Santos et al., 2005). In rats, abnormal auditory brainstem response, cytokine elevation, and apoptosis from cadmium exposure are blocked by administration of antioxidants (Kim et al., 2008). The oxidative effect of cadmium appears to be due to inhibition of complexes II and III of the mitochondrial electron transport chain (Wang et al., 2004).

Paraquat administered subcutaneously to adult rats accumulated only in areas that lie outside the BBB, including AP and pineal (Naylor et al., 1995). Paraquat neurotoxicity, which involves increased tumor necrosis factor (TNF) alpha and increased superoxide production by microglia, is mediated by oxidative stress (Wu et al., 2005). In hepatocytes, herbicides uncouple oxidative phosphorylation, inhibit complexes II and IV, deplete glutathione (GSH), and cause mammalian cell death by inducing lipid peroxidation (Palmeira et al., 1995). Paraquat is suggested as a risk factor for PD (Wu et al., 2005; Peng et al., 2007).

MSG added to food is a common source of concentrated free glutamate (Walker and Lupien, 2000), which in excess is excitotoxic. Glutamic acid decarboxylase levels in brain are noted to be much lower in autism (Fatemi et al., 2002). MSG administered to neonatal rats resulted in widespread neuronal necrosis in the arcuate nucleus (Rascher and Mestres, 1980). Administration of MSG after 1 month of age resulted in injury to the ME—a CVO unprotected by BBB—but arcuate neurons were spared, consistent with closure of the BBB (Peruzzo et al., 2000).

Subcutaneous injections of relatively small amounts of MSG (0.1–0.5 mg/g body weight) in 7 day old mice reduced glutamic acid decarboxylase activity in hippocampus and cerebellum at 60 days (Urena-Guerrero et al., 2003). But greatest MSG toxicity was found in areas outside the BBB, particularly the ME, which receives axon terminals from the nearby arcuate nucleus and other hypothalamic secretory neurons (Meister et al., 1989).

A single subcutaneous dose of MSG to adult rats induced severe ultrastructural alterations in acetylcholine-positive AP neurons, which transport acetylcholinesterase to the NTS (Karcsu et al., 1985). Intraperitoneal administration of MSG to rats resulted in oxidative changes in CVO, including lipid peroxides, which persisted for long periods after exposure (Bawari et al., 1995; Singh et al., 2003).

As reviewed by McGinnis (2001), worrisome levels of inorganic mercury exist in domestic water supplies, carbon-burning emissions, and municipal sludge used as fertilizer—and individual inorganic mercury ingestion can be much greater than expected. Mercury cell chlor-alkali plants are used to produce many food products, including high fructose corn syrup, which may contain mercury (Dufault et al., 2009). Ingested inorganic mercury avidly binds intestine, causing inflammation at low nanomolar concentrations; fractional systemic absorption of ingested inorganic mercury is evidenced by Pink disease, a profound neurological disease in young children who ingested inorganic mercury found in teething powders (McGinnis, 2001). Autopsy reports for Pink disease include reference to vagal degeneration and "small cell" (microglial?) infiltration in the brainstem (Wyllie and Stern, 1931).

By intramuscular injection, inorganic mercury accumulated largely in AP and brainstem motor nuclei (Arvidson, 1992), and was prominent in AP 16 days after injection (Nordberg and Sereniu, 1969). Inorganic mercury added to drinking water of rats concentrated in the motor nuclei of brainstem and deep nuclei of cerebellum (Moller-Madsen and Danscher, 1986).

Organic mercury, as found in fish and as preservative in some vaccines (Poling 2008), passes the BBB readily. Most organic mercury is converted to inorganic mercury for excretion in feces, but some recirculates to increase inorganic mercury concentration in blood (Havarinasab et al., 2007). Once in the brain, inorganic mercury persists for years (Vahter et al., 1994). It is the inorganic form which associates with immune stimulation (Havarinasab et al., 2007) and increased microglia in brain (Geier and Geier, 2007). Notably, amalgam removal decreased plasma and red-cell inorganic mercury levels by 73% (Halbach et al., 2008).

The absence of BBB increases accumulation of inorganic mercury during and after chronic methyl mercury (organic) exposure. Methyl mercury was administered orally for 18 months to adult female primates, and mercury levels were measured in six regions of brain, including pituitary, a CVO lacking BBB. Inorganic mercury concentrations increased on average in the six areas 30-fold at 6 months and 60-fold at 18 months, but by far the highest concentrations of mercury—largely inorganic— were achieved in pituitary. In animals in which methyl mercury was discontinued at 6 months, inorganic levels continued to climb in the pituitary—doubling between 6 and 12 months—but not in regions with BBB. Mercury in control animals was undetectable in most regions, but appeared higher in pituitary. One or two primates in each exposure group had distinctly higher or lower fractions of inorganic mercury across brain regions, assumed secondary to individual variations in demethylation (Vahter et al., 1994).

9.5 FINDINGS CONSISTENT WITH BRAINSTEM PATHOLOGY IN AUTISM

On the basis of clinical observations consistent with pathology of the reticular formation, Rimland proposed brainstem—in spite of its phylogenic antiquity—as site of primary pathology in autism (Rimland, 1964). It has been postulated that inherent developmental flexibility of the serotonergic system, which richly endows the brainstem, might help explain the varied clinical presentation of autism (Cordes, 2005). A detailed psychobiological model has evolved to explain dysregulated social behavior as a consequence of disturbed vagal messenging (Porges et al., 1996). Electroencephalographic studies suggested centrencephalic rather than circumscribed telencephalic damage in autism (Gilberg and Schaumann, 1983). Against this conceptual background, we present findings in autism that are consistent with brainstem pathology, including abnormality of specific CVO.

9.5.1 CLINICAL AND ELECTROPHYSIOLOGICAL BRAINSTEM FINDINGS IN AUTISM

Decreased or absent postrotational nystagmus, and lack of dizziness or nausea after spinning suggested brainstem dysfunction in autism (Ornitz, 1983). Half (15,306/30,676) of the autistic subjects in the ARI survey often or sometimes engaged in "whirling like a top." Abnormal auditory brainstem response in autism also suggests brainstem dysfunction (Klin, 1993; Kwon et al., 2007).

Increased heart-rate variability, failure to habituate to respiratory response, and enhancement of vascular reaction to visual input were interpreted by early autism investigators as evidence of altered function of the reticular formation (Bonvallet and Allen, 1963), which is distributed extensively within the brainstem. More recently, abnormal heart rate, blood pressure, and respiratory activity during task performance were ascribed to abnormal vagal tone (Althaus et al., 2004). Impaired cardiac barore-flex and depressed vagal tone more specifically implicates medullary structures (Ming et al., 2005). Baroreflex is mediated by afferents from the glossopharyngeal nerve IX, which synapse in the NTS, from which excitatory signals to the DMV are relayed via the vagus to slow heart rate.

9.5.2 ABNORMAL BRAINSTEM MORPHOLOGY

Magnetic resonance imaging (MRI) demonstrated hypoplastic brainstem (Courchesne, 1997), smaller midbrain and medulla (Hashimoto et al., 1993), and lesser brainstem gray-matter volume (Jou et al., 2008) in autism. In a classical 1985 survey of the entire brain of an autistic adult, Bauman and Kemper (1985) reported unusual packing density and arborization of neurons of the inferior olive, imme-diately adjacent to DVC. A follow-up series of six brains revealed enlargement of inferior olivary neurons in the younger subjects, and unusually diminished size in adults. Peripheral clustering of the inferior olivary neurons was observed in five of six subjects (Kemper and Bauman, 1993).

Bailey reported variable developmental abnormalities in brainstems of six autistic subjects. Description of a 4 year old male from this cohort is illustrative:

> ... medulla oblongata was large but the pyramids were relatively small. There was mild widening of the sulci of the superior cerebellar vermis...apparent reduplication of the medial accessory olive, and multiple small bilateral groups of ectopic neurons lay lateral to the olives in the inferior cerebellar peduncles. An aberrant tract was present in both sides of the pontine tegmentum...midbrain was unusually small and the periaqueductal grey matter and raphe nuclei appeared disproportionately large... (Bailey et al., 1998).

Two subjects with autistic behaviors had numerous swollen axon terminals ("spheroids") in various motor and sensory nuclei and reticular formation of the medulla, as well as hypothalamus, dorsomedial thalamus, hippocampus, and cere-bral cortex (Weidenheim et al., 2001). Abnormal morphology was evident in neurons of the superior olivary nucleus of the caudal pons in five autistic subjects (Kulesza and Mangunay, 2008).

9.5.3 BIOCHEMICAL ABNORMALITIES IN AUTISM

Melatonin is produced only by a CVO (the pineal). Blood levels of melatonin (Kulman et al., 2000; Nir et al., 1995) and its metabolite (Tordjman et al., 2005) are depressed in autism, and none of 24 autistic subjects examined in one study demon-strated normal circadian variations in melatonin (Kulman et al., 2000). Abnormal melatonin production potentially disrupts neurodevelopment by affecting neuroplas-ticity (Baydas et al., 2002; Yun et al., 2004).

Melatonin is an efficient antioxidant (Allegra et al., 2003), which directly scavenges free radicals (Reiter et al., 2002), stimulates production of antioxidant enzymes (Kotler et al., 1998), and increases activity of antioxidant enzymes (Reiter et al., 1998). Unlike other endogenous antioxidants, melatonin easily crosses BBB (Gupta et al., 2003). Melatonin administration reduced neural lipid peroxidation and levels of degraded glial fibrillar acidic protein in hippocampus, cortex, and cerebellum in experimentally stressed rats (Baydas et al., 2002). In models of oxidative stress—including exposure to cadmium, paraquat, and kainic acid—melatonin blocks lipid peroxidation (Reiter et al., 1998). Melatonin protects against gut ulceration in stressed animals by scavenging free radicals and reducing oxidative damage (Bandyopadhyay et al., 2002).

Groups of autistic children had significantly lower plasma levels of oxytocin (Green et al, 2001; Modahl et al., 1998), failure to demonstrate normal longitudinal increases in oxytocin blood levels (Modahl et al., 1998), and predominance of the nonamidated, physiologically inactive form of oxytocin (Green et al., 2001). Oxytocin synthesis and storage are potentially sensitive to toxicants because oxytocin from synthetic hypothalamic nuclei is transported for storage in the posterior pituitary (no BBB) via axons, which pass through the ME (no BBB) (Larsen et al., 1991).

Patterns of social behavior, communications, and rituals in autism may attribute to altered oxytocin (Carter et al., 1992; Insel, 1997; Insel and Hulihan, 1995; Insel et al., 1999). Deficits in social investigation and memory in oxytocin–knockout mice were rescued by intraventricular administration of oxytocin (Ferguson et al., 2000). Oxytocin infusion also reduced repetitive behaviors in autism (Hollander et al., 2003). Oxytocin is a potent antioxidant at nanomolar concentrations and prevents peroxidation of brain membranes (Moosmann and Behl, 2002).

9.5.4 FEATURES OF REGRESSION IN AUTISM

The three primary somatobehavioral features of regression are explicable on the basis of neurotoxicant-induced impairment of the DVC, and variation in clinical presentation of these features may result from differential degrees of impairment in these minute brainstem structures.

It is widely appreciated that parasympathetic visceromotor fibers of the vagus that originate in the DMV stimulate normal peristalsis, gastroesophogeal sphincter contraction, and secretory function in the gut. It follows that objective signs of constipation and reflux in most regressed subjects, as presented earlier, are consistent with impaired visceromotor signals from the brainstem.

Duodenal biopsies from regressed subjects frequently demonstrated enlarged Paneth's cells full of secretory granules (Horvath et al., 1999) (Figure 9.4). Since section of the vagus nerve blocks release of Paneth's cell granulations (Eletskii et al., 1984), the finding in autism is consistent with impaired visceromotor signals from brainstem. Interestingly, exposure of primates to mercury results in enlarged Paneth's cells full of secretory granules (Chen et al., 1983).

It should be noted that diarrhea—including onset of diarrhea in the regressive period—is prominent in some autistic children. Plausible explanations exist within the model. Overflow diarrhea from stasis proximal to impacted stool is not uncommonly reported by clinicians. Poor vagal tone potentially results in a net softening

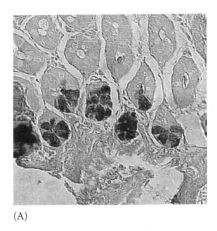
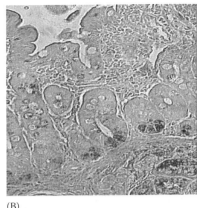

(A)   (B)

FIGURE 9.4   (See color insert following page 200.) Enlargement of Paneth's cells, as indicated by dark staining of secretory granules, was a frequent finding in a series of duodenal biopsies from children with regressed autism (A), as compared to non-autistic controls (B). (Photographs courtesy of Karoly Horvath MD, PhD, Professor of Pediatrics, Thomas Jefferson University, Philadelphia, PA.)

effect on stool if reduction in secretory function results in microbial overgrowth or malabsorption. Alternatively, hypermotility could result from toxicant-induced disinhibition of sympathetic efferents from the NTS.

Impaired vagal signaling is considered sufficient basis for loss of vocalizations during the early stage of speech development. The complex process of phonation— word or nonword—is mediated by vagal motor efferents from DMV to the intrinsic and extrinsic muscles of the larynx, posterior tongue, and tensor palati (the latter is noted to affect opening of the eustachian tube). Importantly, vagal afferents to NTS coordinate the position and shape of the vocal folds and muscles of phonation. "Tone of voice" differences in autism (Paul et al., 2005) are consistent with vagal alteration, which associates with altered pitch (Shaffer et al., 2005).

The model essentially states that altered mechanics of vocalization—dysarthria— can underlie loss of vocalization in autistic regression. The existence of complex cognitive impairments in older autistic subjects does not contradict brainstem-mediated loss of vocalizations, because cognitive impairments in older subjects could result from later changes in brain. The proposed vagal dysarthria should not be confused with classical "motor apraxia of speech," which includes additional glossal and facial signs not seen in autism. The observation of marked improvement in communication with an electronic speech-generating device (Thunberg et al., 2007) is more consistent with brainstem-mediated vocalization deficit than higher cognitive incapacity in some older autistic children. Parents in the ARI survey report that at age 3–5 years, 20% of children with autism (5,880/31,109) were significantly better at correctly pointing to named objects than in saying the names of the same objects.

Frank dysarthria was reported in 12% (3/25) of a cohort of autistic children with identifiable mitochondrial abnormalities (Weissman et al., 2008). Specific data from the ARI parent survey also are consistent with altered mechanical vocalization: of children whose onset of autistic symptoms occurred after 1 year of age, 17% (4,141/23,685) reportedly started talking normally, then had talk replaced by whispering for at least 1 week. Of this subgroup, 1771 children deteriorated to loss of all whispering as well as loss of talking, and another 679 children continued whispering long-term.

Altered function of NTS is a plausible mechanism for loss of social function, because NTS projects secondarily to limbic and cortical areas known to mediate social behavior, arousal, mood, emotion, anxiety, seizure activity, and pain perception (Marvel et al., 2004; Nemeroff et al., 2006). Vagal nerve stimulation for depression is thought to act via innervation of the NTS (Nemeroff et al., 2006), and vagal nerve stimulation for seizure control has been reported to improve significantly varied autistic behaviors (Murphy et al., 2000). As discussed earlier, concurrent CVO-mediated changes in oxytocin may contribute to loss of social skills as well.

It is observed that: (1) social regression often precedes language regression (Goldberg et al., 2003), (2) social regression may be unaccompanied by language regression (Goldberg et al., 2003; Lord et al., 2004), and (3) language regression nearly always is accompanied by social regression (Goldberg et al., 2003; Lord et al., 2004). A cogent explanation for these variations exists within the detailed anatomy of the DVC. NTS predictably is more vulnerable to blood-born toxicants than DMV, because in its caudal portion, the dorsal aspect of NTS is unprotected by BBB (Gross et al., 1990). Although the distances are not great, toxicants must enter the DMV by diffusion from AP (and NTS) entry points.

The model's site specificity allows different toxicants independently to provoke regression by one-time or cumulative insult. Likewise, different toxicants may act in combination or sequentially on CVO to exceed the neurophysiological threshold for regression. The model does not imply entirely normal biochemistry or development of the brainstem or other parts of the brain prior to regression, and in fact encourages consideration of preexisting conditions, which potentially affect the regressive threshold.

In this context, it is interesting that the vulnerable period for thalidomide exposure as risk factor for autism (20–24 days) corresponds to the timing of formation of the medullary motor nuclei (Rodier et al., 1997). Intriguing too is decreased autonomic activation of heart rate (and brainstem auditory evoked potentials) in Faroes Island children as a function of cord-blood levels of mercury (Grandjean et al., 2004). Earlier weakening or maldevelopment of brainstem structures—including influences, which are not modulated directly by BBB—conceivably potentiate regression triggered by toxicant effects on brainstem.

A summary of objective findings in autism, which are consistent with brainstem abnormality or abnormality of brainstem-proximate CVO, is presented in Table 9.1.

9.5.5 OXIDATIVE MECHANISMS

The mechanisms of relevant toxicants are substantially oxidative, so it is appropriate to consider oxidative stress in the context of the proposed model. Greater oxidative stress in blood and urine (Chauhan and Chauhan, 2006; Chauhan et al., 2008;

TABLE 9.1
Reported Findings in Autism, Which Are Consistent with Brainstem Abnormality or Consistent with Abnormality of CVO Found within or Proximate to the Brainstem

Studies	References
Clinical observations	
Excessive thirst	Terai et al. (1999)
Salt-craving and flavor-aversion	ARI parent survey
Tone-of-voice alterations	Paul et al. (2005)
Talk → whisper	ARI parent survey
Electrical speech generation	Thunber et al. (2007)
Secretin effect	Horvath et al. (1998)
Altered postrotatory response	Ornitz (1983)
Cardiac baroreflex	Ming et al. (2005)
Heart rate, respiratory and vascular	Althaus et al. (2004), Bonvallet and Allen (1963)
Electrical studies	
Auditory brainstem response	Klin (1993), Kwon et al. (2007)
Centrencephalic electroencephalograms	Gilberg and Schaumann (1983)
Decreased cardiac parasympathetic tone	Ming et al. (2005)
Vagal nerve stimulation	Murphy et al. (2000)
Magnetic resonance imaging	
Smaller brainstem	Courchesne (1997)
Smaller medulla and midbrain	Hashimoto et al. (1993)
Decreased brainstem gray matter	Jou et al. (2008)
Radiographic studies	
Fecal loading in 100% of regressed cohort	Torrente et al. (2002)
Fecal loading in >50% of mixed cohort	Afzal et al. (2003)
Endoscopic studies	
Esophageal reflux 67% of regressed cohort	Horvath et al. (1999)
Microscopic studies	
Neuronal morphology/clustering inf. olives	Kemper and Bauman (1993)
Neuronal morphology superior olives	Kulesza and Mangunay (2008)
Ectopic neurons and aberrant tracts	Bailey et al. (1998)
Swollen axon terminals in medullary nuclei	Weidenheim et al. (2001)
Paneth's cells enlarged with granules	Horvath et al. (1999)
Biochemical studies	
Abnormal oxytocin production	Green et al. (2001), Modahl et al. (1998)
Abnormal melatonin production	Kulman et al. (2000), Nir et al. (1995), Tordjman et al. (2005)

McGinnis, 2004; Suh et al., 2008; Yao et al., 2006) and greater oxidative modification of hippocampus (Evans et al., 2008), cerebral cortex (Evans et al., 2008; Lopez-Hurtado and Prieto, 2008), and cerebellum (Sajdel-Sulkowska et al., 2008) exists in children already diagnosed with autism. Gastrointestinal inflammation, emotional stress associated with noncommunication, sleep disturbance, and lower production of melatonin and oxytocin may contribute variably to greater oxidative stress after regression.

There is some support—elevated brain-derived neurotrophic factor (BDNF) in cord blood, greater maternal stress during gestation, more perinatal complications—for the suggestion that oxidative stress is heightened prior to regression (McGinnis, 2004, 2007). If oxidative stress were higher in brain prior to regression, then correspondingly lower antioxidant protection in brain would be expected to influence thresholds for brainstem injury by toxicants. Greater peripheral oxidative stress alone plausibly lowers the threshold for CVO-mediated regression, because the cholinergic—especially, muscarinic—nervous system is sensitive to oxidative stress (McGinnis, 2004), and extracranial vagal parasympathetics are exclusively cholinergic.

Cholinergic receptors are inhibited preferentially by oxidants (De Sarno and Pope, 1998), and numbers of cholinergic receptors are reduced under conditions of oxidative stress (Gajewski et al., 1988). Cholinergic receptor activity measured in basal forebrain and parietal cortex was lower in autism (Perry et al., 2001), and it has been suggested that cerebral hypoperfusion in autism results from muscarinic inhibition (McGinnis, 2004). The cholinergic system is essential for brain development, acting as modulator of neuronal proliferation, migration, and differentiation (Roda et al., 2008).

We retrospectively compared acetylcholine (ACh) levels in plasma and CSF from children aged 3–15 who were identifiable as autistic or nonautistic. Mean plasma ACh was much lower in autistic children (192 ± 36 ng/L; $n=94$) than in nonautistic children (464 ± 85 ng/L; $n=66$). Mean ACh in CSF also was lower in an autistic cohort (941 ± 202 ng/L; $n=16$) than a nonautistic cohort (1558 ± 510 ng/L; $n=8$). It is not known whether these levels reflect the state of neurological transmission in autism. Chronic exposure of animals to cadmium or methyl mercury is noted to lower ACh in brain (Hrdina et al., 1976), but existence of any such relationship in autism is speculative.

9.5.6 INFLAMMATORY MECHANISMS IN AUTISM

Microglia are resident immune cells in the brain, which normally influence late embryonic and postnatal brain development by exerting an important "pruning effect." Microglia also release potentially cytotoxic inflammatory cytokines and oxidative factors in response to toxicants or infections. Microglial activation is assumed to relate to the pathogenesis of PD and is associated with neuronal cell loss in many toxic exposures (Mangano and Hayley, 2009). An increase in microglia is seen after exposure to inorganic mercury (Charleston et al., 1994), and in association with inorganic mercury accumulation after organic mercury exposure (Vahter et al., 1994).

Microglial activation in autism is evidenced by greater inflammatory cytokines in CSF and microscopic changes in examined areas of brain (cerebral cortex, cingulate gyrus, cerebellum) (Vargas et al., 2005). As yet, there is no clear understanding of when neuroinflammation begins in autism, how neuroinflammation varies longitudinally, or how variable patterns might reflect etiologies.

Many xenobiotics, including bacterial lipopolysaccharide (LPS), stimulate peripheral mononuclear cells and brain microglia to increase production of TNF, which plays a central role in the cascade of potentially cytotoxic factors in the immune response. In cell cultures, ACh blocks TNF-induced cell activation (Saeed et al., 2005). In PD, TNF is increased in CSF and brain (McCoy et al., 2006). TNF in CSF was also elevated in two autistic cohorts, one exclusively comprised of regressed subjects (Chez et al., 2007); the other with 10 of 12 regressed (Zimmerman et al., 2005). High CSF/blood ratios of TNF, which poorly transits the BBB, implies increased TNF production in the brain, at least in the regressive subgroup (Chez et al., 2007).

LPS poorly transits the BBB. Systemic administration of LPS to adult animals results in immediate and robust TNF production in brain, detectable in neuronal cell bodies, but only at CVO or immediately adjacent structures, and most intensely at the AP and ME. LPS-induced TNF expression in the NTS was modest at 1.5 h, and marked by 18 h. At the same intervals, TNF was absent initially in DMV, then present at 18 h. TNF reached other nuclei, such as hypoglossal IX, by 18 h (Breder et al., 1994). Another study administered LPS and initially found gene encoding for TNF only in CVO, followed by a migratory pattern of TNF-positive cells around CVO at three hours, and finally a ubiquitous presence of TNF-positive cells throughout the brain at 6 h (Nadeau and Rivest, 1999).

Whether TNF plays a significant role in the pathogenesis of autism—as suspected in PD on the basis of animal models (McCoy et al., 2006)—is unproven. Within our model, it is possible that toxicant-induced TNF production by CVO (especially AP and ME, which lack tight barriers to CSF) at time of regression is sufficient basis for large increases in TNF and other inflammatory cytokines in CSF. The toxicants used as examples in our model certainly stimulate TNF production.

Cadmium has been regarded as one of the "inflammation-related xenobiotics" because low concentrations potently stimulate inflammatory cytokines, including TNF, in hepatocytes (Souza et al., 2004). Exposure of neonatal rats provides clear evidence that MSG increases TNF in brain unprotected by BBB, and that the increase is associated with neuronal death, possibly via apoptosis (Chaparro-Huerta et al., 2002). Paraquat-induced TNF has been implicated in pathogenesis of lung disease, and production of TNF in response to LPS by peripheral monocytes is increased by paraquat up to 18-fold (Erroi et al., 1992). An increase of the same order of magnitude in TNF upregulation in response to LPS was reported in peripheral monocytes of a subgroup of autistic children (Jyonouchi et al., 2001), but the finding has not been examined in the context of toxicant exposure.

TNF-alpha actions on AP and NTS substantially disrupt autonomic control of the gut. For instance, by modulating release of glutamate by primary vagal afferents to the NTS, TNF-alpha in animal experiments produced extreme gastric stasis (Hermann and Rogers, 2008). Interestingly, work with experimental colitis suggests that intestinal inflammation may affect adversely survival and function of DMV neurons. Exposure of cultured DMV neurons to TNF diminished cell proliferation, increased apoptosis, and altered calcium response to glutamate (Ammori et al., 2008). Besides endogenous inflammatory factors, viruses also easily may enter at CVO (Banks, 2000).

9.6 FUTURE RESEARCH

Within the current technology, it may be possible to identify brainstem lesions, which can account for regression and other deficits observed in autism. Special attention to thin, unmyelinated "C-fibers" is warranted, since these comprise afferents to NTS and efferents from the DMV, which may be highly sensitive to toxicant exposure. Direct examination of the vagus nerve is needed to rule out extracranial neuropathy in autism, and afford inference about status of the DMV and NTS. When possible, identification of regressed subgroups may afford a useful methodology.

Physical detection of toxicants in brain—especially CVO and brainstem—of subjects with autism is indicated. While tissue half-lives and combined toxicity might obscure etiology in tissue-concentration studies, significant findings in even a subset of the autistic population could be enormously important.

Oxidative residuals of neurotoxicity may be detectable in relevant areas of brain when toxins are not. Lipofuscin, a relatively stable matrix of oxidized lipid and cross-linked protein, was elevated in cerebral cortex in autism (Lopez-Hurtado and Prieto, 2008), suggesting a need for complete lipofuscin mapping. Examination of lipofuscin itself for accumulation of toxicants is an interesting possibility (Opitz et al., 1996). Carboxyethyl pyrrole (CEP) is a promising marker for axonal oxidation in autism (Evans et al., 2008). Distribution of oxidative markers in animal brain after exposures to toxicants may provide a valuable context for interpretation of findings in brain of autistic subjects.

Regional differences in distribution of receptors, inflammatory markers, and oxidative modification are interpretable from the toxicological perspective. For instance, while mercury levels in medulla from whales were considered only mildly elevated in relation to estimated lowest-observable-adverse-effect levels, a significant correlation existed between total mercury concentration and N-methyl-D-aspartate (NMDA) receptor levels (Basu et al., 2009). TNF levels in brainstem structures potentially reflect effects of toxicants. A preliminary study found a significant correlation between concentrations of mercury and 3-nitrotyrosine in cerebellum from subjects with autism (Sajdel-Sulkowska et al., 2008). Suspicion of toxicants as triggers in autism will stimulate a host of creative research methodologies.

REFERENCES

Adams, J.B., Romdalvik, J., Ramanujam, V.M., and Legator, M.S. 2007. Mercury, lead, and zinc in baby teeth of children with autism versus controls. *J. Toxicol. Environ. Health A.* 70:1046–1051.

Afzal, N., Murch, S., Thirrupathy, K., Berger, L., Fagbemi, A., and Heuschkel, R. 2003. Constipation with acquired megarectum in children with autism. *Pediatrics* 112:939–942.

Agnati, L.F., Zoli, M., Stromberg, I., and Fuxe, K. 1995. Intercellular communication in the brain: Wiring versus volume transmission. *Neuroscience* 69:711–726.

Allegra, M., Reiter, R.J., Tan, D.X., Gentile, C., Tesoriere, L., and Livrea, M.A. 2003. The chemistry of melatonin's interaction with reactive species. *J. Pineal Res.* 34:1–10.

Althaus, M., Van Roon, S.M., Lambertus, Mulder, L.J.M., Mulder, G., Aarnoudse, C.C., and Minderaa, R.B. (2004). Autonomic response patterns observed during the performance of an attention-demanding task in two groups of children with autistic-type difficulties in social adjustment. *Psychophysiology* 41:893–904.

Ammori, J.B., Zhang, W.Z., Li, J.Y., Chai, B.X., and Mulholland, M.W. 2008. Effect of intestinal inflammation on neuronal survival and function in the dorsal motor nucleus of the vagus. *Surgery* 144:149–158.

Arvidson, B. 1986. Autoradiographic localization of cadmium in the rat brain. *Neurotoxicology* 7:89–96.

Arvidson, B. 1992. Accumulation of inorganic mercury in lower motoneurons of mice. *Neurotoxicology* 13:277–80.

Arvidson, B. and Tjalve, H. 1986. Distribution of 109Cd in the nervous system of rats after intravenous injection. *Acta Neuropathol.* 69:111–116.

Bailey, A., Luthert, P., Dean, A., Harding, B., Janota, I., Montgomery, M., Rutter, M., and Lantos, P. 1998. A clinicopathological study of autism. *Brain* 121:889–905.

Bandyopadhyay, D., Biswas, K., Bhattacharyya, M., Reiter, R.J., and Banerjee, R.K. 2002. Involvement of reactive oxygen species in gastric ulceration: Protection by melatonin. *Indian J. Exp. Biol.* 2002:693–705.

Banks, W.A. 2000. Protector, prey and perpetrator: The pathophysiology of the blood–brain barrier in neuroAIDS. *NeuroAIDS* 3:1–5.

Bassotti, G., Germani, U., Pagliaricci, S., Plesa, A., Giulietti, O., Mannarino, E., and Morelli, A. 1998. Esophageal manometric abnormalities in Parkinson's disease. *Dysphagia* 13:28–31.

Basu, N., Scheuhammer, A.M., Sonne, C., Letcher, R.J., Born, E.W., and Dietz, R. 2009. Is dietary mercury of toxicological concern to wild polar bears (*Ursus maritimus*)? *Environ. Toxicol. Chem.* 28:133–140.

Bauman, M. and Kemper, T.L. 1985. Histoanatomic observations of the brain in early infantile autism. *Neurology* 35:866–874.

Bawari, M., Babu, G.N., Ali, M.M., and Misra, U.K. 1995. Effect of neonatal monosodium glutamate on lipid peroxidation in adult rat brain. *Neuroreport* 6:650–652.

Baydas, G., Nedzvetsky, V.S., Nerush, P.A., Krichenko, S.V., Demchenko, H.M., and Reiter, R.J. 2002. A novel role for melatonin: Regulation of the expression of cell adhesion molecules in the rat hippocampus and cortex. *Neurosci. Lett.* 326:109–112.

Bernard, S., Enayati, A., Redwood, L., Roger, H., and Binstock, T. 2001. Autism: A novel form of mercury poisoning. *Med. Hypotheses* 56:462–471.

Bonvallet, M. and Allen, M.B. 1963. Prolonged spontaneous and evoked reticular activation following discreet bulbar lesions. *Electroencephal. Clin. Neurophysiol.* 15:969–988.

Braak, H., Ghebremedhin, E., Rub, U., Bratzke, H., and Del Tredici, K., 2004. Stages in the development of Parkinson's related pathology. *Cell. Tissue Res.* 31:121–134.

Breder, C.D., Hazuka, C., Ghayur, T., Klug, C., Huginin, M., Yasuda, K., Teng, M., and Saper, C.B. 1994. Regional induction of tumor necrosis factor alpha expression in the mouse brain after systemic lipopolysaccharide administration. *Proc. Natl. Acad. Sci. U.S.A.* 91:11393–11397.

Broadwell, R.D., Balin, B.J., Salcman, M., and Kaplan, R.S. 1983. Brain–blood barrier? Yes and no. *Proc. Natl. Acad. Sci. U.S.A.* 80:7352–7356.

Carter, C.S., Williams, J.R., Witt, D.M., and Insel, T.R. 1992. Oxytocin and social bonding. *Ann. N.Y. Acad. Sci.* 652:204–211.

Cersosimo, M.G. and Benarroch, E.E. 2008. Neural control of the gastrointestinal tract: Implications for Parkinson disease. *Mov. Disord.* 23:1065–1075.

Chaparro-Huerta, V., Rivera-Cervantes, M.C., Torres-Mendoza, B.M., and Beas-Zarate, C. 2002. Neuronal death and tumor necrosis factor-alpha response to glutamate-induced excitotoxicity in the cerebral cortex of neonatal rats. *Neurosci. Lett.* 333:95–98.

Charleston, J.S., Bolender, R.P., Mottet, N.K., Body, R.L., Vahter, M.E., and Burbacher, T.M. 1994. Increases in the number of reactive glia in the visual cortex of *Macaca fascicularis* following subclinical long-term methylmercury exposure. *Toxicol. Appl. Pharmacol.* 129:196–206.

Chauhan, A. and Chauhan, V. 2006. Oxidative stress in autism. *Pathophysiology* 13:171–181.

Chauhan, A., Sheikh, A.M., and Chauhan, V. 2008. Increased copper-mediated oxidation of membrane phosphatidylethanolamine in autism. *Am. J. Biochem. Biotechnol. (Special Issue on Autism Spectrum Disorders)* 4:101–104.

Chen, W., Body, R.L., and Mottet, N.K. 1983. Biochemical and morphological studies of monkeys chronically exposed to methylmercury. *J. Toxicol. Environ. Health* 12:407–416.

Chez, M.G., Dowling, T., Patel, P.B., Khanna, P., and Kominsky, M. 2007. Elevation of tumor necrosis factor-alpha in cerebrospinal fluid of autistic children. *Pediatr. Neurol.* 36:361–365.

Cordes, S.P. 2005. Molecular genetics of the early development of hindbrain serotonergic neurons. *Clin. Genet.* 68:487–494.

Courchesne, E. 1997. Brainstem, cerebellar and limbic neuroanatomical abnormalities in autism. *Curr. Opin. Neurobiol.* 7:269–278.

Curtis, K.S., Verbalis, J.G., and Stricker, E.M. 1996. Area postrema lesions in rats appear to disrupt rapid feedback inhibition of fluid intake. *Brain Res.* 726:31–38.

Davidovitch, M., Glick, L., Holtzman, G., Tirosh, E., and Safir, M.P. 2000. Developmental regression in autism: Maternal perception. *J Autism Dev. Disord.* 30:113–119.

De Sarno, P. and Pope, R.S. 1998. Phosphoinositide hydrolysis activated by muscarinic or glutamatergic, but not adrenergic, receptors is impaired in ApoE-deficient mice and by hydrogen peroxide and peroxynitrite. *Exp. Neurol.* 152:123–128.

Dufault, R., LeBlanc, B., Schnoll, R., Cornett, C., Schweitzer, L., Wallinga, D., Hightower, J., Patrick, L., and Lukiw, W.J. (2009). Mercury from chlor-alkali plants: Measured concentrations in food product sugar. *Environ. Health* 8:2.

Edwards, G.L., White, B.D., He, B., Dean, R.G., and Martin, R.J. 1997. Elevated hypothalamic neuropeptide Y levels in rats with dorsomedial hindbrain lesions. *Brain Res.* 755:84–90.

Eletskii, I., Kulikov, O.V., and Tsibulevskii, A. 1984. Reactions of Paneth cells of the rat jejunum to section of the vagus nerves (ultrastructural analysis). *Arkh. Anat. Gistol. Embriol.* 86:73–79.

Erroi, A., Bianchi, M., and Ghezzi, P. 1992. The pneumotoxicant paraquat potentiates IL-1 and TNF production by human mononuclear cells. *Agents Actions* 36:66–69.

Evans, T.A., Siedlak, S.L., Lu, L., Fu, X., Wang, Z., McGinnis, W.R., Fakhoury, E., Castellani, R.J., Hazen, S.L., Walsh, W.J., Lewis, A.T., Salomon, R.G., Smith, M.A., Perry, G., and Zhu, X. 2008. The autistic phenotype exhibits a remarkably localized modification of brain protein by products of free radical-induced lipid oxidation. *Am. J. Biochem. Biotechnol. (Special Issue on Autism Spectrum Disorders)* 4:61–72.

Fatemi, S.H., Halt, A.R., Stary, J.M., Kanodia, R., Schulz, S.C., and Realmuto, G.R. 2002. Glutamic acid decarboxylase 65 and 67 kDa proteins are reduced in autistic parietal and cerebellar cortices. *Biol. Psychiatry* 52:805–810.

Ferguson, J.N., Young, L.J., Hearn, E.F., Matzuk, M.M., Insel, T.R., and Winslow, J.T. 2000. Social amnesia in mice lacking the oxytocin gene. *Nat. Genet.* 25:284–288.

Gajewski, M., Laskowska-Bozek, H., Orlewski, P., Maslinski, S., and Ryzewski, J. 1988. Influence of lipid peroxidation and hydrogen peroxide on muscarinic cholinergic receptors and ATP level in rat myocytes and lymphocytes. *Int. J. Tissue React.* 10:281–290.

Geier, D.A. and Geier, M.R. 2007. A case series of children with apparent mercury toxic encephalopathies manifesting with clinical symptoms of regressive autistic disorders. *J. Toxicol. Environ. Health A.* 70:837–851.

Geier, D.A., Kern, J.K., Garver, C.R., Adams, J.B., Audhya, T., Nataf, R., and Geier, M.R. (2008). Biomarkers of environmental toxicity and susceptibility in autism. *J. Neurol. Sci.* 280:101–118.

Geva, R. and Feldman, R. 2008. A neurobiological model for the effects of early brainstem functioning on the development of behavior and emotion regulation in infants: Implications for prenatal and perinatal risk. *J. Child Psychol. Psychiatry* 49:1031–1041.

Gilberg, C. and Schaumann, H. 1983. Epilepsy presenting as infantile autism? Two case studies. *Neuropediatrics* 14:206–212.

Goldberg, E.A. 2004. The link between gastroenterology and autism. *Gastroenterol. Nurs.* 27:16–19.

Goldberg, W.A., Osann, K., Filipek, P.A., Laulhere, T., Jarvis, K., Modahl, C., Flodman, P., and Spence, M.A. 2003. Language and other regression: Assessment and timing. *J. Autism Dev. Disord.* 33:607–616.

Grandjean, P. and Landrigan, P.J. 2006. Developmental neurotoxicity of industrial chemicals. *Lancet* 368:2167–2178.

Grandjean, P., Murata, K., Budtz-Jorgensen, E., and Weihe, P. 2004. Cardiac autonomic activity in methylmercury neurotoxicity: 14-year follow-up of a Faroese birth cohort. *J. Pediatr.* 144:169–176.

Green, L., Fein, D., Modahl, C., Feinstein, C., Waterhouse, L., and Morris, M. 2001. Oxytocin and autistic disorder: Alterations in peptide forms. *Biol. Psychiatry* 50:609–613.

Gross, P.M., Wall, K.M., Pang, J.J., Shaver, S.W., and Wainman, D.S. 1990. Microvascular specializations promoting rapid interstitial solute dispersion in nucleus tractus solitarius. *Am. J. Physiol.* 259:1131–1138.

Gupta, Y.K., Gupta, M., and Kohli, K. 2003. Neuroprotective role of melatonin in oxidative stress vulnerable brain. *Indian J. Physiol. Pharmacol.* 47:373–386.

Halbach, S., Vogt, S., Kohler, W., Felgenhauer, N., Weizl, G., Kremers, L., Silker, T., and Melchart, D. 2008. Blood and urine mercury levels in adult amalgam patients of a randomized controlled trial: Interaction of Hg species in erythrocytes. *Environ. Res.* 107:69–78.

Hansen, R.L., Ozonoff, S., Krakowiak, P., Angkustsiri, K., Jones, C., Deprey, L.J., Le, D.N., Croen, L.A., and Hertz-Picciotto, I. 2008. Regression in autism: Prevalence and associated factors in the CHARGE Study. *Ambul. Pediatr.* 8:25–31.

Hashimoto, T., Tayama, M., Miyazaki, M., Murakawa, K., Shimakawa, S., Yoneda, Y., and Kuroda, Y. 1993. Brainstem involvement in high functioning autistic children. *Acta Neurol. Scand.* 88:123–128.

Havarinasab, X., Bjorn, E., Nielsen, J.B., and Hultman, P. 2007. Mercury species in lymphoid and non-lymphoid tissues after exposure to methyl mercury: Correlation with autoimmune parameters during and after treatment in susceptible mice. *Toxicol. Appl. Pharmacol.* 221:21–28.

Hermann, G.E. and Rogers, R.C. 2008. TNFalpha: A trigger of autonomic dysfunction. *Neuroscientist* 14:53–67.

Hollander, E., Novotny, S., Hanratty, M., Yaffe, R., DeCaria, C.M., Aronowitz, B.R., and Mosovich, S. 2003. Oxytocin infusion reduces repetitive behaviors in adults with autistic and Asperger's disorders. *Neuropsychopharmacology* 28:193–198.

Horvath, K., Papadimitriou, J.C., Rabsztyn, A., Drachenberg, C., and Tildon, J.T. 1999. Gastrointestinal abnormalities in children with autistic disorder. *J. Pediatr.* 135:559–563.

Horvath, K., Stefanatos, G., Sokolski, K.N., Wachtel, R., Nabors, L., and Tildon, J.T. 1998. Improved social and language skills after secretin administration in patients with autism spectrum disorders. *J. Assoc. Acad. Minor. Phys.* 9:9–15.

Hrdina, P.D., Peters, D.A., and Singhai, R.L. 1976. Effects of chronic exposure to cadmium, lead and mercury of brain biogenic amines in rat. *Res. Commun. Chem. Pathol. Pharmacol.* 15:483–493.

Insel, T.R. 1997. A neurobiological basis of social attachment. *Am. J. Psychiatry* 154:726–735.

Insel, T.R. and Hulihan, T.J. 1995. A gender-specific mechanism for pair bonding: Oxytocin and partner preference. *Behav. Neurosci.* 109:782–789.

Insel, T.R., O'Brien, D.J., and Leckman, J.F. 1999. Oxytocin, vasopressin, and autism: Is there a connection? *Biol. Psychiatry* 45:145–157.

Institute of Medicine (2004). Immunization safety review committee: Vaccines and Autism. Washington, DC. http:/www.iom.edu/report.asp?id = 20155

Johnson, A.K. and Edwards, G.L. (1991). Central projections of osmotic and hypervolaemic signals in homeostatic thirst. In *Thirst—Physiological and Psychological Aspects*, eds. D.J. Ramsay and D.A. Booth. New York: Springer-Verlag, pp. 149–175.

Johnson, A.K. and Gross, P.M. 1993. Sensory circumventricular organs and brain homeostatic pathways. *FASEB J.* 7:678–686.

Jou, R.J., Minshew, N.J., Melhem, N.M., Keshavan, M.S., and Hardan, A.Y. 2008. Brainstem volumetric alterations in children with autism. *Psychol. Med.* 24:1–8.

Jyonouchi, H., Sun, S., and Le, H. 2001. Proinflammatory and regulatory cytokine production associated with innate and adaptive immune responses in children with autism spectrum disorders and developmental regression. *J. Neuroimmunol.* 120:170–179.

Kanner, L. 1943. Autistic disturbances of affective contact. *Nervous Child.* 2:217–250.

Karcsu, S., Jancso, G., Kreutzberg, G.W., Toth, L., Kiraly, E., Bacsy, E., and Laszlo, F.A. 1985. A glutamate-sensitive neuronal system originating from the area postrema terminates in and transports acetylcholinesterase to the nucleus of the solitary tract. *J. Neurocytol.* 14:563–578.

Kemper, T.L. and Bauman, M.L. 1993. The contribution of neuropathological studies to the understanding of autism. *Neurol. Clin.* 11:175–187.

Kern, J.K. and Jones, A.M. 2006. Evidence of toxicity, oxidative stress, and neuronal insult in autism. *J. Toxicol. Environ. Health* 9:485–499.

Kim, S.J., Jeong, H.J., Myung, N.Y., Kim, M.C., Lee, J.H., So, H.S., Park, R.K.,Kim, H.J., Um, J.Y., and Hong, S.H. 2008. The protective mechanism of antioxidants in cadmium-induced ototoxicity in vitro and in vivo. *Environ. Health Perspect.* 116:854–862.

Klin, A. 1993. Auditory brainstem responses in autism: Brainstem dysfunction or peripheral hearing loss? *J. Autism Dev. Disord.* 23:15–35.

Kotler, M., Rodriguez, C., Sainz, R.M., Antolin, I., and Mendendez-Pelaez, A. 1998. Melatonin increases gene expression for antioxidant enzymes in rat brain cortex. *J. Pineal Res.* 24:83–89.

Kulesza, R.J. and Mangunay, K. 2008. Morphological features of the medial superior olive in autism. *Brain Res.* 1200:132–137.

Kulman, G., Lissoni, P., Rovelli, F., Roselli, M.G., Brivio, F., and Sequeri, P. 2000. Evidence of pineal endocrine hypofunction in autistic children. *Neurol. Endocrinol. Lett.* 21:31–34.

Kwon, S., Kim, J., Choe, B.H., Ko, C., and Park, S. 2007. Electrophysiological assessment of central auditory processing by auditory brainstem responses in children with autism spectrum disorders. *J. Korean Med. Sci.* 22:656–659.

Larsen, P.J., Moller, M., and Mikkelsen, J.D. 1991. Efferent projections from the periventricular and medial parvicellular subnuclei of the hypothalamic paraventricular nucleus to circumventricular organs of the rat: A *Phaseolus vulgaris*-leucoagglutinin (PHA-L) tracing study. *J. Comp. Neurol.* 306:462–479.

Lathe, R. 2008. Environmental factors and limbic vulnerability in childhood autism. *Am. J. Biochem. Biotechnol.* (*Special Issue on Autism Spectrum Disorders*) 4:183–197.

Lawrence, C.B., Allan, S.M., and Rothwell, N.J. (1998). Interleukin-1beta and the interleukin-1 receptor antagonist act in the striatum to modify excitotoxic brain damage in the rat. *Eur. J. Neurosci.* 10:1188–1195.

Lopez-Hurtado, E. and Prieto, J.J. 2008. A microscopic study of language-related cortex in autism. *Am. J. Biochem. Biotechnol.* (*Special Issue on Autism Spectrum Disorders*) 4:121–129.

Lord, C., Schulman, C., and DiLavore, P. 2004. Regression and word loss in autistic spectrum disorders. *J Child Psychol. Psychiatry* 45:936–955.

Madsen, K.M. and Vestergaard, M. 2004. MMR vaccination and autism: What is the evidence for a causal association? *Drug Safety* 27:831–840.

Mangano, E.N. and Hayley, S. (2009). Inflammatory priming of the substantia nigra influences the impact of later paraquat exposure: Neuroimmune sensitization of neurodegeneration. *Neurobiol. Aging* 30:1361–1378.

Marvel, F.A., Chen, C.C., Badr, N., Gaykema, R.P., and Goehler, L.E. 2004. Reversible inactivation of the dorsal vagal complex blocks lipopolysaccharide-induced social withdrawal and c-Fos expression in central autonomic nuclei. *Brain Behav. Immun.* 18:123–134.

McCoy, M.K., Martinez, T.N., Ruhn, K.A., Szymkowski, D.E., Smith, C.G., Botterman, B.R., Tansey, K.E., and Tansey, M.G. 2006. Blocking soluble tumor necrosis factor signaling with dominant-negative tumor necrosis factor inhibitor attenuates loss of dopaminergic neurons in models of Parkinson's disease. *J. Neurosci.* 26:9365–9375.

McGinnis, W.R. 2001. Mercury and autistic gut disease. *Environ Health Perspect.* 109:A303–304.

McGinnis, W.R. 2004. Oxidative stress in autism. *Altern. Ther. Health Med.* 10:22–36.

McGinnis, W.R. 2007. Could oxidative stress from psychosocial stress affect neurodevelopment in autism? *J Autism Dev. Disord.* 37:993–994.

Meister, B., Ceccatelli, S., Hokfelt, T., Anden, N.E., Anden, M., and Theodorsson, E. 1989. Neurotransmitters, neuropeptides and binding sites in the rat mediobasal hypothalamus: Effects of monosodium glutamate (MSG) lesions. *Neurochem. Int.* 76:343–368.

Mendez-Armenta, M., Villeda-Hernandez, J., Barroso-Moguel, R., Nava-Ruiz, C., Jimenez-Capdeville, M.E., and Rios, C. 2003. Brain regional lipid peroxidation and metallothionein levels of developing rats exposed to cadmium and dexamethasone. *Toxicol. Lett.* 144:151–157.

Ming, X., Brimacombe, M., Malek, J.H., Jani, N., and Wagner, G.C. 2008. Autism spectrum disorders and identified toxic land fills: Co-occurrence across states. *Environ. Health Insights* 2:55–59.

Ming, X., Julu, P.O.O., Brimacombe, M., Connor, S., and Daniels, M.L. 2005. Reduced cardiac parasympathetic activity in children with autism. *Brain Dev.* 27:509–516.

Modahl, C., Green, L., Fein, D., Morris, M., Waterhouse, L., Feinstein, C., and Levin, H. 1998. Plasma oxytocin levels in autistic children. *Biol. Psychiatry* 43:270–277.

Moller-Madsen, B. and Danscher, G. 1986. Localization of mercury in CNS of the rat. I. Mercuric chloride ($HgCl_2$) per os. *Environ. Res.* 1:29–43.

Moosmann, B. and Behl, C. 2002. Secretory peptide hormones are biochemical antioxidants: Structure–activity relationship. *Mol. Pharmacol.* 61:260–268.

Murphy, J.V., Wheless, J.W., and Schmoll, C.M. 2000. Left vagal nerve stimulation in six patients with hypothalamic hamartomas. *Pediatr. Neurol.* 23:167–168.

Nadeau, S. and Rivest, S. 1999. Regulation of the gene encoding tumor necrosis factor alpha (TNF-alpha) in the rat brain and pituitary in response in different models of systemic immune challenge. *Neuropathol. Exp. Neurol.* 58:61–77.

Naylor, J.L., Widdowson, P.S., Simpson, M.G., Farnworth, M., Ellis, M.K., and Lock, E.A. 1995. Further evidence that the blood/brain barrier impedes paraquat entry into the brain. *Hum. Exp. Toxicol.* 14:587–594.

Nelson, K.B. and Bauman, M.L. 2003. Thimerosal and autism? *Pediatrics* 111:674–679.

Nemeroff, C.B., Mayberg, H.S., Krahl, S.E., McNamara, J., Frazer, A., Henry, T.R., George, M.S., Charney, D.S., and Brannan, S.K. 2006. VNS therapy in treatment-resistant depression: Clinical evidence and putative neurobiological mechanisms. *Neuropsychopharmacology* 31:1345–1355.

Nir, I., Meir, D., Zilber, N., Knowlber, H., Hadjez, J., and Lerner, Y. 1995. Brief report: Circadian melatonin, thyroid-stimulating hormone, prolactin, and cortisol levels in serum of young adults with autism. *J Autism Dev. Disord.* 25:641–654.

Nordberg, G.F. and Sereniu, F. 1969. Distribution of inorganic mercury in the guinea pig brain. *Acta Pharmacol. Toxicol.* 27:269–283.

Onyango, I.G. 2008. Mitochondrial dysfunction and oxidative stress in Parkinson's disease. *Neurochem. Res.* 33:589–597.

Opitz, H., Schweinsberg, F., Grossmann, T., Wendt-Gallitelli, M.F., and Meyermann, R. 1996. Demonstration of mercury in the human brain and other organs 17 years after metallic mercury exposure. *Clin. Neuropathol.* 15:139–144.

Ornitz, E.M. 1983. The functional neuroanatomy of infantile autism. *Int. J. Neurosci.* 19:85–124.

Palmeira, C.M., Moreno, A.J., and Madeira, V.M. 1995. Thiols metabolism is altered by the herbicides paraquat, dinoseb and 2,4-D: A study in isolated hepatocytes. *Toxicol. Lett.* 81:115–123.

Palmer, R.F., Blanchard, S., and Wood, R. 2009. Proximity to point sources of environmental mercury release as a predictor of autism prevalence. *Health Place* 15:18–24.

Paul, R., Augustyn, A., Klin, A., and Volkmar, F.R. 2005. Perception and production of prosody by speakers with autism spectrum disorder. *J. Autism Dev. Disord.* 35:205–220.

Peele, D.B., Farmer, J.D., and MacPhail, R.C. 1988. Behavioral consequences of chelator administration in acute cadmium toxicity. *Fundam. Appl. Toxicol.* 11:416–428.

Peng, J., Peng, L., Stevenson, F.F., Doctorow, W.R., and Anderson, J.K. 2007. Iron and paraquat as synergistic environmental risk factors in sporadic Parkinson's disease accelerate age-related neurodegeneration. *J. Neurosci.* 27:6914–6922.

Perry, E.K., Lee, M.L, Martin-Ruiz, C.M., Court, J.A., Volsen, S.G., Merrit, J., Folly, E., Iversen, P.E., Bauman, M.L., Perry, R.H., and Wenk, G.L. 2001. Cholinergic activity in autism: Abnormalities in the cerebral cortex and basal fore brain. *Am. J. Psychiatry* 158:1058–1066.

Peruzzo, B., Pastor, F.E., Blazquez, J.L., Schobitz, K., Pelaez, B., Amat, P., and Rodriguez, E.M. 2000. A second look at the barriers of the medial basal hypothalamus. *Exp. Brain Res.* 132:10–26.

Poling, J.S. 2008. Vaccines and autism revisited. *N. Engl. J. Med.* 359:655.

Porges, W.W., Doussard-Roosevelt, J.A., Portales, A.L., and Greenspan, S.I. 1996. Infant regulation of the vagal "brake" predicts child behavior problems: A psychobiological model of social behavior. *Dev. Psychobiol.* 8:697–712.

Rascher, K. and Mestres, P. 1980. Reaction of the hypothalamic ventricular lining following systemic administration of MSG. *Scan Electron Microsc.* 3:457–464.

Reiter, R.J., Guerrero, J.M., Garcia, J.J., and Acuna-Castroviejo, D. 1998. Reactive oxygen intermediate, molecular damage, and aging. Relation to melatonin. *Ann. N.Y. Acad. Sci.* 854:41–424.

Reiter, R.J., Tan, D.X., Mayo, J.C., Sainz, R.M., and Lopez-Burillo, S. 2002. Melatonin, longevity and health in the aged: An assessment. *Free Radic. Res.* 36:1323–1329.

Rimland, B. 1964. *Infantile Autism*, New York: Meredith Publishing Company.

Rimland, B. and McGinnis, W. 2002. Vaccines and autism. *Lab. Med.* 33:708–716.

Roda, E., Coccini, T., Acerbi, D., Castoldi, A., Bernocchi, G., and Manzo, L. 2008. Cerebellum cholinergic muscarinic receptor (subtype-2 and -3) and cytoarchitecture after developmental exposure to methylmercury: An immunohistological study in rat. *J. Chem. Neuroanat.* 35:285–294.

Rodier, P.M., Ingram, J.L., Tisdale, B., and Croog, V.J. 1997. Linking etiologies in humans and animal models: Studies of autism. *Reprod. Toxicol.* 11:417–422.

Saeed, R.W., Varma, S., Nemeroff, T.P., Sherry, B., Balakhaneh, D., Huston, J., Tracey, K.J., Al-Abed, Y., and Metz, C.N. 2005. Cholinergic stimulation blocks endothelial cell activation and leukocyte recruitment during inflammation. *J. Exp. Med.* 201:1113–1123.

Sajdel-Sulkowska, E.M., Lipinksi, B., Windom, H., Audhya, T., and McGinnis, W. 2008. Oxidative stress in autism: Elevated cerebellar 3-nitrotyrosine levels. *Am. J. Biochem. Biotechnol.* (*Special Issue on Autism Spectrum Disorders*) 4:73–84.

Santos, F.W., Zeni, G., Rocha, J.B., Weis, S.N., Fachinetto, J.M., Favero, A.M., and Noguiera, C.W. 2005. Diphenyl diselenide reverses cadmium-induced oxidative damage on mice tissues. *Chem. Biol. Interact.* 151:159–165.

Shaffer, M.J., Jackson, C.E., Szabo, C.A., and Simpson, C.B. 2005. Vagal nerve stimulation: Clinical and electrophysiological effects on vocal fold function. *Ann. Otol. Rhinol. Laryngol.* 114:7–14.

Singh, P., Mann, K.A., Mangat, H.K., and Kaur, G. 2003. Prolonged glutamate excitotoxicity: Effects on mitochondrial antioxidants and antioxidant enzymes. *Mol. Cell. Biochem.* 243:139–145.

Souza, V., Escobar Md Mdel, C., Gomez-Quiroz, L., Bucio, L., Hernandez, E., Cossio, E.C., and Gutierrez-Ruiz, M.C. 2004. Acute cadmium exposure enhances AP-1 DNA binding and induces cytokines expression and heat shock protein in HepG2 cells. *Toxicology* 197:213–228.

Spellman, S.J. and Warner, H.A. 1977. Parkinsonism and the gut. *Prim. Care* 4:447–462.

Suh, J.H., Walsh, W.J., McGinnis, W.R., Lewis, A., and Ames, B.N. 2008. Altered sulfur amino acid metabolism in immune cells of children diagnosed with autism. *Am. J. Biochem. Biotechnol. (Special Issue on Autism Spectrum Disorders)* 4:105–113.

Tanguay, P.E. and Edwards, R.M. 1982. Electrophysiological studies of autism: The whisper of the bang. *J. Autism Dev. Disord.* 12:177–184.

Terai, K., Munesue, T., and Hiratani, M. 1999. Excessive water drinking behavior in autism. *Brain Dev.* 21:103–106.

Thunberg, G., Ahlsen, E., and Sandberg, A.D. 2007. Children with autistic spectrum disorders and speech-generating devices: Communication in different activities at home. *Clin. Linguist Phonology* 21:457–479.

Tordjman, S., Anderson, G.M., Pichard, N., Charbuy, H., and Touitou, Y. 2005. Noctural excretion of 6-sulphatoxymelatonin in children and adolescents with autistic disorder. *Biol. Psychiatry* 57:134–138.

Torrente, F., Ashwood, R.D., Day, R., Machado, N., Furlano, R.I., Anthony, A., Davies, S.E., Wakefield, A.J., Thomson, M.A., Walker-Smith, J.A., and Murch, S.H. 2002. Small intestinal enteropathy with epithelial IgG and complement deposition in children with regressive autism. *Mol. Psychiatry* 7:375–382.

Tuchman, R.F. and Rapin, I. 1997. Regression in pervasive developmental disorders: Seizures and epileptiform electroencephalogram correlates. *Pediatrics* 99:560–566.

Urena-Guerrero, M.E., Lopez-Perez, S.J., and Beas-Zarate, C. 2003. Neonatal monosodium glutamate treatment modifies glutamic acid decarboxylase activity during rat brain postnatal development. *Neurochem. Int.* 42:269–276.

Vahter, M., Mottet, N.K., Friberg, L., Lind, B., Shen, D.D., and Burbacher, T. 1994. Speciation of mercury in the primate blood and brain following long-term exposure to methyl mercury. *Toxicol. Appl. Pharmacol.* 124:221–229.

Vargas, D.L., Nascimbene, C., Krishnan, C., Zimmerman, A.W., and Pardo, C.A. 2005. Neuroglial activation and neuroinflammation in the brain of patients with autism. *Ann. Neurol.* 57:67–81.

Vitkovic, L., Konsman, J.P., Bockaert, J., Dantzer, R., Homburger, V., and Jacque, C. 2000. Cytokine signals propagate through the brain. *Mol. Pscyhiatry* 5:604–615.

Wakefield, A.J., Murch, S.H., Anthony, A., Linnell, J., Casson, D.M., Malik, M., Berelowitz, W., Dhillon, A.P., Thomson, M.A., Harvey, P., Valentine, A., Davies, S.E., and Walker-Smith, J.A. 1998. Illeal-lymphoid-nodular hyperplasia, non-specific colitis, and pervasive developmental disorder in children. *Lancet* 351:637–641.

Wakefield, A.J., Thomson, M.A., Walker-Smith, J.A., and Murch, S.H. 2002. Small intestinal enteropathy with epithelial IgG and complement deposition in children with regressive autism. *Mol. Psychiatry* 7:375–382.

Walker, R. and Lupien, J.R. (2000). The safety evaluation of monosodium glutamate. *J. Nutr.* 130:1049S–10452S.

Wang, Y., Fang, J., Leonard, S.S., and Rao, K.M. 2004. Cadmium inhibits the electron transfer chain and induces reactive oxygen species. *Free Radic. Biol. Med.* 36:1434–1443.

Weidenheim, K.M., Goodman, L., Dickson, D.W., Gillberg, C., Rastam, M., and Rapin, I. 2001. Etiology and pathophysiology of autistic behavior: Clues from two cases with an unusual variant of neuroaxonal dystrophy. *J. Child Neurol.* 16:809–819.

Weissman, J.R., Kelly, R.I., Bauman, M.L., Cohen, B.H., Murray, K.F., Mitchell, R.L., Kern, R.L., and Natowicz, M.R. 2008. Mitochondrial disease in autism spectrum disorder patients: A cohort analysis. *Public Library of Science (PloS ONE)* 3:1–6.

Werner, E. and Dawson, G. 2005. Validation of the phenomenon of autistic regression using home videotapes. *Arch. Gen. Psychiatry* 62:889–895.

Windham, G.C., Zhang, L., Gunier, R., Croen, L.A., and Grether, J.K. 2006. Autism spectrum disorders in relation to distribution of hazardous air pollutants in the San Francisco Bay area. *Environ. Health Perspect.* 114:1438–1444.

Wislocki, G.B. and Putnam, T.J. 1920. Note on the anatomy of the areae postremae. *Anat. Rec.* 19:281–287.

Wu, X.F., Block, M.L., Zhang, W., Qin, L., Wilson, B., Zhang, W.Q., Veronesi, B., and Hong, J.S. 2005. The role of microglia in paraquat-induced dopaminergic neurotoxicity. *Antioxid. Redox Signal.* 7:654–661.

Wyllie, W.G. and Stern, R.O. 1931. Pink disease: Its morbid anatomy, with a note on treatment. *Arch. Dis. Child* 6:137–156.

Yang, B., Goulet, M., Boismenu, R., and Ferguson, A.V. 2004. Secretin depolarizes nucleus tractus solitarius neurons through activation of a nonselective cationic conductance. *Am. J. Physiol. Regul. Comp. Physiol.* 286:927–934.

Yao, W., Walsh, W.J., McGinnis, W.R., and Pratico, D. 2006. Altered vascular phenotype in autism: Correlation with oxidative stress. *Arch. Neurol.* 63:1161–1164.

Yun, A.J., Bazar, K.A., and Lee, P.Y. 2004. Pineal attrition, loss of cognitive plasticity, and onset of puberty during the teen years: Is it a modern maladaptation exposed by evolutionary displacement? *Med. Hypotheses* 63:939–950.

Zimmerman, A.W., Jyonouchi, H., Comi, A.M., Connors, S.L., Milstien, S., Varsou, A., and Heyes, M.P. 2005. Cerebrospinal fluid and serum markers of inflammation in autism. *Pediatr. Neurol.* 33:195–201.

10 Abnormalities in Membrane Lipids, Membrane-Associated Proteins, and Signal Transduction in Autism

Ved Chauhan* and Abha Chauhan

Department of Neurochemistry, New York State Institute for Basic Research in Developmental Disabilities, Staten Island, NY 10314, USA

CONTENTS

* Corresponding author: Tel.: +1-718-494-5257; fax: +1-718-698-7916; e-mail: ved.chauhan@omr.state.ny.us

Membrane lipids play an important role in the control of cellular functions. In this chapter, we present evidence that autism spectrum disorders (ASD) are associated with abnormalities in lipid metabolism, membrane-associated proteins, and signal transduction. Altered levels of amino-glycerophospholipids (AGP) in the membrane, increased peroxidation of lipids, and decreased membrane fluidity in autism suggest that membrane signaling may be affected in autism. Increased phospholipase A_2 (PLA_2) activity in the blood and lymphoblasts of autistic subjects suggests that this lipid-metabolizing enzyme may be affected in autism. If membrane lipids abnormalities occur in autism, then lipid rafts, membrane domains with a strong affinity for signaling molecules, may also be involved in the etiology of autism. An association of phosphatidylinositol 3-kinase (PI3K) gene in autism; decreased activity of protein kinase C (PKC); increased activity of protein kinase A (PKA) in the lymphoblasts from autistic subjects; altered brain levels of Bcl2 and p53 involved in apoptosis; inflammation and altered levels of cytokines; and mutational changes in the proteins involved in cell signaling such as neuroligins, Pten, SHANK3, Wnt, reelin, and voltage-dependent calcium channels suggest impairment in signal transduction in autism. These abnormalities in the signal system may account for some of the structural changes and cognitive deficits in the brains of individuals with autism.

10.1   INTRODUCTION

Autism spectrum disorders (ASD), also known as pervasive developmental disorders (PDDs), cause severe and pervasive impairment in language, cognition, and socialization. These disorders include autism (severe form), pervasive developmental disorder—not otherwise specified (PDD-NOS), and a much milder form, Asperger syndrome. They also include two rare disorders: Rett syndrome and childhood disintegrative disorder. Autism is a heterogeneous disorder, both etiologically and phenotypically. Within this autism spectrum, there are variations in the severity of the disorder, the level of cognitive functioning, the presence or absence of associated medical conditions such as seizures or other neurological disorders, and whether or not there is a history of regression from apparent normal development. Etiologically, autism is generally considered to be a polygenetic disorder resulting from interactions of alleles at several loci (Sutcliffe, 2008).

The genetic predisposition of autism may be obvious, but there is limited knowledge of causative or secondary abnormalities in the biochemical pathways in autism. The concept of membrane abnormalities as a cause of neurodevelopmental disorders was suggested by Horrobin (1999). Phospholipids make up the bulk of all internal and external neuronal membranes. Alteration in membrane lipids can result in defective membrane functions and therefore may have a wide impact on learning and behavior. Some of the important membrane functions associated with phospholipids that are essential for the proper functioning of the cells include generation of intracellular second messengers, i.e., inositoltriphosphate (IP_3) and diacylglycerol (DG), by receptor-coupled cleavage of phosphoinositides, and maintenance of fluid environment by unsaturated fatty acids. In addition, phosphoinositides are cofactors of protein-phosphorylating enzymes such as Akt/protein kinase B (Kisseleva, Cao, and Majerus, 2002) and endocytosis (Ikonomov et al., 2002). Sphingomyelin generates sphingosine, an intracellular messenger (van Blitterswijk et al., 2003). Most neuronal membrane proteins such as receptors and receptor-coupled enzymes are embedded in or attached to phospholipid membranes. The quaternary structure of protein and, therefore, the function of protein depend on the precise composition of the immediate phospholipid environment. Alterations in membrane lipid metabolism, such as composition of fatty acids, oxidation of lipids, and/or altered levels of phospholipids in the membrane, will affect the functions of proteins that are involved in signal transduction. It is pertinent to mention that the fluid mosaic model of membrane, which described membrane as a lipid bilayer in which proteins are diffused freely, has been modified substantially. Membrane compartmentalization occurs by lipid–lipid, lipid–protein, and membrane–cytoskeletal interactions (Nicolau et al., 2006), and alterations in membrane composition will affect all of these interactions, and thus signal transduction. In this chapter, we present evidence that suggests a role of abnormalities in membrane biochemistry and signal transduction in autism.

10.2   ABNORMALITIES IN MEMBRANE AMINO-GLYCEROPHOSPHOLIPIDS IN AUTISM

We previously reported that the levels of phosphatidylethanolamine (PE) were decreased while phosphatidylserine (PS) were increased in the erythrocyte membranes from children with autism as compared to typically developing siblings (Chauhan et al., 2004b). PE and PS belong to a class of phospholipids known as amino-glycerophospholipids (AGP). In addition to the erythrocyte membrane, AGP were also affected in the blood plasma in autism. As shown in Figure 10.1, a significant increase in plasma levels of AGP was observed in autism subjects (mean$\pm$SE$=0.2022\pm0.021$) as compared to typically developing siblings (mean$\pm$SE$=0.1575\pm0.017$) (Chauhan et al., 2004b). The acidic lipids are localized mainly on the cytoplasmic side of the membrane. During apoptosis and also in oxidative stress, normal symmetry of the membrane is lost, and PE and PS are externalized (Jain, 1984; Matsura et al., 2005). Externalization of PS also plays an important role in the aggregation of platelets (Bucki et al., 2001). It remains to be studied whether orientation of these lipids in the membrane is affected in autism. Alterations in brain energy and phospholipid metabolism in autism have also been suggested to correlate with the neuropsychologic and language deficits (Minshew et al., 1993).

10.3   MEMBRANE FLUIDITY AND ROLE OF FATTY ACIDS IN AUTISM

Membrane fluidity refers to the viscosity of the lipid bilayer of a cell membrane. The phospholipids of membrane contain fatty acids of varying lengths and saturation. Shorter-chain fatty acids and ones with greater unsaturation are less stiff, less viscous,

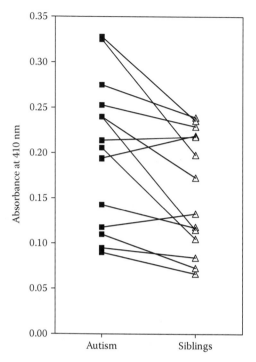

FIGURE 10.1 Increased AGP content in the plasma of autism subjects as compared to typically developing sibling controls. Total lipids extracted from the plasma samples of 14 children with autism (■) and their 14 nonautistic siblings (△) were labeled with trinitrobenzene sulfonic acid (TNBS), and absorbance of the samples read at 410 nm. (Reproduced from Chauhan, V. et al., *Life Sci.*, 74, 1635, 2004b. With permission.)

and have lower melting points. We have observed that fluidity of the erythrocyte membrane from children with autism is significantly lower than that of normal siblings (Chauhan et al, 2005). These results suggest that membranes are more rigid in autism. Biomembranes are generally in the fluid liquid-crystalline phase and maintenance of optimal membrane fluidity is critical to biological functions. It has a marked effect on membrane properties, modulating the activity of membrane-bound enzymes and other membrane-associated molecules such as ion channels and receptors (Houslay and Stanley, 1982). The activities of integral membrane proteins are markedly affected by the physical state of the lipids in which they are embedded. For example, fluid membranes have a greater number of insulin receptors and more responsive receptors, resulting in heightened sensitivity to insulin (Neufeld and Corbo, 1984). Rigid membrane adversely affects the function of tissues throughout the body, including the brain. In autistic subjects with developmental regression, Bu et al. (2006) observed increased levels of ω-9 fatty acids, i.e., eicosenoic acid (20:1n9) and erucic acid (22:1n9) when compared with typically developing controls. In addition, an increase in eicosadienoic acid (20:2n6) and a decrease in palmietaidic acid (trans,16:1n7t) were observed in autistic children with clinical regression compared to those with early onset autism. The above evidence on decreased fluidity of the erythrocyte membrane, and alterations in the fatty acid composition in autism suggest that abnormalities in fatty acid metabolism may be involved in this disorder.

The composition of fatty acids in the membrane phospholipids can be influenced by the dietary intake of polyunsaturated fatty acids, the status of oxidative stress, and/or the action of phospholipase A_2 (PLA_2), an enzyme that removes the sn-2 fatty acids of phospholipids. It is known that dietary ω-3 fatty acids affect osmotic fragility and membrane fluidity (Hagve, Lie, and Gronn, 1993). Such effects may be responsible for the decreased blood viscosity and improved microcirculation observed after feeding ω-3 fatty acids to animals (Young and Conquer, 2005).

Long-chain ω-3 fatty acids such as eicosapentaenoic acid (EPA) and docosahexaenoic acid (DHA) have important structural roles as components of cellular membranes. Both DHA and EPA are linked with many aspects of neural function including neurotransmission, membrane fluidity, ion channel, enzyme regulation, and gene expression (Young and Conquer, 2005). If unsaturated fatty acids are more in our diet, the cell membrane becomes more fluid. DHA is the most unsaturated of all fatty acids, and it helps in fluid cell membranes. The incorporation of EPA and DHA into membrane phospholipids increases after ingestion of large amounts of ω-3 fatty acids.

Epidemiological studies suggest that dietary consumption of EPA and DHA, commonly found in fish or fish oil, may decrease the risk for certain neuropsychiatric disorders. Decreased blood levels of ω-3 fatty acids have been reported in several neuropsychiatric conditions, including attention deficit (hyperactivity) disorder, Alzheimer's disease, schizophrenia, and depression (Young and Conquer, 2005). Supplementation studies, using individual or a combination of ω-3 fatty acids, suggest that certain symptoms associated with some of these disorders may improve with ω-3 fatty acid supplementation (Young and Conquer, 2005). Recently, Amminger et al. (2007) reported an advantage of dietary supplementation of ω-3 fatty acids for the hyperactivity and stereotypy of individuals with behavioral disorders.

10.4 PHOSPHOLIPASE A_2 AND AUTISM

PLA_2 hydrolyzes the sn-2 fatty acids of phospholipids, giving rise to polyunsaturated fatty acids and lysophospholipids. The released fatty acid, i.e., arachidonic acid is a major source of the production of prostaglandins and leukotrienes. Chromosomal linkage studies with genetic markers have provided possible genetic links to autism. Multiple genes have been postulated to be involved in the etiology of ASD (reviewed in Abrahams and Geschwind, 2008; Lamb et al., 2000). Several studies have suggested that loci D1S1675 (Risch et al., 1999), D6S283-D6S261 (Philippe et al., 1999), D7S530-D7S684 (International Molecular Genetic Study of Autism Consortium, 1998), and D13S800 (Barrett et al., 1999) are potential gene sites for autism. While these studies point to the involvement of different loci in autism, overlapping loci on chromosome 7 have been detected in all these studies. Therefore, PLA_2 (7q31-located at D7S530-D7S684 loci on chromosome 7) may be involved in the etiology of autism.

We have observed that PLA_2 activity is higher in lymphoblasts from autism subjects than from control subjects (Chauhan and Chauhan, 2008; Chauhan et al., 2007). Ward (2000) also observed significantly higher concentrations of PLA_2 in the erythrocytes from patients with regressive autism and classical autism/Asperger disorder than from control subjects. Interestingly, supplementation with EPA in patients with classical autism or Asperger disorder resulted in significantly reduced PLA_2 concentrations compared to nontreated individuals.

The role of PLA_2 in the etiology of several other neurodevelopmental disorders has also been documented previously (Bell et al., 2004). It has been suggested that genetic inheritance may cause phospholipid abnormalities in dyslexia that are somewhat similar to those found in schizophrenia (Horrobin and Bennett, 1999). PLA_2 levels were reported to be significantly higher in dyslexic-type adults and schizophrenics than in control subjects (MacDonell et al., 2000).

Two functional candidate genes (phospholipase genes) have been identified: phospholipase Cβ2 (PLCβ2) and PLA_2, group IVB (cytosolic; PLA2G4B). Molecular genetic studies have suggested a reading disability (RD, dyslexia) susceptibility locus on chromosome 15q (Morris et al., 2004). The locus was mapped to the region surrounding D15S994 and D15S944, which is located within PLCβ2 and is 1.6 Mb from PLA2G4B, thus suggesting a role of phospholipases in neurodevelopmental disorders.

10.5 POLYPHOSPHOINOSITIDES AND AUTISM

Phosphatidylinositol (PI), PI 4-phosphate (PI 4P), PI 4,5-P_2, PI 3P, PI 3,4-P_2, and PI 3,4,5-P_3 belong to a group of lipids collectively known as phosphoinositides. The amount of these lipids is generally less than 1% of total lipids, but they are essential lipids in signal transduction. Phospholipase C–mediated cleavage of PI 4,5-P_2 produces two intracellular messengers: DG, an activator of protein kinase C (PKC), and IP_3, a calcium mobilizer (Chauhan et al., 1990). Phosphatidylinositol 3-kinase (PI3K) phosphorylates PI, PI 4P, and PI 4,5-P_2 at the 3-OH group of inositol ring, giving rise to PI 3P, PI 3,4-P_2, and PI 3,4,5-P_3. Extensive evidence from our group and other groups has shown that PIP_2 and PIP_3 are potent activators of PKC (Chauhan and Brockerhoff, 1988; Chauhan, Chauhan, and Brockerhoff, 1991; Chauhan et al., 1989, 1991; Derman et al., 1997; Lee and Bell, 1991; Singh et al., 1993; Toker et al., 1994). The 3-OH-phosphorylated phosphoinositides also have an important function in the activation of protein kinase B/Akt (enzyme involved in apoptosis), and also in membrane trafficking. An association of inositol polyphosphate-1-phosphatase (INPP1), phosphoinositide-3-kinase catalytic gamma polypeptide (PIK3CG), and tuberous sclerosis complex 2 (TSC2) gene variants with autistic disorder and its implications for phosphatidylinositol signaling in autism were suggested by Serajee et al. (2003). In addition to lipid moiety of phosphoinositides, its water-soluble part, i.e., myo-inositol was also altered in autism (Serajee et al., 2003). A decrease in concentration of myo-inositol in autism compared to typically developing controls was reported. The additional role of phosphoinositides in autism is discussed in Section 10.9.

10.6   PROTEIN KINASES AND AUTISM

Intracellular signaling is carried out by the phosphorylation of proteins by protein kinases. These protein kinases have specific requirement for activation, e.g., PKC requires calcium, PS and DG; protein kinase A requires cAMP; and protein kinase B requires PIP_3. We studied the activities of Ca^{2+}/Mg^{2+}-ATPase (which regulates intracellular calcium concentration) in the erythrocytes, and of protein-phosphorylating enzymes, namely, PKC and PKA, in lymphoblasts from autism and controls subjects (Chauhan et al., 2007). The activity of membrane Ca^{2+}/Mg^{2+}-ATPase was higher in autism subjects than in controls. The results suggested that intracellular calcium levels might be increased in autism. Interestingly, basal intracellular calcium levels were observed to be higher in the lymphoblasts from autism subjects than in lymphoblasts from control subjects. Since imbalance in calcium homeostasis can affect the activity of PKC in autism, we also measured the PKC activity in lymphoblasts from autism and control subjects. PKC activity was decreased in both cytosolic and membrane fractions in autism as compared to controls. On the other hand, the activity of cAMP-dependent PKA was increased in autistic lymphoblasts as compared to control lymphoblasts. Recently, Lintas et al. (2008) reported an association between autism and PRKCB1 gene variants, pointing towards the role of PKCβ in altered epithelial permeability, and demonstrating a significant downregulation of brain PRKCB1 gene expression in autism. Our data on levels of intracellular calcium, activities of Ca^{2+}/Mg^{2+}-ATPase, PKC, and PKA strongly support that signal transduction may be abnormal in autism (Chauhan et al., 2007).

10.7   LIPOPROTEIN, CHOLESTEROL, AND AUTISM

The family of low-density lipoprotein (LDL) receptors represents a collection of membrane receptors that have been remarkably conserved throughout evolution. These multifunctional receptors known to regulate cholesterol transport are gaining attention in neuroscience due to their ability to transduce a diversity of extracellular signals across the membrane. Their roles in modulating synaptic plasticity and in hippocampus-specific learning and memory have recently come to light. In addition, genetic, biochemical, and behavioral studies have implicated these signaling systems in a number of neurodegenerative and neuropsychiatric disorders involving loss of cognitive ability, such as Alzheimer's disease, schizophrenia, and autism (reviewed in Qiu, Korwek, and Weeber, 2006).

The results of several genomic screens suggest the presence of an autism susceptibility locus on chromosome 19p13.2–q13.4. The apolipoprotein E (apoE) gene on chromosome 19 encodes for a protein, apoE, whose different isoforms (E2, E3, E4) influence neuronal growth. ApoE participates in lipid transport and metabolism, repair, growth, and maintenance of axons and myelin during neuronal development. Persico et al. (2004) reported a linkage/association between reelin (RELN) gene polymorphisms and autistic disorder. ApoE participates in the reelin signaling pathway by competitively antagonizing reelin binding to ApoE receptor 2 and to very-low-density lipoprotein receptors (VLDL). ApoE2 displays the lowest receptor binding affinity compared with ApoE3 and ApoE4. The linkage/association was assessed between primary autism and ApoE alleles in 223 complete trios, from 119 simplex Italian families, and 44 simplex/29 multiplex Caucasian-American families. Statistically significant disequilibrium favored the transmission of epsilon2 alleles to autistic offspring, over epsilon3 and epsilon4 (Persico et al., 2004). However, the study by Raiford et al. (2004) did not find an association between apoE and autism.

In blood, lipids are transported by lipoproteins. Corbett et al. (2007) reported a potential role for dyslipidemia in the pathogenesis of some forms of ASD. Using two-dimensional electrophoresis and analyzing 6348 peptide components of serum, apolipoprotein (apo) B-100 had an effect size >0.99, with a $p < 0.05$ and a Mascot identification score of 30 or greater, for autism compared to controls. In addition, apo B-100 and apo A-IV were higher in children with high-functioning autism compared to low-functioning autism.

Some alterations of lipids in autism may also be linked to secondary abnormalities. For example, Smith-Lemli-Opitz syndrome (SLOS), a genetic condition of impaired cholesterol biosynthesis, is associated with autism (Tierney et al., 2001). It has been suggested that in addition to SLOS, there may be other disorders of sterol metabolism or homeostasis associated with ASD (Tierney et al., 2006). However, the incidence of SLOS and other sterol disorders among individuals with ASD is not known.

10.8 CALCIUM AND CALCIUM ION CHANNELS IN AUTISM

Calcium is a vital intracellular signaling molecule. The concentration of intracellular calcium is low in the resting cell; however, its levels rise from low nanomolar to micromolar levels after receptor-coupled stimulation of the cell. The receptor-coupled increase in intracellular levels of calcium is important for neuronal survival, differentiation, migration, and synaptogenesis (Aamodt and Constantine-Paton, 1999; Cline, 2001; Komuro and Rakic, 1998; Moody and Bosma, 2005; Represa and Ben Ari, 2005; Spitzer, Root, and Borodinsky, 2004). Defects in these developmental processes can lead to some of the neuroanatomical abnormalities, such as increases in cell-packing density, decreases in neuron size and arborization, and alterations in connectivity, that are associated with ASD patients (Courchesne et al., 2005; DiCicco-Bloom et al., 2006). Voltage-gated calcium channels mediate calcium influx in response to membrane depolarization and regulate intracellular processes such as contraction, secretion, neurotransmission, and gene expression. Their activity is essential for coupling electrical signals in the cell surface to physiological events in cells.

Functional mutations in genes encoding voltage-gated Ca^{2+} channels have been suggested as a possible cause of ASD (Hemara-Wahanui et al., 2005; Splawski et al., 2004, 2006). Point mutations in the gene encoding the L-type voltage-gated Ca^{2+} channel $Ca_V1.2$ (CACNA1C) cause Timothy syndrome, a multisystem disorder that includes cardiac abnormalities and autism (Splawski et al., 2004, 2005). $Ca_V1.2$ plays an important role in the activation of transcription factors, such as cAMP-response-element-binding protein (CREB) and myocyte enhancer factor 2 (MEF2), involving neuronal survival and dendritic arborization (West et al., 2001). The mutations associated with Timothy syndrome prevent voltage-dependent inactivation of $Ca_V1.2$, which causes the channels to have longer open periods and to carry more Ca^{2+} than wild-type channels (Splawski et al., 2004, 2005). Similar evidence of calcium involvement in autism comes from a mutation in CACNA1F, which encodes the L-type voltage-gated Ca^{2+} channel $Ca_V1.4$. It was reported to cause autistic symptoms in a New Zealand family of patients who have stationary night blindness (Hemara-Wahanui et al., 2005; Hope et al., 2005).

ASD-associated mutations have been identified not only in genes encoding Ca^{2+} channels themselves but also in genes encoding ion channels whose activity is directly modulated by Ca^{2+}. Several point mutations in SCN1A and SCN2A genes, which encode the voltage-activated Na^+ channels $Na_V1.1$ and $Na_V1.2$, respectively, are associated with childhood epilepsy and autism (Weiss et al., 2003). Mutations in a C-terminal region of other voltage-gated Na^+ channels reduce the amount of channel inactivation, raising the possibility that excessive ion channel activity leads to ASD (Glaaser et al., 2006; Kim et al., 2004). Another report suggests that there is also an association between a Ca^{2+}-activated K^+ channel (BKCa) and ASD (Laumonnier et al., 2006). Disruption of the BKCa gene KCNMA1 led to haploinsufficiency and reduced BKCa activity. The reported decrease in BKCa channel activity, together with the reduced inactivation of voltage-gated Ca^{2+} channels in individuals with autism, suggests that some forms of autism are due to abnormally sustained increases in intracellular Ca^{2+} levels.

Glutamate receptors are ligand-gated Ca^{2+} channels that are important in many activity-dependent developmental processes. Polymorphisms in GRIN2A, which encodes a NMDA receptor subunit, have also been associated with ASD (Barnby et al., 2005). ASD-associated polymorphisms were reported in the gene encoding subunit 2 of the kainate ionotropic glutamate receptor (GRIK2) and in metabotropic glutamate receptor genes (Jamain et al., 2002; Serajee et al., 2003). The transcription factor ARX is expressed in several cell types throughout the forebrain and is thought to regulate the development of gamma-aminobutyric acid (GABA)-ergic neurons in the basal ganglia and cortex (Friocourt et al., 2006). Mutations of ARX can lead to epilepsy, movement disorders, cortical malformations, mental retardation, and in some cases, autism (Stromme et al., 2002; Turner et al., 2002).

Wingless-type mouse memory tumor virus (MMTV) integration site family member (Wnt) proteins form a family of highly conserved secreted signaling molecules that regulate cell-to-cell interactions during embryogenesis. The role of WNT2 has also been implicated in ASDs. Two families with mutations in WNT2 have been identified, and a polymorphism in an upstream region of WNT2 has been associated with families defined by severe language abnormalities (Wassink et al., 2001). Increases in Ca^{2+} concentrations have recently been shown to enhance the synthesis and release of Wnt through activity of the Ca^{2+}-regulated transcription factor CREB (Wayman et al., 2006). Considering the pivotal role of calcium in cellular signaling, it is possible that calcium may have a wide role in the etiology of ASD.

10.9 ROLE OF MEMBRANE-ASSOCIATED PROTEINS SUCH AS PTEN, NEUROLIGINS, SHANK3, REELIN, AND SEROTONIN RECEPTORS IN AUTISM

Figure 10.2 represents the mechanism by which membrane-associated proteins participate in the cellular signaling. Growth factor binds to its receptor and activates PI3K,

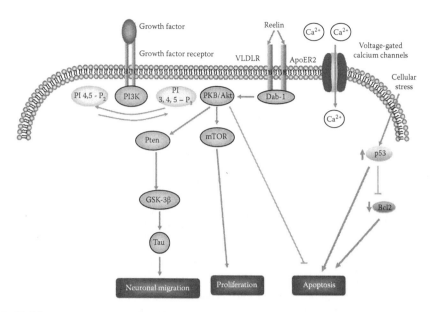

FIGURE 10.2 (See color insert following page 200.) Participation of growth factor receptors, reelin, voltage-gated calcium channels, p53, and Bcl2 in neuronal migration, proliferation, and apoptosis. Growth factor binds to its receptor and activated phosphatidylinositol 3-kinase (PI3K), which converts phosphatidylinositol 4,5-bisphosphate (PI 4, 5-P_2) to phopsphatidylinositol 3, 4, 5-trisphosphate (PI 3, 4, 5-P_3). PI 3, 4, 5-P_3 is an activator of protein kinase B (also known as Akt) that triggers proliferation pathways by activating the mammalian target of rapamycin (mTOR). Akt also activates phosphatase and tensin homolog on chromosome 10 (Pten), which dephosphorylates PI 3, 4, 5-P_3 to PI 4, 5-P_2. Pten activates glycogen synthase kinase-3β (GSK-3β), which phosphorylates tau protein involved in neuronal migration. Reelin binds to very low-density lipoprotein receptor (VLDLR) and apolipoprotein E receptor 2 (ApoER2), which activate Disabled-1 protein (Dab-1). Dab-1 activates the Akt involved in neuronal migration and proliferation. Cellular stress, on the other hand, affects the activities of p53 and Bcl2, proteins involved in apoptosis.

which converts PI 4,5-P_2 (PIP$_2$) to PI 3,4,5-P_3 (PIP$_3$). PIP$_3$ is an activator of PKB (also known as Akt) that triggers proliferation of the cell. Akt also activates phosphatase and tensin homolog on chromosome 10 (Pten), which dephosphorylates PIP$_3$ to PIP$_2$ and may initiate apoptotic signaling. Pten activates glycogen synthase kinase-3β (GSK-3β), which phosphorylates tau protein, a cytoskeletal protein. Phosphorylation of tau protein is important for neuronal migration. Reelin binds to VLDL receptor (VLDLR) and apolipoprotein E receptor 2 (apoER2), and it activates Disabled-1 protein (Dab1) that also activates PKB. Calcium channels are important for controlled and fast requirement of intracellular calcium, which is vital for the biological activities of numerous proteins. Cellular stress initiates pathways leading to apoptosis by decreasing the levels of p53 (a proapoptotic protein) and decreasing the levels of Bcl2 (an antiapoptotic protein).

In Figure 10.3, the role of neuroligins (Nlgn), neurexins (Nrxns), as well as SH3 and multiple ankyrin repeat domains 3 (SHANK3) proteins in cellular signaling are

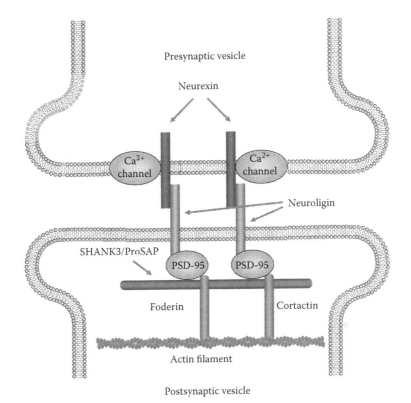

Presynaptic vesicle

Postsynaptic vesicle

FIGURE 10.3 (See color insert following page 200.) Interaction of neurexin and neuroligins. Neurexins participate in synaptic transmission by affecting calcium channels. They also interact with neuroligins of postsynaptic vesicles. Neuroligin controls the actin assembly by interacting with postsynaptic density protein 95 (PSD-95), which further interacts with SHANK3. SHANK3/PSD-95 interact with foderin and cortactin, which bind to actin filament.

described. Neurexins in presynaptic vesicles interact with neuroligins at the postsynaptic vesicles, and neuroligins further interact with shank3 through postsynaptic density protein 95 (PSD95). SHANK3 also interacts with actin filaments with the help of foderin and cortactin.

Serotonin (5-hydroxytryptamine, i.e., 5HT) is a calming neurotransmitter that is produced from the amino acid tryptophan in nerve cells. Its reuptake transporters and receptors are shown in Figure 10.4. Imbalance of serotonin metabolism affects mood and behavior. Selective serotonin reuptake inhibitors (SSRIs) such as fluoxetine (Prozac) have been widely used for mood and behavioral problems. They block serotonin from entering the neuron and keep it active for longer periods of time in the synaptic gaps.

The potential role of these proteins in autism is discussed below.

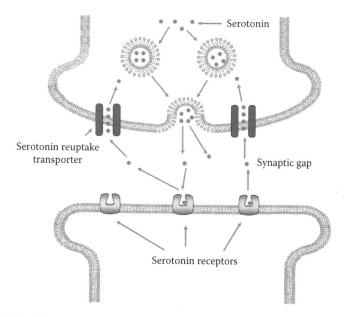

FIGURE 10.4   (See color insert following page 200.) Serotonin and its receptors, and serotonin reuptake transporter. Serotonin molecules from the presynaptic vesicles are released into the synaptic gap, where they are internalized by serotonin receptors into the postsynaptic vesicles. Serotonin molecules are also retaken from synaptic gaps to the presynaptic vesicle by the serotonin reuptake transporters. An imbalance of the uptake and reuptake system in serotonin causes brain dysfunctions.

10.9.1   POTENTIAL ROLE OF PTEN AND PI3K/AKT PATHWAY IN AUTISM

Pten is involved in mechanisms that control development of neuronal and synaptic structures and, subsequently, synaptic function (Fraser et al., 2008). Pten mutations have been reported in autistic individuals with macrocephaly (Butler et al., 2005; Goffin et al., 2001; Zori et al., 1998). Several reports have suggested that germline mutations in Pten can lead to multiple hamartoma syndromes and syndromes clinically characterized by autism associated with macrocephaly (Buxbaum et al., 2007; Greer and Wynshaw-Boris, 2006; Herman et al., 2007; Kwon et al., 2006). In addition, mutations in Pten have been linked to other brain disorders such as macrocephaly, seizure, Lhermitte-Duclos disease, and mental retardation (Waite and Eng, 2002). Pten seems to have a wide range of implications in autism, although further studies are warranted.

While Pten hydrolyzes the 3′ phosphate group of PIP_3 (Maehama and Dixon, 1998), PI3K catalyzes the phosphorylation of the 3′ hydroxyl group of phosphoinositides, resulting in Akt activation. Upon activation, Akt phosphorylates proteins that are involved in signal transduction such as TSC 2 gene product tuberin, GSK3β, and the proapoptotic protein BAD (Luo, Manning, and Cantley, 2003). Alterations in the PI3K/Akt pathway have been linked to many brain disorders. Decreased levels of Akt are associated with schizophrenia (Emamian et al., 2004), and in individuals with TSC mutations exhibiting central nervous system disorders, including autism (Wiznitzer, 2004). The PI3K/Akt pathway has also been linked to fear conditioning in rats (Lin et al., 2001). Bcl2, an antiapoptotic protein, is one of the downstream targets modulated by Akt. Activated Akt stimulates changes in Bcl2 expression, resulting in antiapoptotic effects in hippocampal neurons (Matsuzaki et al., 1999).

10.9.2 Neuroligins and Autism

Neuroligins are transmembrane proteins expressed on the postsynaptic cell that bind to neurexins, which are presynaptic transmembrane proteins, and they appear to play a crucial role in maintaining the functionality of the brain's synaptic circuitry (Figure 10.3). Synapses provide essential connections between nerve cells in the brain that enable signals to be transmitted. Neural connections require precise organization of the presynaptic and postsynaptic neurons. Nrxns and Nlgns perform important functions in synaptic transmission (Missler et al., 2003; Varoqueaux et al., 2006) and differentiation of synaptic contacts (Graf et al., 2004; Scheiffele et al., 2000), and both Nrxns and Nlgns have been identified as candidate genes for autism (Jamain et al., 2003; Szatmari et al., 2007). The family of human neuroligins consists of five genes (NLGN1 at chromosome 3q26, NLGN2 at 17p13, NLGN3 at Xq13, NLGN4 at Xp22, and NLGN4Y at Yq11). Recent studies reported polymorphisms in neuroligin-3 (NLGN3) and neuroligin-4 (NLGN4) genes in ASD (Talebizadeh et al., 2006; Ylisaukko-oja et al., 2005).

The role of genetic variants of NLGN has been controversial. One missense variant, p.I679V in NLGN4Y gene, was identified in an individual with autism, as well as his father, who had learning disabilities (Yan et al., 2008). Talebizadeh et al. (2006) observed that splice variants of NLGN3 and NLGN4 genes might lead to ASD. Yamakawa et al. (2007) reported that syntrophin-gamma2 (SNTG2) binds to NLGN 4X and NLGN 4Y, and that the binding is affected by the autism-related mutations. On the other hand, Wermter et al. (2008) reported that there is no evidence for the involvement of NLGN3 and NLGN4X genetic variants with high-functioning autistic individuals. Further research is warranted to clarify the role of neuroligins in autism.

10.9.3 SHANK3 and Autism

The SHANK3 gene is located on chromosome 22. SHANK3 (also known as ProSAP2) regulates the structural organization of dendritic spines and is a binding partner of neuroligins. Jeffries et al. (2005) reported that SHANK3 is a candidate gene for autism and abnormal brain development. Durand et al. (2007) reported that a mutation of a single copy of SHANK3 on chromosome 22q13 could result in language and/or social communication disorders. A recent report suggests that SHANK1 (SH3 and multiple ankyrin repeat domains 1) mutant mice exhibit altered postsynaptic density (PSD) protein composition; reduced size of dendritic spines; smaller, and thinner PSDs; and weaker basal synaptic transmission (Hung et al., 2008). Behaviorally, mutant mice had increased anxiety-related behavior and impaired contextual fear memory, suggesting the importance of SHANK1 for synapse structure and function in vivo, and a role for SHANK1 in specific cognitive processes, a feature that may be relevant to ASD in humans. Considering the involvement of SHANK3 in dendritic spine formation and its binding to Nlgn, it is possible that SHANK3 may play an important role in the etiology of autism.

10.9.4 REELIN AND AUTISM

Several genome-wide screens have indicated the presence of an autism susceptibility locus within the distal long arm of chromosome 7 (7q). Mapping at 7q22 within this region showed a candidate gene reelin (RELN). RELN encodes a signaling protein that plays a pivotal role in the migration of several neuronal cell types and in the development of neural connections. Reelin modulates synaptic plasticity by enhancing the induction and maintenance of long-term potentiation (D'Arcangelo, 2005; Weeber et al., 2002). It also stimulates dendrite (Niu et al., 2004) and dendritic spine (Niu, Yabut, and D'Arcangelo, 2008) development and regulates the continuing migration of neuroblasts generated in adult neurogenesis sites such as subventricular and subgranular zones.

Several studies have suggested impairments in reelin signaling in autism. Fatemi et al. (2001) reported that dysregulation of reelin and Bcl-2 may be responsible for some of the brain structural changes and behavioral abnormalities observed in autism. Fatemi, Stary, and Egan (2002) also reported reduced levels of reelin in the blood of autistic subjects. Serajee, Zhong, and Huq (2006) studied 34 single nucleotide polymorphisms (SNPs) in the RELN gene, with an average spacing between the SNPs of 15 kb, for evidence of an association with autism, and observed significant differences in the transmission of the alleles of exon 22 and intron 59 SNP to autistic subjects, suggesting a role for the RELN gene in susceptibility to autism. In addition, Fatemi et al. (2005) reported reductions in reelin protein and mRNA as well as Disabled 1 (Dab 1, a gene encoding a key regulator of reelin signaling) mRNA and elevations in reelin receptor, i.e., VLDLR mRNA. Family-based association analyses showed a significant association for the 5′-UTR repeat (PDT p-value = 0.002), suggesting the potential of RELN as an important contributor to genetic risk in autism (Skaar et al., 2005). While most of the studies suggest a role of reelin in the etiology of autism, a few studies did not find any link between reelin and the etiology of autism. Krebs et al. (2002) suggested that GGC polymorphism of the RELN gene is unlikely to be a major susceptibility factor in autism and/or genetic heterogeneity. In another study, case–control and affected sib–pair findings did not support role for RELN in susceptibility to ASD, but the more powerful family-based association study demonstrated that RELN alleles with larger numbers of CGG repeats may play a role in the etiology of some cases of ASD, especially in children without delayed phrase speech (Zhang et al., 2002). Further research is warranted to assess the precise role of RELN in autism.

10.9.5 SEROTOGENIC RECEPTORS AND AUTISM

In the central nervous system, serotonin, i.e., 5HT plays an important role as a neurotransmitter in the modulation of anger, aggression, mood, sleep, appetite, and metabolism. Serotonin has broad activities in the brain, and genetic variations in serotonin receptors and the serotonin transporter, which facilitates reuptake of serotonin into presynapses, have been implicated in neurological diseases. Increased platelet serotonin levels have been consistently found in a cohort of autistic subjects. Suggested mechanisms for hyperserotonemia in autism are increased synthesis of serotonin by tryptophan hydroxylase, increased uptake into platelets through 5HT transporter (5HTt), diminished release from platelets through 5HT2A receptor (5HT2Ar), and decreased metabolism by monoamine oxidase (MAOA) (Hranilovic et al., 2008). Recent studies suggest that serotonin transporter (SERT)–binding capacity measured by single-photon emission computed tomography (SPECT) is disturbed in autism (Makkonen et al., 2008; McDougle, 2008).

The serotogenic system is also affected in prenatal viral infection, which also has an association with neurodevelopmental disorders such as schizophrenia and autism. Winter et al. (2008) reported disruption of serotonergic system after prenatal viral infection that may be attributed to potential modeling disruptions occurring in patients with schizophrenia and autism. Hranilovic et al. (2007) have reported a significant negative relationship between platelets serotonin levels and speech development, indicating the relationship between the peripheral 5HT concentrations and verbal abilities in autistic subjects. However, no association of polymorphic variants of the serotonin transporter (5-HTT) gene-linked polymorphic region (5-HTTLPR) with ASD was observed (Zhong et al., 1999). Further research is warranted to confirm the role of serotonin in the etiology of autism.

10.9.6 Evidence of Altered Levels of Bcl2 and p53 (Markers of Apoptosis) in the Brains of Autism Subjects

Bcl2 derives its name from *B-cell lymphoma 2*. Bcl2 is membrane-bound antiapoptotic protein with a neuroprotective role in the central nervous system (Lin et al., 1996). The p53 tumor suppressor protein (tumor protein 53) plays a central role in controlling cell growth and apoptotic cell death in response to cellular stress and DNA damage (Araki et al., 2000). In autism, many areas of the brain show abnormalities in autism, including loss of pyramidal neurons and granule cells in the hippocampus as well as significant loss and atrophy of Purkinje cells in the cerebellum (Bauman and Kemper, 2005; Fatemi and Halt, 2001; Ritvo et al., 1986). Emerging evidence suggests that apoptotic mechanisms may be responsible for causing neuropsychiatric disorders such as schizophrenia (Jarskog et al., 2000) and autism (Araghi-Niknam and Fatemi, 2003; Fatemi and Halt, 2001; Fatemi et al., 2001). In particular, significant reduction in the levels of Bcl2 (a membrane-bound antiapoptotic protein) and a concomitant increase in p53 levels have been reported in cerebellum (Araghi-Niknam and Fatemi, 2003; Fatemi and Halt, 2001; Fatemi et al., 2001), parietal cortex (Fatemi and Halt, 2001; Fatemi et al., 2001), and superior frontal cortex of autism subjects (Araghi-Niknam and Fatemi, 2003). It is not known whether altered levels of Bcl2 and p53 in autism are due to previous prenatal or postnatal environmental insults or alternatively because of ongoing neurodegeneration. The above studies indicate that apoptosis may be involved in the pathogenesis of autism.

10.10 OXIDATIVE STRESS, INFLAMMATION, AND CELL SIGNALING

During oxidative stress, free radicals, i.e., reactive oxygen species (ROS) and reactive nitrogen species (RNS), react with proteins, lipids, and nucleic acids and affect their functions, leading to cell death. ROS plays crucial role in both normal and pathological cell signaling processes such as calcium homeostasis, kinase activity, and gene regulation (Esposito et al., 2004). Oxidative stress controls the activities of receptor and nonreceptor types of protein tyrosine kinases (Hardwick and Sefton, 1995; Kharbanda et al., 1995; Pu et al., 1996), ras (Lander et al., 1996), protein tyrosine phosphatases (Garcia-Morales et al., 1990; George and Parker, 1990), protein kinase C (Gopalakrishna, Chen, and Gundimeda, 1993), and transcription factors such as NF-AT (Abate et al., 1990) and NF-kB (Hayashi, Ueno, and Okamoto, 1993; Staal et al., 1990). Among these factors, transcriptional factors are most important because of their role in different phases of brain development and wiring. Transcriptional factors are central in cross-talk among cells and signaling molecules. Oxidative stress leads to an increase in Fos expression, an event linked to apoptosis and reduced synaptic plasticity. On the other hand, oxidative stress leads to decreased levels of Jun D, a protein that upregulates antioxidant response element (ARE)–mediated expression and induces the detoxifying enzymes in response to oxidative insults. ROS can also increase the expression of p53 and Fas (Mao et al., 2006). p53 and Fas can, in turn, lead to increased ROS production, indicating a feed-forward mechanism to ensure the death of cells committed to die. Therefore, oxidative damage of membrane lipids/proteins may result in abnormal cellular signaling.

10.10.1 OXIDATIVE STRESS IN AUTISM

Oxidative stress–induced production of lipid peroxides and their by-products is known to result in the loss of membrane functions and integrity (Jain, 1984). Lipid peroxidation is a chain reaction between polyunsaturated fatty acids and ROS, producing lipid peroxides and hydrocarbon polymers that are both highly toxic to the cell (Horton and Fairhurst, 1987; Jain, 1984; Tappel, 1973). In a recent review article, we have gathered evidence of oxidative stress in autism (Chauhan and Chauhan, 2006). We previously reported that lipid peroxidation is increased in the plasma of children with autism as compared to their developmentally normal siblings (Chauhan et al., 2004a). Malonyldialdehyde (MDA) is an end product of peroxidation of polyunsaturated fatty acids and related esters, and therefore, is used as a marker of lipid peroxidation (Jain, 1984). The plasma MDA contents measured by reaction with thiobarbituric acid (TBA) were higher in 87% of autism subjects (Chauhan et al., 2004a). Recently, we also observed increased lipid peroxidation in cerebellum and temporal cortex of brain in autism (Chauhan et al., 2009). MDA levels were significantly increased by 124% in the cerebellum and by 256% in the temporal cortex in autism as compared to control subjects.

Other studies also indicated increased levels of other lipid peroxidation and protein oxidation markers in autism, thus confirming increased oxidative stress in autism. Zoroglu et al. (2004) reported increased TBA-reactive substances in the erythrocytes of autism subjects as compared to normal controls. Ming et al. (2005) reported increased excretion of 8-isoprostane-F2alpha in the urine of children with autism. Isoprostanes are produced from the free radical oxidation of arachidonic acid through nonenzymatic oxidation of cell membrane lipids. Evans et al. (2008) reported increased levels of lipid-derived oxidative protein modification, i.e., carboxyethyl pyrrole and iso[4]levuglandin E2–protein adducts, in the autistic brain, primarily in the white matter. Sajdel-Sulkowska et al. (2008) reported increased levels of 3-nitrotyrosine (a specific marker for oxidative damage of protein) in the cerebella of autistic subjects. Lipofuscin, a matrix of oxidized lipid and cross-linked protein, forms as a result of oxidative injury in the tissues. Density of lipofuscin was observed to be greater in cortical brain areas concerned with social behavior and communication in autism (Lopez-Hurtado and Prieto, 2008).

Several studies have suggested alterations in the enzymes that play a vital role in the defense mechanism against damage by ROS in autism. In autism, decreased activity of glutathione peroxidase (GPx) in plasma (Yorbik et al., 2002) and in erythrocytes (Pasca et al., 2006; Yorbik et al., 2002), reduced levels of total glutathione and lower redox ratio of reduced glutathione (GSH) to oxidized glutathione (GSSG) in plasma (James et al., 2004), decreased catalase activity in red blood cells (Zoroglu et al., 2004), and decreased superoxide dismutase (SOD) activity in plasma, all point toward oxidative stress. On the contrary, Sogut et al. (2003) reported unchanged plasma SOD activity and increased GPx activity in autism.

Ceruloplasmin (a copper-transporting protein) and transferrin (an iron-transporting protein) are major antioxidant proteins that are synthesized in several tissues including brain (Arnaud, Gianazza, and Miribel, 1988; Loeffler et al., 1995). Ceruloplasmin inhibits the peroxidation of membrane lipids catalyzed by metal ions such as Fe and Cu (Gutteridge, Richmond, and Halliwell, 1979). It also acts as ferroxidase and SOD, and it protects polyunsaturated fatty acids in red blood cell membranes from active oxygen radicals (Arnaud, Gianazza, and Miribel, 1988). We reported reduced levels of serum ceruloplasmin and transferrin in children with autism as compared to their unaffected siblings (Chauhan et al., 2004a). The transferrin levels were observed to be lower in 16 of 19 (84%) children with autism as compared to their unaffected siblings, while ceruloplasmin levels were lower in 13 of 19 (68%) children with autism as compared to their developmentally normal siblings (Chauhan et al., 2004a). It was of particular interest to observe that the levels of ceruloplasmin and transferrin were reduced more markedly in children with autism who had lost acquired language skills (Chauhan et al., 2004a). Children who had not lost language skills had levels similar to that seen in the typically developing siblings. These results suggest that there is an altered regulation of transferrin and ceruloplasmin in children with regressive autism. Such alterations may lead to abnormal iron and copper metabolism in autism, which may have a pathological role in autism. Some preliminary studies have suggested altered serum Cu/Zn ratios in autism (McGinnis, 2004).

We recently reported that there might be a link between decreased levels of PE in the membrane and copper-mediated oxidation of lipids (Chauhan, Sheikh, and Chauhan, 2008). We studied the effect of copper on the oxidation of liposomes composed of mouse brain lipids, and also on the lymphoblasts from autism and control subjects. Among the various metal cations (copper, iron, calcium, cadmium, and zinc), only copper was found to oxidize PE, while having no effect on other phospholipids. The action of copper on PE oxidation was time-dependent. Copper oxidized PE in a concentration-dependent manner. No difference was observed between copper-mediated oxidation of diacyl-PE and alkenyl-PE (plasmalogen). Copper-mediated oxidation of PE in autistic lymphoblasts was higher than in control lymphoblasts. Taken together, our studies suggest that ceruloplasmin and copper may be involved in the oxidative stress, and in reducing the levels of membrane PE in autism.

10.10.2   Cytokines, Inflammation, and Autism

A number of studies have implicated oxidative stress as a major upstream component in the signaling cascade involved in activation of redox-sensitive transcription factors and proinflammatory gene expression, leading to inflammatory response (Parola et al., 1999; Uchida et al., 1999) Cytokines are glycoproteins that are involved in cell signaling and are used extensively in cellular communication. Cytokines are critical to the development and functioning of both the innate and adaptive immune response. They are often secreted by immune cells that have encountered a pathogen, thereby activating and recruiting further immune cells to increase the system's response to the pathogen. Cytokines are also involved in several developmental processes during embryogenesis. Several investigators have reported peripheral immune abnormalities in autism (Ashwood and Wakefield, 2006; Jyonouchi et al., 2005; Korvatska et al., 2002; Pardo, Vargas, and Zimmerman, 2005; Singh et al., 1991; Vojdani et al., 2008; Warren et al., 1986; Yonk et al., 1990; Zimmerman et al., 2005). It is also known that cytokines and chemokines play roles as mediators of inflammatory reactions in the central nervous system and in the processes of neuronal–neuroglia interactions that modulate the neuroimmune system. In a recent study, we examined the activation levels of cytokines including the proinflammatory cytokines (IL-6, IL-1β, TNF-α, and GM-CSF), Th1 cytokines (IL-2 and IFN-γ), Th2 cytokines (IL-4, IL-5, and IL-10), and the chemokine IL-8 in the brains of ASD patients and compared with age- and gender-matched normal subjects (Li et al., 2009). Our results showed that TNF-α, IL-6, GM-CSF, IFN-γ, and IL-8 were significantly increased in the brains of ASD patients compared with the control subjects. However, the Th2 cytokines (Il-4, IL-5, and IL-10) showed no significant difference. Th1/Th2 ratio was also significantly elevated in ASD patients. In addition, we found that regulatory IL-10 was not increased in compensatory response to the increased Th1 cytokines in ASD patients (Li et al., 2009). Other groups have also reported that there are abnormalities in immune responses in the central nervous system of individuals with autism (Pardo, Vargas, and Zimmerman, 2005b; Vargas et al., 2005; Vojdani et al., 2008), suggesting that neuroinflammation may have implications in the pathogenesis of autism.

10.11   LIPID RAFTS AND DISORDERS OF THE BRAIN

A new and fairly rapid development in the field of lipid rafts is changing the general view on how membrane complexity takes place. Lipid rafts are microdomains within the membrane that are defined by their cholesterol and sphingomyelin content. Although research on lipid raft and its association with ASD is lacking, this chapter would not be complete without postulating a role of lipid raft in neurodevelopmental disorders. A recent review describes the role of the raft microdomain in neurodevelopment (Allen, Halverson-Tamboli, and Rasenick, 2007). Drugs for treating mood disorders (unipolar depression and bipolar disorder) and schizophrenia tend to accumulate in lipid raft (Eisensamer et al., 2005), and affect the signaling of raft-associated proteins. Although chronic antidepressant treatment does not alter membrane cholesterol content, treatment with chemically distinct antidepressants results in the movement of Gαs (but not other G proteins) out of lipid rafts and into closer association with adenyl cyclase (Donati and Rasenick, 2005; Menkes et al., 1983; Toki, Donati, and Rasenick, 1999). This may contribute to the increased cAMP and synaptic changes that are observed after chronic antidepressant treatment (Donati and Rasenick, 2003).

Lipid raft has been reported to be involved in several neurodegenerative diseases. Lipid rafts may function as platforms for the production of neurotoxic proteins, such as amyloid beta-protein in Alzheimer's disease (Ehehalt et al., 2003) and prion protein in transmissible spongiform encephalopathies (Taylor and Hooper, 2006), which may then be poised to modulate raft-associated signaling cascade. There is enough information in the literature on the role of lipid rafts in neurotransmitter signaling. Allen, Halverson-Tamboli, and Rasenick (2007) have proposed that lipid rafts of the membrane are vehicles for neurotransmitter signaling, through a clustering of receptors and components of receptor-activated signaling cascades. Ionotropic neurotransmitter receptors (ligand-gated ion channels) are localized in lipid rafts (Allen, Halverson-Tamboli, and Rasenick, 2007). The binding of receptors and neurotransmitters takes place in lipid rafts (Burger, Gimpl, and Fahrenholz, 2000; Sooksawate and Simmonds, 2001). Lipid rafts also contribute in the trafficking of ionotropic receptors (Hering, Lin, and Sheng, 2003; Pediconi et al., 2004). G-protein-coupled neurotransmitter receptors (GPCR) signaling complexes are present in lipid rafts (Neubig, 1994), and lipid rafts are involved in GPCR trafficking. In addition, lipid rafts have been shown to regulate the functions of G-proteins, thereby affecting the function of phospholipase and calcium signaling, a process of pathway for neurotansmitter-mediated cellular signaling (reviewed in Allen, Halverson-Tamboli, and Rasenick, 2007). Considering the important role that is played by raft microdomains in signal transduction, it is postulated that these lipid rafts may also be involved in abnormal signaling in autism.

10.12   CONCLUSIONS

In this chapter, we have gathered evidence on how membrane lipids and proteins may be involved in the development of autism. Genetic and environmental factors are the most important factors in the etiology of autism. If we look into the down stream target of these factors, i.e., membrane and proteins function, it becomes apparent that membrane is the intermediate link between genetic/environmental factors and the functions of proteins. Other signaling molecules that are directly or indirectly connected to lipids such as reelin, SHANK3, Wnt, neuroligins, Bcl2 and Pten can also contribute significantly to the etiology of autism.

REFERENCES

Aamodt, S. M. and M. Constantine-Paton (1999). The role of neural activity in synaptic development and its implications for adult brain function. *Adv. Neurol.* 79:133–144.

Abate, C., L. Patel, F. J. Rauscher III, and T. Curran (1990). Redox regulation of fos and jun DNA-binding activity in vitro. *Science* 249:1157–1161.

Abrahams, B. S. and D. H. Geschwind (2008). Advances in autism genetics: On the threshold of a new neurobiology. *Nat. Rev. Genet.* 9:341–355.

Allen, J. A., R. A. Halverson-Tamboli, and M. M. Rasenick (2007). Lipid raft microdomains and neurotransmitter signaling. *Nat. Rev. Neurosci.* 8:128–140.

Amminger, G. P., G. E. Berger, M. R. Schafer, C. Klier, M. H. Friedrich, and M. Feucht (2007). Omega-3 fatty acids supplementation in children with autism: a double-blind randomized, placebo-controlled pilot study. *Biol. Psychiatry* 61:551–553.

Araghi-Niknam, M. and S. H. Fatemi (2003). Levels of Bcl-2 and P53 are altered in superior frontal and cerebellar cortices of autistic subjects. *Cell Mol. Neurobiol.* 23:945–952.

Araki, N., T. Morimasa, T. Sakai, H. Tokuoh, S. Yunoue, M. Kamo, K. Miyazaki, K. Abe, H. Saya, and A. Tsugita (2000). Comparative analysis of brain proteins from p53-deficient mice by two-dimensional electrophoresis. *Electrophoresis* 21:1880–1889.

Arnaud, P., E. Gianazza, and L. Miribel (1988). Ceruloplasmin. *Methods Enzymol.* 163:441–452.

Ashwood, P. and A. J. Wakefield (2006). Immune activation of peripheral blood and mucosal CD3 +lymphocyte cytokine profiles in children with autism and gastrointestinal symptoms. *J. Neuroimmunol.* 173:126–134.

Barnby, G., A. Abbott, N. Sykes, A. Morris, D. E. Weeks, R. Mott, J. Lamb, A. J. Bailey, and A. P. Monaco (2005). Candidate-gene screening and association analysis at the autism-susceptibility locus on chromosome 16p: Evidence of association at GRIN2A and ABAT. *Am. J. Hum. Genet.* 76:950–966.

Barrett, S., J. C. Beck, R. Bernier, E. Bisson, T. A. Braun, T. L. Casavant, D. Childress, S. E. Folstein, M. Garcia, M. B. Gardiner, S. Gilman, J. L. Haines, K. Hopkins, R. Landa, N. H. Meyer, J. A. Mullane, D. Y. Nishimura, P. Palmer, J. Piven, J. Purdy, S. L. Santangelo, C. Searby, V. Sheffield, J. Singleton, and S. Slager et al. (1999). An autosomal genomic screen for autism. Collaborative linkage study of autism. *Am. J. Med. Genet.* 88:609–615.

Bauman, M. L. and T. L. Kemper (2005). Neuroanatomic observations of the brain in autism: A review and future directions. *Int. J. Dev. Neurosci.* 23:183–187.

Bell, J. G., E. E. Mackinlay, J. R. Dick, D. J. MacDonald, R. M. Boyle, and A. C. Glen (2004). Essential fatty acids and phospholipase A2 in autistic spectrum disorders. *Prostaglandins Leukot. Essent. Fatty Acids* 71:201–204.

Bu, B., P. Ashwood, D. Harvey, I. B. King, J. V. Water, and L. W. Jin (2006). Fatty acid compositions of red blood cell phospholipids in children with autism. *Prostaglandins Leukot. Essent. Fatty Acids* 74:215–221.

Bucki, R., P. A. Janmey, R. Vegners, F. Giraud, and J. C. Sulpice (2001). Involvement of phosphatidylinositol 4,5-bisphosphate in phosphatidylserine exposure in platelets: Use of a permeant phosphoinositide-binding peptide. *Biochemistry* 40:15752–15761.

Burger, K., G. Gimpl, and F. Fahrenholz (2000). Regulation of receptor function by cholesterol. *Cell Mol. Life Sci.* 57:1577–1592.

Butler, M. G., M. J. Dasouki, X. P. Zhou, Z. Talebizadeh, M. Brown, T. N. Takahashi, J. H. Miles, C. H. Wang, R. Stratton, R. Pilarski, and C. Eng (2005). Subset of individuals with autism spectrum disorders and extreme macrocephaly associated with germline PTEN tumour suppressor gene mutations. *J. Med. Genet.* 42:318–321.

Buxbaum, J. D., G. Cai, P. Chaste, G. Nygren, J. Goldsmith, J. Reichert, H. Anckarsater, M. Rastam, C. J. Smith, J. M. Silverman, E. Hollander, M. Leboyer, C. Gillberg, A. Verloes, and C. Betancur (2007). Mutation screening of the PTEN gene in patients with autism spectrum disorders and macrocephaly. *Am. J. Med. Genet. B Neuropsychiatr. Genet.* 144B:484–491.

Chauhan, A., H. Brockerhoff, H. M. Wisniewski, and V. P. Chauhan (1991). Interaction of protein kinase C with phosphoinositides. *Arch. Biochem. Biophys.* 287:283–287.

Chauhan, A. and V. Chauhan (2006). Oxidative stress in autism. *Pathophysiology* 13:171–181.

Chauhan, A., V. Chauhan, W. T. Brown, and I. Cohen (2004a). Oxidative stress in autism: Increased lipid peroxidation and reduced serum levels of ceruloplasmin and transferrin—the antioxidant proteins. *Life Sci.* 75:2539–2549.

Chauhan, A., V. Chauhan, I. L. Cohen, and W. T. Brown (2005). Increased lipid peroxidation and membrane rigidity in autism: Relationship with behavior abnormalities. In *Oxidative Stress in Autism Symposium,* Institute for Basic Research in Developmental Disabilities, Staten Island, NY, June 16, 2005.

Chauhan, A., V. P. Chauhan, and H. Brockerhoff (1991). Activation of protein kinase C by phosphatidylinositol 4,5-bisphosphate: Possible involvement in Na^+/H^+ antiport down-regulation and cell proliferation. *Biochem. Biophys. Res. Commun.* 175:852–857.

Chauhan, A., V. P. Chauhan, D. S. Deshmukh, and H. Brockerhoff (1989). Phosphatidylinositol 4,5-bisphosphate competitively inhibits phorbol ester binding to protein kinase C. *Biochemistry* 28:4952–4956.

Chauhan, A., B. Muthaiyah, M. M. Essa, T. W. Brown, J. Wegiel, and V. Chauhan (2009). Increased lipid peroxidation in cerebellum and temporal cortex in autism. International Meeting for Autism Research, Chicago, IL, May 8, 2009.

Chauhan, A., A. M. Sheikh, and V. Chauhan (2008). Increased copper-mediated oxidation of membrane phosphatidylethanolamine in autism. *Am. J. Biochem. Biotechnol. (Special issue on Autism Spectrum Disorders)* 4:95–100.

Chauhan, V. and A. Chauhan (2008). Aberrant signal transduction and membrane abnormalities in autism. 6th International Meeting for Autism Research (IMFAR), London, UK.

Chauhan, V., A. Chauhan, I. L. Cohen, W. T. Brown, and A. Sheikh (2004b). Alteration in amino-glycerophospholipids levels in the plasma of children with autism: A potential biochemical diagnostic marker. *Life Sci.* 74:1635–1643.

Chauhan, V., A. Chauhan, I. L. Cohen, and A. M. Sheikh (2007). Abnormalities in signal transduction in autism. 6th International Meeting for Autism research (IMFAR), Seattle, WA.

Chauhan, V. P. and H. Brockerhoff (1988). Phosphatidylinositol-4,5-bisphosphate may antecede diacylglycerol as activator of protein kinase C. *Biochem. Biophys. Res. Commun.* 155:18–23.

Chauhan, V. P., A. Chauhan, D. S. Deshmukh, and H. Brockerhoff (1990). Lipid activators of protein kinase C. *Life Sci.* 47:981–986.

Cline, H. T. (2001). Dendritic arbor development and synaptogenesis. *Curr. Opin. Neurobiol.* 11:118–126.

Corbett, B. A., A. B. Kantor, H. Schulman, W. L. Walker, L. Lit, P. Ashwood, D. M. Rocke, and F. R. Sharp (2007). A proteomic study of serum from children with autism showing differential expression of apolipoproteins and complement proteins. *Mol. Psychiatry* 12:292–306.

Courchesne, E., E. Redcay, J. T. Morgan, and D. P. Kennedy (2005). Autism at the beginning: Microstructural and growth abnormalities underlying the cognitive and behavioral phenotype of autism. *Dev. Psychopathol.* 17:577–597.

D'Arcangelo, G. (2005). Apoer2: A reelin receptor to remember. *Neuron* 47:471–473.

Derman, M. P., A. Toker, J. H. Hartwig, K. Spokes, J. R. Falck, C. S. Chen, L. C. Cantley, and L. G. Cantley (1997). The lipid products of phosphoinositide 3-kinase increase cell motility through protein kinase C. *J. Biol. Chem.* 272:6465–6470.

DiCicco-Bloom, E., C. Lord, L. Zwaigenbaum, E. Courchesne, S. R. Dager, C. Schmitz, R. T. Schultz, J. Crawley, and L. J. Young (2006). The developmental neurobiology of autism spectrum disorder. *J. Neurosci.* 26:6897–6906.

Donati, R. J. and M. M. Rasenick (2003). G protein signaling and the molecular basis of antidepressant action. *Life Sci.* 73:1–17.

Donati, R. J. and M. M. Rasenick (2005). Chronic antidepressant treatment prevents accumulation of gsalpha in cholesterol-rich, cytoskeletal-associated, plasma membrane domains (lipid rafts). *Neuropsychopharmacology* 30:1238–1245.

Durand, C. M., C. Betancur, T. M. Boeckers, J. Bockmann, P. Chaste, F. Fauchereau, G. Nygren, M. Rastam, I. C. Gillberg, H. Anckarsater, E. Sponheim, H. Goubran-Botros, R. Delorme, N. Chabane, M. C. Mouren-Simeoni, P. de Mas, E. Bieth, B. Roge, D. Heron, L. Burglen, C. Gillberg, M. Leboyer, and T. Bourgeron (2007). Mutations in the gene encoding the synaptic scaffolding protein SHANK3 are associated with autism spectrum disorders. *Nat. Genet.* 39:25–27.

Ehehalt, R., P. Keller, C. Haass, C. Thiele, and K. Simons (2003). Amyloidogenic processing of the Alzheimer beta-amyloid precursor protein depends on lipid rafts. *J. Cell. Biol.* 160:113–123.

Eisensamer, B., M. Uhr, S. Meyr, G. Gimpl, T. Deiml, G. Rammes, J. J. Lambert, W. Zieglgansberger, F. Holsboer, and R. Rupprecht (2005). Antidepressants and antipsychotic drugs colocalize with 5-HT3 receptors in raft-like domains. *J. Neurosci.* 25:10198–10206.

Emamian, E. S., D. Hall, M. J. Birnbaum, M. Karayiorgou, and J. A. Gogos (2004). Convergent evidence for impaired AKT1-GSK3beta signaling in schizophrenia. *Nat. Genet.* 36:131–137.

Esposito, F., R. Ammendola, R. Faraonio, T. Russo, and F. Cimino (2004). Redox control of signal transduction, gene expression and cellular senescence. *Neurochem. Res.* 29:617–628.

Evans, T. A., S. L. Siedlak, L. Lu, X. Fu, Z Wang, W. R. McGinnis, E. Fakhoury, R. J. Castellani, S. L. Hazen, W. J. Walsh, A. T. Lewis, R. G. Salomon, M. A. Smith, G. Perry, and X. Zhu (2008). The autistic phenotype exhibits a remarkably localized modification of brain protein by products of free radical-induced lipid oxidation. *Am. J. Biochem. Biotechnol. (Special Issue on Autism Spectrum Disorders)* 4:61–72.

Fatemi, S. H. and A. R. Halt (2001). Altered levels of Bcl2 and p53 proteins in parietal cortex reflect deranged apoptotic regulation in autism. *Synapse* 42:281–284.

Fatemi, S. H., A. R. Halt, J. M. Stary, G. M. Realmuto, and M. Jalali-Mousavi (2001). Reduction in anti-apoptotic protein Bcl-2 in autistic cerebellum. *Neuroreport* 12:929–933.

Fatemi, S. H., A. V. Snow, J. M. Stary, M. Araghi-Niknam, T. J. Reutiman, S. Lee, A. I. Brooks, and D. A. Pearce (2005). Reelin signaling is impaired in autism. *Biol. Psychiatry* 57:777–787.

Fatemi, S. H., J. M. Stary, and E. A. Egan (2002). Reduced blood levels of reelin as a vulnerability factor in pathophysiology of autistic disorder. *Cell Mol. Neurobiol.* 22:139–152.

Fraser, M. M., I. T. Bayazitov, S. S. Zakharenko, and S. J. Baker (2008). Phosphatase and tensin homolog, deleted on chromosome 10 deficiency in brain causes defects in synaptic structure, transmission and plasticity, and myelination abnormalities. *Neuroscience* 151:476–488.

Friocourt, G., K. Poirier, S. Rakic, J. G. Parnavelas, and J. Chelly (2006). The role of ARX in cortical development. *Eur. J. Neurosci.* 23:869–876.

Garcia-Morales, P., Y. Minami, E. Luong, R. D. Klausner, and L. E. Samelson (1990). Tyrosine phosphorylation in T cells is regulated by phosphatase activity: Studies with phenylarsine oxide. *Proc. Natl. Acad. Sci. U.S.A.* 87:9255–9259.

George, R. J. and C. W. Parker (1990). Preliminary characterization of phosphotyrosine phosphatase activities in human peripheral blood lymphocytes: Identification of CD45 as a phosphotyrosine phosphatase. *J. Cell Biochem.* 42:71–81.

Glaaser, I. W., J. R. Bankston, H. Liu, M. Tateyama, and R. S. Kass (2006). A carboxyl-terminal hydrophobic interface is critical to sodium channel function. Relevance to inherited disorders. *J. Biol. Chem.* 281:24015–24023.

Goffin, A., L. H. Hoefsloot, E. Bosgoed, A. Swillen, and J. P. Fryns (2001). Pten mutation in a family with Cowden syndrome and autism. *Am. J. Med. Genet.* 105:521–524.

Gopalakrishna, R., Z. H. Chen, and U. Gundimeda (1993). Nitric oxide and nitric oxide-generating agents induce a reversible inactivation of protein kinase C activity and phorbol ester binding. *J. Biol. Chem.* 268:27180–27185.

Graf, E. R., X. Zhang, S. X. Jin, M. W. Linhoff, and A. M. Craig (2004). Neurexins induce differentiation of GABA and glutamate postsynaptic specializations via neuroligins. *Cell* 119:1013–1026.

Greer, J. M. and A. Wynshaw-Boris (2006). Pten and the brain: Sizing up social interaction. *Neuron* 50:343–345.

Gutteridge, J. M., R. Richmond, and B. Halliwell (1979). Inhibition of the iron-catalysed formation of hydroxyl radicals from superoxide and of lipid peroxidation by desferrioxamine. *Biochem. J.* 184:469–472.

Hagve, T. A., O. Lie, and M. Gronn (1993). The effect of dietary *N*–3 fatty acids on osmotic fragility and membrane fluidity of human erythrocytes. *Scand. J. Clin. Lab Invest. Suppl* 215:75–84.

Hardwick, J. S. and B. M. Sefton (1995). Activation of the Lck tyrosine protein kinase by hydrogen peroxide requires the phosphorylation of Tyr-394. *Proc. Natl. Acad. Sci. U.S.A.* 92:4527–4531.

Hayashi, T., Y. Ueno, and T. Okamoto (1993). Oxidoreductive regulation of nuclear factor kappa B. Involvement of a cellular reducing catalyst thioredoxin. *J. Biol. Chem.* 268:11380–11388.

Hemara-Wahanui, A., S. Berjukow, C. I. Hope, P. K. Dearden, S. B. Wu, J. Wilson-Wheeler, D. M. Sharp, P. Lundon-Treweek, G. M. Clover, J. C. Hoda, J. Striessnig, R. Marksteiner, S. Hering, and M. A. Maw (2005). A CACNA1F mutation identified in an X-linked retinal disorder shifts the voltage dependence of Cav1.4 channel activation. *Proc. Natl. Acad. Sci. U.S.A.* 102:7553–7558.

Hering, H., C. C. Lin, and M. Sheng (2003). Lipid rafts in the maintenance of synapses, dendritic spines, and surface AMPA receptor stability. *J. Neurosci.* 23:3262–3271.

Herman, G. E., E. Butter, B. Enrile, M. Pastore, T. W. Prior, and A. Sommer (2007). Increasing knowledge of PTEN germline mutations: Two additional patients with autism and macrocephaly. *Am. J. Med. Genet. A* 143:589–593.

Hope, C. I., D. M. Sharp, A. Hemara-Wahanui, J. I. Sissingh, P. Lundon, E. A. Mitchell, M. A. Maw, and G. M. Clover (2005). Clinical manifestations of a unique X-linked retinal disorder in a large New Zealand family with a novel mutation in CACNA1F, the gene responsible for CSNB2. *Clin. Experiment. Ophthalmol.* 33:129–136.

Horrobin, D. F. (1999). The phospholipid concept of psychiatric disorders to the neurodevelopmental concept of schizophrenia. In *Phospholipid Spectrum Disorder in Psychiatry*, eds. M. Peet, I. Glen, and D. F. Horrobin, Maurius Press, Cavnforth, UK, pp. 3–20.

Horrobin, D. F. and C. N. Bennett (1999). New gene targets related to schizophrenia and other psychiatric disorders: Enzymes, binding proteins and transport proteins involved in phospholipid and fatty acid metabolism. *Prostaglandins Leukot. Essent. Fatty Acids* 60:141–167.

Horton, A. A. and S. Fairhurst (1987). Lipid peroxidation and mechanisms of toxicity. *Crit. Rev. Toxicol.* 18:27–79.

Houslay, M. D. and K. K. Stanley (1982). *Dynamics of Biological Membranes: Influence on Synthesis, Structure and Function.* Chichester and New York: Wiley.

Hranilovic, D., Z. Bujas-Petkovic, R. Vragovic, T. Vuk, K. Hock, and B. Jernej (2007). Hyperserotonemia in adults with autistic disorder. *J. Autism Dev. Disord.* 37:1934–1940.

Hranilovic, D., R. Novak, M. Babic, M. Novokmet, Z. Bujas-Petkovic, and B. Jernej (2008). Hyperserotonemia in autism: The potential role of 5HT-related gene variants. *Coll. Antropol.* 32, Suppl 1:75–80.

Hung, A. Y., K. Futai, C. Sala, J. G. Valtschanoff, J. Ryu, M. A. Woodworth, F. L. Kidd, C. C. Sung, T. Miyakawa, M. F. Bear, R. J. Weinberg, and M. Sheng (2008). Smaller dendritic spines, weaker synaptic transmission, but enhanced spatial learning in mice lacking Shank1. *J. Neurosci.* 28:1697–1708.

Ikonomov, O. C., D. Sbrissa, T. Yoshimori, T. L. Cover, and A. Shisheva (2002). PIKfyve Kinase and SKD1 AAA ATPase define distinct endocytic compartments. Only PIKfyve expression inhibits the cell-vacuolating activity of *Helicobacter pylori* VacA toxin. *J. Biol. Chem.* 277:46785–46790.

International Molecular Genetic Study of Autism Consortium (1998). A full genome screen for autism with evidence for linkage to a region on chromosome 7q. *Hum. Mol. Genet.* 7:571–578.

Jain, S. K. (1984). The accumulation of malonyldialdehyde, a product of fatty acid peroxidation, can disturb aminophospholipid organization in the membrane bilayer of human erythrocytes. *J. Biol. Chem.* 259:3391–3394.

Jamain, S., C. Betancur, H. Quach, A. Philippe, M. Fellous, B. Giros, C. Gillberg, M. Leboyer, and T. Bourgeron (2002). Linkage and association of the glutamate receptor 6 gene with autism. *Mol. Psychiatry* 7:302–310.

Jamain, S., H. Quach, C. Betancur, M. Rastam, C. Colineaux, I. C. Gillberg, H. Soderstrom, B. Giros, M. Leboyer, C. Gillberg, and T. Bourgeron (2003). Mutations of the X-linked genes encoding neuroligins NLGN3 and NLGN4 are associated with autism. *Nat. Genet.* 34:27–29.

James, S. J., P. Cutler, S. Melnyk, S. Jernigan, L. Janak, D. W. Gaylor, and J. A. Neubrander (2004). Metabolic biomarkers of increased oxidative stress and impaired methylation capacity in children with autism. *Am. J. Clin. Nutr.* 80:1611–1617.

Jarskog, L. F., J. H. Gilmore, E. S. Selinger, and J. A. Lieberman (2000). Cortical bcl-2 protein expression and apoptotic regulation in schizophrenia. *Biol. Psychiatry* 48:641–650.

Jeffries, A. R., S. Curran, F. Elmslie, A. Sharma, S. Wenger, M. Hummel, and J. Powell (2005). Molecular and phenotypic characterization of ring chromosome 22. *Am. J. Med. Genet. A* 137:139–147.

Jyonouchi, H., L. Geng, A. Ruby, and B. Zimmerman-Bier (2005). Dysregulated innate immune responses in young children with autism spectrum disorders: Their relationship to gastrointestinal symptoms and dietary intervention. *Neuropsychobiology* 51:77–85.

Kharbanda, S., R. Ren, P. Pandey, T. D. Shafman, S. M. Feller, R. R. Weichselbaum, and D. W. Kufe (1995). Activation of the c-Abl tyrosine kinase in the stress response to DNA-damaging agents. *Nature* 376:785–788.

Kim, J., S. Ghosh, H. Liu, M. Tateyama, R. S. Kass, and G. S. Pitt (2004). Calmodulin mediates Ca^{2+} sensitivity of sodium channels. *J. Biol. Chem.* 279:45004–45012.

Kisseleva, M. V., L. Cao, and P. W. Majerus (2002). Phosphoinositide-specific inositol polyphosphate 5-phosphatase IV inhibits Akt/protein kinase B phosphorylation and leads to apoptotic cell death. *J. Biol. Chem.* 277:6266–6272.

Komuro, H. and P. Rakic (1998). Orchestration of neuronal migration by activity of ion channels, neurotransmitter receptors, and intracellular Ca^{2+} fluctuations. *J. Neurobiol.* 37:110–130.

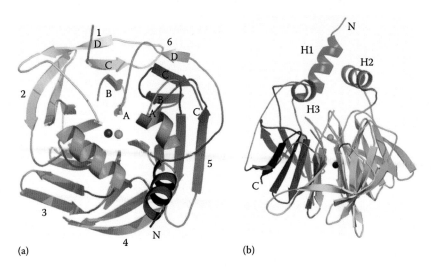

(a)   (b)

FIGURE 6.2 Overall structure of PON1. (a) View of the six-bladed-propeller from above. Shown are the N- and C-termini, and the two calcium atoms in the central tunnel of the propeller (the "catalytic calcium" or Ca1, green (left); the "structural calcium" or Ca2, red (right)). (b) A side view of the propeller. At the top of the propeller, there are three helices H1–H3 which determine the PONs' cell distribution, translocation and secretion (H1), and protein–lipid and protein–protein interactions (H2 and H3). (Reproduced from Harel, M. et al., *Nat. Struct. Mol. Biol.*, 11, 412, 2004. With permission.)

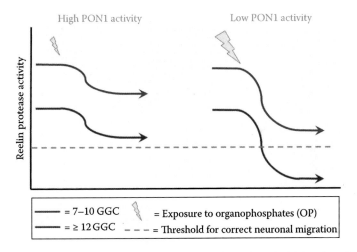

FIGURE 6.3 The gene × environment model for autism. The model involves the Reelin (RELN) and Paraoxonase 1 (PON1) genes, and prenatal exposure to organophosphates (OP). RELN variants carrying either "normal" (7–10 repeats) or "long" (≥12 repeats) GGC alleles genetically determine whether levels of reelin are normal or reduced, respectively. In principle, both conditions are compatible with normal neurodevelopment. However, prenatal exposure to OP can transiently inhibit the proteolytic activity of reelin, which might then fall below the threshold required for correct neuronal migration, also depending on baseline levels of RELN gene expression determined genetically and epigenetically. In addition, exposure to identical doses of OP can affect reelin to a different extent depending on the amount and affinity spectrum of the OP- inactivating enzyme paraoxonase produced by the PON1 alleles of each individual. (Reproduced from Persico, A.M. and Bourgeron, T., *Trends Neurosci.*, 29, 349, 2006. With permission.)

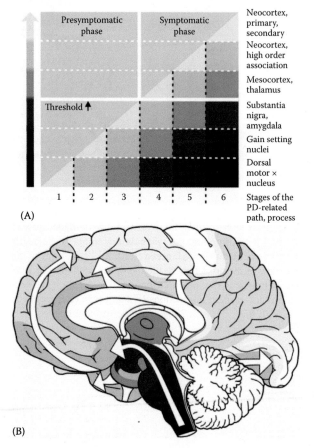

	Presymptomatic phase		Symptomatic phase			
						Neocortex, primary, secondary
						Neocortex, high order association
						Mesocortex, thalamus
Threshold ↑						Substantia nigra, amygdala
						Gain setting nuclei
						Dorsal motor × nucleus
1	2	3	4	5	6	Stages of the PD-related path, process

(A)

(B)

FIGURE 9.3 The ascending pathology of Parkinson's disease occurs in six recognizable stages, beginning in the DMV of the medulla. Progressive shading in table (A) corresponds to the like-shaded anatomic regions represented in diagram (B). (From Braak, H. et al., *Cell. Tissue Res.*, 31, 121, 2004. With permission.)

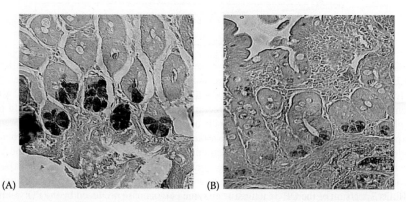

(A) (B)

FIGURE 9.4 Enlargement of Paneth's cells, as indicated by dark staining of secretory granules, was a frequent finding in a series of duodenal biopsies from children with regressed autism (A), as compared to non-autistic controls (B). (Photographs courtesy of Karoly Horvath MD, PhD, Professor of Pediatrics, Thomas Jefferson University, Philadelphia, PA.)

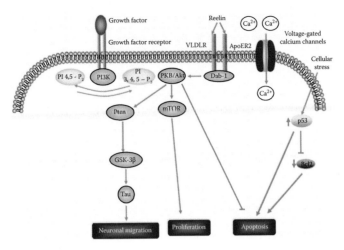

FIGURE 10.2 Participation of growth factor receptors, reelin, voltage-gated calcium channels, p53, and Bcl2 in neuronal migration, proliferation, and apoptosis. Growth factor binds to its receptor and activated phosphatidylinositol 3-kinase (PI3K), which converts phosphatidylinositol 4,5-bisphosphate (PI 4, 5-P_2) to phopsphatidylinositol 3, 4, 5-trisphosphate (PI 3, 4, 5-P_3). PI 3, 4, 5-P_3 is an activator of protein kinase B (also known as Akt) that triggers proliferation pathways by activating the mammalian target of rapamycin (mTOR). Akt also activates phosphatase and tensin homolog on chromosome 10 (Pten), which dephosphorylates PI 3, 4, 5-P_3 to PI 4, 5-P_2. Pten activates glycogen synthase kinase-3β (GSK-3β), which phosphorylates tau protein involved in neuronal migration. Reelin binds to very low-density lipoprotein receptor (VLDLR) and apolipoprotein E receptor 2 (ApoER2), which activate Disabled-1 protein (Dab-1). Dab-1 activates the Akt involved in neuronal migration and proliferation. Cellular stress, on the other hand, affects the activities of p53 and Bcl2, proteins involved in apoptosis.

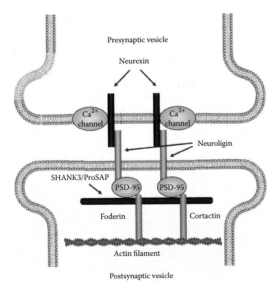

FIGURE 10.3 Interaction of neurexin and neuroligins. Neurexins participate in synaptic transmission by affecting calcium channels. They also interact with neuroligins of postsynaptic vesicles. Neuroligin controls the actin assembly by interacting with postsynaptic density protein 95 (PSD-95), which further interacts with SHANK3. SHANK3/PSD-95 interact with foderin and cortactin, which bind to actin filament.

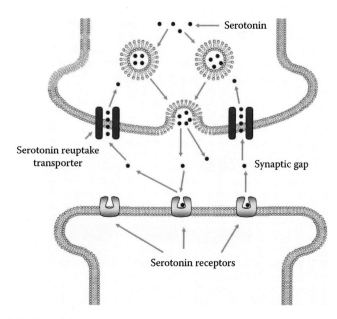

FIGURE 10.4 Serotonin and its receptors, and serotonin reuptake transporter. Serotonin molecules from the presynaptic vesicles are released into the synaptic gap, where they are internalized by serotonin receptors into the postsynaptic vesicles. Serotonin molecules are also retaken from synaptic gaps to the presynaptic vesicle by the serotonin reuptake transporters. An imbalance of the uptake and reuptake system in serotonin causes brain dysfunctions.

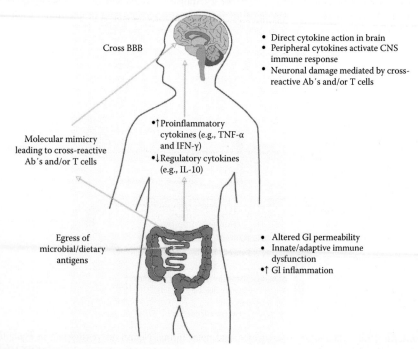

FIGURE 14.1 Possible mechanism by which GI dysfunction may trigger autistic behaviors in children with autism and GI disturbance.

Korvatska, E., Water J. Van de, T. F. Anders, and M. E. Gershwin (2002). Genetic and immunologic considerations in autism. *Neurobiol. Dis.* 9:107–125.

Krebs, M. O., C. Betancur, S. Leroy, M. C. Bourdel, C. Gillberg, and M. Leboyer (2002). Absence of association between a polymorphic GGC repeat in the 5′ untranslated region of the reelin gene and autism. *Mol. Psychiatry* 7:801–804.

Kwon, C. H., B. W. Luikart, C. M. Powell, J. Zhou, S. A. Matheny, W. Zhang, Y. Li, S. J. Baker, and L. F. Parada (2006). Pten regulates neuronal arborization and social interaction in mice. *Neuron* 50:377–388.

Lamb, J. A., J. Moore, A. Bailey, and A. P. Monaco (2000). Autism: Recent molecular genetic advances. *Hum. Mol. Genet.* 9:861–868.

Lander, H. M., A. J. Milbank, J. M. Tauras, D. P. Hajjar, B. L. Hempstead, G. D. Schwartz, R. T. Kraemer, U. A. Mirza, B. T. Chait, S. C. Burk, and L. A. Quilliam (1996). Redox regulation of cell signaling. *Nature* 381:380–381.

Laumonnier, F., S. Roger, P. Guerin, F. Molinari, R. M'rad, D. Cahard, A. Belhadj, M. Halayem, A. M. Persico, M. Elia, V. Romano, S. Holbert, C. Andres, H. Chaabouni, L. Colleaux, J. Constant, J. Y. Le Guennec, and S. Briault (2006). Association of a functional deficit of the BKCa channel, a synaptic regulator of neuronal excitability, with autism and mental retardation. *Am. J. Psychiatry* 163:1622–1629.

Lee, M. H. and R. M. Bell (1991). Mechanism of protein kinase C activation by phosphatidylinositol 4,5-bisphosphate. *Biochemistry* 30:1041–1049.

Li, X., Chauhan, A., A.M. Sheikh, S. Patil, V. Chauhan, X-M. Li, L. Ji, T. Brown, and M. Malik (2009). Elevated immune response in the brain of autistic patients. *J. Neuroimmunol.* 207:111–116.

Lin, C. H., S. H. Yeh, C. H. Lin, K. T. Lu, T. H. Leu, W. C. Chang, and P. W. Gean (2001). A role for the PI-3 kinase signaling pathway in fear conditioning and synaptic plasticity in the amygdala. *Neuron* 31:841–851.

Lin, E. Y., A. Orlofsky, H. G. Wang, J. C. Reed, and M. B. Prystowsky (1996). A1, a Bcl-2 family member, prolongs cell survival and permits myeloid differentiation. *Blood* 87:983–992.

Lintas, C., R. Sacco, K. Garbett, K. Mirnics, R. Militerni, C. Bravaccio, P. Curatolo, B. Manzi, C. Schneider, R. Melmed, M. Elia, T. Pascucci, S. Puglisi-Allegra, K. L. Reichelt, and A. M. Persico (2008). Involvement of the PRKCB1 gene in autistic disorder: Significant genetic association and reduced neocortical gene expression. *Mol. Psychiatry.* 13: 1–14.

Loeffler, D. A., J. R. Connor, P. L. Juneau, B. S. Snyder, L. Kanaley, A. J. DeMaggio, H. Nguyen, C. M. Brickman, and P. A. LeWitt (1995). Transferrin and iron in normal, Alzheimer's disease, and Parkinson's disease brain regions. *J. Neurochem.* 65:710–724.

Lopez-Hurtado, E. and Prieto J.J. (2008). A microscopic study of language-related cortex in autism. *Am. J. Biochem. Biotechnol.* (*Special Issue on Autism Spectrum Disorders*) 4:130–145.

Luo, J., B. D. Manning, and L. C. Cantley (2003). Targeting the PI3K-Akt pathway in human cancer: Rationale and promise. *Cancer Cell* 4:257–262.

MacDonell, L. E., F. K. Skinner, P. E. Ward, A. I. Glen, A. C. Glen, D. J. Macdonald, R. M. Boyle, and D. F. Horrobin (2000). Increased levels of cytosolic phospholipase A2 in dyslexics. *Prostaglandins Leukot. Essent. Fatty Acids* 63:37–39.

Maehama, T. and J. E. Dixon (1998). The tumor suppressor, PTEN/MMAC1, dephosphorylates the lipid second messenger, phosphatidylinositol 3,4,5-trisphosphate. *J. Biol. Chem.* 273:13375–13378.

Makkonen, I., R. Riikonen, H. Kokki, M. M. Airaksinen, and J. T. Kuikka (2008). Serotonin and dopamine transporter binding in children with autism determined by SPECT. *Dev. Med. Child Neurol.* 50:593–597.

Mao, Y., G. Song, Q. Cai, M. Liu, H. Luo, M. Shi, G. Ouyang, and S. Bao (2006). Hydrogen peroxide-induced apoptosis in human gastric carcinoma MGC803 cells. *Cell Biol. Int.* 30:332–337.

Matsura, T., A. Togawa, M. Kai, T. Nishida, J. Nakada, Y. Ishibe, S. Kojo, Y. Yamamoto, and K. Yamada (2005). The presence of oxidized phosphatidylserine on Fas-mediated apoptotic cell surface. *Biochim. Biophys. Acta* 1736:181–188.

Matsuzaki, H., M. Tamatani, N. Mitsuda, K. Namikawa, H. Kiyama, S. Miyake, and M. Tohyama (1999). Activation of Akt kinase inhibits apoptosis and changes in Bcl-2 and Bax expression induced by nitric oxide in primary hippocampal neurons. *J. Neurochem.* 73:2037–2046.

McDougle, C. J. (2008). Serotonin and dopamine transporter binding in children with autism. *Dev. Med. Child Neurol.* 50:565.

McGinnis, W. R. (2004). Oxidative stress in autism. *Altern. Ther. Health Med.* 10:22–36.

Menkes, D. B., M. M. Rasenick, M. A. Wheeler, and M. W. Bitensky (1983). Guanosine triphosphate activation of brain adenylate cyclase: Enhancement by long-term antidepressant treatment. *Science* 219:65–67.

Ming, X., T. P. Stein, M. Brimacombe, W. G. Johnson, G. H. Lambert, and G. C. Wagner (2005). Increased excretion of a lipid peroxidation biomarker in autism. *Prostaglandins Leukot. Essent. Fatty Acids* 73:379–384.

Minshew, N. J., G. Goldstein, S. M. Dombrowski, K. Panchalingam, and J. W. Pettegrew (1993). A preliminary ^{31}P MRS study of autism: Evidence for undersynthesis and increased degradation of brain membranes. *Biol. Psychiatry* 33:762–773.

Missler, M., W. Zhang, A. Rohlmann, G. Kattenstroth, R. E. Hammer, K. Gottmann, and T. C. Sudhof (2003). Alpha-neurexins couple Ca^{2+} channels to synaptic vesicle exocytosis. *Nature* 423:939–948.

Moody, W. J. and M. M. Bosma (2005). Ion channel development, spontaneous activity, and activity-dependent development in nerve and muscle cells. *Physiol. Rev.* 85:883–941.

Morris, D. W., D. Ivanov, L. Robinson, N. Williams, J. Stevenson, M. J. Owen, J. Williams, and M. C. O'Donovan (2004). Association analysis of two candidate phospholipase genes that map to the chromosome 15q15.1–15.3 region associated with reading disability. *Am. J. Med. Genet. B Neuropsychiatr. Genet.* 129B:97–103.

Neubig, R. R. (1994). Membrane organization in G-protein mechanisms. *FASEB J.* 8:939–946.

Neufeld, N. D. and L. M. Corbo (1984). Membrane fluid properties of cord blood mononuclear leucocytes: Association with increased insulin receptors. *Pediatr. Res.* 18:773–778.

Nicolau, D. V., Jr., K. Burrage, R. G. Parton, and J. F. Hancock (2006). Identifying optimal lipid raft characteristics required to promote nanoscale protein–protein interactions on the plasma membrane. *Mol. Cell. Biol.* 26:313–323.

Niu, S., A. Renfro, C. C. Quattrocchi, M. Sheldon, and G. D'Arcangelo (2004). Reelin promotes hippocampal dendrite development through the VLDLR/ApoER2-Dab1 pathway. *Neuron* 41:71–84.

Niu, S., O. Yabut, and G. D'Arcangelo (2008). The Reelin signaling pathway promotes dendritic spine development in hippocampal neurons. *J. Neurosci.* 28:10339–10348.

Pardo, C. A., D. L. Vargas, and A. W. Zimmerman (2005). Immunity, neuroglia and neuroinflammation in autism. *Int. Rev. Psychiatry* 17:485–495.

Parola, M., G. Bellomo, G. Robino, G. Barrera, and M. U. Dianzani (1999). 4-Hydroxynonenal as a biological signal: Molecular basis and pathophysiological implications. *Antioxid. Redox. Signal.* 1:255–284.

Pasca, S. P., B. Nemes, L. Vlase, C. E. Gagyi, E. Dronca, A. C. Miu, and M. Dronca (2006). High levels of homocysteine and low serum paraoxonase 1 arylesterase activity in children with autism. *Life Sci.* 78:2244–2248.

Pediconi, M. F., C. E. Gallegos, E. B. Los Santos, and F. J. Barrantes (2004). Metabolic cholesterol depletion hinders cell-surface trafficking of the nicotinic acetylcholine receptor. *Neuroscience* 128:239–249.

Persico, A. M., L. D'Agruma, L. Zelante, R. Militerni, C. Bravaccio, C. Schneider, R. Melmed, S. Trillo, F. Montecchi, M. Elia, M. Palermo, D. Rabinowitz, T. Pascucci, S. Puglisi-Allegra, K. L. Reichelt, L. Muscarella, V. Guarnieri, J. M. Melgari, M. Conciatori, and F. Keller (2004). Enhanced APOE2 transmission rates in families with autistic probands. *Psychiatr. Genet.* 14:73–82.

Philippe, A., M. Martinez, M. Guilloud-Bataille, C. Gillberg, M. Rastam, E. Sponheim, M. Coleman, M. Zappella, H. Aschauer, L. Van Maldergem, C. Penet, J. Feingold, A. Brice, and M. Leboyer (1999). Genome-wide scan for autism susceptibility genes. Paris Autism Research International Sibpair Study. *Hum. Mol. Genet.* 8:805–812.

Pu, M., A. A. Akhand, M. Kato, M. Hamaguchi, T. Koike, H. Iwata, H. Sabe, H. Suzuki, and I. Nakashima (1996). Evidence of a novel redox-linked activation mechanism for the Src kinase which is independent of tyrosine 527-mediated regulation. *Oncogene* 13:2615–2622.

Qiu, S., K. M. Korwek, and E. J. Weeber (2006). A fresh look at an ancient receptor family: Emerging roles for low density lipoprotein receptors in synaptic plasticity and memory formation. *Neurobiol. Learn. Mem.* 85:16–29.

Raiford, K. L., Y. Shao, I. C. Allen, E. R. Martin, M. M. Menold, H. H. Wright, R. K. Abramson, G. Worley, G. R. DeLong, J. M. Vance, M. L. Cuccaro, J. R. Gilbert, and M. A. Pericak-Vance (2004). No association between the APOE gene and autism. *Am. J. Med. Genet. B Neuropsychiatr. Genet.* 125B:57–60.

Represa, A. and Y. Ben Ari (2005). Trophic actions of GABA on neuronal development. *Trends Neurosci.* 28:278–283.

Risch, N., D. Spiker, L. Lotspeich, N. Nouri, D. Hinds, J. Hallmayer, L. Kalaydjieva, P. McCague, S. Dimiceli, T. Pitts, L. Nguyen, J. Yang, C. Harper, D. Thorpe, S. Vermeer, H. Young, J. Hebert, A. Lin, J. Ferguson, C. Chiotti, S. Wiese-Slater, T. Rogers, B. Salmon, P. Nicholas, P. B. Petersen, C. Pingree, W. McMahon, D. L. Wong, L. L. Cavalli-Sforza, H. C. Kraemer, and R. M. Myers (1999). A genomic screen of autism: Evidence for a multilocus etiology. *Am. J. Hum. Genet.* 65:493–507.

Ritvo, E. R., B. J. Freeman, A. B. Scheibel, T. Duong, H. Robinson, D. Guthrie, and A. Ritvo (1986). Lower Purkinje cell counts in the cerebella of four autistic subjects: Initial findings of the UCLA-NSAC Autopsy Research Report. *Am. J. Psychiatry* 143:862–866.

Sajdel-Sulkowska, E. M., B. Lipinski, H. Windom, T. Audhya, and W. R. McGinnis (2008). Oxidative stress in autism: Elevated cerebellar 3-nitrotyrosine levels. *Am. J. Biochem. Biotechnol. (Special Issue on Autism Spectrum Disorders)* 4:73–84.

Scheiffele, P., J. Fan, J. Choih, R. Fetter, and T. Serafini (2000). Neuroligin expressed in nonneuronal cells triggers presynaptic development in contacting axons. *Cell* 101:657–669.

Serajee, F. J., R. Nabi, H. Zhong, and A. H. Mahbubul Huq (2003). Association of INPP1, PIK3CG, and TSC2 gene variants with autistic disorder: Implications for phosphatidylinositol signaling in autism. *J. Med. Genet.* 40:e119.

Serajee, F. J., H. Zhong, and A. H. Mahbubul Huq (2006). Association of Reelin gene polymorphisms with autism. *Genomics* 87:75–83.

Serajee, F. J., H. Zhong, R. Nabi, and A. H. Huq (2003). The metabotropic glutamate receptor 8 gene at 7q31: Partial duplication and possible association with autism. *J. Med. Genet.* 40:e42.

Singh, S. S., A. Chauhan, H. Brockerhoff, and V. P. Chauhan (1993). Activation of protein kinase C by phosphatidylinositol 3,4,5-trisphosphate. *Biochem. Biophys. Res. Commun.* 195:104–112.

Singh, V. K., R. P. Warren, J. D. Odell, and P. Cole (1991). Changes of soluble interleukin-2, interleukin-2 receptor, T8 antigen, and interleukin-1 in the serum of autistic children. *Clin. Immunol. Immunopathol.* 61:448–455.

Skaar, D. A., Y. Shao, J. L. Haines, J. E. Stenger, J. Jaworski, E. R. Martin, G. R. DeLong, J. H. Moore, J. L. McCauley, J. S. Sutcliffe, A. E. Ashley-Koch, M. L. Cuccaro, S. E. Folstein, J. R. Gilbert, and M. A. Pericak-Vance (2005). Analysis of the RELN gene as a genetic risk factor for autism. *Mol. Psychiatry* 10:563–571.

Sogut, S., S. S. Zoroglu, H. Ozyurt, H. R. Yilmaz, F. Ozugurlu, E. Sivasli, O. Yetkin, M. Yanik, H. Tutkun, H. A. Savas, M. Tarakcioglu, and O. Akyol (2003). Changes in nitric oxide levels and antioxidant enzyme activities may have a role in the pathophysiological mechanisms involved in autism. *Clin. Chim. Acta* 331:111–117.

Sooksawate, T. and M. A. Simmonds (2001). Effects of membrane cholesterol on the sensitivity of the GABA(A) receptor to GABA in acutely dissociated rat hippocampal neurones. *Neuropharmacology* 40:178–184.

Spitzer, N. C., C. M. Root, and L. N. Borodinsky (2004). Orchestrating neuronal differentiation: Patterns of Ca^{2+} spikes specify transmitter choice. *Trends Neurosci.* 27:415–421.

Splawski, I., K. W. Timothy, N. Decher, P. Kumar, F. B. Sachse, A. H. Beggs, M. C. Sanguinetti, and M. T. Keating (2005). Severe arrhythmia disorder caused by cardiac L-type calcium channel mutations. *Proc. Natl. Acad. Sci. U.S.A.* 102:8089–8096.

Splawski, I., K. W. Timothy, L. M. Sharpe, N. Decher, P. Kumar, R. Bloise, C. Napolitano, P. J. Schwartz, R. M. Joseph, K. Condouris, H. Tager-Flusberg, S. G. Priori, M. C. Sanguinetti, and M. T. Keating (2004). Ca(V)1.2 calcium channel dysfunction causes a multisystem disorder including arrhythmia and autism. *Cell* 119:19–31.

Splawski, I., D. S. Yoo, S. C. Stotz, A. Cherry, D. E. Clapham, and M. T. Keating (2006). CACNA1H mutations in autism spectrum disorders. *J. Biol. Chem.* 281:22085–22091.

Staal, F. J., M. Roederer, L. A. Herzenberg, and L. A. Herzenberg (1990). Intracellular thiols regulate activation of nuclear factor kappa B and transcription of human immunodeficiency virus. *Proc. Natl. Acad. Sci. U.S.A.* 87:9943–9947.

Stromme, P., M. E. Mangelsdorf, M. A. Shaw, K. M. Lower, S. M. Lewis, H. Bruyere, V. Lutcherath, A. K. Gedeon, R. H. Wallace, I. E. Scheffer, G. Turner, M. Partington, S. G. Frints, J. P. Fryns, G. R. Sutherland, J. C. Mulley, and J. Gecz (2002). Mutations in the human ortholog of Aristaless cause X-linked mental retardation and epilepsy. *Nat. Genet.* 30:441–445.

Sutcliffe, J. S. (2008). Genetics. Insights into the pathogenesis of autism. *Science* 321:208–209.

Szatmari, P., A. D. Paterson, L. Zwaigenbaum, W. Roberts, J. Brian, X. Q. Liu, J. B. Vincent, J. L. Skaug, A. P. Thompson, L. Senman, L. Feuk, C. Qian, S. E. Bryson, M. B. Jones, C. R. Marshall, S. W. Scherer, V. J. Vieland, C. Bartlett, L. V. Mangin, R. Goedken, A. Segre, M. A. Pericak-Vance, M. L. Cuccaro, J. R. Gilbert, H. H. Wright, R. K. Abramson, C. Betancur, T. Bourgeron, C. Gillberg, M. Leboyer, J. D. Buxbaum, K. L. Davis, E. Hollander, J. M. Silverman, J. Hallmayer, L. Lotspeich, J. S. Sutcliffe, J. L. Haines, S. E. Folstein, J. Piven, T. H. Wassink, V. Sheffield, D. H. Geschwind, M. Bucan, and W. T. Brown et al. (2007). Mapping autism risk loci using genetic linkage and chromosomal rearrangements. *Nat. Genet.* 39:319–328.

Talebizadeh, Z., D. Y. Lam, M. F. Theodoro, D. C. Bittel, G. H. Lushington, and M. G. Butler (2006). Novel splice isoforms for NLGN3 and NLGN4 with possible implications in autism. *J. Med. Genet.* 43(5):e21.

Tappel, A. L. (1973). Lipid peroxidation damage to cell components. *Fed. Proc.* 32:1870–1874.

Taylor, D. R. and N. M. Hooper (2006). The prion protein and lipid rafts. *Mol. Membr. Biol.* 23:89–99.

Tierney, E., I. Bukelis, R. E. Thompson, K. Ahmed, A. Aneja, L. Kratz, and R. I. Kelley (2006). Abnormalities of cholesterol metabolism in autism spectrum disorders. *Am. J. Med. Genet. B Neuropsychiatr. Genet.* 141B:666–668.

Tierney, E., N. A. Nwokoro, F. D. Porter, L. S. Freund, J. K. Ghuman, and R. I. Kelley (2001). Behavior phenotype in the RSH/Smith-Lemli-Opitz syndrome. *Am. J. Med. Genet.* 98:191–200.

Toker, A., M. Meyer, K. K. Reddy, J. R. Falck, R. Aneja, S. Aneja, A. Parra, D. J. Burns, L. M. Ballas, and L. C. Cantley (1994). Activation of protein kinase C family members by the novel polyphosphoinositides PtdIns-3,4-P2 and PtdIns-3,4,5-P3. *J. Biol. Chem.* 269:32358–32367.

Toki, S., R. J. Donati, and M. M. Rasenick (1999). Treatment of C6 glioma cells and rats with antidepressant drugs increases the detergent extraction of G(s alpha) from plasma membrane. *J. Neurochem.* 73:1114–1120.

Turner, G., M. Partington, B. Kerr, M. Mangelsdorf, and J. Gecz (2002). Variable expression of mental retardation, autism, seizures, and dystonic hand movements in two families with an identical ARX gene mutation. *Am. J. Med. Genet.* 112:405–411.

Uchida, K., M. Shiraishi, Y. Naito, Y. Torii, Y. Nakamura, and T. Osawa (1999). Activation of stress signaling pathways by the end product of lipid peroxidation. 4-Hydroxy-2-nonenal is a potential inducer of intracellular peroxide production. *J. Biol. Chem.* 274:2234–2242.

van Blitterswijk, W. J., A. H. van der Luit, R. J. Veldman, M. Verheij, and J. Borst (2003). Ceramide: Second messenger or modulator of membrane structure and dynamics? *Biochem. J.* 369:199–211.

Vargas, D. L., C. Nascimbene, C. Krishnan, A. W. Zimmerman, and C. A. Pardo (2005). Neuroglial activation and neuroinflammation in the brain of patients with autism. *Ann. Neurol.* 57:67–81.

Varoqueaux, F., G. Aramuni, R. L. Rawson, R. Mohrmann, M. Missler, K. Gottmann, W. Zhang, T. C. Sudhof, and N. Brose (2006). Neuroligins determine synapse maturation and function. *Neuron* 51:741–754.

Vojdani, A., E. Mumper, D. Granpeesheh, L. Mielke, D. Traver, K. Bock, K. Hirani, J. Neubrander, K. N. Woeller, N. O'Hara, A. Usman, C. Schneider, F. Hebroni, J. Berookhim, and J. McCandless (2008). Low natural killer cell cytotoxic activity in autism: The role of glutathione, IL-2 and IL-15. *J. Neuroimmunol.* 205:148–154.

Waite, K. A. and C. Eng (2002). Protean PTEN: Form and function. *Am. J. Hum. Genet.* 70:829–844.

Ward, P. E. (2000). Potential diagnostic aids for abnormal fatty acid metabolism in a range of neurodevelopmental disorders. *Prostaglandins Leukot. Essent. Fatty Acids* 63:65–68.

Warren, R. P., N. C. Margaretten, N. C. Pace, and A. Foster (1986). Immune abnormalities in patients with autism. *J. Autism Dev. Disord.* 16:189–197.

Wassink, T. H., J. Piven, V. J. Vieland, J. Huang, R. E. Swiderski, J. Pietila, T. Braun, G. Beck, S. E. Folstein, J. L. Haines, and V. C. Sheffield (2001). Evidence supporting WNT2 as an autism susceptibility gene. *Am. J. Med. Genet.* 105:406–413.

Wayman, G. A., S. Impey, D. Marks, T. Saneyoshi, W. F. Grant, V. Derkach, and T. R. Soderling (2006). Activity-dependent dendritic arborization mediated by CaM-kinase I activation and enhanced CREB-dependent transcription of Wnt-2. *Neuron* 50:897–909.

Weeber, E. J., U. Beffert, C. Jones, J. M. Christian, E. Forster, J. D. Sweatt, and J. Herz (2002). Reelin and ApoE receptors cooperate to enhance hippocampal synaptic plasticity and learning. *J. Biol. Chem.* 277:39944–39952.

Weiss, L. A., A. Escayg, J. A. Kearney, M. Trudeau, B. T. MacDonald, M. Mori, J. Reichert, J. D. Buxbaum, and M. H. Meisler (2003). Sodium channels SCN1A, SCN2A and SCN3A in familial autism. *Mol. Psychiatry* 8:186–194.

Wermter, A. K., I. Kamp-Becker, K. Strauch, G. Schulte-Korne, and H. Remschmidt (2008). No evidence for involvement of genetic variants in the X-linked neuroligin genes NLGN3 and NLGN4X in probands with autism spectrum disorder on high functioning level. *Am. J. Med. Genet. B Neuropsychiatr. Genet.* 147B:535–537.

West, A. E., W. G. Chen, M. B. Dalva, R. E. Dolmetsch, J. M. Kornhauser, A. J. Shaywitz, M. A. Takasu, X. Tao, and M. E. Greenberg (2001). Calcium regulation of neuronal gene expression. *Proc. Natl. Acad. Sci. U.S.A.* 98:11024–11031.

Winter, C., T. J. Reutiman, T. D. Folsom, R. Sohr, R. J. Wolf, G. Juckel, and S. H. Fatemi (2008). Dopamine and serotonin levels following prenatal viral infection in mouse—Implications for psychiatric disorders such as schizophrenia and autism. *Eur. Neuropsychopharmacol.* 18:712–716.

Wiznitzer, M. (2004). Autism and tuberous sclerosis. *J. Child Neurol.* 19:675–679.

Yamakawa, H., S. Oyama, H. Mitsuhashi, N. Sasagawa, S. Uchino, S. Kohsaka, and S. Ishiura (2007). Neuroligins 3 and 4X interact with syntrophin-gamma2, and the interactions are affected by autism-related mutations. *Biochem. Biophys. Res. Commun.* 355:41–46.

Yan, J., J. Feng, R. Schroer, W. Li, C. Skinner, C. E. Schwartz, E. H. Cook, Jr., and S. S. Sommer (2008). Analysis of the neuroligin 4Y gene in patients with autism. *Psychiatr. Genet.* 18:204–207.

Ylisaukko-oja, T., K. Rehnstrom, M. Auranen, R. Vanhala, R. Alen, E. Kempas, P. Ellonen, J. A. Turunen, I. Makkonen, R. Riikonen, T. Nieminen-von Wendt, L. von Wendt, L. Peltonen, and I. Jarvela (2005). Analysis of four neuroligin genes as candidates for autism. *Eur. J. Hum. Genet.* 13:1285–1292.

Yonk, L. J., R. P. Warren, R. A. Burger, P. Cole, J. D. Odell, W. L. Warren, E. White, and V. K. Singh (1990). CD4+ helper T cell depression in autism. *Immunol. Lett.* 25:341–345.

Yorbik, O., A. Sayal, C. Akay, D. I. Akbiyik, and T. Sohmen (2002). Investigation of antioxidant enzymes in children with autistic disorder. *Prostaglandins Leukot. Essent. Fatty Acids* 67:341–343.

Young, G. and J. Conquer (2005). Omega-3 fatty acids and neuropsychiatric disorders. *Reprod. Nutr. Dev.* 45:1–28.

Zhang, H., X. Liu, C. Zhang, E. Mundo, F. Macciardi, D. R. Grayson, A. R. Guidotti, and J. J. Holden (2002). Reelin gene alleles and susceptibility to autism spectrum disorders. *Mol. Psychiatry* 7:1012–1017.

Zhong, N., L. Ye, W. Ju, W. T. Brown, J. Tsiouris, and I. Cohen (1999). 5-HTTLPR variants not associated with autistic spectrum disorders. *Neurogenetics* 2:129–131.

Zimmerman, A. W., H. Jyonouchi, A. M. Comi, S. L. Connors, S. Milstien, A. Varsou, and M. P. Heyes (2005). Cerebrospinal fluid and serum markers of inflammation in autism. *Pediatr. Neurol.* 33:195–201.

Zori, R. T., D. J. Marsh, G. E. Graham, E. B. Marliss, and C. Eng (1998). Germline PTEN mutation in a family with Cowden syndrome and Bannayan-Riley-Ruvalcaba syndrome. *Am. J. Med. Genet.* 80:399–402.

Zoroglu, S. S., F. Armutcu, S. Ozen, A. Gurel, E. Sivasli, O. Yetkin, and I. Meram (2004). Increased oxidative stress and altered activities of erythrocyte free radical scavenging enzymes in autism. *Eur. Arch. Psychiatry Clin. Neurosci.* 254:143–147.

11 Mitochondrial Component of Calcium Signaling Abnormality in Autism

J. Jay Gargus[1,2,]*

[1]Department of Physiology and Biophysics and
[2]Division of Human Genetics, Department of
Pediatrics, School of Medicine, University of
California, Irvine, Irvine, CA 92697, USA

CONTENTS

11.1 Introduction 208
11.2 Mitochondrial DNA Mutations in Autism 209
11.3 Functional Mitochondrial Defects in Autism 210
11.4 Mitochondria are Central Participants in Calcium Homeostasis.............. 211
11.5 Timothy Syndrome Causes Autism via a Defect in Calcium
　　　Channel Function 212
11.6 Other Defects in the Calcium Signaling Pathway in Autism.................... 214
11.7 Calcium Signaling Dysfunction Causes Defects in Neurosecretion.......... 215
11.8 Family of Autism-Related Diseases with Defective Neuronal
　　　Calcium Signaling.. 216
11.9 Pharmacogenetic Calcium Signaling Abnormalities 218
11.10 Conclusion.. 218
Acknowledgment 219
References.. 219

There are several suggestions in the literature that oxidative stress and mitochondrial function are abnormal in autism. However, these defects produce such global perturbations of cellular homeostasis that it is difficult to discern the critical pathway leading to the disease phenotype. Resolving this pathway is important

* Corresponding author: Tel.: +1-949-824-7702; fax: +1-949-824-1762; e-mail: jjgargus@uci.edu

since it provides the most promising target for novel drug development. Since most reactive oxygen species (ROS) arise as by-products of electron transport and oxidative phosphorylation, primary mitochondrial defects are a likely source of ROS. Certainly, genetic defects in mitochondrial function do impose a massive oxidative stress. In the same fashion in which there have been many hints of abnormal ROS levels in autism, many disparate clues have recently come to suggest that abnormal neuronal calcium signaling also plays a role in autism. This is a process recently recognized to be under mitochondrial regulation and capable of disrupting neuronal synaptic function and hence behavior. Therefore, a body of evidence now suggests that calcium signaling abnormalities are a fundamental pathway perturbed in autism, with many lesions arising from primary defects in mitochondrial function, but with other lesions primarily perturbing other components of the calcium signaling pathway and only secondarily impairing mitochondrial function.

11.1   INTRODUCTION

The autistic spectrum disorders (ASD) all share the same characteristic core deficits in social interaction, communication, and behavior; however, they remain a group of developmental disorders that are only behaviorally, not yet pathophysiologically, defined. The high heritability of ASD is assurance that genes and the biochemical pathways they subserve underlie the phenotype, but to date these pathways remain elusive. There are several suggestions in the literature that oxidative stress and mitochondrial dysfunction are abnormal in autism, likely in turn impacting a variety of downstream processes (Chauhan and Chauhan, 2006; Gargus and Imtiaz, 2008; James et al., 2006). But since these impacts on cellular homeostasis are so broad, it remains difficult to discern those pathways most directly connected to the critical phenotypes of autism, and therefore those that would appear the most promising targets for novel drug development. Oxidative stress produces oxidative damage in a cell, tissue, or organ caused by the reactive oxygen species (ROS), such as free radicals and peroxide, interacting with an array of critical endogenous biomolecules. Is this ROS damage etiologically important in the neurological phenotype, or does it merely serve the role of a useful correlative biomarker? Since most ROS arise as by-products from essential metabolic reactions, with electron transport and oxidative phosphorylation of the mitochondria accounting for the vast majority, primary mitochondrial defects are a likely source. Certainly genetic defects in mitochondrial function do impose a huge endogenous oxidative stress (Esposito et al., 1999; Subramaniam et al., 2008). But while they cause an increase in ROS, they also impose a dramatic deficiency in the cell's essential ATP energy supply and in the other essential cellular processes subserved by the mitochondria, such as maintenance of the membrane potential and calcium homeostasis. Just as there have been many hints of abnormal ROS levels in autism, many genetic and biophysical clues have recently come to suggest that abnormal neuronal calcium signaling may also play a role in autism (Gargus, 2009). While calcium homeostasis and signaling are intensely studied biophysical phenomena that are well recognized to play a central role in many aspects of excitable cell biology and synaptic physiology (Flavell and Greenberg, 2008), their role in disease processes is only beginning to emerge (Bezprozvanny and Gargus, 2008). Likewise the coordinating role mitochondria play in these processes has only recently been recognized (Szabadkai and Duchen, 2008). In this chapter, evidence will be presented that calcium signaling abnormalities are a critical and fundamental pathway perturbed in autism, with many lesions arising from primary defects in mitochondrial function, but other lesions perturbing this calcium signaling being independent of a direct impact on the mitochondria.

11.2   MITOCHONDRIAL DNA MUTATIONS IN AUTISM

Arguably the most specific way to show the primacy of a mitochondrial defect in disease is to show a heritable functional mutation in the small segment of the genome carried on the mitochondrial chromosome, the mtDNA, since its encoded proteins only contribute to the mitochondrial membranes. But only a few isolated case reports of mitochondrial DNA mutations in autism have been reported. One patient had the G8363A mutation in the mtDNA tRNA$_{Lys}$ gene documented in blood and skeletal muscle (Graf et al., 2000), and five patients had large mtDNA deletions (Fillano et al., 2002). But these were not typical autism patients as the predominant component of their more severe phenotype was seizures. However, another study has shown that it is very difficult to identify mtDNA mutations in standard, nonsyndromic forms of ASD (Pons et al., 2004). In this study, the investigators explicitly documented the A3243G mtDNA mutation in families with autism. This mutation was originally recognized to cause the MELAS phenotype, an acronym for "mitochondrial encephalomyopathy, lactic acidosis and strokes." Pons et al. (2004) showed that the mothers of four patients with autism had detectable levels of the mutant mtDNA. This mutation was shown to be heteroplasmic, meaning that there were two populations of mtDNA, the wild-type (WT) normal copy, and the mutant copy. Since all cells have hundreds of mitochondria and each mitochondrion has multiple mtDNA molecules, mixed heteroplasmic mitochondrial populations can support cell survival even when the mutation causes a very severe functional defect. However, at low levels of heteroplasmy, it becomes extremely difficult to molecularly detect the mutation against a much higher abundance of the WT molecule. Therefore, while these investigators could detect the mother's mtDNA mutation in two affected sons as well as in their mothers, no mutation could be detected, even using five different tissues in the analysis, in the two remaining children with autism whose mothers carried a heteroplasmic mutation. This may well reflect current technical limitations for detecting low levels of heteroplasmy. This problem is being addressed by emerging techniques that have already broadened the spectrum of recognizable mitochondrial disease (Bannwarth et al., 2008). By providing a more complete picture of phenotypes produced by low levels of heteroplasmic mutations that underlie modest defects in mitochondrial function, such techniques hold the potential to assess the full impact of mtDNA mutations in autism. At this point the data suggest, however, that we likely have only a significant underestimate of this impact.

11.3 FUNCTIONAL MITOCHONDRIAL DEFECTS IN AUTISM

The mtDNA encodes only 13 of the thousands of proteins required to produce functional mitochondria. The remainder of the mitochondrial proteins are encoded by genes on the nuclear chromosomes (nDNA). The role of modest mitochondrial defects in autism has been shown most commonly by demonstration of altered mitochondrial function in subsets of children with autism and a syndrome of energy deficiency, some associated with specific nDNA lesions (Gargus and Imtiaz, 2008). In a large retrospective study of cases of typical nonsyndromic autism, a biochemical profile of mitochondrial energy deficiency was observed for the cohort with autism (Filipek et al., 2004). The signature observed in this group of typical patients with autism included a reduced plasma total and free carnitine ($P<0.001$), moderate hyperammonemia ($P<0.001$), and chronic lactic acidosis. The lactic acidosis was associated with a plasma lactate that itself was only modestly abnormal, but there was an elevated plasma lactate/pyruvate ratio that was predominated by the abnormal pyruvate values. This lactate/pyruvate ratio was confirmed to be a chronic lactic acidosis since it was accompanied by an elevated plasma alanine level ($P<0.001$). Importantly, individual patients were not sufficiently abnormal to be resolved with statistical significance, but rather a large cohort was required to provide the analytical power to discern these group differences (Filipek et al., 2004). Subsequently, a comparably sized Portuguese population study revealed remarkably similar findings: most patients with autism had an increased lactate/pyruvate ratio, but only 20% had a statistically significant elevated lactate, even fewer (<7%) had a functional mitochondrial defect ascertained at muscle biopsy, and none had an identifiable mtDNA mutation (Oliveira et al., 2005). Further epidemiological evaluation of the Portuguese study revealed functional mitochondrial disorders to be the second most common autism-associated disorder, accounting for 5% of cases (Oliveira et al., 2007).

Rare chromosomal rearrangements have the well established ability to link complex phenotypes to specific chromosomal loci, and the most common chromosomal rearrangement seen in autism is an inverted duplication of chromosome 15q11-q13 (Cook et al., 1997). The extra chromosomal material is generally maternal, and carried as an extra marker chromosome, implicating imprinted genes at this locus (Schanen, 2006), but the specific dosage-sensitive gene(s) causing the syndrome remains to be discovered. Filipek and coworkers reported two such children with autism and a maternal 15q-inverted duplication marker chromosome as well as a panel of biochemical signs of mild mitochondrial dysfunction, including elevated serum lactate, pyruvate, ammonia, and alanine, an elevated urinary lactic acid, a secondary carnitine deficiency, and a biopsy-proven partial deficiency of mitochondrial respiratory complex III (Filipek et al., 2003). A similar pattern of biochemical signs of modest mitochondrial energy deficiency have been observed in the syndromic form of ASD caused by mutations in *MECP2* that produce Rett syndrome. Rett syndrome patients were shown to have modest lactic acidosis and hyperammonemia (Eeg-Olofsson et al., 1990) and the mouse model shown to have functional defects in mitochondrial respiratory complex III (Kriaucionis et al., 2006). Likewise, another important syndromic form of ASD is tuberous sclerosis, caused by dominant mutations in either *TSC1* or *TSC2*. The protein products of these two genes heteromultimerize to regulate TOR, a key calcium-sensitive regulator of mitochondrial function whose name arises from the fact that it is the target of rapamycin (Chen et al., 2008; Liu and Butow, 2006). While magnetic resonance spectroscopy (MRS) has been shown to detect elevated central nervous system (CNS) lactate in this disease (Yapici et al., 2007), peripheral biochemical markers of mitochondrial energy deficiency have yet to be reported. In addition, linkage and association studies have revealed autism susceptibility loci at 1p, 2q, 3q, 5p, 7q, 9q, 11p, 15q, 16p, 17q, and Xq; however, none makes a major contribution to the common disease risk, each accounting for <1%, and while many hypothetical candidates have been proposed, no specific susceptibility genes in the loci have been proven (Abrahams and Geschwind, 2008).

Recently, linkage and association studies in nonsyndromic autism have focused attention on mitochondrial dysfunction caused by variation in *SLC25A12*. This gene on 2q24 encodes the brain-specific isoform of the mitochondrial calcium-regulated aspartate/glutamate carrier. In a large study, nine candidate genes in this region were scanned for autism-associated single nucleotide polymorphisms (SNPs) and two SNPs, located in introns 3 and 16 of *SLC25A12*, were found associated with the disease (Ramoz et al., 2004). The same risk haplotype at these two SNPs was then confirmed to be linked and associated with the disease in 197 families (Ramoz et al., 2004). Subsequent studies confirmed that autism was associated with other SNPs within the locus, although none appeared to be functional (Segurado et al., 2005). More recently, a study of postmortem brain tissue from six patients with autism and matched controls showed significantly increased transport activity by the product of the *SLC25A12* gene in autism. However, no mutations or polymorphisms were found associated with the disease (Palmieri et al., 2008). Furthermore, all of the excess enzyme activity found in brain samples from patients with autism was calcium-dependent and was found to be associated with elevated cytosolic calcium levels in tissue from subjects with autism (Palmieri et al., 2008). They found that controlling for the calcium levels, transport activity was identical in isolated mitochondria from patients and controls. They therefore concluded that the critical link to this altered mitochondrial metabolism observed in the brains of patients with autism was in fact caused by altered calcium homeostasis, although it was never directly studied.

11.4 MITOCHONDRIA ARE CENTRAL PARTICIPANTS IN CALCIUM HOMEOSTASIS

As discussed above, calcium plays a central role in mitochondrial function. Mitochondria produce a transmembrane proton electrochemical potential ($\Delta\mu_H^+$), via electron transport along the inner membrane's chain of respiratory complexes. Therefore, $\Delta\mu_H^+$ is the primary energy currency of the mitochondria. It is used to either synthesize ATP or to carry out the coupled transport of other chemical species including calcium. The accumulation of calcium is an important mitochondrial function, and quantitatively calcium transported into the mitochondria represents the major cytosolic reserve. Therefore, a major demand placed on mitochondrial calcium transport collapses $\Delta\mu_H^+$ and has the same net effects on the mitochondrial currency available for ATP synthesis as a primary defect in mitochondrial electron transport or oxidative phosphorylation.

Until recently, the endoplasmic reticulum (ER) had been thought to contain the only dynamic pool of ionized calcium that participates in a host of cellular signaling functions. This intracellular store of calcium could be rapidly released via intrinsic ER channels, the inositol 1,4,5-triphosphate receptors (IP$_3$R) and the ryanodine receptors (RyR). Once released, this calcium would activate a host of kinases, ion channels, and transcription factors, and then be resequestered via the ER's calcium ATPase (SERCA). The importance of this pathway in health and disease is best shown in the pharmacogenetic malignant hyperthermia syndrome (MHS) (Gargus, 2008a, 2009), and there are suggestions of a variant of this disorder in a rare endophenotype of autism (Gargus and Imtiaz, 2008). In genetically susceptible individuals with MHS, the cytosolic calcium pool is hypersensitive. Therefore, general anesthesia triggers a massive release of cytosolic calcium. This in turn produces the hallmarks of the syndrome—muscle rigidity directly from calcium activation of the contractile proteins through a process referred to as excitation–contraction coupling, and then lactic acidosis, hypercapnea, hypoxemia, and hyperthermia, as the mitochondria struggle to resequester the calcium load. Three genes are known to carry MHS susceptibility alleles, but additional MHS loci remain to be defined. The known MHS genes encode: the sarcoplasmic reticulum ryanodine receptor calcium release channel (*RYR1*) causing MHS type 1, the sarcolemmal sodium channel (*SCN4A*) causing MHS type 2, and the sarcolemmal calcium channel (*CACNA1S*) causing MHS type 5. In neurons, these same channels and paralogous channels participate in the related process of excitation–secretion coupling that drives neurotransmission, a process in which defects are implicated in autism (see below).

While mitochondria have long been known to sequester the vast majority of intracellular calcium, only recently, the dynamic nature of this mitochondrial calcium pool has been recognized (Spat et al., 2008; Szabadkai and Duchen, 2008). The mitochondria are now known to actively communicate with the ER calcium signaling apparatus in the generation of rapid calcium signals, forming a bidirectional link between energy metabolism and cellular signals transmitted via changes in the cytosolic-free calcium ion concentration (Danial et al., 2003; Hayashi and Su, 2007; Patterson et al., 2005). It is therefore likely that the modest abnormalities of mitochondrial energetics observed in autism will result in and/or be caused by abnormal calcium signaling (Gargus, 2009). In fact, we have observed a presentation of the constellation of MHS in two siblings with functional mitochondrial defects, congenital hypotonia, and autism. They do not have a *RYR1* allele that accounts for most MHS, and one child has a muscle biopsy-proven partial respiratory complex 3 deficiency, while the other's muscle biopsy reveals only mitochondrial hyperproliferation, a nonspecific indication of weak mitochondrial dysfunction. Their primary genetic lesion remains to be discovered (Gargus and Imtiaz, 2008).

11.5 TIMOTHY SYNDROME CAUSES AUTISM VIA A DEFECT IN CALCIUM CHANNEL FUNCTION

The calcium ion is one of the most ancient, universal, and versatile biological signaling molecules, known to regulate physiological systems at every level from membrane potential and ion transporters to kinases and transcription factors (Berridge et al., 2000). Disruptions of intracellular calcium homeostasis underlie a host of emerging diseases, the calciumopathies (Bezprozvanny and Gargus, 2008; Stutzmann et al., 2006). Cytosolic calcium signals originate either as extracellular calcium enters a cell through plasma membrane ion channels, or, as discussed above, from the release of an intracellular calcium store in the ER via IP_3R and RyR channels. Therefore to a large extent, calciumopathies represent a subset of the ion channel diseases, the channelopathies (Gargus, 2003, 2005). They include the mitochondria, in addition, as the major intracellular calcium repository that dynamically participates with the ER stores in calcium signaling.

The importance of calcium signaling abnormalities in autism is most saliently brought into focus through the lens of Timothy syndrome (TS). TS is predominated by the lethal cardiac arrhythmia syndrome referred to as long QT (LQT) because of its characteristic electrocardiographic (EKG) findings (Splawski et al., 2004, 2005). LQT, a channelopathy disease, has been extensively reviewed and has now been shown to be caused by mutations in all of the cardiac ion channels that contribute to the ventricular action potential (Gargus, 2005, 2008a; Priori and Napolitano, 2006). The pathogenic alleles in these eight ion channel loci all prolong the repolarization of the working myocardium, prolonging the QT interval and setting the stage for a fatal arrhythmia. Like most of the other LQT mutations, TS (also called LQT8) is a simple monogenic dominant channelopathy. It additionally produces extracardiac symptoms such as an invariant syndactyly. Other organ systems are often affected as well, so that immune deficiency, intermittent hypoglycemia, and seizures occur in a significant portion of cases as well. Surprisingly, over 80% of the patients also have autism (Splawski et al., 2004, 2005). The same specific allele of *CACNA1C*, a gene that encodes the "cardiac-expressed" voltage-gated calcium channel, was found to cause TS in 12 de novo unrelated cases (Splawski et al., 2004). This channel is a close paralog of the MHS5 channel discussed above, so lessons learned from that disease should be informative. The specific recurrent de novo mutation, G406R, is located in the minor alternatively spliced exon 8A of the gene. Two other alleles in this locus cause a very similar syndrome but without the syndactyly. These are found in exon 8, not 8A, suggesting cutaneous expression of only the minor transcript (Splawski et al., 2005). The two exons are mutually exclusive, with the vast majority of the mRNA containing exon 8, and both exons encoding the same protein domain. One of the exon 8 alleles produces exactly the same G406R missense as the classic TS mutation, but causes a severe early lethal disease, likely because of the higher abundance of this transcript isoform. The other allele in this exon was only found in a mosaic individual, suggesting that most mutations in this gene are not compatible with viability (Gargus, 2003).

Since so much is understood about the pathogenesis of LQT and the biophysics of the ion channels involved, and it is so clear that one specific "mild" mutation in a calcium channel causes this syndrome and autism, TS might well be the finely honed scalpel that has been long sought to reveal the pathophysiology underlying the enigma of autism. The TS mutant channel expressed in the heart is expressed in the neurons of the brain, and it must cause the symptoms in both organs since TS is a simple monogenic disease of both phenotypes. Since the TS channel conducts a major component of the inward calcium current underlying the depolarized QT interval, a lengthening of the QT to produce the LQT characteristic of the syndrome suggests that excess current is conducted by the mutant channel. This is supported by the finding that a loss-of-function allele at this locus causes the short QT Brugada syndrome (Antzelevitch et al., 2007) and by pharmacology, since the channel blocker verapamil is used to treat TS, and the channel opener Bay K 8644 can mimic the TS arrhythmia (Jacobs et al., 2006; Sicouri et al., 2007). The mutant and normal wild-type (WT) versions of the channel have been expressed in vitro and kinetic analysis has been applied to dissecting the molecular defect biophysically (Antzelevitch et al., 2007; Barrett and Tsein, 2008). It is clear that the major effect of the TS mutation is to alter the speed with which the opened conducting channel returns to a nonconducting conformation, a process called channel inactivation. The channel inactivation arising from changes in the membrane potential are slowed, as would be predicted from the cardiac findings, but a separate mechanism of the inactivation regulated by the calcium signal itself is greatly accelerated. The net result of the mutant is a very rapid inactivation of 50% of the current, and then a very slow inactivation of the remainder (Barrett and Tsein, 2008). Therefore, it remains to be determined exactly which aspect is key to neuronal dysfunction and how downstream signaling is perturbed by this altered neuronal mechanism to produce the characteristic phenotype of autism. Nonetheless, these biophysical findings greatly extend the pathophysiology of autism and begin to render it a neurobiological rather than strictly behavioral phenotype. This brightens the prospect that new molecular targets can be discovered against which new generations of drugs can be developed in this disease.

11.6   OTHER DEFECTS IN THE CALCIUM SIGNALING PATHWAY IN AUTISM

While the TS mutation is highly informative, clearly it does not account for even a tiny fraction of the cases with classical autism. There are, however, additional suggestions that the calcium signaling pathway illuminated by the TS mutation is germane to autism. As discussed above, such a pathway clearly has the ability to integrate the mitochondrial lesions of autism into a consensus signaling pathophysiology. Furthermore, mutations in *CACNA1H*, a paralog of the TS/ LQT8 and MHS5 channels, have been found in familial autism (Splawski et al., 2006). These rare mutations behave more like those contributing to a multigenic disease, such as most cases of autism appear to be, since they do not neatly segregate with the disease as would be the case for a monogenic factor. So while they appear to contribute susceptibility to autism pathogenesis, they are insufficient to cause monogenic disease.

As a further suggestion that the pathophysiology of classical calcium signaling diseases such as MHS might be informative in autism, mutations in a paralog of the MHS2 and LQT3 sodium channel genes, *SCN1A* have been found in rare cases of familial autism (Weiss et al., 2003). This neuronal sodium channel gene had previously been shown to contribute pathogenic alleles to the seizure syndromes generalized epilepsy with febrile seizures plus (GEFS+) and severe myoclonic epilepsy of infancy (SMEI) (Ma and Gargus, 2007) as well as to the migraine syndrome familial hemiplegic migraine (FHM3) (Dichgans et al., 2005; Gargus and Tournay, 2007). It is particularly intriguing that the autism-associated alleles are quite different from the seizure alleles, which produce a more severe lesion in the channel protein, but that they are very similar to the mutations found in the FHM3 families (Gargus and Tournay, 2007). Both FHM3 and autism alleles perturb the same regions of the channel protein, and they are those intracellular regions that interact with calmodulin, a bound protein subunit of the channel that confers calcium sensitivity to its regulation (Gargus, 2009).

Recently in a large survey of consanguineous Middle Eastern families with autism, the technique of microarray homozygosity mapping identified one family that segregated a homozygous deletion of *SCN7A* (Morrow et al., 2008). This gene lies adjacent to *SCN1A* within the sodium channel gene cluster on chromosome 2 and it is rapidly evolving, having arisen from *SCN1A* by endoduplication (Plummer and Meisler, 1999). Its mRNA is neuronally expressed; however, no function of the putative ion channel it encodes has yet been observed (Saleh et al., 2005). It therefore becomes a promising candidate gene that reinforces a neuronal excitation–secretion coupling MHS-like calcium signaling pathogenesis in autism.

11.7 CALCIUM SIGNALING DYSFUNCTION CAUSES DEFECTS IN NEUROSECRETION

As discussed above, neuronal calcium signaling culminates in the release of neurotransmitter vesicles into the synaptic cleft via the process of excitation–secretion coupling. Also discussed above was the syndromic form of autism found in Rett syndrome, shown to be caused by mutations in *MECP2*. Such mutations in mutant mouse models reveal behavioral changes reminiscent of autism (Moretti et al., 2005). In addition, neuronal function studied in the mouse *MECP2* knock-out Rett model revealed that excitatory, but not inhibitory, synapses showed less spontaneous activity than control. This observation suggests a defect in the calcium-dependent processes of excitatory neurosecretion and synaptic vesicle trafficking (Nelson et al., 2006). In a consistent fashion, mutations in neuroligins, postsynaptic cell-adhesion molecules that participate in synaptic function, have been found in rare patients with autism and have been implicated in the disease (Jamain et al., 2003; Sudhof, 2008). The studies of the neuroligin *NGLN3* mutant (R451C allele) mouse model also showed impaired social interactions, enhanced spatial learning abilities, but in this case inhibitory synaptic transmission was increased with no apparent effect on excitatory synapses (Tabuchi et al., 2007). Deletion of *NGLN3*, in contrast, did not cause such changes, indicating that the pathogenic allele is a gain-of-function mutation. Therefore, both the Rett and the *NGLN3* mouse models reveal an increased ratio of inhibitory/excitatory synaptic transmission and serve to suggest that such a neuronal defect contributes to autism. Mutations have also been found in patients with autism in the genes that encode proteins that interact with the neuroligins. These genes include *NRXN1* (Yan et al., 2008), *SHANK3* (Durand et al., 2007), and *CNTNAP2* (Arking et al., 2008). Together with the mitochondrial and ion channel defects, these lesions begin to build a case that autism pathogenesis involves calcium signaling defects that culminate in defective excitation–secretion coupling, synaptic vesicle trafficking, and neurosecretion.

11.8 FAMILY OF AUTISM-RELATED DISEASES WITH DEFECTIVE NEURONAL CALCIUM SIGNALING

A number of common highly heritable diseases have long been recognized to be comorbid with autism—seizures, migraine, and bipolar disease (BPD) being the most prominent (Gargus, 2009; McElroy, 2004; Pellock, 2004). While there are many competing theories for such familial clustering of comorbid conditions, an important consideration is that these superficially distinct common diseases share some fundamental heritable components of vulnerability, likely arising from shared subsets of susceptibility-conferring loci. On the other hand, while these common diseases, like autism, are overwhelmingly multigenic, the strongest clues to understanding these phenotypes are still provided by analysis of rare monogenic forms of these diseases. This is particularly clear for the seizure and migraine phenotypes (Dodick and Gargus, 2008; Gargus, 2006; Gargus and Shih, 2007). The monogenic seizure and migraine diseases are all caused by ion channel mutations and have a common channelopathy pathogenesis. The mutations all produce constitutionally hyperexcitable neurons that are susceptible to periodic decompensations, much like the LQT heart or the MHS muscle (Gargus, 2006, 2008a). For example, the gene families (*FHM1/CACNA1A*, *FHM2/ATP1A2*, and *FHM3/SCN1A*), the mutational lesions and the integrated pathophysiology underlying familial hemiplegic migraine, are all strikingly homologous to those in LQT and MHS, and provide a robust platform for understanding the pathogenesis of the calcium channel autism syndrome, TS/LQT8. The *FHM3* and *FHM1* genes are paralogs of the sodium and calcium channel genes that contribute to MHS (*MHS2* and *MHS5*, respectively) and to LQT (*LQT3* and *LQT8*, respectively). The close relationship of the FHM3 and autism alleles of *FHM3/SCN1A* has been discussed above. *FHM1* encodes the neuronal P/Q calcium channel that participates in excitatory neurosecretion. In vitro expression of *FHM1* alleles of *CACNA1A* in murine pain fiber neurons showed that the mutant alleles cause a dominant-negative loss of the P/Q calcium channels. Additionally, this loss allows other calcium channel types to be overexpressed in their place, further perturbing nerve function (Barett et al., 2005; Cao et al., 2004, 2005; Tao and Cao, 2008). This finding, however, remains controversial since other investigators found conflicting results in their FHM1 models (Kaja et al., 2005; Tottene et al., 2002). FHM2 is a channelopathy caused by mutations that functionally alter an ion pump, not a channel (Segall et al., 2004, 2005). The FHM2 gene encodes the $\alpha 2$ subunit of the Na, K- ATPase, a plasmalemmal enzyme that consumes over 30% of the cell's ATP energy to create the transmembrane ion gradients that allow the ion channels to function. As a major consumer of mitochondrial ATP energy and a sustainer of channel function, this mechanism sits in an intriguing junction of multiple pathways. The enzyme transports sodium and potassium; it does not transport calcium, however, preliminary studies on in vitro expression of FHM2 alleles have shown that these dominant ATP1A2 ion pump mutants primarily produce alterations in neuronal calcium signaling and do so by suppressing calcium release from ER stores via IP_3R (Gargus, 2008b; Smith et al., 2009). Therefore, all three FHM loci, like the three known MHS loci, encode membrane proteins that participate in calcium signaling. It is of note while the FHM2 and MHS1 loci encode quite distinct proteins; both serve as links to the release of ER calcium stores. Therefore, each syndrome involves a sodium and calcium channel plus a link to release of the ER calcium stores. Finally, this pathway seems to extend to the mitochondria since recent studies have directly shown that for murine *CACNA1A* seizure alleles in the *FHM1* locus, pathogenesis is through a pathway that involves disruptions in calcium signaling leading to induced mitochondrial dysfunction that is ultimately capable of causing apoptosis (Bawa and Abbott, 2008).

There are no simple monogenic forms of BPD, however, an illustration of how calcium signaling pathogenesis extends into behavioral neuropsychiatric syndromes is revealed by the recent discovery that the same *CACNA1C* locus mutated in TS/LQT8 was found to be the sole replicated significant association found in two large genome-wide association studies (GWAS) of BPD (Sklar et al., 2008). The SNP markers that were found to be associated with BPD were all in intron 3 of the gene, but their effect has yet to be functionally characterized. Similarly, SNP variants in *BCL2*, an autosomal gene encoding an antiapoptotic integral mitochondrial membrane protein that controls calcium signaling and contributes to the modulation of many cellular functions including gene expression and synaptic plasticity, was found to be associated with BPD and additionally to cause functional defects in calcium signaling in vitro and in mouse models (Du et al., 2008; Einat et al., 2005). The *BCL2* variant associated with increased risk for BPD decreased BCL2 protein levels, increased baseline cytosolic calcium levels, and elevated IP_3R agonist-stimulated cytosolic calcium release and apoptosis.

Finally, calcium signaling abnormalities have been revealed in the monogenic mitochondrial migraine syndromes, monogenic neurodegenerative diseases, such as Huntington disease, and in multigenic neurodegenerative diseases such as Alzheimer and Parkinson disease. Migraine is a common symptom of mitochondrial encephalomyopathy (Finsterer, 2006) and these mitochondrial migraine syndromes are the only migraine syndromes recognized to be caused by major-effect loci other than FHM. These mitochondrial syndromes include disease caused by the classic mtDNA mutations, such as the point mutations underlying mitochondrial encephalomyopathy, lactic acidosis, and strokes (MELAS), or the more recently resolved autosomal nDNA mutations, such as those causing cerebral autosomal dominant arteriopathy with subcortical infarcts and leukoencephalopathy (CADASIL) or in *POLG*, the autosomal gene encoding mitochondrial DNA polymerase γ (Finsterer, 2006; Gladstone and Dodick, 2005; Hudson and Chinnery, 2006; Porter et al., 2005). Huntington disease is caused by dominant polyglutamine-expansion mutations in *HTT*, encoding huntingtin. Evaluation of striatal GABAergic neurons from mouse models expressing full-length human huntingtin revealed that the toxic polyglutamine-expanded huntingtin increased mitochondrial depolarizations in response to *N*-methyl-D-aspartate (NMDA) receptor calcium signals, leading to apoptosis (Fernandes et al., 2007; Zhang et al., 2008). An analysis of calcium signaling abnormalities in brain slices of Alzheimer disease transgenic mouse models highlight the critical roles of calcium signaling in the neuronal pathophysiology, with some studies pointing to direct presenilin-induced ER calcium release (Nelson et al., 2007; Tu et al., 2006), others to presenilin-linked disruptions in RyR calcium signaling (Stutzmann et al., 2007), and still others to presenilin-linked disruptions in IP_3R

calcium signaling (Cheung et al., 2008). The presenilin mutations are rare monogenic causes of the disease, however, mitochondrial dysfunction secondary to oxidative stress seems to be an important contributor to common forms of the disease as well as to Parkinson disease (Yang et al., 2008). In the case of Parkinson disease, the importance of the TS-related calcium channel CACNA1D in pacemaker activity of the substantia nigra dopaminergic neurons that are vulnerable in this disease seems critical. The demands the calcium signals driven by this pacemaker channel place on mitochondria create the age-dependent vulnerability characteristic of the disease, and blockers of this channel spare the mitochondria and are neuroprotective in a murine model (Surmeier, 2007).

11.9 PHARMACOGENETIC CALCIUM SIGNALING ABNORMALITIES

Despite the presence of constitutively defective ion channels in most of the simple monogenic channelopathy diseases such as those causing seizures, MHS, FHM, or LQT, healthful homeostasis predominates the majority of the time. Periodic decompensations occur, and a number of monogenic calcium signaling diseases are recognized to be vulnerable to environmental triggers. Classically such an interaction is referred to as a pharmacogenetic syndrome. Clearly MHS fits the classical definition of such a disease, since the anesthesia trigger is required to manifest the disease in the genetically susceptible individuals. LQT is essentially the same, since the fatal arrhythmia is generally triggered by a massive adrenergic release that occurs as part of the "fight or flight" response. Here the offending trigger "drug" is endogenously synthesized epinephrine, so while not classically pharmacogenetic, it is transparently related. From this perspective, it is reasonable to note that a classic technique to trigger calcium signaling through IP$_3$R is the use of thimerosal (Kaplin et al., 1994), a sulfhydryl oxidizing reagent that is known as a preservative once used in vaccines. Likewise several drugs, but most notably valproate (DeVivo et al., 1998), cause a carnitine deficiency syndrome similar to that seen in the energy-deficient endophenotype of autism (Filipek et al., 2004; Gargus and Imtiaz, 2008), and this drug is one of the few drugs that produces a pharmacogenetic syndrome in human and rodents of autism (Arndt et al., 2005; Schneider and Przewlocki, 2005; Wagner et al., 2006).

11.10 CONCLUSION

Just as clues began to accumulate several years ago that mitochondrial function and ROS production are abnormal in autism, many new disparate clues have come to suggest that abnormal neuronal calcium signaling may serve as the scaffold that unites these and newly recognized genetic lesions into a consensus pathophysiology of autism with a more mechanistic neurobiological underpinning. This evidence now suggests that calcium signaling abnormalities are a fundamental pathway perturbed in autism, with the multigenic disease architecture including primary defects in mitochondrial function, but also other lesions perturbing this calcium signaling pathway independent of a direct impact on the mitochondria. Aspects of this same pathway are beginning to be recognized in other complex neurobehavioral diseases, and hopefully extensions of the work though metabolomics, physiomics, and work in model systems will provide new windows to extend this work to the promotion of new targets for novel drug discovery in autism (Gargus and Imtiaz, 2007).

ACKNOWLEDGMENT

Supported in part by grants to J.J.G. from the National Institutes of Health, the Doris Duke Charitable Foundation and National Alliance for Autism Research/Autism Speaks. The author has no conflicting financial interests.

REFERENCES

Abrahams, B.S. and Geschwind, D.H. (2008). Advances in autism genetics: On the threshold of a new neurobiology. *Nat. Rev. Genet.* 9: 341–355.

Antzelevitch, C., Pollevick, G.D., Cordeiro, J.M., Casis, O., Sanguinetti, M.C., Aizawa, Y., Guerchicoff, A., Pfeiffer, R., Oliva, A., Wollnik, B., Gelber, P., Bonaros, E.P. Jr, Burashnikov, E., Wu, Y., Sargent, J.D., Schickel, S., Oberheiden, R., Bhatia, A., Hsu, L.F., Haïssaguerre, M., Schimpf, R., Borggrefe, M., and Wolpert, C. (2007). Loss-of-function mutations in the cardiac calcium channel underlie a new clinical entity characterized by ST-segment elevation, short QT intervals, and sudden cardiac death. *Circulation* 115: 442–449.

Arking, D.E., Cutler, D.J., Brune, C.W., Teslovich, T.M., West, K., Ikeda, M., Rea, A., Guy, M., Lin, S., Cook, E.H., and Chakravarti, A. (2008). A common genetic variant in the neurexin superfamily member CNTNAP2 increases familial risk of autism. *Am. J. Hum. Genet.* 82: 160–164.

Arndt, T.L., Stodgell, C.J., and Rodier P.M. (2005). The teratology of autism. *Int. J. Dev. Neurosci.* 23: 189–199.

Bannwarth, S., Procaccio, V., Rouzier, C., Fragaki, K., Poole, J., Chabrol, B., Desnuelle, C., Pouget, J., Azulay, J.P., Attarian, S., Pellissier, J.F., Gargus, J.J., Abdenur, J.E., Mozaffar, T., Calvas, P., Labauge, P., Pages, M., Wallace, D.C., Lambert, J.C., and Paquis-Flucklinger, V. (2008). Rapid identification of mitochondrial DNA (mtDNA) mutations in neuromuscular disorders by using surveyor strategy. *Mitochondrion* 8: 136–145.

Barrett, C.F., Cao, Y.Q., and Tsien, R.W. (2005). Gating deficiency in a familial hemiplegic migraine type 1 mutant P/Q-type calcium channel. *J. Biol. Chem.* 280: 24064–24071.

Barrett, C.F. and Tsien, R.W. (2008). The Timothy syndrome mutation differentially affects voltage- and calcium-dependent inactivation of CaV1.2 L-type calcium channels. *Proc. Natl. Acad. Sci. U.S.A.* 105: 2157–2162.

Bawa, B. and Abbott, L.C. (2008). Analysis of calcium ion homeostasis and mitochondrial function in cerebellar granule cells of adult CaV 2.1 calcium ion channel mutant mice. *Neurotox. Res.* 13: 1–18.

Berridge, M.J., Lipp, P., and Bootman, M.D. (2000). The versatility and universality of calcium signalling. *Nat. Rev. Mol. Cell Biol.* 1: 11–21.

Bezprozvanny, I. and Gargus, J.J. (2008). Calcium signaling disease. *J. Gen. Physiol.* 132: 1a–32a.

Cao, Y.Q., Piedras-Rentería, E.S., Smith, G.B., Chen, G., Harata, N.C., and Tsien, R.W. (2004). Presynaptic Ca^{2+} channels compete for channel type-preferring slots in altered neurotransmission arising from Ca^{2+} channelopathy. *Neuron* 43: 387–400.

Cao, Y.Q. and Tsien, R.W. (2005). Effects of familial hemiplegic migraine type 1 mutations on neuronal P/Q-type Ca^{2+} channel activity and inhibitory synaptic transmission. *Proc. Natl. Acad. Sci U.S.A.* 102: 2590–2595.

Chauhan, A. and Chauhan, V. (2006). Oxidative stress in autism. *Pathophysiology* 13: 171–181.

Chen, C., Liu, Y., Liu, R., Ikenoue, T., Guan, K.L., Liu, Y., and Zheng, P. (2008). TSC-mTOR maintains quiescence and function of hematopoietic stem cells by repressing mitochondrial biogenesis and reactive oxygen species. *J. Exp. Med.* 205: 2397–2408.

Cheung, K.H., Shineman, D., Müller, M., Cárdenas, C., Mei, L., Yang, J., Tomita, T., Iwatsubo, T., Lee, V.M., and Foskett, J.K. (2008). Mechanism of Ca^{2+} disruption in Alzheimer's disease by presenilin regulation of InsP3 receptor channel gating. *Neuron* 58: 871–883.

Cook, E.H. Jr, Lindgren, V., Leventhal, B.L., Courchesne, R., Lincoln, A., Shulman, C., Lord, C., and Courchesne, E. (1997). Autism or atypical autism in maternally but not paternally derived proximal 15q duplication. *Am. J. Hum. Genet.* 60: 928–934.

Danial, N.N., Gramm, C.F., Scorrano, L., Zhang, C.Y., Krauss, S., Ranger, A.M., Datta, S.R., Greenberg, M.E., Licklider, L.J., Lowell, B.B., Gygi, S.P., and Korsmeyer, S.J. (2003). BAD and glucokinase reside in a mitochondrial complex that integrates glycolysis and apoptosis. *Nature* 424: 952–956.

DeVivo, D., Bohan, T., Coulter, D., Dreifuss, F., Greenwood, R., Nordli, D. J., Shields, W., Stafstrom, C., and Tein, I. (1998). L-Carnitine supplementation in childhood epilepsy: Current perspectives. *Epilepsia* 39: 1216–1225.

Dichgans, M., Freilinger, T., Eckstein, G., Babini, E., Lorenz-Depiereux, B., Biskup, S., Ferrari, M.D., Herzog, J., van den Maagdenberg, A.M., Pusch, M., and Strom, T.M. (2005). Mutation in the neuronal voltage-gated sodium channel SCN1A in familial hemiplegic migraine. *Lancet* 366: 371–377.

Dodick, D.W. and Gargus, J.J. (2008). Why migraines strike. *Sci. Am.* 299: 56–63.

Du, J., Marchado-Vierira, R., Pivovarova, N.B., Chen, G., Andrews, S.B., and Manji, H.K. (2008). Calcium dysregulation in bipolar disorder: A critical role for Bcl-2 gene polymorphisms in human subjects. *J. Gen. Physiol.* 132: 32a.

Durand, C.M., Betancur, C., Boeckers, T.M., Bockmann, J., Chaste, P., Fauchereau, F., Nygren, G., Rastam, M., Gillberg, I.C., Anckarsäter, H., Sponheim, E., Goubran-Botros, H., Delorme, R., Chabane, N., Mouren-Simeoni, M.C., de Mas, P., Bieth, E., Rogé, B., Héron, D., Burglen, L., Gillberg, C., Leboyer, M., and Bourgeron, T. (2007). Mutations in the gene encoding the synaptic scaffolding protein SHANK3 are associated with autism spectrum disorders. *Nat. Genet.* 39: 25–27.

Eeg-Olofsson, O., al-Zuhair, A.G., Teebi, A.S., Daoud, A.S., Zaki, M., Besisso, M.S., and Al-Essa, M.M. (1990). Rett syndrome: A mitochondrial disease? *J. Child Neurol.* 5: 210–214.

Einat, H., Yuan, P., and Manji, H.K. (2005). Increased anxiety-like behaviors and mitochondrial dysfunction in mice with targeted mutation of the Bcl-2 gene: Further support for the involvement of mitochondrial function in anxiety disorders. *Behav. Brain Res.* 165: 172–180.

Esposito, L.A., Melov, S., Panov, A., Cottrell, B.A., and Wallace, D.C. (1999). Mitochondrial disease in mouse results in increased oxidative stress. *Proc. Natl. Acad. Sci. U.S.A.* 96: 4820–4825.

Fernandes, H.B., Baimbridge, K.G., Church, J., Hayden, M.R., and Raymond, L.A. (2007). Mitochondrial sensitivity and altered calcium handling underlie enhanced NMDA-induced apoptosis in YAC128 model of Huntington's disease. *J. Neurosci.* 27: 13614–13623.

Filipek, P.A., Juranek, J., Nguyen, M.T., Cummings, C., and Gargus, J.J. (2004). Relative carnitine deficiency in autism. *J. Autism Dev. Disord.* 34: 615–623.

Filipek, P.A., Juranek, J., Smith, M., Mays, L.Z., Ramos, E.R., Bocian, M., Masser-Frye, D., Laulhere, T.M., Modahl, C., Spence, M.A., and Gargus, J.J. (2003). Mitochondrial dysfunction in autistic patients with 15q inverted duplication. *Ann. Neurol.* 53: 801–804.

Fillano, J.J., Goldenthal, M.J., Rhodes, C.H., and Marín-García, J. (2002). Mitochondrial dysfunction in patients with hypotonia, epilepsy, autism and developmental delay: HEADD syndrome. *J. Child Neurol.* 17: 435–439.

Finsterer, J. (2006). Central nervous system manifestations of mitochondrial disorders. *Acta Neurol. Scand.* 114: 217–238.

Flavell, S.W. and Greenberg, M.E. (2008). Signaling mechanisms linking neuronal activity to gene expression and plasticity of the nervous system. *Annu. Rev. Neurosci* 31: 563–590.

Gargus, J.J. (2003). Unraveling monogenic channelopathies and their implications for complex polygenic disease. *Am. J. Hum. Genet.* 72: 785–803.

Gargus, J.J. (2005). Receptor, transporter and ion channel diseases. In: *Encyclopedia of Molecular Cell Biology and Molecular Medicine.* R.A. Meyers, eds. Wiley-VCH, Weinheim, Vol. 11, pp. 637–711.

Gargus, J.J. (2006). Ion channel functional candidate genes in multigenic neuropsychiatric disease. *Biol. Psychiatry* 60: 177–185.

Gargus, J.J. (2008a). Receptor, transporter and ion channel diseases. In: *Neurobiology.* R.A. Meyers, eds. Wiley-VCH, Weinheim, Vol. 2, pp. 669–742.

Gargus, J.J. (2008b). Calcium signaling abnormalities in familial hemiplegic migraine, type 2 (FHM2), a window into autism and polygenic neuropsychiatric channelopathies. *J. Gen. Physiol.* 132: 19a–20a.

Gargus, J.J. (2009). Genetic calcium signaling abnormalities in the CNS: Seizures, migraine and autism. The Year in Human & Medical Genetics 2009. *Annals of the New York Academy of Sciences* 1151: 133–156.

Gargus, J.J. and Imtiaz, F. (2008). Mitochondrial energy-deficient endophenotype in autism. *Am. J. Biochem. Biotechnol. (Special Issue on Autism Spectrum Disorders)* 4: 198–207.

Gargus, J.J. and Shih, C.H. (2007). Monogenic migraine syndromes highlight novel drug targets. *Drug Dev. Res.* 68: 432–440.

Gargus, J.J. and Tournay, A. (2007). Novel mutation confirms seizure locus SCN1A is also FHM3 migraine locus. *Ped. Neurol.* 37: 407–410.

Gladstone, J.P. and Dodick, D.W. (2005). Migraine and cerebral white matter lesions: When to suspect cerebral autosomal dominant arteriopathy with subcortical infarcts and leukoencephalopathy (CADASIL). *Neurologist* 11: 19–29.

Graf, W.D., Marin-Garcia, J., Gao, H.G., Pizzo, S., Naviaux, R.K., Markusic, D., Barshop, B.A., Courchesne, E., and Haas, R.H. (2000). Autism associated with the mitochondrial DNA G8363A transfer RNALys mutation. *J. Child Neurol.* 15: 357–361.

Hayashi, T. and Su, T.P. (2007). Sigma-1 receptor chaperones at the ER-mitochondrion interface regulate Ca^{2+} signaling and cell survival. *Cell* 131: 596–610.

Hudson, G. and Chinnery, P.F. (2006). Mitochondrial DNA polymerase-gamma and human disease. *Hum. Mol. Genet.* 15: R244–R252.

Jacobs, A., Knight, B.P., McDonald, K.T., and Burke, M.C. (2006). Verapamil decreases ventricular tachyarrhythmias in a patient with Timothy syndrome (LQT8). *Heart Rhythm* 3: 967–970.

Jamain, S., Quach, H., Betancur, C., Råstam, M., Colineaux, C., Gillberg, I.C., Soderstrom, H., Giros, B., Leboyer, M., Gillberg, C., and Bourgeron, T., and Paris Autism Research International Sibpair Study (2003). Mutations of the X-linked genes encoding neuroligins NLGN3 and NLGN4 are associated with autism. *Nat. Genet.* 34: 27–29.

James, S.J., Melnyk, S., Jernigan, S., Cleves, M.A., Halsted, C.H., Wong, D.H., Cutler, P., Bock, K., Boris, M., Bradstreet, J.J., Baker, S.M., and Gaylor, D.W. (2006). Metabolic endophenotype and related genotypes are associated with oxidative stress in children with autism. *Am. J. Med. Genet. B. Neuropsychiatr. Genet.* 141B: 947–956.

Kaja, S., van de Ven, R.C., Broos, L.A., Veldman, H., van Dijk, J.G., Verschuuren, J.J., Frants, R.R., Ferrari, M.D., van den Maagdenberg, A.M., and Plomp J.J. (2005). Gene dosage-dependent transmitter release changes at neuromuscular synapses of CACNA1A R192Q knockin mice are non-progressive and do not lead to morphological changes or muscle weakness. *Neuroscience* 135: 81–95.

Kaplin, A.I., Ferris, C.D., Voglmaier, S.M., and Snyder, S.H. (1994). Purified reconstituted inositol 1,4,5-trisphosphate receptors. Thiol reagents act directly on receptor protein. *J. Biol. Chem.* 269: 28972–28978.

Kriaucionis, S., Paterson, A., Curtis, J., Guy, J., Macleod, N., and Bird, A. (2006). Gene expression analysis exposes mitochondrial abnormalities in a mouse model of Rett syndrome. *Mol. Cell Biol.* 26: 5033–5042.

Liu, Z. and Butow, R.A. (2006). Mitochondrial retrograde signaling. *Annu. Rev. Genet.* 40: 159–185.

Ma, S. and Gargus, J.J. (2007). The genetics of neuronal channelopathies. In: *Encyclopedia of Life Sciences*. Wiley, Chichester.

McElroy, S.L. (2004). Diagnosing and treating comorbid (complicated) bipolar disorder. *J. Clin. Psychiatry* 65: Suppl 15: 35–44.

Moretti, P., Bouwknecht, J.A., Teague, R., Paylor, R., and Zoghbi, H.Y. (2005). Abnormalities of social interactions and home-cage behavior in a mouse model of Rett syndrome. *Hum. Mol. Genet.* 14: 205–220.

Morrow, E.M., Yoo, S.Y., Flavell, S.W., Kim, T.K., Lin, Y., Hill, R.S., Mukaddes, N.M., Balkhy, S., Gascon, G., Hashmi, A., Al-Saad, S., Ware, J., Joseph, R.M., Greenblatt, R., Gleason, D., Ertelt, J.A., Apse, K.A., Bodell, A., Partlow, J.N., Barry, B., Yao, H., Markianos, K., Ferland, R.J., Greenberg, M.E., and Walsh, C.A. (2008). Identifying autism loci and genes by tracing recent shared ancestry. *Science* 321: 218–223.

Nelson, E.D., Kavalali, E.T., and Monteggia, L.M. (2006). MeCP2-dependent transcriptional repression regulates excitatory neurotransmission. *Curr. Biol.* 16: 710–716.

Nelson, O., Tu, H., Lei, T., Bentahir, M., de Strooper, B., and Bezprozvanny, I. (2007). Familial Alzheimer disease-linked mutations specifically disrupt Ca^{2+} leak function of presenilin 1. *J. Clin. Invest.* 117: 1230–1239.

Oliveira, G., Ataíde, A., Marques, C., Miguel, T.S., Coutinho, A.M., Mota-Vieira, L., Gonçalves, E., Lopes, N.M., Rodrigues, V., Carmona da Mota, H., and Vicente, A.M. (2007). Epidemiology of autism spectrum disorder in Portugal: Prevalence, clinical characterization, and medical conditions. *Dev. Med. Child Neurol.* 49: 726–733.

Oliveira, G., Diogo, L., Grazina, M., Garcia, P., Ataíde, A., Marques, C., Miguel, T., Borges, L., Vicente, A.M., and Oliveira, C.R. (2005). Mitochondrial dysfunction in autism spectrum disorders: A population-based study. *Dev. Med. Child Neurol.* 47: 185–189.

Palmieri, L., Papaleo, V., Porcelli, V., Scarcia, P., Gaita, L., Sacco, R., Hager, J., Rousseau, F., Curatolo, P., Manzi, B., Militerni, R., Bravaccio, C., Trillo, S., Schneider, C., Melmed, R., Elia, M., Lenti, C., Saccani, M., Pascucci, T., Puglisi-Allegra, S., Reichelt, K.L., and Persico, A.M. (2008). Altered calcium homeostasis in autism-spectrum disorders: evidence from biochemical and genetic studies of the mitochondrial aspartate/glutamate carrier AGC1. *Mol. Psychiatry* 2008 Jul 8 [Epub ahead of print].

Patterson, R.L., van Rossum, D.B., Kaplin, A.I., Barrow, R.K., and Snyder, S.H. (2005). Inositol 1,4,5-trisphosphate receptor/GAPDH complex augments Ca^{2+} release via locally derived NADH. *Proc. Natl. Acad. Sci. U.S.A.* 102: 1357–1359.

Pellock, J.M. (2004). Understanding co-morbidities affecting children with epilepsy. *Neurology* 62 (5 Suppl. 2):S17–S23.

Plummer, N.W. and Meisler, M.H. (1999). Evolution and diversity of mammalian sodium channel genes. *Genomics* 57: 323–331.

Pons, R., Andreu, A.L., Checcarelli, N., Vilà, M.R., Engelstad, K., Sue, C.M., Shungu, D., Haggerty, R., de Vivo, D.C., and DiMauro, S. (2004). Mitochondrial DNA abnormalities and autistic spectrum disorders. *J. Pediatr.* 144: 81–85.

Porter, A., Gladstone, J.P., and Dodick, D.W. (2005). Migraine and white matter hyperintensities. *Curr. Pain Headache Rep.* 9: 289–293.

Priori, S.G. and Napolitano, C. (2006). Role of genetic analyses in cardiology. Part I: Mendelian diseases: Cardiac channelopathies. *Circulation* 113: 1130–1135.

Ramoz, N., Reichert, J.G., Smith, C.J., Silverman, J.M., Bespalova, I.N., Davis, K.L., and Buxbaum, J.D. (2004). Linkage and association of the mitochondrial aspartate/glutamate carrier SLC25A12 gene with autism. *Am. J. Psychiatry* 161: 662–669.

Saleh, S., Yeung, S.Y., Prestwich, S., Pucovsky, V., and Greenwood, I. (2005). Electrophysiological and molecular identification of voltage-gated sodium channels in murine vascular myocytes. *J. Physiol.* 568(Pt. 1): 155–169.

Schanen, N.C. (2006). Epigenetics of autism spectrum disorders. *Hum. Mol. Genet.* 15: Spec No 2: R138–R150.

Schneider, T. and Przewlocki, R. (2005). Behavioral alterations in rats prenatally exposed to valproic acid: Animal model of autism. *Neuropsychopharmacology* 30: 80–89.

Segall, L., Scanzano, R., Kaunisto, M.A., Wessman, M., Palotie, A. Gargus, J.J., and Blostein, R. (2004). Kinetic alterations due to a missense mutation in the Na,K-ATPase α2 subunit cause familial hemiplegic migraine type 2. *J. Biol. Chem.* 279: 43692–43696.

Segall, L., Mezzetti, A., Scanzano, R., Gargus, J.J., Purisima, E., and Blostein, R. (2005). Alterations in the α2 isoform of the Na,K-ATPase associated with familial hemiplegic migraine type 2. *Proc. Nat. Acad. Sci. U.S.A.* 102: 11106–11111.

Segurado, R., Conroy, J., Meally, E., Fitzgerald, M., Gill, M., and Gallagher, L. (2005). Confirmation of association between autism and the mitochondrial aspartate/glutamate carrier SLC25A12 gene on chromosome 2q31. *Am. J. Psychiatry* 162: 2182–2184.

Sicouri, S., Timothy, K.W., Zygmunt, A.C., Glass, A., Goodrow, R.J., Belardinelli, L., and Antzelevitch, C. (2007). Cellular basis for the electrocardiographic and arrhythmic manifestations of Timothy syndrome: effects of ranolazine. *Heart Rhythm* 4: 638–647.

Sklar, P., Smoller, J.W., Fan, J., Ferreira, M.A., Perlis, R.H., Chambert, K., Nimgaonkar, V.L., McQueen, M.B., Faraone, S.V., Kirby, A., de Bakker, P.I., Ogdie, M.N., Thase, M.E., Sachs, G.S., Todd-Brown, K., Gabriel, S.B., Sougnez, C., Gates, C., Blumenstiel, B., Defelice, M., Ardlie, K.G., Franklin, J., Muir, W.J., McGhee, K.A., MacIntyre, D.J., McLean, A., VanBeck, M., McQuillin, A., Bass, N.J., Robinson, M., Lawrence, J., Anjorin, A., Curtis, D., Scolnick, E.M., Daly, M.J., Blackwood, D.H., Gurling, H.M., and Purcell, S.M. (2008). Whole-genome association study of bipolar disorder. *Mol. Psychiatry* 13: 558–569.

Smith, I.F., Shih, C, Blostein, R, Parker, I., and Gargus, J.J. (2009). Role of Na/K pump in regulation of IP3R calcium channel demonstrated by familial hemiplegic migraine (FHM2) mutations. The Royal Society Meeting on Membrane Transport in Flux: The Ambiguous Interface Between Channels and Pumps. London, May 19, 20, 2008. *Phil. Trans. Royal Soc. B.* (in press).

Spät, A., Szanda, G., Csordás, G., and Hajnóczky, G. (2008). High- and low-calcium-dependent mechanisms of mitochondrial calcium signalling. *Cell Calcium* 44: 51–63.

Splawski, I., Timothy, K.W., Decher, N., Kumar, P., Sachse, F.B., Beggs, A.H., Sanguinetti, M.C., and Keating, M.T. (2005). Severe arrhythmia disorder caused by cardiac L-type calcium channel mutations. *Proc. Natl. Acad. Sci. U.S.A.* 102: 8089–8096.

Splawski, I., Timothy, K.W., Sharpe, L.M., Decher, N., Kumar, P., Bloise, R., Napolitano, C., Schwartz, P.J., Joseph, R.M., Condouris, K., Tager-Flusberg, H., Priori, S.G., Sanguinetti, M.C., and Keating, M.T. (2004). Ca(V)1.2 calcium channel dysfunction causes a multisystem disorder including arrhythmia and autism. *Cell* 119: 19–31.

Splawski, I., Yoo, D.S., Stotz, S.C., Cherry, A., Clapham, D.E., and Keating, M.T. (2006). CACNA1H mutations in autism spectrum disorders. *J. Biol. Chem.* 281: 22085–22091.

Stutzmann, G.E., Smith, I., Caccamo, A., Oddo, S., Laferla, F.M., and Parker, I. (2006). Enhanced ryanodine receptor recruitment contributes to Ca^{2+} disruptions in young, adult, and aged Alzheimer's disease mice. *J. Neurosci.* 26: 5180–5189.

Stutzmann, G.E., Smith, I., Caccamo, A., Oddo, S., Parker, I., and Laferla, F. (2007). Enhanced ryanodine-mediated calcium release in mutant PS1-expressing Alzheimer's mouse models. *Ann. N.Y. Acad. Sci.* 1097: 265–277.

Subramaniam, V., Golik, P., Murdock, D.G., Levy, S., Kerstann, K.W., Coskun, P.E., Melkonian, G.A., and Wallace, D.C. (2008). MITOCHIP assessment of differential gene expression in the skeletal muscle of Ant1 knockout mice: Coordinate regulation of OXPHOS, antioxidant, and apoptotic genes. *Biochim. Biophys. Acta* 1777: 666–675.

Südhof, T.C. (2008). Neuroligins and neurexins link synaptic function to cognitive disease. *Nature* 455: 903–911.

Surmeier, D.J. (2007). Calcium, ageing, and neuronal vulnerability in Parkinson's disease. *Lancet Neurol.* 6: 933–938.

Szabadkai, G. and Duchen, M.R. (2008). Mitochondria: The hub of cellular Ca^{2+} signaling. *Physiology* 23: 84–94.

Tabuchi, K., Blundell, J., Etherton, M.R., Hammer, R.E., Liu, X., Powell, C.M., and Südhof, T.C. (2007). Neuroligin-3 mutation implicated in autism increases inhibitory synaptic transmission in mice. *Science* 318: 71–76.

Tao, J. and Cao, Y.Q. (2008). Voltage-gated Ca^{2+} channels in trigeminal nociceptive processing. *J. Gen. Physiol.* 132: 22a.

Tottene, A., Fellin, T., Pagnutti, S., Luvisetto, S., Striessnig, J., Fletcher, C., and Pietrobon, D. (2002). Familial hemiplegic migraine mutations increase $Ca^{(2+)}$ influx through single human CaV2.1 channels and decrease maximal CaV2.1 current density in neurons. *Proc. Natl. Acad. Sci. U.S.A.* 99: 13284–13289.

Tu, H., Nelson, O., Bezprozvanny, A., Wang, Z., Lee, S.F., Hao, Y.H., Serneels, L., De Strooper, B., Yu, G., and Bezprozvanny, I. (2006). Presenilins form ER Ca^{2+} leak channels, a function disrupted by familial Alzheimer's disease-linked mutations. *Cell* 126: 981–993.

Wagner, G.C., Reuhl, K.R., Cheh, M., McRae, P., and Halladay, A.K. (2006). A new neurobehavioral model of autism in mice: Pre- and postnatal exposure to sodium valproate. *J. Autism Dev. Disord.* 36: 779–793.

Weiss, L.A., Escayg, A., Kearney, J.A., Trudeau, M., MacDonald, B.T., Mori, M., Reichert, J., Buxbaum, J.D., and Meisler, M.H. (2003). Sodium channels SCN1A, SCN2A and SCN3A in familial autism. *Mol. Psychiatry* 8: 186–194.

Yan, J., Noltner, K., Feng, J., Li, W., Schroer, R., Skinner, C., Zeng, W., Schwartz, C.E., and Sommer, S.S. (2008). Neurexin 1alpha structural variants associated with autism. *Neurosci. Lett.* 438: 368–370.

Yang, J.L., Weissman, L., Bohr, V.A., and Mattson, M.P. (2008). Mitochondrial DNA damage and repair in neurodegenerative disorders. *DNA Repair* 7: 1110–1120.

Yapici, Z., Dörtcan, N., Baykan, B.B., Okan, F., Dinçer, A., Baykal, C., Eraksoy, M., and Roach, S. (2007). Neurological aspects of tuberous sclerosis in relation to MRI/MR spectroscopy findings in children with epilepsy. *Neurol. Res.* 29: 449–454.

Zhang, H., Li, Q., Graham, R.K., Slow, E., Hayden, M.R., and Bezprozvanny, I. (2008). Full length mutant huntingtin is required for altered Ca^{2+} signaling and apoptosis of striatal neurons in the YAC mouse model of Huntington's disease. *Neurobiol. Dis.* 31: 80–88.

12 Inflammation and Neuroimmunity in the Pathogenesis of Autism: Neural and Immune Network Interactions

Carlos A. Pardo-Villamizar[1],* and Andrew W. Zimmerman[2,3,4]

[1]Division of Neuroimmunology and Neuroinfectious Disorders, Department of Neurology and Departments of [2]Neurology and [3]Psychiatry and Behavioral Sciences, Johns Hopkins University School of Medicine, Baltimore, MD 21287, USA

[4]Department of Neurology and Developmental Medicine, Kennedy Krieger Institute, Baltimore, MD 21205, USA

CONTENTS

* Corresponding author: Tel.: +1-410-614-4548; fax: +1-410-502-6736; e-mail: cpardov1@jhmi.edu

225

The role of the immune system and inflammation in the pathogenesis and pathophysiology of autism spectrum disorders (ASDs) is controversial. It is very clear now that the interaction of the immune system with the central nervous system (CNS) is critical for normal neurological and behavioral functions. Recent studies support the view that immune responses are involved in the modeling of the CNS during prenatal and postnatal stages, and that neuroimmune activity may disrupt normal neurodevelopment and contribute to the neuropathological abnormalities found in ASDs. This review focuses on the most recent research that links immunological factors, inflammation, and neuroimmune responses with autism. The findings include maternal autoantibodies against fetal neural epitopes, the activation of neuroglia and neuroimmune pathways and abnormalities in systemic immune responses in children with autism. These immunological factors influence two important stages of the CNS function: early brain development and neuronal organization, and later neuronal and synaptic physiology. A better understanding of the role of immunity and neuroinflammation in the pathogenesis of autism may have important clinical and therapeutic implications. Future studies should focus on the actions of neuroimmune factors during brain development in the pathogenesis of autism.

12.1   INTRODUCTION

Autism spectrum disorders (ASD) are neurodevelopmental disorders with neurobehavioral manifestations that involve communication, social interaction, and behavioral abnormalities (Rapin and Tuchman, 2008). It is increasingly clear that immunological factors and immune dysregulation are important in the pathogenesis and persistence of neurobehavioral abnormalities in ASD (Ashwood, Wills, and Van de, 2006; Pardo, Vargas, and Zimmerman, 2005). In addition, evidence from the effects of maternal viral infections during pregnancy (Chess, Fernandez, and Korn, 1978), an excess of autoimmune disorders in mothers of subjects with ASD or their families (Comi et al., 1999), and the effects of environmental factors on the immune system supports the view that various types of disturbances of immune function are important in the pathogenesis of ASD and in the perpetuation of their associated behavioral and neurological abnormalities. Growing evidence of immunological abnormalities in patients with ASD (Ashwood, Wills, and Van de, 2006) also indicates that, in addition to the spectrum of neurological and behavioral problems exhibited by patients with ASD, other systems, including the immune system and gastrointestinal tract, are also affected. The causes and effects of these immune system abnormalities in autism are unknown but could be critical for maintaining, if not also initiating, some of the abnormalities in central nervous system (CNS) function. These abnormalities likely have both polygenic and environmental bases that will have important clinical and therapeutic implications. Current evidence suggests that neurobiological abnormalities in ASD are associated with changes in cytoarchitectural and neuronal organization that may be determined by genetic, environmental, immunological, and toxic factors (DiCicco-Bloom et al., 2006; Pardo and Eberhart, 2007). Since neuroimmune pathways and CNS cell populations, such as the neuroglia (astroglia and microglia), play central roles during brain development, in cortical organization, neuronal function, and the modulation of immune responses, it is quite possible that these factors, acting in concert with host immunogenetic factors, contribute to the pathogenesis of ASD.

12.2   CONCEPT OF INFLAMMATION

Inflammatory responses represent the main mechanism by which the immune system reacts to challenges by either exogenous or intrinsic factors that disturb homeostasis in the human body. Inflammation comprises a complex network of interacting cells of the immune system and chemical mediators that act locally in all areas of the body in response to those challenges. Inflammation has been viewed traditionally as a defense mechanism to resist or prevent infection, react to tissue injury, or limit the development of cellular or organ dysfunction. This concept has been enlarged recently by new evidence that supports critical roles for inflammation for maintaining cellular viability, initiating pathways of tissue repair and growth, and the sculpting of new organs and functional systems during development (Christiaens et al., 2008; Griffiths, Neal, and Gasque, 2007; Hagberg and Mallard, 2005; Medzhitov, 2008). Although the traditional concept of inflammation has focused on the cellular reactions mediated by leukocytes in areas of tissue damage, this simplistic approach is no longer sufficient as increasing evidence suggests that the main mechanisms of inflammatory responses by the immune system consist of a complex network of interactions between the innate and adaptive immune responses that exert well-coordinated control in development, homeostasis, and reaction to the dysfunction of specific organ systems and the internal environment (Medzhitov, 2008). Although the functional dichotomy of the innate and adaptive systems is a way to understand the immune response, it is also clear that there is a continuous overlap of these two mechanisms of immune action, with the innate responses being less specific but more consistent in maintaining homeostasis and function, and the adaptive response being more specific and focused on reactions to particular deleterious challenges. Thus, inflammation is not necessarily limited to the cellular reaction to injury mediated by leukocytes, but rather it consists of well-coordinated responses by cellular elements as well as several types of chemical mediators such as cytokines, chemokines, and others that maintain tissue homeostasis and function (Barton, 2008). Although inflammation is mostly homeostatic and beneficial, it is clear that deviations of immune system responses may also generate dysfunction and damage such as those that occur in autoimmune disorders (e.g., systemic lupus erythematous or multiple sclerosis), exaggerated responses to infection (e.g., acute disseminated encephalomyelitis), or exogenous challenges (e.g., postvaccinal reactions) (Blanco et al., 2008; Medzhitov, 2008).

12.2.1 IMMUNOLOGICAL RESPONSES IN THE CNS

Although the CNS had been considered an immune-privileged structure, several studies have recently demonstrated that such a concept is no longer valid (Zipp and Aktas, 2006). Recent studies support the view that the immune and CNSs have constant interactions between them that preserve their homeostasis and function (Griffiths, Neal, and Gasque, 2007; Ransohoff, 2002). Both systems are highly hierarchical in structure and maintain their functions based on complex interactions among specialized cells and chemical mediators. While the central role of the immune response in the CNS is to react to tissue injury and maintain an active process of surveillance for the detection of infection and noxious factors, there is growing evidence that the immune system in the brain also contributes to fundamental processes of brain modeling and plasticity (Bauer, Rauschka, and Lassmann, 2001). Because of the diversity in the microenvironments and cellular processes involved in immune and nervous system activity, the elements and mechanisms involved in neuroimmune responses in the CNS are different than those that operate in non-CNS tissues. Some of these mechanisms are modulated by the interplay of chemical mediators such as cytokines and chemokines as well as immune cells (e.g., leukocytes and monocytes), together with elements of the CNS such as neurons, neurotransmitters, neuroglia, and blood vessels (Ransohoff, 2002). In the CNS environment, neuroglial cell populations and the blood–brain barrier (BBB) function as a neurovascular-immune unit that facilitates the continuous functional association of the CNS with the immune system and constitutes the main modulator of neuroimmune interactions (Abbott, Ronnback and Hansson, 2006; Kim et al., 2006).

12.2.2 WHAT IS NEUROINFLAMMATION?

Inflammation in the CNS (neuroinflammation) is a host mechanism that involves elements of the immune and nervous systems in response to the injury, infection, or dysfunction of the CNS and its components. Neuroinflammation involves the interplay of elements of innate and adaptive immunity such as cellular responses by monocytes, B or T cells; mediators such as cytokines, chemokines, and their receptors; complement and other chemical modulators, along with elements of the CNS such as neuroglia, BBB, and neurochemical mediators (e.g., neurotransmitters and metalloproteinases) (Griffiths, Neal, and Gasque, 2007; Infante-Duarte et al., 2008; Tilleux and Hermans, 2007). Similar to immune activation in other organs or tissues, neuroinflammation may involve both innate and adaptive types of immune responses. Most of the adaptive neuroimmune responses are triggered by infectious processes (e.g., viral encephalitis) or external injury to the CNS (e.g., head trauma) and involve the disruption of the BBB, the infiltration of T cells into the brain and spinal cord structures, or the production of specific antibodies that target CNS antigens or other proteins involved in disease processes. Innate neuroimmune responses involve mostly intrinsic responses by neuroglia, such as microglial and astroglial activation, along with increased expression by CNS cells, neurons, neuroglia, and elements of the BBB; and cytokines, chemokines, and other neuroimmune mediators (e.g., metalloproteinases, Toll-like receptors [TLR], and microRNA) (Baltimore et al., 2008; Cardona et al., 2008; Charo and Ransohoff, 2006; Page-McCaw, Ewald, and Werb, 2007; Ransohoff, Liu, and Cardona, 2007). Innate neuroimmune responses occur in neurodegenerative diseases with abnormalities of CNS homeostasis such as those that occur in metabolic and seizure disorders. Frequently, both innate and adaptive neuroimmune responses occur concomitantly; however, they also may have distinctive pathogenic roles at different stages of neurological dysfunction. There is a growing controversy about whether the roles of neuroinflammatory responses are deleterious or protective in the setting of neurological dysfunction or injury, and it is now evident from different experimental approaches that neuroinflammation may play dual roles, both in providing neuroprotection as well as producing injury in the CNS (Griffiths, Neal, and Gasque, 2007; Skaper, 2007; Tilleux and Hermans, 2007).

12.3 HOW DO IMMUNE FACTORS AND INFLAMMATION INFLUENCE ASD?

Although ASDs are not recognized as classical immune mediated disorders, there is increasing interest in examining the role of the immune system and inflammation in the development and persistence of the complex neurological and behavioral abnormalities seen in these disorders. From early brain development to adulthood, immune responses are involved in mechanisms of neurodevelopmental plasticity, neuronal and cortical organization, synaptic function and adaptive synaptic plasticity, and critical stages of brain function that determine neurological and behavioral activity (Pardo, 2008; Pardo, Vargas, and Zimmerman, 2005). There is also recent evidence in humans that maternal environmental factors such as autoantibodies directed to the fetal brain may influence immune responses during fetal brain development (Braunschweig et al., 2007; Singer et al., 2008; Zimmerman et al., 2007) and lead, in experimental animals, to the development of neuropathological abnormalities and behaviors similar to those present in ASD (Patterson, 2002).

12.3.1 INFLUENCE OF THE IMMUNE SYSTEM ON BRAIN DEVELOPMENT AND THE PATHOGENESIS OF ASD

Brain development is a complex and dynamic process in which different molecular pathways overlap with each other and change over time to produce a well-organized and compartmentalized structure. The development of the cerebral cortex, for example, involves highly complex and coordinated phases of cellular organization that includes four overlapping stages: neurogenesis, fate determination, migration, and differentiation, which finally result in the highly organized architecture and circuitry that characterize the mammalian neocortex. The role of neuroimmune factors is critical for all processes of neuronal migration, axonal growth, neuronal positioning, cortical lamination, as well as dendritic and synaptic formation. All elements of the neuroimmune network—including astrocytes and microglia; immune mediators such as cytokines, chemokines, and soluble factors produced by neuroglia (e.g., growth factors and neurotrophins); as well as other classical immune pathways such as those associated with the major histocompatibility complex (e.g., MHC class I) and complement—participate in mechanisms of neurodevelopment during intrauterine and postnatal stages. Therefore, a dual role, developmental and immunological, is now a well-recognized feature of all elements of neuroimmune responses (Boulanger and Shatz, 2004; Tonelli, Postolache, and Sternberg, 2005).

Because the disorganization of cortical neurons, abnormalities in mini-columnar organization and subcortical white matter, as well as brain growth abnormalities are the dominant features of the neuropathology of ASD (Bauman and Kemper, 2005; Casanova, 2007), it is likely that the critical period of pathogenesis in autism occurs during fetal brain development and the first year of life (Pardo, 2008; Pardo and Eberhart, 2007). During this critical pathogenic period, neurodevelopmental processes such as neuronal migration, cortical lamination, synaptic and dendritic modeling, and the establishment of neuronal and cortical networks are influenced not only by genetic factors, but also by important neuroimmune mechanisms that involve astrocytes and microglia; interactions of cytokines, chemokines, and their receptors; the developmental expression of TLRs; and complement activation (Bauer, Kerr, and Patterson, 2007; Lagercrantz and Ringstedt, 2001; Stevens et al., 2007). These neurobiological processes, along with the influence of the neuroimmune system, are crucial for the development of neurological and behavioral trajectories, such as social cognition, language and communication, and motor development (Pardo and Eberhart, 2007). Disturbances of specific neurobiological trajectories triggered by abnormalities in the maternal environment or by genetic influences may eventually translate into abnormal patterns of neurodevelopment and behaviors that characterize ASD. In addition to their actions during the period of pathogenesis, neuroimmune responses also may be activated during post-pathogenic stages during which neurological regression, abnormal neuronal activity (e.g., seizures), and aberrant neural networks may trigger such responses as the part of deleterious responses or even as the part of neuroprotective pathways. It is unclear at present, whether neuroimmune responses or neuroinflammation are common occurrences in the brain of patients with ASD during postnatal stages or adulthood; however, our neuroimmunopathological studies suggest that a chronic stage of immune activation or neuroinflammation occurs at least in subsets of patients with ASD. The presence of these changes is not determined by the age or duration of the disorder, and in the postmortem brain tissues we examined, it appears to be an ongoing, long-term neuropathological process (Vargas et al., 2005).

12.3.2 Cytokines and Chemokines in Brain Development

Along with the neuroglia, another important element of the neuroimmune response that contributes to brain development is a complex network of cytokines, chemokines, and their receptors. Both cytokines and chemokines are well-known mediators of immunological activity, maturation, and the trafficking of immune cells and responses to injury (Engelhardt and Ransohoff, 2005; Ransohoff, Liu, and Cardona, 2007). Although few human studies are available, neuropathological studies have demonstrated that subsets of chemokines are present in the CNS and exert their modulatory and developmental functions on neurons, neuroglia, and BBB by inter-acting with membrane receptors, even at early stages of brain development (Rostene, Kitabgi, and Parsadaniantz, 2007). Some chemokines are critical for neuroimmune function and are involved early in neurodevelopment. For example, CCL2 (also known as macrophage chemoattractant protein-1, MCP-1) and CCL5 (also known as RANTES) are important cues for processes of microglial migration and the coloni-zation of the CNS (Rezaie, Cairns and Male, 1997). Experimental models in rodents have demonstrated the crucial function of CXCL12 (also known as stromal derived factor-1, SDF-1) and its receptor, and CXCR4 in mechanisms of cerebellar develop-ment, neuronal migration, and axonal pathfinding (Lazarini et al., 2003; Ma et al., 1998; Stumm and Hollt, 2007; Zou et al., 1998). CXCL12 appears to have an impor-tant function in mechanisms that control migration of Cajal–Retzius cells, important sources of the glycoprotein *reelin* and other factors that support radial glia in the critical process of cortical lamination (Paredes et al., 2006). Functional disturbances in reelin and Cajal–Retzius cells result in abnormalities of neuronal positioning, cortical lamination, and the columnar organization of the cortical neurons, puta-tive factors that may contribute to the neuropathological abnormalities in autism (Fatemi et al., 2005). Similarly, cytokines have been recognized as important fac-tors during brain development (Pousset, 1994; Pousset, Fournier, and Keane, 1997). Cytokines traditionally recognized as "pro-inflammatory," such IL-6, TNF-α, and IL-1β, as well as "anti-inflammatory" cytokines, such as TGF-β, are involved in pathways that contribute to CNS development (Bauer, Kerr, and Patterson, 2007; Munoz-Fernandez and Fresno, 1998; Nakashima and Taga, 2002; Taga and Fukuda, 2005). The TGF-β cytokine family, for example, is involved in essential nervous tissue remodeling, including cell-cycle control, regulation of early development and differentiation, neuron survival, and astrocyte differentiation (Gomes, Sousa, and Romao, 2005). Cytokines such as IL-6 appear to mediate long-lasting changes in the transcription and behavior of adult offspring following maternal immune activation during gestation (Smith et al., 2007).

12.3.3 Maternal Environment and Effects of Immune Responses on Neurodevelopment in the Pathogenesis of ASD

There is growing evidence that the maternal immune environment affects the devel-oping fetal CNS and determines specific patterns of inflammation-mediated brain and behavioral pathology (Hagberg and Mallard, 2005; Meyer, Yee, and Feldon, 2007; Meyer et al., 2006). The most exciting line of research that links maternal immunological factors in the pathogenesis of ASD comes from the demonstration of maternal autoantibodies in the serum of some mothers of patients with autism (Braunschweig et al., 2007; Singer et al., 2008; Zimmerman et al., 2007) and their presence correlates with a history of early developmental regression in their off-spring (Braunschweig et al., 2007). Two different groups of researchers have dem-onstrated the presence of antibodies that cross-react with fetal, but not adult, neural antigens. These findings suggest that, at least in a subset of patients with autism, the potential passive transfer of maternal antibodies during fetal life may have played a pathogenic role in the presence of the disorder. It is unclear, however, what the specific targets of these autoantibodies are or what triggers their production. Following an earlier study by Dalton et al. (2003), both groups have successfully transferred the recently described serum anti-fetal brain antibodies from mothers of children with autism into animal models during gestation, and demonstrated behavioral changes suggesting features of autism in the offspring of mice (Morris et al., 2008) and monkeys (Martin et al., 2008).

Another recent topic of increasing interest focuses on the potential role of immunotoxicants and nutritional factors that activate maternal immune responses and which in turn may affect early stages of brain development. There is growing evidence for effects of environmental toxins such as herbicides and other environmental chemicals on either maternal or fetal immune activation that may produce developmental brain disarrangements associated with the neurological and behavioral problems observed in ASD (Dietert and Dietert, 2008; Roman, 2007). We have observed neuroinflammation following the experimental neonatal exposure of rats (analogous to early third trimester in humans) to terbutaline, a β-2 adrenergic receptor agonist and drug for asthma that is commonly used for tocolysis (slowing premature labor) (Zerrate et al., 2007), as well as in the brain of murine offspring following the gestational transfer of human maternal anti-fetal brain antibodies (Morris et al., 2008). These observations support the relevance of maternal immune states and are consistent with descriptions of an increased frequency of autoimmune disorders in mothers and families of subjects with autism (Comi et al., 1999; Croen et al., 2005; Molloy et al., 2006; Mouridsen et al., 2007; Sweeten et al., 2003). Immunogenetic susceptibility factors, particularly in maternal human leukocyte antigens (HLA), will be discussed in Section 12.4.

In addition to the epidemiological and immune evidence from studies in human subjects, experimental models of maternal infections and immune challenges have demonstrated the effects of immune responses on the development of neurobiological and behavioral abnormalities consistent with neuropsychiatric disorders such as autism and schizophrenia (Patterson, 2002, 2007). Although different gestational periods of vulnerability may determine specific outcomes, it appears that infection-associated immunological events in early stages of fetal life may have a greater impact than later stages on the occurrence and progression of neurodevelopmental abnormalities (Bach et al., 2008; Meyer, Yee, and Feldon, 2007). In animal models, the disruption of normal cytokine and chemokine developmental pathways, triggered by either infections or immune challenges, appears to modify the expression patterns of these immune mediators in the fetal brain. In turn, these altered patterns determine the development of neuropathological changes and the various forms of behavioral dysfunction that emerge later in life (Meyer et al., 2006; Shi et al., 2003; Smith et al., 2007). Interleukin-6, a well-known pro-inflammatory cytokine during adulthood, appears to be a key factor in the development of pathogenic effects from maternal immune challenges (Smith et al., 2007). Other immune regulators such as bone morphogenetic proteins and TGF-β also appear to play important roles during stages of maternal immune reactions that challenge the developing fetal brain (Jonakait, 2007). These experimental observations point out that future studies on the pathogenesis of ASD should focus on a more detailed analysis of maternal infections as potential risk factors associated with the development of these disorders.

12.3.4   NEUROGLIA AND NEUROINFLAMMATORY RESPONSES DURING ADULTHOOD

In the CNS, neuroglial cells such as astrocytes and microglia, along with perivascular macrophages and endothelial cells, are important for maintaining normal neuronal function and homeostasis (Aloisi, 2001; Bauer, Rauschka, and Lassmann, 2001; Bessis et al., 2007; Dong and Benveniste, 2001; Neumann, 2001; Prat et al., 2001; Trapp et al., 2007; Williams and Hickey, 2002). As such, these CNS elements are also involved in immune function and the interaction of the immune and nervous systems. Neuroglial cells also contribute in a number of ways to the regulation of immune responses and neuronal activity in the CNS. Both microglia and astrocytes are involved in crucial neurobiological functions and contribute extensively to processes of cortical organization, neuroaxonal guidance, and synaptic plasticity (Fields and Stevens-Graham, 2002; Murai and Van Meyel, 2007). Astrocytes, for example, play an important role in the detoxification of excess excitatory amino acids (Nedergaard, Takano, and Hansen, 2002), the maintenance of the integrity of the BBB (Prat et al., 2001), the production of neurotrophic factors (Bauer et al., 2001), and the metabolism of glutamate (Nedergaard, Takano, and Hansen, 2002; Tilleux and Hermans, 2007). Under normal homeostatic conditions, astrocytes facilitate neuronal survival by producing growth factors and mediating the uptake and removal of excitotoxic neurotransmitters, such as glutamate, from the synaptic microenvironment (Nedergaard, Takano, and Hansen, 2002; Ransom et al., 2003). Both astroglia and microglia are involved in pathogenic inflammatory mechanisms that are common to diverse disorders of the CNS and are important factors in the neuroimmune response that occurs in response to the disruption of homeostasis in the CNS. During neuroglial activation secondary to injury or neuronal dysfunction, astrocytes and microglia produce several factors that modulate inflammatory responses. For example, they secrete pro-inflammatory cytokines, chemokines, and metalloproteinases that can magnify and accelerate immune reactions within the CNS (Bauer, Rauschka, and Lassmann, 2001; Benn, Halfpenny, and Scolding, 2001; Rosenberg, 2002). Microglial cells, for example, are involved in synaptic stripping, cortical plasticity, as well as immune surveillance (Aloisi, 2001; Ambrosini and Aloisi, 2004; Graeber, Bise, and Mehraein, 1993; Trapp et al., 2007). Perivascular astrocytes and microglia modulate BBB activity and secrete factors that regulate the trafficking of immune cells into the CNS.

In several degenerative and immune-mediated disorders of the CNS, such as Alzheimer's disease (AD), HIV dementia, epilepsy, schizophrenia, and multiple sclerosis, astroglia and microglia associated with innate neuroimmune responses are central to the pathogenic mechanisms of neurodegeneration and appear to mediate important processes that lead to neuronal dysfunction (Aloisi, 2001; Golde, 2002). For example, in HIV dementia, microglial activation and infiltration by macrophages contribute to the neuronal damage responsible for the dementia (Kaul, Garden, and Lipton, 2001). In other disorders such as epilepsy, and particularly in Rasmussen's syndrome, a rare pediatric epileptic disorder, both astroglial and microglial reactions occur in parallel to adaptive neuroimmune responses mediated by the T-cell infiltration of the cerebral cortex (Pardo et al., 2004). In neurodegenerative disorders such as Parkinson's disease (PD) and AD, the role of the neuroimmune response has

been exposed as a critical part of the cascade of molecular and cellular events leading to either the dysfunction of specific neuronal populations, such as nigral cells
in PD, or the processing and degradation of amyloid in AD (Blasko and Grubeck-
Loebenstein, 2003; McGeer and McGeer, 2002; Nagatsu and Sawada, 2005). Several
studies have shown that microglia are activated and increased in number in schizophrenia, both in postmortem tissue and on positron emission tomography, which
may result from several possible underlying metabolic disturbances (Radewicz et al.,
2000; van Berckel et al., 2008; Wierzba-Bobrowicz et al., 2005). Clinical similarities
with schizophrenia raise the possibility of using analogous approaches to diagnostic
imaging in autism. Because of the central importance of neuroinflammatory pathways and neuroglia in response to neuronal dysfunction and their pathogenic roles in
diverse neurological disorders, we have hypothesized that neuroimmune responses
and neuroinflammation are associated with the pathogenic mechanisms involved in
cortical and neuronal dysfunction observed in ASD. Neuroinflammation in autism
may lend itself to treatment trials using anti-inflammatory drugs, which have shown
some benefit in PD and AD, as well as schizophrenia (Muller et al., 2002; Vlad
et al., 2008; Wahner et al., 2007).

12.3.5 Neuroglia, Neuroinflammation, and Synaptic Plasticity

Neuroglia are fundamental components of communication in neuronal networks by
the virtue of their contribution to the modulation of synaptic and dendritic function and by the generation of responses to neuronal activity. These functions are
facilitated by complex neuroglia–neuronal interactions in which both microglia and
astroglia maintain a dynamic structural and functional association with synapses
and dendrites (Volterra and Meldolesi, 2005). Neuronal–neuroglia interactions are
regionally specific and occur in all regions of the CNS. Astroglia exhibit extensive
and elaborate interplay with both presynaptic and postsynaptic structures in a highly
organized way, as individual astrocytes are associated with specific microdomains
and local circuits. In the hippocampus, for example, individual astrocytes maintain a
functional association with a specific neuronal territory that modulates the physiology
of a well-defined subset of synapses. It has been calculated that in the hippocampus, an individual astrocyte domain may modulate the function of 140,000 synapses
(Bushong et al., 2002; Kirov and Harris, 1999). Similarly, Bergmann glia in the cerebellum have specific local interactions with individual synapses in discrete microdomains (Grosche et al., 1999). Recent morphological and neurophysiological studies
have also demonstrated that individual astroglia in the cerebral cortex interact with
specific islands of functional synapses and that a single astrocyte may enwrap from
4 to 8 neurons and establish contacts with 300 to 600 dendrites (Halassa et al., 2007).
Astroglial responses to neuronal activity are facilitated by calcium signaling, triggered by factors that include glutamate and ATP, and also involve purinergic receptors and gap-junctional signaling (Scemes and Giaume, 2006). The demonstration
of the functional role of calcium signaling in the gliotransmitter environment has
exposed the critical role of astrocytes in modulating synaptic function (Nedergaard,
Ransom, and Goldman, 2003; Volterra and Meldolesi, 2005). The secretion of astroglial factors with neuromodulatory function is central to the regulation of synaptic

efficacy and long-term synaptic plasticity (Montana et al., 2006; Panatier et al., 2006; Pascual et al., 2005). Among these factors, cytokines such as TNF-α appear to be involved in mechanisms of glia-mediated homeostasis during the activity-dependent remodeling of the developing and established neuronal circuits that follow brain injury (Beattie et al., 2002; Stellwagen and Malenka, 2006). These observations support the important role of the gliotransmitter environment in the modulation of neuronal function.

12.3.6 Chronic Neuroimmune Reactions in ASD

Although most of the focus of the role of neuroinflammation is directed to the critical periods of prenatal and postnatal development, there is growing evidence that neuroimmune reactions are also involved in neuropathological and behavioral disturbances during postnatal stages and into the adulthood of patients with autism. Our neuropathological studies of postmortem brain tissues from patients with autism demonstrate an active and ongoing neuroinflammatory process in the cerebral cortex and white matter, characterized by astroglial and neuroglial activation. These findings support a role for neuroimmune responses in the pathogenesis and persistence of abnormalities in ASD (Vargas et al., 2005). Since both astroglia and microglia are involved in pathogenic inflammatory mechanisms common to many different disorders of the CNS, it is possible that different factors (e.g., genetic susceptibility, maternal factors, and prenatal environmental exposures) may trigger the development of these neuroglial reactions. Furthermore, more detailed studies of immune factors performed by protein array techniques have demonstrated that cytokines/chemokines such as MCP-1, IL-6, and TGFβ1, which are mainly derived from activated neuroglia, are the most prevalent cytokines in brain tissues (Vargas et al., 2005). Similar observations are also seen in the cerebrospinal fluid from patients with autism. These findings strongly support the hypothesis that neuroimmune reactions are part of the neuropathological processes in ASD and are among the factors that contribute to CNS dysfunction in ASD. However, the significance of the neuroinflammatory response to the specific neuropathologies and behavioral disruptions in ASD and its relevance to the etiology of ASD requires further exploration.

12.4 INFLAMMATION AND IMMUNOGENETICS IN ASD

12.4.1 Genetic Susceptibility and Immune Responses in Neurological Disease

A critical issue in the natural history of a disease is the influence that the immune system and immunogenetic host factors may have on its pathogenesis. The pathogenic mechanisms of many neurological diseases, including neurodegenerative and neuroimmunological disorders, are influenced by the spectrum and functions of the proteins associated with immunological pathways. The expression of proteins such as MHC or its HLA, cytokines, chemokines, and integrins is closely associated with the function of these immunological pathways and may determine the patterns of susceptibility and severity of disease. Allelic variations in regulatory regions of cytokine genes, point mutations, or single nucleotide substitutions have been shown to affect gene transcription and levels of cytokine expression and to produce interindividual variation in cytokine production (Meenagh et al., 2002). Single nucleotide polymorphisms (SNPs) and haplotypes of cytokine and chemokine genes produce genetic differences in cytokine expression that predispose to disease or confer resistance in immune-mediated disorders by influencing the strength and duration of the immune response (Bidwell et al., 1999, 2001; Haukim et al., 2002). The clinical outcomes of autoimmune, inflammatory, and neurodegenerative disorders appear to be influenced by the balance between pro-inflammatory and anti-inflammatory pathways, modulated by cytokines and chemokines. This relationship has been supported by numerous reports of the association of some cytokine alleles and expression phenotypes with immune-mediated or autoimmune disorders (Bidwell et al., 1999, 2001; Haukim et al., 2002). The association of SNPs of genes associated with inflammation has been investigated in inflammatory and neurodegenerative disorders such as AD and PD, as well as neuroinflammatory disorders such as multiple sclerosis and HIV-associated dementia (Crusius et al., 1995; Epplen et al., 1997; Gonzalez et al., 2002; Hakansson et al., 2005a,b; Mycko et al., 1998). These polymorphisms may modify the natural history of the disease by producing increased or decreased susceptibility to immune-mediated responses or other pathogenic factors. For example, one polymorphism of the MCP-1 gene (A-2518G) is associated with an increased risk of developing HIV dementia (Gonzalez et al., 2002), early onset of PD (Nishimura et al., 2003), increased resistance to antipsychotic therapy in schizophrenic patients (Mundo et al., 2005), and increased levels of MCP-1 in serum in AD patients (Fenoglio et al., 2004; Pola et al., 2004). In other disorders, SNPs of cytokine genes have been shown to be protective against the onset or increased severity of disease. For example, a polymorphism in position 1082 of the IL-10 gene promoter has been shown to be protective against severe forms of multiple sclerosis, with the effect increasing over the years (Luomala et al., 2003). More recently, the potential association of a SNP of IL-6 has been associated with the development of PD (Hakansson et al., 2005a,b).

12.4.2   ROLE OF MHC ON SUSCEPTIBILITY IN ASD

At present the clearest evidence for the importance of immunogenetic factors in autism is derived from studies of HLA typing in families. Increased frequencies of HLA DR4, DR13, A2, and B44 have been reported in children with autism (Daniels et al., 1995; Lee et al., 2006; Torres et al., 2002, 2006). Studies of HLA in simplex families indicated that mothers and their sons in a geographically defined group had a significantly higher frequency of DR4 than normal control subjects, when compared to a nationally distributed multiplex sample (Lee et al., 2006). Furthermore, no HLA linkage was found in a series of multiplex families, which may have other genetic etiologies for autism (Rogers et al., 1999). Since HLA DR4 is frequently associated with autoimmune disorders such as rheumatoid arthritis, it may signify increased susceptibility in mothers to form immune responses in response to fetal antigens, a situation that may be analogous to Rh isoimmunization in hemolytic disease of the newborn. There may also be regional susceptibility due to environmental factors, since autoimmune disorders reported in mothers have varied among studies from different areas (Comi et al., 1999; Molloy et al., 2006; Mouridsen et al., 2007; Sweeten et al., 2003). Recent studies of HLA in sets of parents, grandparents, and children with autism have demonstrated the selective transmission of HLA DR4 from maternal grandparents to the mother, with greater frequency than from the mother to her child with autism (Johnson et al., 2008). This enlarges our concept of a specific type of susceptibility in which the mother becomes the "genetic patient" in an immune interaction with her fetus. This is one possible immunogenetic mechanism for autism that requires further investigation. Future studies of other potential immunogenetic factors should also focus on defining the presence of specific SNPs and haplotypes in cytokines, chemokines, their receptors, and other immune factors, such as complement, integrins, and matrix metalloproteinases.

12.5 CONCLUSION

Inflammation and immune factors may influence the pathogenesis and perpetuation of pathophysiological events that lead to ASD by their effect on brain development as well as CNS function during adulthood. Because specific immune challenges may occur during neurodevelopment, immunological and neuroimmune responses that follow such challenges, whether environmental, maternal, or neurogenetic, may constitute critical pathogenic factors in the development of ASD. The role of immune factors and neuroinflammation are still uncertain but could be critical in maintaining, if not also in initiating, some of the abnormalities present in the CNS in ASD. A better understanding of the role of the immune system and neuroimmune reactions in the pathogenesis of ASD may have important clinical and therapeutic implications.

ACKNOWLEDGMENTS

Dr. Pardo is supported by the Peter Emch Fund for Autism Research, the Bart A. McLean Fund for Neuroimmunology Research, Cure Autism Now, and NIH-NIDA (K08-DA16160). Dr. Zimmerman is supported by the Hussman Foundation.

REFERENCES

Abbott, N. J., L. Ronnback, and E. Hansson. 2006. Astrocyte-endothelial interactions at the blood-brain barrier. *Nat. Rev.* 7:41–53.
Aloisi, F. 2001. Immune function of microglia. *Glia* 36:165–179.
Ambrosini, E. and F. Aloisi. 2004. Chemokines and glial cells: A complex network in the central nervous system. *Neurochem. Res.* 29:1017–1038.
Ashwood, P., S. Wills, and J. Van de Water. 2006. The immune response in autism: A new frontier for autism research. *J. Leukoc. Biol.* 80:1–15.
Bach, J. P., B. Rinn, B. Meyer, R. Dodel, and M. Bacher. 2008. Role of MIF in inflammation and tumorigenesis. *Oncology* 75:127–133.
Baltimore, D., M. P. Boldin, R. M. O'Connell, D. S. Rao, and K. D. Taganov. 2008. MicroRNAs: New regulators of immune cell development and function. *Nat. Immunol.* 9:839–845.
Barton, G. M. 2008. A calculated response: Control of inflammation by the innate immune system. *J. Clin. Invest.* 118:413–420.

Bauer, J., H. Rauschka, and H. Lassmann. 2001. Inflammation in the nervous system: The human perspective. *Glia* 36:235–243.

Bauer, S., B. J. Kerr, and P. H. Patterson. 2007. The neuropoietic cytokine family in development, plasticity, disease and injury. *Nat. Rev.* 8:221–232.

Bauman, M. L. and T. L. Kemper. 2005. Structural brain automy in autism: What is the evidence? In *The Neurobiology of Autism*, M. L. Bauman and T. L. Kemper (Eds.). Baltimore, MD: The Johns Hopkins University Press, pp. 136–149.

Beattie, E. C., D. Stellwagen, W. Morishita, J. C. Bresnahan, B. K. Ha, M. Von Zastrow, M. S. Beattie, and R. C. Malenka. 2002. Control of synaptic strength by glial TNFalpha. *Science* 295:2282–2285.

Benn, T., C. Halfpenny, and N. Scolding. 2001. Glial cells as targets for cytotoxic immune mediators. *Glia* 36:200–211.

Bessis, A., C. Bechade, D. Bernard, and A. Roumier. 2007. Microglial control of neuronal death and synaptic properties. *Glia* 55:233–238.

Bidwell, J., L. Keen, G. Gallagher, R. Kimberly, T. Huizinga, M. F. McDermott, J. Oksenberg, J. McNicholl, F. Pociot, C. Hardt, and S. D'Alfonso. 2001. Cytokine gene polymorphism in human disease: On-line databases, supplement 1. *Genes Immun.* 2:61–70.

Bidwell, J. L., N. A. Wood, H. R. Morse, O. O. Olomolaiye, L. J. Keen, and G. J. Laundy. 1999. Human cytokine gene nucleotide sequence alignments: Supplement 1. *Eur. J. Immunogenet.* 26:135–223.

Blanco, P., A. K. Palucka, V. Pascual, and J. Banchereau. 2008. Dendritic cells and cytokines in human inflammatory and autoimmune diseases. *Cytokine Growth Factor Rev.* 19:41–52.

Blasko, I. and B. Grubeck-Loebenstein. 2003. Role of the immune system in the pathogenesis, prevention and treatment of Alzheimer's disease. *Drugs Aging* 20:101–113.

Boulanger, L. M. and C. J. Shatz. 2004. Immune signalling in neural development, synaptic plasticity and disease. *Nat. Rev.* 5:521–531.

Braunschweig, D., P. Ashwood, P. Krakowiak, I. Hertz-Picciotto, R. Hansen, L. A. Croen, I. N. Pessah, and J. Van de Water. 2007. Autism: Maternally derived antibodies specific for fetal brain proteins. *Neurotoxicology* 29:226–231.

Bushong, E. A., M. E. Martone, Y. Z. Jones, and M. H. Ellisman. 2002. Protoplasmic astrocytes in CA1 stratum radiatum occupy separate anatomical domains. *J. Neurosci.* 22:183–192.

Cardona, A. E., M. Li, L. Liu, C. Savarin, and R. M. Ransohoff. 2008. Chemokines in and out of the central nervous system: Much more than chemotaxis and inflammation. *J. Leukoc. Biol.* 84:587–594.

Casanova, M. F. 2007. The neuropathology of autism. *Brain Pathol.* 17:422–433.

Charo, I. F. and R. M. Ransohoff. 2006. The many roles of chemokines and chemokine receptors in inflammation. *N. Engl. J. Med.* 354:610–621.

Chess, S., P. Fernandez, and S. Korn. 1978. Behavioral consequences of congenital rubella. *J. Pediatr.* 93:699–703.

Christiaens, I., D. B. Zaragoza, L. Guilbert, S. A. Robertson, B. F. Mitchell, and D. M. Olson. 2008. Inflammatory processes in preterm and term parturition. *J. Reprod. Immunol.* 79:50–57.

Comi, A. M., A. W. Zimmerman, V. H. Frye, P. A. Law, and J. N. Peeden. 1999. Familial clustering of autoimmune disorders and evaluation of medical risk factors in autism. *J. Child Neurol.* 14:388–394.

Croen, L. A., J. K. Grether, C. K. Yoshida, R. Odouli, and J. Van de Water. 2005. Maternal autoimmune diseases, asthma and allergies, and childhood autism spectrum disorders: A case-control study. *Arch. Pediatr. Adolesc. Med.* 159:151–157.

Crusius, J. B., A. S. Pena, B. W. van Oosten, G. Bioque, A. Garcia, C. D. Dijkstra, and C. H. Polman. 1995. Interleukin-1 receptor antagonist gene polymorphism and multiple sclerosis. *Lancet* 346:979.

Dalton, P., R. Deacon, A. Blamire, M. Pike, I. McKinlay, J. Stein, P. Styles, and A. Vincent. 2003. Maternal neuronal antibodies associated with autism and a language disorder. *Ann. Neurol.* 53:533–537.

Daniels, W. W., R. P. Warren, J. D. Odell, A. Maciulis, R. A. Burger, W. L. Warren, and A. R. Torres. 1995. Increased frequency of the extended or ancestral haplotype B44-SC30-DR4 in autism. *Neuropsychobiology* 32:120–123.

DiCicco-Bloom, E., C. Lord, L. Zwaigenbaum, E. Courchesne, S. R. Dager, C. Schmitz, R. T. Schultz, J. Crawley, and L. J. Young. 2006. The developmental neurobiology of autism spectrum disorder. *J. Neurosci.* 26:6897–6906.

Dietert, R. R. and J. M. Dietert. 2008. Potential for early-life immune insult including developmental immunotoxicity in autism and autism spectrum disorders: Focus on critical windows of immune vulnerability. *J. Toxicol. Environ. Health B Crit. Rev.* 11:660–680.

Dong, Y. and E. N. Benveniste. 2001. Immune function of astrocytes. *Glia* 36:180–190.

Engelhardt, B. and R. M. Ransohoff. 2005. The ins and outs of T-lymphocyte trafficking to the CNS: Anatomical sites and molecular mechanisms. *Trends Immunol.* 26:485–495.

Epplen, C., S. Jackel, E. J. Santos, M. D'Souza, D. Poehlau, B. Dotzauer, E. Sindern, M. Haupts, K. P. Rude, F. Weber, J. Stover, S. Poser, W. Gehler, J. P. Malin, H. Przuntek, and J. T. Epplen. 1997. Genetic predisposition to multiple sclerosis as revealed by immunoprinting. *Ann. Neurol.* 41:341–352.

Fatemi, S. H., A. V. Snow, J. M. Stary, M. Araghi-Niknam, T. J. Reutiman, S. Lee, A. I. Brooks, and D. A. Pearce. 2005. Reelin signaling is impaired in autism. *Biol. Psychiatry* 57:777–787.

Fenoglio, C., D. Galimberti, C. Lovati, I. Guidi, A. Gatti, S. Fogliarino, M. Tiriticco, C. Mariani, G. Forloni, C. Pettenati, P. Baron, G. Conti, N. Bresolin, and E. Scarpini. 2004. MCP-1 in Alzheimer's disease patients: A-2518G polymorphism and serum levels. *Neurobiol. Aging* 25:1169–1173.

Fields, R. D. and B. Stevens-Graham. 2002. New insights into neuron-glia communication. *Science* 298:556–562.

Golde, T. E. 2002. Inflammation takes on Alzheimer disease. *Nat. Med.* 8:936–938.

Gomes, F. C., V. O. Sousa, and L. Romao. 2005. Emerging roles for TGF-beta1 in nervous system development. *Int. J. Dev. Neurosci.* 23:413–424.

Gonzalez, E., B. H. Rovin, L. Sen, G. Cooke, R. Dhanda, S. Mummidi, H. Kulkarni, M. J. Bamshad, V. Telles, S. A. Anderson, E. A. Walter, K. T. Stephan, M. Deucher, A. Mangano, R. Bologna, S. S. Ahuja, M. J. Dolan, and S. K. Ahuja. 2002. HIV-1 infection and AIDS dementia are influenced by a mutant MCP-1 allele linked to increased monocyte infiltration of tissues and MCP-1 levels. *Proc. Natl. Acad. Sci. U.S.A.* 99:13795–13800.

Graeber, M. B., K. Bise, and P. Mehraein. 1993. Synaptic stripping in the human facial nucleus. *Acta Neuropathol.* 86:179–181.

Griffiths, M., J. W. Neal, and P. Gasque. 2007. Innate immunity and protective neuroinflammation: New emphasis on the role of neuroimmune regulatory proteins. *Int. Rev. Neurobiol.* 82:29–55.

Grosche, J., V. Matyash, T. Moller, A. Verkhratsky, A. Reichenbach, and H. Kettenmann. 1999. Microdomains for neuron-glia interaction: Parallel fiber signaling to Bergmann glial cells. *Nat. Neurosci.* 2:139–143.

Hagberg, H. and C. Mallard. 2005. Effect of inflammation on central nervous system development and vulnerability. *Curr. Opin. Neurol.* 18:117–123.

Hakansson, A., L. Westberg, S. Nilsson, S. Buervenich, A. Carmine, B. Holmberg, O. Sydow, L. Olson, B. Johnels, E. Eriksson, and H. Nissbrandt. 2005a. Interaction of polymorphisms in the genes encoding interleukin-6 and estrogen receptor beta on the susceptibility to Parkinson's disease. *Am. J. Med. Genet. B Neuropsychiatr. Genet.* 133:88–92.

Hakansson, A., L. Westberg, S. Nilsson, S. Buervenich, A. Carmine, B. Holmberg, O. Sydow, L. Olson, B. Johnels, E. Eriksson, and H. Nissbrandt. 2005b. Investigation of genes coding for inflammatory components in Parkinson's disease. *Mov. Disord.* 20:569–573.

240 Autism: Oxidative Stress, Inflammation, and Immune Abnormalities

Halassa, M. M., T. Fellin, H. Takano, J. H. Dong, and P. G. Haydon. 2007. Synaptic islands defined by the territory of a single astrocyte. *J. Neurosci.* 27:6473–6477.

Haukim, N., J. L. Bidwell, A. J. Smith, L. J. Keen, G. Gallagher, R. Kimberly, T. Huizinga, M. F. McDermott, J. Oksenberg, J. McNicholl, F. Pociot, C. Hardt, and S. D'Alfonso. 2002. Cytokine gene polymorphism in human disease: On-line databases, supplement 2. *Genes Immun.* 3:313–330.

Infante-Duarte, C., S. Waiczies, J. Wuerfel, and F. Zipp. 2008. New developments in understanding and treating neuroinflammation. *J. Mol. Med.* 86:975–985.

Johnson, W. G., M. Sreenath, S. Buyske, and E. S. Stenroos. 2008. Teratogenic alleles in autism and other neurodevelopmental disorders. In *Autism: Current Theories and Evidence*, A. W. Zimmerman (Ed.). Totowa, NJ: Humana Press, pp. 41–68.

Jonakait, G. M. 2007. The effects of maternal inflammation on neuronal development: Possible mechanisms. *Int. J. Dev. Neurosci.* 25:415–425.

Kaul, M., G. A. Garden, and S. A. Lipton. 2001. Pathways to neuronal injury and apoptosis in HIV-associated dementia. *Nature* 410:988–994.

Kim, J. H., J. H. Kim, J. A. Park, S. W. Lee, W. J. Kim, Y. S. Yu, and K. W. Kim. 2006. Blood-neural barrier: Intercellular communication at glio-vascular interface. *J. Biochem. Mol. Biol.* 39:339–345.

Kirov, S. A. and K. M. Harris. 1999. Dendrites are more spiny on mature hippocampal neurons when synapses are inactivated. *Nat. Neurosci.* 2:878–883.

Lagercrantz, H. and T. Ringstedt. 2001. Organization of the neuronal circuits in the central nervous system during development. *Acta Paediatr.* 90:707–715.

Lazarini, F., T. N. Tham, P. Casanova, F. Arenzana-Seisdedos, and M. Dubois-Dalcq. 2003. Role of the alpha-chemokine stromal cell-derived factor (SDF-1) in the developing and mature central nervous system. *Glia* 42:139–148.

Lee, L. C., A. A. Zachary, M. S. Leffell, C. J. Newschaffer, K. J. Matteson, J. D. Tyler, and A. W. Zimmerman. 2006. HLA-DR4 in families with autism. *Pediatr. Neurol.* 35:303–307.

Luomala, M., T. Lehtimaki, H. Huhtala, M. Ukkonen, T. Koivula, M. Hurme, and I. Elovaara. 2003. Promoter polymorphism of IL-10 and severity of multiple sclerosis. *Acta Neurol. Scand.* 108:396–400.

Ma, Q., D. Jones, P. R. Borghesani, R. A. Segal, T. Nagasawa, T. Kishimoto, R. T. Bronson, and T. A. Springer. 1998. Impaired B-lymphopoiesis, myelopoiesis, and derailed cerebellar neuron migration in C. *Proc. Natl. Acad. Sci. U.S.A.* 95:9448–9453.

Martin, L. A., P. Ashwood, D. Braunschweig, M. Cabanlit, J. Van de Water, and D. G. Amaral. 2008. Stereotypies and hyperactivity in rhesus monkeys exposed to IgG from mothers of children with autism. *Brain Behav. Immun.* 22:806–816.

McGeer, P. L. and E. G. McGeer. 2002. Local neuroinflammation and the progression of Alzheimer's disease. *J. Neurovirol.* 8:529–538.

Medzhitov, R. 2008. Origin and physiological roles of inflammation. *Nature* 454:428–435.

Meenagh, A., F. Williams, O. A. Ross, C. Patterson, C. Gorodezky, M. Hammond, W. A. Leheny, and D. Middleton. 2002. Frequency of cytokine polymorphisms in populations from western Europe, Africa, Asia, the Middle East and South America. *Hum. Immunol.* 63:1055–1061.

Meyer, U., M. Nyffeler, A. Engler, A. Urwyler, M. Schedlowski, I. Knuesel, B. K. Yee, and J. Feldon. 2006. The time of prenatal immune challenge determines the specificity of inflammation-mediated brain and behavioral pathology. *J. Neurosci.* 26:4752–4762.

Meyer, U., B. K. Yee, and J. Feldon. 2007. The neurodevelopmental impact of prenatal infections at different times of pregnancy: The earlier the worse? *Neuroscientist* 13:241–256.

Molloy, C. A., A. L. Morrow, J. Meinzen-Derr, G. Dawson, R. Bernier, M. Dunn, S. L. Hyman, W. M. McMahon, J. Goudie-Nice, S. Hepburn, N. Minshew, S. Rogers, M. Sigman, M. A. Spence, H. Tager-Flusberg, F. R. Volkmar, and C. Lord. 2006. Familial autoimmune thyroid disease as a risk factor for regression in children with autism spectrum disorder: A CPEA study. *J. Autism Dev. Disord.* 36:317–324.

Montana, V., E. B. Malarkey, C. Verderio, M. Matteoli, and V. Parpura. 2006. Vesicular transmitter release from astrocytes. *Glia* 54:700–715.

Morris, C. M., M. Pletnikov, A. W. Zimmerman, and H. S. Singer. 2008. Maternal antibodies and the placental-fetal IgG transfer theory. In *Autism: Current Theories and Evidence*, A. W. Zimmerman (Ed.). Totowa, NJ: Humana Press, pp. 309–328.

Mouridsen, S. E., B. Rich, T. Isager, and N. J. Nedergaard. 2007. Autoimmune diseases in parents of children with infantile autism: A case-control study. *Dev. Med. Child Neurol.* 49:429–432.

Muller, N., M. Riedel, C. Scheppach, B. Brandstatter, S. Sokullu, K. Krampe, M. Ulmschneider, R. R. Engel, H. J. Moller, and M. J. Schwarz. 2002. Beneficial antipsychotic effects of celecoxib add-on therapy compared to risperidone alone in schizophrenia. *Am. J. Psychiatry* 159:1029–1034.

Mundo, E., A. C. Altamura, S. Vismara, R. Zanardini, S. Bignotti, R. Randazzo, C. Montresor, and M. Gennarelli. 2005. MCP-1 gene (SCYA2) and schizophrenia: A case-control association study. *Am. J. Med. Genet.* 132B(1):1–4.

Munoz-Fernandez, M. A. and M. Fresno. 1998. The role of tumour necrosis factor, interleukin 6, interferon-gamma and inducible nitric oxide synthase in the development and pathology of the nervous system. *Prog. Neurobiol.* 56:307–340.

Murai, K. K. and D. J. Van Meyel. 2007. Neuron glial communication at synapses: Insights from vertebrates and invertebrates. *Neuroscientist* 13:657–666.

Mycko, M., W. Kowalski, M. Kwinkowski, A. C. Buenafe, B. Szymanska, E. Tronczynska, A. Plucienniczak, and K. Selmaj. 1998. Multiple sclerosis: The frequency of allelic forms of tumor necrosis factor and lymphotoxin-alpha. *J. Neuroimmunol.* 84:198–206.

Nagatsu, T. and M. Sawada. 2005. Inflammatory process in Parkinson's disease: Role for cytokines. *Curr. Pharm. Des.* 11:999–1016.

Nakashima, K. and T. Taga. 2002. Mechanisms underlying cytokine-mediated cell-fate regulation in the nervous system. *Mol. Neurobiol.* 25:233–244.

Nedergaard, M., B. Ransom, and S. A. Goldman. 2003. New roles for astrocytes: Redefining the functional architecture of the brain. *Trends Neurosci.* 26:523–530.

Nedergaard, M., T. Takano, and A. J. Hansen. 2002. Beyond the role of glutamate as a neurotransmitter. *Nat. Rev. Neurosci.* 3:748–755.

Neumann, H. 2001. Control of glial immune function by neurons. *Glia* 36:191–199.

Nishimura, M., S. Kuno, I. Mizuta, M. Ohta, H. Maruyama, R. Kaji, and H. Kawakami. 2003. Influence of monocyte chemoattractant protein 1 gene polymorphism on age at onset of sporadic Parkinson's disease. *Mov. Disord.* 18:953–955.

Page-McCaw, A., A. J. Ewald, and Z. Werb. 2007. Matrix metalloproteinases and the regulation of tissue remodelling. *Nat. Rev. Mol. Cell Biol.* 8:221–233.

Panatier, A., D. T. Theodosis, J. P. Mothet, B. Touquet, L. Pollegioni, D. A. Poulain, and S. H. Oliet. 2006. Glia-derived D-serine controls NMDA receptor activity and synaptic memory. *Cell* 125:775–784.

Pardo C. A. 2008. Can neuroinflammation influence the development of autism spectrum disorders? In *Autism: Current Theories and Evidence*, A. W. Zimmerman (Ed.). Totowa, NJ: Humana Press, pp. 329–346.

Pardo, C. A. and C. G. Eberhart. 2007. The neurobiology of autism. *Brain Pathol.* 17:434–447.

Pardo, C. A., D. L. Vargas, and A. W. Zimmerman. 2005. Immunity, neuroglia and neuroinflammation in autism. *Int. Rev. Psychiatry* 17:485–495.

Pardo, C. A., E. P. Vining, L. Guo, R. L. Skolasky, B. S. Carson, and J. M. Freeman. 2004. The pathology of Rasmussen syndrome: Stages of cortical involvement and neuropathological studies in 45 hemispherectomies. *Epilepsia* 45:516–526.

Paredes, M. F., G. Li, O. Berger, S. C. Baraban, and S. J. Pleasure. 2006. Stromal-derived factor-1 (CXCL12) regulates laminar position of Cajal-Retzius cells in normal and dysplastic brains. *J. Neurosci.* 26:9404–9412.

Pascual, O., K. B. Casper, C. Kubera, J. Zhang, R. Revilla-Sanchez, J. Y. Sul, H. Takano, S. J. Moss, K. McCarthy, and P. G. Haydon. 2005. Astrocytic purinergic signaling coordinates synaptic networks. *Science* 310:113–116.

Patterson, P. H. 2002. Maternal infection: Window on neuroimmune interactions in fetal brain development and mental illness. *Curr. Opin. Neurobiol.* 12:115–118.

Patterson, P. H. 2007. Neuroscience. Maternal effects on schizophrenia risk. *Science* 318:576–577.

Pola, R., A. Flex, E. Gaetani, A. S. Proia, P. Papaleo, A. D. Giorgio, G. Straface, G. Pecorini, M. Serricchio, and P. Pola. 2004. Monocyte chemoattractant protein-1 (MCP-1) gene polymorphism and risk of Alzheimer's disease in Italians. *Exp. Gerontol.* 39:1249–1252.

Pousset, F. 1994. Developmental expression of cytokine genes in the cortex and hippocampus of the rat central nervous system. *Brain Res.* 81:143–146.

Pousset, F., J. Fournier, and P. E. Keane. 1997. Expression of cytokine genes during ontogenesis of the central nervous system. *Ann. N.Y. Acad. Sci.* 814:97–107.

Prat, A., K. Biernacki, K. Wosik, and J. P. Antel. 2001. Glial cell influence on the human blood-brain barrier. *Glia* 36:145–155.

Radewicz, K., L. J. Garey, S. M. Gentleman, and R. Reynolds. 2000. Increase in HLA-DR immunoreactive microglia in frontal and temporal cortex of chronic schizophrenics. *J. Neuropathol. Exp. Neurol.* 59:137–150.

Ransohoff, R. M. 2002. The chemokine system in neuroinflammation: An update. *J. Infect. Dis.* 186(Suppl. 2):S152–S156.

Ransohoff, R. M., L. Liu, and A. E. Cardona. 2007. Chemokines and chemokine receptors: Multipurpose players in neuroinflammation. *Int. Rev. Neurobiol.* 82:187–204.

Ransom, B., T. Behar, and M. Nedergaard. 2003. New roles for astrocytes (stars at last). *Trends Neurosci.* 26:520–522.

Rapin, I. and R. F. Tuchman. 2008. Autism: Definition, neurobiology, screening, diagnosis. *Pediatr. Clin. North Am.* 55:1129–1146, viii.

Rezaie, P., N. J. Cairns, and D. K. Male. 1997. Expression of adhesion molecules on human fetal cerebral vessels: Relationship to microglial colonisation during development. *Brain Res. Dev. Brain Res.* 104:175–189.

Rogers, T., L. Kalaydjieva, J. Hallmayer, P. B. Petersen, P. Nicholas, C. Pingree, W. M. McMahon, D. Spiker, L. Lotspeich, H. Kraemer, P. McCague, S. Dimiceli, N. Nouri, T. Peachy, J. Yang, D. Hinds, N. Risch, and R. M. Myers. 1999. Exclusion of linkage to the HLA region in ninety multiplex sibships with autism. *J. Autism Dev. Disord.* 29:195–201.

Roman, G. C. 2007. Autism: Transient in utero hypothyroxinemia related to maternal flavonoid ingestion during pregnancy and to other environmental antithyroid agents. *J. Neurol. Sci.* 262:15–26.

Rosenberg, G. A. 2002. Matrix metalloproteinases in neuroinflammation. *Glia* 39:279–291.

Rostene, W., P. Kitabgi, and S. M. Parsadaniantz. 2007. Chemokines: A new class of neuromodulator? *Nat. Rev.* 8:895–903.

Scemes, E. and C. Giaume. 2006. Astrocyte calcium waves: What they are and what they do. *Glia* 54:716–725.

Shi, L., S. H. Fatemi, R. W. Sidwell, and P. H. Patterson. 2003. Maternal influenza infection causes marked behavioral and pharmacological changes in the offspring. *J. Neurosci.* 23:297–302.

Singer, H. S., C. M. Morris, C. D. Gause, P. K. Gillin, S. Crawford, and A. W. Zimmerman. 2008. Antibodies against fetal brain in sera of mothers with autistic children. *J. Neuroimmunol.* 194:165–172.

Skaper, S. D. 2007. The brain as a target for inflammatory processes and neuroprotective strategies. *Ann. N.Y. Acad. Sci.* 1122:23–34.

Smith, S. E., J. Li, K. Garbett, K. Mirnics, and P. H. Patterson. 2007. Maternal immune activation alters fetal brain development through interleukin-6. *J. Neurosci.* 27:10695–10702.

Stellwagen, D. and R. C. Malenka. 2006. Synaptic scaling mediated by glial TNF-alpha. *Nature* 440:1054–1059.

Stevens, B., N. J. Allen, L. E. Vazquez, G. R. Howell, K. S. Christopherson, N. Nouri, K. D. Micheva, A. K. Mehalow, A. D. Huberman, B. Stafford, A. Sher, A. M. Litke, J. D. Lambris, S. J. Smith, S. W. John, and B. A. Barres. 2007. The classical complement cascade mediates CNS synapse elimination. *Cell* 131:1164–1178.

Stumm, R. and V. Hollt. 2007. CXC chemokine receptor 4 regulates neuronal migration and axonal pathfinding in the developing nervous system: Implications for neuronal regeneration in the adult brain. *J. Mol. Endocrinol.* 38:377–382.

Sweeten, T. L., S. L. Bowyer, D. J. Posey, G. M. Halberstadt, and C. J. McDougle. 2003. Increased prevalence of familial autoimmunity in probands with pervasive developmental disorders. *Pediatrics* 112:e420.

Taga, T. and S. Fukuda. 2005. Role of IL-6 in the neural stem cell differentiation. *Clin. Rev. Allergy Immunol.* 28:249–256.

Tilleux, S. and E. Hermans. 2007. Neuroinflammation and regulation of glial glutamate uptake in neurological disorders. *J. Neurosci. Res.* 85:2059–2070.

Tonelli, L. H., T. T. Postolache, and E. M. Sternberg. 2005. Inflammatory genes and neural activity: Involvement of immune genes in synaptic function and behavior. *Front. Biosci.* 10:675–680.

Torres, A. R., A. Maciulis, E. G. Stubbs, A. Cutler, and D. Odell. 2002. The transmission disequilibrium test suggests that HLA-DR4 and DR13 are linked to autism spectrum disorder. *Hum. Immunol.* 63:311–316.

Torres, A. R., T. L. Sweeten, A. Cutler, B. J. Bedke, M. Fillmore, E. G. Stubbs, and D. Odell. 2006. The association and linkage of the HLA-A2 class I allele with autism. *Hum. Immunol.* 67:346–351.

Trapp, B. D., J. R. Wujek, G. A. Criste, W. Jalabi, X. Yin, G. J. Kidd, S. Stohlman, and R. Ransohoff. 2007. Evidence for synaptic stripping by cortical microglia. *Glia* 55:360–368.

van Berckel, B. N., M. G. Bossong, R. Boellaard, R. Kloet, A. Schuitemaker, E. Caspers, G. Luurtsema, A. D. Windhorst, W. Cahn, A. A. Lammertsma, and R. S. Kahn. 2008. Microglia activation in recent-onset schizophrenia: A quantitative (R)-[11C]PK11195 positron emission tomography study. *Biol. Psychiatry* 64:820–822.

Vargas, D. L., C. Nascimbene, C. Krishnan, A. W. Zimmerman, and C. A. Pardo. 2005. Neuroglial activation and neuroinflammation in the brain of patients with autism. *Ann. Neurol.* 57:67–81.

Vlad, S. C., D. R. Miller, N. W. Kowall, and D. T. Felson. 2008. Protective effects of NSAIDs on the development of Alzheimer disease. *Neurology* 70:1672–1677.

Volterra, A. and J. Meldolesi. 2005. Astrocytes, from brain glue to communication elements: The revolution continues. *Nat. Rev.* 6:626–640.

Wahner, A. D., J. M. Bronstein, Y. M. Bordelon, and B. Ritz. 2007. Nonsteroidal anti-inflammatory drugs may protect against Parkinson disease. *Neurology* 69:1836–1842.

Wierzba-Bobrowicz, T., E. Lewandowska, W. Lechowicz, T. Stepien, and E. Pasennik. 2005. Quantitative analysis of activated microglia, ramified and damage of processes in the frontal and temporal lobes of chronic schizophrenics. *Folia Neuropathol.* 43:81–89.

Williams, K. C. and W. F. Hickey. 2002. Central nervous system damage, monocytes and macrophages, and neurological disorders in AIDS. *Annu. Rev. Neurosci.* 25:537–562.

Zerrate, M. C., M. Pletnikov, S. L. Connors, D. L. Vargas, F. J. Seidler, A. W. Zimmerman, T. A. Slotkin, and C. A. Pardo. 2007. Neuroinflammation and behavioral abnormalities after neonatal terbutaline treatment in rats: Implications for autism. *J. Pharmacol. Exp. Ther.* 322:16–22.

Zimmerman, A. W., S. L. Connors, K. J. Matteson, L. C. Lee, H. S. Singer, J. A. Castaneda, and D. A. Pearce. 2007. Maternal antibrain antibodies in autism. *Brain Behav. Immun.* 21:351–357.

Zipp, F. and O. Aktas. 2006. The brain as a target of inflammation: Common pathways link inflammatory and neurodegenerative diseases. *Trends Neurosci.* 29:518–527.

Zou, Y. R., A. H. Kottmann, M. Kuroda, I. Taniuchi, and D. R. Littman. 1998. Function of the chemokine receptor CXCR4 in haematopoiesis and in cerebellar development. *Nature* 393:595–599.

13 Possible Impact of Innate Immunity on Autism

*Harumi Jyonouchi**

Department of Pediatrics, University of Medicine
and Dentistry of New Jersey, Newark, NJ 07028, USA

CONTENTS

* Corresponding author: Tel.: +1-973-972-1414; fax: +1-973-972-5895; e-mail: jyanouha@umdnj.edu

13.1   INTRODUCTION

Autism spectrum disorders (ASD) are complex developmental disorders with largely unknown etiology. Although recent progress in genetics have defined various disorders that manifest autistic features, this may account for up to 10%–15% of ASD, usually manifested as severe classical autism. For the remaining ASD patients, the diagnosis of ASD is solely based on subjective behavioral symptoms, which can vary markedly time to time during development. The presence of comorbidities also affects their behavioral symptoms. Gastrointestinal (GI) inflammation, one of the most common comorbidities in ASD, likely affects mood, irritability, and concentration simply because of abdominal discomfort. Recent studies indicate the presence of more complex mechanisms affecting the brain via gut neuro-immune network, as detailed later.

Apart from GI symptoms, a subset of ASD children presents with frequent childhood infections including otitis media, rhinosinusitis, and upper respiratory-tract infection. However, conventional immune workup is often unrevealing in such ASD children. Subtle immune abnormalities have been described in ASD children, although the effects of such abnormalities are unclear. Nevertheless, recent studies may indicate the possible impact of innate immunity on the onset and/or progress of ASD in some but not all ASD children.

In this chapter, the overview of innate immunity in the GI tract and in the central nervous system (CNS) is discussed first, and then immune abnormalities reported in the GI tract and in the CNS in autism are discussed. Lastly, the possible impact of innate immunity on neuro-immune interactions in autism is discussed.

13.2   INNATE IMMUNITY: AN OVERVIEW

In addition to the obvious host immune defense that eliminates foreign pathogens, the immune system exerts surveillance against aberrant cell growth and tissue injury and facilitates tissue repair. In other words, the immune system orchestrates to maintain homeostasis and the integrity of our body. To carry out such a complex task, the immune system is composed by various components, which may overlap in their functions. Immune responses can be grossly divided into two components: innate immunity and adaptive immunity. The innate immunity acts as the first line of immune defense sensing the deviation of immune homeostasis such as pathogen invasion. Innate immune cells sense pathogen-derived molecular patterns (PAMPs) via specific receptors called pattern recognition receptors (PRRs). Toll-like receptors (TLRs) are the first family of PRRs characterized (Zedler and Faist, 2006). PRRs can also sense molecular patterns derived from injured tissue (the so-called danger-signals) and can initiate immune reaction, a process which appears to be vital for wound healing (Zedler and Faist, 2006). It is now well recognized that the innate immunity bridges subsequent adaptive immune responses that then reciprocally affect innate immune responses. Namely, PRR-mediated signaling activates antigen (Ag)-presenting cells (APCs) by up-regulating the expression of major histocompatibility complex (MHC)/ co-stimulatory molecules, augmenting the Ag processing, and facilitating the migration of APCs to the lymphoid organs (Teitelbaum and Allan Walker, 2005).

The innate immunity is exerted in an Ag-independent manner and components of innate immunity are genetically predetermined. Thus, the innate immunity can function at birth and may play more significant roles in the first years of life before Ag-dependent adaptive immunity fully develops. However, such characteristics of innate immunity may be accompanied by a possibility of being more vulnerable to subtle genetic variation than adaptive immunity.

13.2.1 INNATE IMMUNITY IN THE GUT MUCOSA

The structures essential for composing the mucosal immune system include the epithelial cell monolayer and gut-associated lymphoid tissue (GALT), primarily composed of Peyer's patches (PP) and lamina propria (LP).

13.2.1.1 The Epithelium

The gut epithelium plays a crucial role in innate immune defense in the gut mucosa. However, the intestinal epithelial barrier is functionally immature in newborns as evidenced in higher intestinal permeability than in adults. Molecules expressed by epithelial cells are also important for the barrier function. The glycosylation patterns of oligosaccharides expressed on epithelial cells are reported to change after birth (Dai et al., 2000; Teitelbaum and Allan Walker, 2005), which make the intestinal epithelial cells less susceptible to complement-mediated cell lyses and also appear to affect colonization patterns of microbes. Impaired intestinal epithelial barrier function in patients with protein-losing enteropathy was implicated in the specific loss of heparan sulfate proteoglycans from the basolateral surface of intestinal epithelial cells (Murch et al., 1996; Westphal et al., 2000). The importance of heparan sulfate proteoglycans was further supported in rodent models deficient of these molecules (Bode et al., 2008).

In addition to their barrier functions, epithelial cells play a major role in gut innate defense partly by producing active mediators. Anti-microbial peptides, which are mainly produced by Paneth cells clustered at the bottom of the intestinal crypts, serve as broad-spectrum antibiotics killing both gram-positive and gram-negative bacteria (Porter et al., 2002). This is also true for respiratory epithelial cells but they also produce interferon-β (IFN-β), a critical factor for innate defense against viral pathogens (Wark et al., 2005). In contrast, colonic epithelial cells are also thought to contribute to the maintenance of homeostasis in the colon where microbes cohabit at high concentrations. The colonic epithelium was shown to express TLR9 on the cell surface in rodents (Lee et al., 2007, 2008). The TLR9 expressed apically in the epithelium is reported to compromise on the inflammatory cascade induced by several TLRs expressed basolaterally (Lee et al., 2007, 2008). The TLR9-deficient mice exhibited more severe epithelial ulceration in colitis induced by dextran sodium sulfate (Lee et al., 2008).

13.2.1.2   GALT

The LP located beneath the intestinal epithelium serves as a meshwork of connective tissue containing plasma blasts, T cells, and various innate immune cells including dendritic cells (DCs), mast cells, macrophages, and granulocytes (neutrophils and eosinophils). The presence of abundant mast cells in the LP during infancy and early childhood is thought to be important for mucosal immune defense against extracellular parasites. In addition, mast cells are also indicated to have a role in tolerance induction against macronutrients (Lu et al., 2006). However, the excessive mast-cell activation can cause various abdominal symptoms by the release of mediators including histamine.

PPs are lymphoid aggregates composed of B-cell follicles, surrounding inter-follicular CD4$^+$ and CD8$^+$ T cells and Ag-presenting innate immune cells (DCs, macrophages, etc.) intervening beneath the follicle-associated epithelium. DCs composed of various subsets are abundant in the subepithelial dome (Wershil and Furuta, 2008). Activated DCs can migrate to mesenteric lymph nodes or LPs and can exert stimulatory and modulatory actions, bridging innate immunity and adaptive immunity (Coombes et al., 2007). The production of tumor necrosis factor (TNF)-α and the expression of TNF-α receptors are important for the development of PPs (Fu and Chaplin, 1999).

The presentation of luminal Ags is affected by the dose of Ag and the presence or absence of adjuvant effects. Pathogenic bacteria produce microbial byproducts, which can stimulate innate immune cells including gut APCs and serve as the major source of adjuvant (Abreu et al., 2005; Franchi et al., 2006). In contrast, a commensal flora often down-regulate APC activation (Smith and Nagler-Anderson, 2005).

13.2.1.3   Effector T-Cell Subsets

To maintain intestinal homeostasis, multiple subsets of T cells are present in the intestinal mucosa including effector subsets of T-helper (Th) cells including Th1, Th2, and Th17; regulatory T (Treg)-cell subsets; and CD8$^+$ T cells. The functions of effector T cells are suboptimal in neonates and most of them are naive T cells that are sensitized with exposure to gut luminal Ags and their responses to naive Ags are under the influence of innate immune responses in the gut mucosa. Th1 and Th2 cells are well established with distinct cytokine production patterns and their roles in immune defense; Th1 cells produce IFN-γ and activate macrophages in defense against intracellular organisms, while Th2 cells promote immunoglobulin E (IgE)-mediated immune defense producing Th2 cytokines (IL [interleukin]-4, IL-5, and IL-13). Th17 cells are characterized by the production of distinct cytokines (IL-17A, IL-17F, and IL-22) and appear important for defense against fungal and certain bacterial pathogens (Bettelli et al., 2007; Harrington et al., 2005; Schmidt-Weber et al., 2007). It has been shown that IL-17A not only augments T-cell priming but also activates innate immune cells (fibroblasts, macrophages, endothelial cells, and epithelial cells), resulting in the production of potent inflammatory mediators (IL-1, IL-6, TNF-α, iNOS, chemokines, etc.) and subsequent neutrophilic inflammation (Bettelli et al., 2007; Schmidt-Weber et al., 2007). The key differentiation factors for Th17 cells are IL-6 and IL-1β in humans (Acosta-Rodriguez et al., 2007; McGeachy and Cua, 2008) and recent studies also indicate a role of IL-23 and TGF-β (Manel et al., 2008; McGeachy and Cua, 2008). IL-23 also serves as a survival factor for Th17 cells, while IL-27 suppresses the development of Th17 cells (Batten et al., 2006; Stumhofer et al., 2006). Th17 cells with their potent proinflammatory natures have been implicated in autoimmune conditions including multiple sclerosis, rheumatoid arthritis, and inflammatory bowel disease (IBD) (Bettelli et al., 2007; Schmidt-Weber et al., 2007). Recently decreased plasma levels of IL-23 but not IL-17 were reported in children with autism in comparison with age-matched normal controls in studies employing 40 autistic children and 20 controls (Enstrom et al., 2008). However, it is unclear how this finding is associated with a potential role of Th17 cells in autism. The enumeration of Th17 cells and ideally the assessment of Th17 cell functions will be informative for further addressing a potential role of Th17 cell in autism. The differentiation of effector T-cell subsets is profoundly affected by innate immune responses, especially cytokine concentrations in the microenvironment, and is discussed in Sections 13.2.1.4 and 13.2.1.5.

13.2.1.4 Treg Cells

The intestinal immune homeostasis is partly maintained by active immune suppression. The major cells involved in this process are Treg cells. Thymus-derived, naturally occurring Treg cells are known to play a role in maintaining self-tolerance in the periphery (Torgerson and Ochs, 2007; Wildin et al., 2001). However, in the gut mucosa, other types of regulatory T cells called induced or adaptive Treg (aTreg) cells appear to play a crucial role in the induction and maintenance of immune tolerance. They are thought to be derived from naive T cells, following Ag exposure in the presence of IL-2 and TGF-β (Chatila et al., 2008). Treg cells are characterized by the expression of CD4, CD25[high], Foxp3, cytotoxic T-lymphocyte associated Ag 4, and glucocorticoid-induced TNF receptor-related protein. Milk protein–specific aTreg cells have been reported to be present in children who have outgrown non-IgE-mediated food allergy (NFA) against cow's milk protein (Karlsson et al., 2004). The Foxp3[-] IL-10[+] T regulatory type 1 cells are also thought to have derived from naive T-cell upon Ag exposure (Chatila, 2005). They were initially recognized in patients with severe combined immunodeficiency following hematopoietic stem cell (Bacchetta et al., 1994), and also are known to be abundant in the intestine (Chatila, 2005).

It is of note that suppressive Treg cells can reciprocally differentiate into proinflammatory Th17 cells and vice versa in both rodents and humans depending on microenvironment. The high concentration of IL-6 overrides differentiation signal by TGF-β preferring Th17 differentiation, while retinoic acid, a metabolite of vitamin A, inhibits IL-6-driven Th17 cell differentiation and greatly augments Treg cell differentiation in the presence of TGF-β (Bettelli et al., 2007; Denning et al., 2007; Mucida et al., 2007). These findings indicate the importance of cytokines produced by innate immune cells. This may be especially true in the first few years of life when shaping T-cell responses in the later life.

13.2.1.5 Effects of Innate Immunity

Innate immune responses in the gut can augment and also suppress subsequent adaptive immunity. Lipopolysaccharide (LPS), an endotoxin, is produced by both pathogenic microbes and commensal floras and sensed by TLR4, a well-known PRR. In the small intestine where bacterial density is low, intestinal epithelial cells respond to LPS by producing proinflammatory cytokines (Hornef et al., 2002, 2003). In the colon where bacteria exist at high density, colonic epithelial cells are much less responsive to LPS rendering the state of endotoxin tolerance (Abreu et al., 2005; Smith and Nagler-Anderson, 2005). They also become less responsive to other TLR-mediated signaling (cross-tolerance). The TLR expression on macrophages and DCs in the small intestine is also down-regulated under normal conditions, preventing excessive inflammatory responses (Hausmann et al., 2002; Smith et al., 2001). Apically expressed TLR9 in the colonic epithelium also mediates inhibitory signaling (Lee et al., 2007, 2008).

The above-described innate immune defense is genetically predetermined and full-term babies are fully capable of mounting innate immune defense. However, Ag-specific, adaptive immune responses are slow to develop. During the first few months of life, the rapid expansion of Ag-specific T and B cells occurs (de Vries et al., 2000). During this period, the subtle changes in innate immune responses can significantly affect the development of GALT and may make certain individuals more prone to aberrant responses to immune insults.

13.2.1.5.1 Genetic Factors

As noted above, the genetically predetermined innate immune defense renders genetic variation (polymorphism) more influential in clinical manifestations as shown in IBD patients. Nucleotide oligomerizing domain 2 (Nod2), a member of PRRs called a Nod-like receptor family, recognizes a component of proteoglycans (PGN), muranyl dipeptide common to most bacterial PGN (Abreu et al., 2005; Franchi et al., 2006; Meylan et al., 2006). Intracellular Nod2 is highly up-regulated in monocytes and Paneth cells and can also be induced on intestinal epithelial cells by TNF-α and IFN-γ (Lala et al., 2003; Rosenstiel et al., 2003). Genetic variation in Nod2 is associated with increased susceptibility to various inflammatory conditions, most notably Crohn's disease (CD), at least in Caucasians (Abreu et al., 2005; Franchi et al., 2006; Rodriguez-Bores et al., 2007). Human CD-associated Nod2 variants exhibit reduced or loss of activity in cell lines, indicating that a deficit in sensing bacterial presence likely triggers abnormal inflammatory responses (Inohara et al., 2003; Ogura et al., 2001). Other multiple genetic factors involved in innate immunity are also included in candidate genes in the development of IBD (Rodriguez-Bores et al., 2007).

13.2.1.5.2 Environmental Factors

13.2.1.5.2.1 Commensal Flora   The lack of the commensal flora or the TLR4 signaling via endotoxin produced by the commensal flora is reported to augment immune responses to food Ags in both animal models and humans (Bashir et al., 2004). The restoration of oral tolerance in germ-free mice by feeding the mice LPS, a TLR4 agonist, has also been reported (Wannemuehler et al., 1982). This is partly attributed to the fact that LPS enhances the suppressive activity of TLR4$^+$CD4$^+$CD45RB^{low}CD25$^+$ Treg cells (Caramalho et al., 2003). A prolonged exposure to LPS or TLR2 stimulants also leads to tolerance and cross-tolerance to other PAMPs in intestinal epithelial cell lines (Otte et al., 2004). Likewise, other TLR agonists derived from the commensal flora also appear to be important in maintaining proper communication between the gut mucosal immune system and the commensal intestinal flora (Abreu et al., 2005; Kelly et al., 2005, Lee et al., 2007, 2008).

In addition to anti-inflammatory effects mediated by the host-immune system, the commensal flora can exert direct anti-inflammatory actions. *Bacteroides thetaiotaomicron* was shown to restrict the signaling induced by flagellin, a TLR5 agonist, and flagellated pathogens. These microbes block downstream signaling associated with NF-κB activation by promoting the nuclear export of transcriptionally active RelA (Kelly et al., 2004). This effect of *B. thetaiotanomicron* may partly explain why the gut tolerates large amounts of flagellated, potentially inflammatory commensal bacteria. In addition, other commensal bacteria were shown to block the activation of NF-κB by inhibiting IκB-α ubiquitination (Neish et al., 2000).

13.2.1.5.2.2 Micronutrients As described in Section 13.2.1.4, a novel role for retinoic acid, the metabolite of vitamin A, in the gut mucosal immunity has been shown. Unlike spleen DCs, LP DCs augment de novo generation of Foxp3$^+$ Treg cells, but their actions are dependent on TGF-β and retinoic acid (Denning et al., 2007; Mucida et al., 2007; Sun et al., 2007) and inhibited by IL-6. Reciprocally, retinoic acid antagonizes IL-6 in Th17 differentiation (Denning et al., 2007; Mucida et al., 2007; Sun et al., 2007). Retinoic acid was also known to imprint gut-homing specificity on T cells (Iwata et al., 2004) and it was reported that retinoic acid induces Foxp3$^+$ Treg cells expressing gut-homing receptors at high levels in both humans and mice (Kang et al., 2007).

Another emerging important regulator in mucosal immunity is adenosine that is likely derived from injured cells/tissues and can be also generated from extracellular nucleotides by ectoenzymes CD39 and CD73 (Sitkovsky et al., 2008). Treg cells were shown to express CD39 and CD73 and adenosine renders Treg cells to produce suppressive cytokines (IL-10 and TGF-β). These findings indicate that Treg cells play a role in restoring homeostasis in sterile tissue injury (Deaglio et al., 2007; Sitkovsky et al., 2008). Adenosine is also reported to exert anti-inflammatory effects independent of Treg cells (Sitkovsky et al., 2008). These findings indicate the importance of micronutrients in the gut mucosal homeostasis.

13.2.2 INNATE IMMUNITY IN THE CNS

As opposed to the gut, the brain is tightly regulated to maintain homeostasis by limiting the influence of external stimuli to protect mostly nonrenewable neuronal cells. The CNS immune system is also quite opposite to the gut immune system in terms of much less exposure to Ag stimuli largely due to the presence of the blood brain barrier (BBB), scant lymphoid tissue without lymphatic drainage, and limited numbers of APCs. The CNS is poorly equipped to mount the immune responses, but recent studies indicate the importance of innate immune cells in the CNS.

13.2.2.1   Innate Immune Cells in the CNS

Microglial cells are thought to be the resident macrophages in the brain and exert the first line of defense in the CNS parenchyma as a sensor of the CNS microenvironment. However, they also play a physiological role in the brain development/functions such as cortical plasticity and synaptic stripping (Davoust et al., 2008; Marin-Teva et al., 2004; Roumier et al., 2004). The quiescent microglial cells are distinguished from other macrophage lineage cells in their morphology extending microglial processes into the parenchyma (Davoust et al., 2008). This may allow them to detect changes in the microenvironment. The quiescent microglial cells are also distinguished from other macrophages with the low expression of cell surface markers including CD45, MHC II, and Fc receptor, rendering them poorly capable of Ag presentation and phagocytosis (Davoust et al., 2008). Upon activation, the microglial cells change into the similar morphology of other macrophages with the retraction of ramifications and start exerting functions of macrophages including phagocytosis, the presentation of Ag, and the production of inflammatory mediators. They can also proliferate, causing microgliosis in various pathological conditions (Streit et al., 1999).

In addition to the microglial cells, other types of macrophages are also present in the CNS–CNS associated macrophages. These include perivascular macrophages, meningeal macrophages, and choroid plexus macrophages. They express CD45[high] and MHCII[+]. In the inflamed CNS, peripheral blood monocytes and/or myeloid progenitors may be recruited to compose bone marrow–derived microglial (BMDM) cells (Davoust et al., 2008; Djukic et al., 2006; Rodriguez et al., 2007). In the rodent model of Alzheimer's disease, BMDM cells are reported to be more effective in clearing amyloid plaques (Simard et al., 2006).

Astrocytes, oligodenrocytes, and neuronal cells can also participate in innate immune responses in addition to their physiological roles. Astrocytes and brain endothelial cells interact to regulate water and electrolyte metabolism in the brain (Abbott et al., 2006). Astrocytes produce neurotropic factors such as glutamate in response to neurotransmitters or other neuronal signaling (Vesce et al., 2007; Zlokovic, 2008). They also acts as a "salt sensor" affecting local neuronal activity in response to changes in local lactate levels (Shimizu et al., 2007).

These innate immune cells are sensing PAMPs and danger signals via PRRs. Among PRRs, TLRs are most extensively studied in the brain. Multiple studies revealed mRNA and/or protein expression of TLR1–TLR8 in microglial cells (Crack and Bray, 2007; Olson and Miller, 2004). Some TLRs are also reported to be expressed on astrocytes (Crack and Bray, 2007). Perivascular and choroids plexus macrophages constitutively express CD14 and TLR4, which render them to sense circulating LPS in the absence of BBB (Laflamme and Rivest, 2001); TLR4 ligands to LPS with CD14 as a cofactor. In rodent models of endotoxemia, it was shown that the initial detection of LPS by these macrophages trigger the rapid up-regulation of CD14 in parenchymal microglial cells (Glezer et al., 2007). The transcription of multiple genes associated with innate immune responses takes place upon signaling that is mainly mediated by the NF-κB pathway (Glezer et al., 2007; Gosselin and Rivest, 2007). In this model, TLR2 is also involved in the production of the second wave of TNF-α and IL-12. TNF-α appears important for priming microglial cells (Glezer et al., 2007). Such innate inflammatory responses need to be tightly regulated considering largely nonrenewable neuronal tissues. These regulatory mechanisms include the production of counter-regulatory cytokines (IL-10, TGF-β, etc.) and the release of glucocorticoids (GCs) (Glezer et al., 2007; Haddad, 2008). Acute innate inflammatory responses in the brain may be protected by rapidly resolving and phagocytosing the excitotoxic damage in acute brain injury models (Gosselin and Rivest, 2007). The protective action of acute innate responses in the brain is also supported by the absence of neuronal damage with the single injection of LPS in the endotoxemia model (Gosselin and Rivest, 2007) and also by the augmented repair of myelin induced by LPS (Glezer et al., 2006).

However, the chronic activation of innate immunity is likely neurotoxic as indicated in various neurodegenerative diseases causing the production of reactive oxygen and nitrogen species, the recruitment of peripheral blood leukocytes and lymphocytes, the impairment of BBB, or other damages. BMDM cells are thought to be preferentially recruited at the site of neuronal insults and BMDM cells can penetrate even intact BBB and expand (Davoust et al., 2008), but their role in neurodegenerative diseases are not well understood.

13.2.2.2   Role of Treg Cells in the CNS Homeostasis

In addition to the above-described regulatory mechanisms in the innate immunity, Treg cells also known to play a role in controlling actions of effector stage T and B cells recruited to the site of neuronal insult/inflammatory in the brain (O'Connor and Anderton, 2008). The effector cells may not only be specific for pathogens invaded to the CNS, but may also be auto-reactive to neuronal tissues. In rodent models of multiple sclerosis (MS), the accumulation of Treg cells has been reported in the recovery stage (Kohm et al., 2006; Korn et al., 2007; Liu et al., 2006). These CNS Treg cells are distinguished from other Treg cells by their strong ability to proliferate, and they may be recruited in an Ag-independent manner by the CNS (O'Connor and Anderton, 2008; O'Connor et al., 2007). It is reported that Treg cells in MS patients is deficient in their function to suppress the proliferation of IFN-γ-producing Th cells, although normal numbers of Treg cells are present in the CNS (Astier and Hafler, 2007; O'Connor and Anderton, 2008; Venken et al., 2008). Treg cells differentiation and proliferation are dependent on cytokines produced by innate immune cells such as TGF-β in the microenvironment. Thus, innate immune cells may be important for supporting regulatory actions of Treg cells in the CNS as shown in the GI mucosa.

13.2.2.3   Neuro-Immune Network

An intricate neuro-immune interaction persists throughout one's life beginning in the stage of embryogenesis. This interaction is thought to be especially critical in the first few years of life. The disruption of this intricate network can lead to pathological condition in the CNS with the developing brain possibly being the most vulnerable.

13.2.2.3.1   Cytokines

In addition to PAMPs, numerous studies report the effects of cytokines on the CNS. Cytokine produced outside the brain can affect the CNS; neuronal tissues are one of the target organs. They may directly affect the brain at the level of brain parenchyma crossing the BBB or entering the brain area lacking the BBB (Goncharova and Tarakanov, 2007). They may also indirectly affect the brain via peripheral nervous systems and also via secondary messengers induced by cytokines (Goncharova and Tarakanov, 2007). For example, IL-2 can penetrate the intact BBB and affect cell growth and survival, the release of multiple mediators, and neuronal activities via IL-2 receptor expressed on neuronal and glial cells (Goncharova and Tarakanov, 2007). Proinflammatory cytokines released by innate immune responses (IL-1β, IL-6, and TNF-α) are known to cause "sickness behaviors" affecting multiple aspects of the CNS functions (Goncharova and Tarakanov, 2007; Gosselin and Rivest, 2007). A part of their actions may be attributed to their regulation of the activity of the serotonin transporter via p38 mitogen-activated protein-kinase pathway (Zhu et al., 2006). IL-1 is also implicated in long-term memory (Goeb et al., 2006; Pickering and O'Connor, 2007). Type 1 IFNs are also known to affect multiple CNS functions. It is well known that a high dose of exogenous type I IFNs can cause depression (Goeb et al., 2006).

These cytokines are also produced by the brain-resident innate immune cells as described in Section 13.2.2.1. TNF-α and IL-1β have been implicated in neurotoxic effects observed in neuronal damages (Gosselin and Rivest, 2007). IL-1β induces the production of reactive oxygen/nitrogen species, modulate activities of metalloproteinases, and increase the synaptic release of nitric oxide. TNF-α triggers the recruitment of neutrophils and monocytes to the site of inflammation and augments their phagocytic functions to eliminate pathogens and tissue debris. Such effects can not only be neuroprotective but also be neurotoxic.

Reciprocally, the CNS affects cytokine network by releasing various mediators such as GCs. For example, acute stress responses via hypophysis-pituitary-adrenal (HPA) axis limit excessive immune responses and restore immune homeostasis. However, chronic stress responses lead to the chronic production of GCs and catecholamines (CAs), which can dysregulate immune functions. Evidence indicates that both GCs and CAs render Th2-skewed responses by suppressing the production of IL-12 by APC; IL-12 is the key cytokine for Th1 differentiation (Blotta et al., 1997; Elenkov, 2008). GCs are also reported to up-regulate the production of IL-4, IL-10, and IL-13 by Th2 cells (Blotta et al., 1997; Elenkov, 2008). Both GCs and CAs affect the production of proinflammatory cytokines by macrophage-monocyte lineage cells (Elenkov, 2008). The cholinergic signaling provides anti-inflammatory action to leukocytes via cholinergic receptors (Franco et al., 2007). Evidence indicates that anti-inflammatory signaling via HPA axis and cholinergic nervous system is dysregulated in the IBD patients as evidenced by markedly reduced 5-hydroxyindoleacetic acid (5-HT) production (Franco et al., 2007).

13.3   EVIDENCE OF INNATE IMMUNE ABNORMALITIES IN AUTISM

13.3.1   GI System

In addition to the behavioral symptoms, certain medical conditions are present in many but not all the ASD children. One of the most common comorbidities in ASD children is GI symptoms (Ashwood and Wakefield, 2006; Ashwood et al., 2004; Horvath et al., 1999; White, 2003). This led to the speculation of GI pathology in the onset and progress of autism. Proposed abnormalities may be more or less associated with "presumed," impaired gut mucosal innate immunity in autistic children.

13.3.1.1 Intestinal Permeability

As discussed in Section 13.2.1, gut epithelial cells are thought to play multiple roles in the gut mucosal innate immunity not only serving as an epithelial barrier but also producing multiple mediators. In the view of the high frequency of GI symptoms, the dysfunction of intestinal epithelial barrier has been hypothesized in ASD children—"leaky gut hypothesis" (White, 2003). This hypothesis postulated that impaired gut permeability in autistic children permits the entry of macromolecules like milk protein, causing the sensitization of gut mucosal immune system and subsequent food allergy (FA). It is also postulated that such macromolecules entered to the blood stream affect the CNS directly. However, it is unclear whether impaired gut permeability is present prior to the onset of GI symptoms or altered permeability is a result of gut mucosal inflammation. It should be noted that children with NFA have been reported to exhibit impaired intestinal permeability that resolves after the implementation of the restricted diet avoiding offending food (Dupont and Heyman, 2000). Recent study in 14 autistic children with current or previous GI complaints found no evidence of changes in intestinal permeability (Robertson et al., 2008).

13.3.1.2 Dysbiosis

Intestinal commensal flora also plays a role in maintaining intestinal homeostasis as discussed in Section 13.2.1.5.2. There have been anecdotal reports of the onset of autism following the administration of antibiotics and the subsequent appearance of GI symptoms. It was hypothesized that antimicrobial administration led to the disruption of commensal flora and the colonization of bacteria producing neurotoxin. In open-label trial, the administration of oral vancomycin in 10 children with regressive autism resulted in short-term improvement in their behavioral symptoms (Sandler et al., 2000). Two studies that examined the constitution of gut microflora in ASD children reported differences from normal controls. One study examined 7 children with regression autism and documented GI symptoms as well as 4 control children and their results revealed significant difference in the upper and the lower intestinal floras between autistic and control children (Finegold et al., 2002). Another study examined 58 ASD children, 15 normal siblings, and 10 unrelated healthy children. The authors reported a higher incidence of *Clostridium histolyticum* group in ASD children; most of ASD children had the history of multiple antibiosis and significant GI symptoms (Parracho et al., 2005). In these studies, it is possible that other factors such as previous frequent antibiosis and the restricted diet on which many ASD children were already placed at the time of the study entry may have affected the results. The careful selection of the study subjects with appropriate case controls may shed a light whether dysbiosis has any role in the pathogenesis of autism.

13.3.1.3 Autism Colitis

Secondary to the high prevalence of GI symptoms in ASD children, abnormalities of GI mucosa has been implicated in the development of autism. Macroscopic (ileocolonic lymphoid nodular hyperplasia [LNH]) and histological findings indicating mild GI mucosal inflammation have been reported in ASD children (Furlano et al., 2001; Wakefield et al., 2000, 2005). Immunohistochemical studies of biopsy specimen from ASD children revealed higher numbers of CD3+CD8+ T cells in the epithelium as well as higher numbers of CD3+ T cells and CD19+ B cells in the LP as compared to those from normal controls (Ashwood et al., 2003). In children with regressive autism, Torrente et al. (2002) reported lymphocytic colitis that is characterized with epithelial IgG and complement deposition. LNH can be observed in normal children and the significance of "autism colitis" appears still controversial. However, one study indicated significantly higher prevalence of LNH in the ileum and colon in ASD children than controls; LNH appears to be not affected by the diet or age at the time of colonoscopy (Wakefield et al., 2005).

In subsequent studies, these authors report the up-regulation of proinflammatory cytokines in the intestinal mucosa. It was reported that LP CD3+ T cells in the duodenum express higher IL-2, TNF-α, and IFN-γ, but less IL-10 and also the higher expression of TNF-α and IFN-γ by LP CD3+ T cells in the colon in ASD children with GI symptoms (Ashwood and Wakefield, 2006; Ashwood et al., 2004). In 18 ASD children with GI symptoms, authors reported increased expression of TNF-α and IFN-γ and less expression of IL-10 by CD3+ T cells in both intestinal mucosa and peripheral blood as compared to normal controls (Ashwood and Wakefield, 2006).

On the other hand, other studies failed to reveal any difference between ASD children and normal controls in the concentration of proinflammatory cytokines (IL-6, IL-8, and IL-1β) in the GI mucosa (DeFelice et al., 2003) or in the stool concentration of calprotectin or rectal nitric oxide: these are nonspecific markers of GI inflammation. Such conflicting results may be partly attributed to the small numbers of study subjects, although most of the studies focus on ASD children with GI symptoms. It still remains to be seen whether "autism colitis" is present or such GI inflammation may be associated with other immune abnormalities such as FA. Unfortunately, in all these studies, the presence or absence of IgE-mediated FA or NFA has not been addressed.

How is the GI inflammation documented in ASD children associated with innate immune abnormalities? Innate immunity is crucial for maintaining immune homeostasis. If there exists aberrant innate immune responses in the gut mucosa as indicated in the peripheral blood of a subset of ASD children (Jyonouchi et al., 2002, 2005b), these ASD children may be vulnerable to GI inflammation triggered by immune insults, developing chronic inflammation as postulated in patients with Crohn's disease.

13.3.1.4 Food Allergy

As detailed in the previous section, young children are more vulnerable to sensitization to common food proteins due to the immature gut mucosal immune system. Secondary to the high frequency of GI symptoms in ASD children, the presence of FA has been suspected. Previously reported immunological abnormalities such as increase in the higher production of Th2 cytokines without stimuli and the higher frequency of Th cells expressing Th2 cytokines suggested the higher prevalence of atopy in ASD children (Gupta et al., 1998; Molloy et al., 2006). However, to my knowledge, there has been no report documenting the high prevalence of atopy in ASD children.

TABLE 13.1
Prevalence of Atopic Disorders

Study Group	Atopic Disorders	AR + AC	AD	Atopic Asthma
ASD children	34/123 (27.6%)	34/123 (27.6%)	10/123 (8.1%)	6/123 (4.9%)
ROM/CRS[a]	3/25 (12.0%)	3/25 (12.0%)	0/25 (0%)	3/25 (12.0%)[a]
FA	6/27 (22.2%)	4/27 (14.8%)	4/27 (14.8%)	3/27 (11.1%)
Control	10/46 (21.7%)	10/46 (21.7%)	3/46 (6.5%)	7/46 (15.2%)[a]

Note: AC, allergic conjunctivitis; AD, allergic dermatitis; AR, allergic rhinitis.
[a] Among ROM/CRS patients and controls, 16 and 2 children were diagnosed with non-atopic asthma, respectively.

One study examining 30 autistic children reports the higher frequency of skin prick test reactivity in their study population, but it is unclear whether these children demonstrated corresponding clinical features; authors report normal IgE levels and no asthma symptoms in these autistic children (Bakkaloglu, 2007). In 123 ASD children evaluated in the Pediatric Allergy/Immunology clinic at our institution, we found no evidence of the high prevalence of atopy (Table 13.1). These ASD children were evaluated by standard diagnostic measures for atopic disorders including the measurement of allergen-specific IgE and skin prick testing. Likewise, we did not find the high frequency of IgE-mediated FA in ASD children evaluated in our clinic.

Various dietary intervention measures have been tried on the basis of anecdotal reports despite the lack of evidence of IgE-mediated FA. Among such dietary intervention measures, a casein-free, gluten-free (cf/gf) diet appears most popular with frequent beneficial effects per parental reports. However, prospective studies addressing the effects of the cf/gf diet revealed conflicting results (Elder et al., 2006; Knivsberg et al., 2002). This may be partly attributed to the random selection of the study subject without proper workup for FA. These studies may have been formulated to test the "leaky gut hypothesis."

In our previous studies, we hypothesized that GI symptoms frequently seen in ASD children can be partly explained by NFA and immune reactivity to food proteins can be detected by measuring the production of TNF-α and other inflammatory cytokines by peripheral blood mononuclear cells (PBMCs) as reported in NFA children (Benlounes et al., 1999). Our results revealed the presence of cellular immune reactivity to common dietary proteins (mainly milk protein) in young ASD children with GI symptoms (Jyonouchi et al., 2005a). We also found that such immune reactivity to food protein was correlated with aberrant responses to LPS (TLR4 agonist) by PBMCs (Jyonouchi et al., 2005b). However, NFA may be playing a lesser role in GI symptoms in older ASD children, since most children likely outgrow NFA condition with the maturation of the gut immune system and the establishment of oral tolerance. We also observed the less prevalence of NFA in older (>6 years) ASD children (unpublished observation).

Given our findings, it is possible that aberrant innate immune responses may provoke undesired immune reactivity against commensal flora in ASD children as observed in IBD patients. In the studies of children who underwent the elimination diet, we found the decline of the cellular reactivity to milk proteins but persistent reactivity to candida Ag, a representative microbial luminal Ag (Jyonouchi et al., 2007). Taken together, our data indicate a role of NFA in GI symptoms in some ASD children in association with aberrant innate immune responses.

In summary, there exist convincing data supporting the presence of chronic GI inflammation in ASD children, but the etiology of GI inflammation, which is likely affected by multiple genetic and environmental factors, is still not well understood. NFA can partly explain the GI symptoms and beneficial effects of dietary interventions in some ASD children. However, aberrant innate immune responses, if present as suggested by our data, likely affect immune reactivity not only to food protein but also to commensal flora. Apparent effects of oral vancomycin and altered commensal flora reported in ASD children may be explained partly by aberrant innate immune responses. Further studies will be required to understand a role of innate immunity in the GI symptoms observed in ASD children.

13.3.2   CNS

Autism has been considered as a heterogeneous neuro-developmental disorder defined by behavioral symptoms and in a majority of patients, the development of autism is likely affected by multiple genetic and possibly environmental factors starting from fetal life. A role of the immune system in the brain pathology has been controversial secondary to the lack of clear evidence of immune reactions unlike other neurodegenerative diseases. However, recent studies indicate the evidence of chronic mild inflammation in the CNS in autism patients.

13.3.2.1   CNS Inflammation

Ongoing inflammation in the CNS in autism has been suggested by several investigators with findings of elevated inflammatory markers in cerebrospinal fluid (CSF). In 12 children with autism, decreased quinolinic acid and neopterin but increased biopterin were reported along with the increase in soluble tumor necrosis factor receptor II (Zimmerman et al., 2005). Others also reported increased levels of TNF-α in both CSF and serum in 10 children with regressive autism (Chez et al., 2007). Elevated cerebellar 3-nitrotyrosine, a marker of oxidative stress, was also reported in 9 autistic children (Sajdel-Sulkowska et al., 2008). Such findings are consistent with active neuro-inflammatory process evidenced by the activation of microglial cells and astrocytes in the cerebral cortex, white matter, and cerebellum in autopsied brains in 11 autistic patients (Vargas et al., 2005). In their studies, they also reported the up-regulation of protein levels of macrophage chemoattractant protein (MCP)-1 and TGF-β1 in the brain tissue along with elevated levels of MCP-1 in CSF. Authors report that the major source of inflammatory cytokines is likely activated astrocytes. Since the numbers of patients in these studies are relatively limited and these study subjects appear to have overt clinical symptoms indicating inflammation, it is uncertain whether such inflammatory processes can be observed in all the autistic children. Nevertheless, it is likely that a subset of autistic children can reveal the evidence of ongoing inflammation involving innate immune cells in the CNS.

13.3.2.2 Mechanisms of Chronic CNS Inflammation

As a cause of "presumed" CNS inflammation, several possibilities have been postulated. These include impaired responses to oxidative stresses and auto-inflammatory/autoimmune conditions. If such mechanisms are present, it may be reasonable to assume that such changes can be detected in the periphery. Several authors have reported changes in serum parameters either indicating oxidative stress (Chauhan and Chauhan, 2006; Corbett et al., 2008; Deth et al., 2008; James et al., 2006) or dysregulated adaptive and innate immune responses (Ashwood et al., 2006, 2008; Sweeten et al., 2003b, 2004). Effects of multiple environmental factors on genetically susceptible individuals (xenobiotics) have been implicated in the development of autism as detailed in Section 13.4.2. A role of mitochondrial dysfunction has been suspected in association with the evidence of increase in oxidative stress in autistic children (Oliveira et al., 2007; Poling et al., 2006). However, it is unclear whether impaired oxidative stress can solely explain reported inflammatory processes in the brain.

The presence of autoantibodies against brain tissues has also been reported as reviewed by Ashwood et al. (Ashwood and Wakefield, 2006; Ashwood et al., 2006). Interestingly, one study reports the higher presence of anti-brain antibodies in autistic children as well as their unaffected siblings (Singer et al., 2006). Epidemiological studies indicate the higher prevalence of autoimmune diseases in parents of children with autism (Mouridsen et al., 2007; Sweeten et al., 2003a). These findings led to the hypothesis that maternally derived anti-brain antibodies have a role in the development of autism. Several authors report the presence of antibodies against fetal brain in sera of mothers with autistic children including antibodies against myelin basic protein and glial acidic fibrillary protein (Croen et al., 2008; Singer et al., 2008; Zimmerman et al., 2007). Others reported that maternal mid-pregnancy autoantibodies to fetal brain may be an early marker for autism (Croen et al., 2008). Then how do these maternal autoantibodies affect fetal and infantile brain? Most of these autoantibodies are IgG in isotype and how these autoantibodies can access to the CNS is unclear in the presence of BBB. It is also unclear how the presence of maternal autoantibodies is associated with frequent comorbidities such as GI symptoms in ASD children.

In summary, evidence is slowly accumulating indicating the presence of ongoing inflammation in the CNS in some, if not all, autistic children involving innate immune cells. However, mechanisms leading to ongoing inflammation are unclear.

13.4 POSSIBLE IMPACT OF INNATE IMMUNITY ON NEURO-IMMUNE INTERACTIONS IN AUTISM

Autism was once thought to be a static encephalopathy caused by structural and genetic abnormalities. However, clinical features in autistic children indicate otherwise. That is, a high frequency of comorbidities such as GI symptoms and sleep disturbance indicates chronic inflammatory condition involving other organ systems. Various studies reported the evidence of ongoing inflammation and chronic oxidative stress not only in the CNS but also in the periphery in autistic children (Ashwood and Wakefield, 2006; Ashwood et al., 2008; Chauhan et al., 2004; Deth et al., 2008; James et al., 2006; Pardo and Eberhart, 2007; Pardo et al., 2005; Vargas et al., 2005;

Zimmerman et al., 2005). Autism without clearly defined metabolic/genetic causes is better to be considered as a chronic multisystem disease(s) under the influence of multiple genetic and environmental factors.

It is generally agreed that there are at least two types of ASD in terms of the disease development: ASD children whose abnormal cognitive development is evident from birth (classical autism) and those who reveal developmental regression generally between 18 and 24 months of age following an apparent span of normal development (regressive autism) (Lainhart et al., 2002). The diagnosis of autism may not be definite, and some ASD children drop the diagnosis of autism, which may occur spontaneously or possibly in response to therapeutic measures (Fein et al., 2005; Kelley et al., 2006; Kleinman et al., 2008; Sutera et al., 2007). What kind of biological abnormalities can lead to the above described clinical features of ASD affecting the multiple organ systems? In this section, postulated mechanisms that may explain many aspects of complex clinical features of ASD are discussed focusing on potential roles of innate immunity.

13.4.1 IMPAIRED SIGNALING OF NEUROTRANSMITTERS

13.4.1.1 Cholinergic Neurotransmission

Cholinergic signaling plays a vital role in many aspects of brain functions and its dysregulation has been implicated in various neurological diseases. The decreased protein expression of $\alpha 3$, $\alpha 4$, and $\beta 2$ nicotinic acetylcholine receptor (nAChR) has been reported in cerebral cortex and the cerebellum of autopsied brains from adult autistic patients (Martin-Ruiz et al., 2004). As for the immune system, the cholinergic neurotransmission plays an important physiological role in down-regulating inflammatory responses (de Jonge and Ulloa, 2007). In rodent models of sepsis, the vagal nerve stimulation attenuates inhibitory responses partly through down-regulating the production of proinflammatory cytokines via $\alpha 7$nAChR (de Jonge and Ulloa, 2007). In the brain, both neuronal and glial cells express nAChR. On the other hand, it was reported that in rat embryonic brain cells, TLR agonist and CD40 ligand (CD154) promote excess cholinergic differentiation from undifferentiated progenitors (Ni et al., 2007); as stated previously, both neuronal and glial cells express TLRs. Nicotinic agonists have been investigated for their potential therapeutic effects on neurodegenerative diseases, since nicotine itself has significant toxicity (de Jonge and Ulloa, 2007). The cholinergic neurotransmission is inhibited by various chemicals, including organic phosphates and nicotinoids, that one may be exposed in daily life. It was proposed that low but chronic exposure to such chemicals may be associated with impaired cholinergic neurotransmission in some autistic children with genetic vulnerability. However, the role of exposure to such toxic chemicals in the development of autism is not well understood.

13.4.1.2 GABA Neurotransmission

The gamma-aminobutyric acid (GABA) receptors (GABR) transmit excitatory responses in adult brains, but they function differently during the development of neuronal maturation. Impaired GABAergic circuits have been implicated in many neuro-developmental disorders including autism (Di Cristo, 2007). Polymorphisms of GABRγ1 and other genes located on chromosome 15q11–13 are reported to be risk factors for autism (Ashley-Koch et al., 2006; Vincent et al., 2006). On the other hand, Tochigi et al. (2007) reported no association between GABR genes in 15q11–13 and autism in a Japanese population. In the periphery, GABA also serves as a neurotransmitter as well as a hormone like factor in both peripheral nervous system and endocrine organs. For example, GABA increases insulin secretion (Gladkevich et al., 2006).

In type 1 diabetes, a T-cell-mediated organ-specific autoimmune disease, GABA expression is down-regulated with the presence of autoantibodies against GABA and glutamic acid decarboxylate (GAD) 65 that catalyzes glutamate to GABA and carbon dioxide by decarboxylation (Gladkevich et al., 2006). GAD65 autoantibody is also known to be present in patients with stiff person's syndrome (SPS), a rare autoimmune neurological disorder. In SPS patients, others report the presence of autoantibody against GABAA-receptor (Raju et al., 2006). Innate immune cells do also express GABAA receptors and selective GABAA receptor agonist was shown to activate macrophages independent of TLRs in vitro and in vivo (Lubick et al., 2007). Environmental exposures to chemicals that inhibit GABA neurotransmission can thus potentially cause various symptoms affecting nervous, endocrine, and immune systems in genetically vulnerable individuals. However, it is not known how such environmental exposure has a role in the development of autism.

13.4.1.3 Ca²⁺ Signaling

Ca^{2+} signaling is fundamental in cell biology and the impaired Ca^{2+} signaling causes a chronic illness affecting multiple organs. Timothy syndrome arises from a single nucleotide change that leads to a mutation in the pore-forming subunit of the L-type Ca^{2+} channel Ca(V)1.2 (Splawski et al., 2004). Their clinical features are characterized by autistic features, severe cardiac arrhythmia, and developmental abnormalities (Splawski et al., 2004). The immune system is also profoundly dependent on Ca^{2+} signaling along with neuronal cells on its function and development. However, little is known regarding any evidence of impaired Ca^{2+} signaling in autism without defined etiology. In the Allergy/Immunology Clinic, we have evaluated over 200 ASD children and did not find any patient indicating impaired Ca^{2+} signaling in the immune system. However, subtle changes in the Ca^{2+} signaling may not be detectable in conventional immune workup. It remains to be seen how potentially impaired Ca^{2+} signaling affects the development of autism.

13.4.1.4 β2 Adrenergic Receptor

The prenatal stimulation of the β2 adrenergic receptor with the use of terbutaline, a β2 agonist and a tocolytic agent, has also been implicated in the increased risk of autism in genetically susceptible individuals (Cheslack-Postava et al., 2007). When terbutaline was administered to rats equivalent to ages of the second and third trimesters of humans, microglial activation was observed, supporting possible effects of a tocolytic agent in autism in susceptible individuals (Zerrate et al., 2007). However, β2 agonists have been used by pregnant women suffering from asthma, without any known adverse effects on offspring. This may be due to a minute amount of β2 agonist entering the blood stream when inhaled as opposed to a large dose of β2 agonist administered intravenously when used as a tocolytic agent.

13.4.2 A Redox/Methylation Hypothesis

As described in the previous sections, the evidence of chronic oxidative stress has been described in ASD children (Deth et al., 2008). It has been hypothesized that altered methionine synthase, which is an effective defense mechanism against oxidative stress in the acute stage but not in chronic condition by affecting DNA methylation and dopamine receptor phospholipid methylation, may be associated with the development of autism along with impaired responses to oxidative stress (Deth et al., 2008). Individuals with genetic susceptibility to xenobiotics will be affected in such conditions. The risk of autism is implicated in environmental exposure to heavy metals and xenobiotics in this hypothesis. However, epidemiological studies failed to reveal a causal association between early exposure to mercury from thimerosal-containing vaccines and immunoglobulins and deficits in neuropsychological functioning at the age of 7–10 years (Thompson et al., 2007). It is possible that such risk may only be objectively found in individuals with defined genetic susceptibility. Likewise, xenobiotics can affect the immune system and alter gene expression by inhibiting DNA methylation, but how the low dose of chronic environmental exposure to xenobiotics can impact the immune system is not well understood.

13.4.3 Effects of Immune Insult

13.4.3.1 Insult In Utero

As indicated in the previous section, the immune system can reciprocally affect neurotransmitter signaling. Thus, immune insults mediated by cytokines and other mediators can profoundly affect the development of brain and other organ systems in vulnerable period. It has been known that maternal infection during pregnancy is a risk factor in neuro-developmental disorders including autism (Arndt et al., 2005). The effects of maternal infection in utero have been studied in animal models, often using TLR agonists such as LPS (endotoxin), mimicking infection-induced innate immune responses without using live pathogens. By using TLR3 agonist mimicking viral infection in rodents, others reported multiple neuro-pathological symptom clusters in adulthood (Meyer et al., 2008a,b; Pessah et al., 2008). Authors reported that abnormalities found depended on the precise timing of prenatal immune insult (Meyer et al., 2008b).

Such effects of innate immune activation in this model are likely affected by genetic susceptibility. This was indicated by the attenuated effects of TLR3 agonist in their model in transgenic mice over-expressing IL-10, a counter-regulatory cytokine (Meyer et al., 2008b). Others also revealed the similar effects of nonpathogenic immune insult in utero in rodents using cytokines as a source of immune insults (Smith et al., 2007). During pregnancy, maternal infection does not necessarily induce fetal infection, but inflammatory mediators induced by innate immune responses can affect fetal brain via inflammatory mediators such as LPS or other means. These findings indicate that maternal innate immune responses, if excessive, can affect lasting effects in the CNS of offspring.

In animal models with maternal viral infection (influenza), deleterious effects on brain structure and functions have also been reported when mice were infected in the late second trimester (Fatemi et al., 2008). As shown in models using a TLR3 agonist, infection with influenza in the late second trimester revealed significant changes in the expression of genes implicated with autism and schizophrenia in the brain in addition to brain atrophy (Fatemi et al., 2008). Interestingly, authors also reported altered levels of serotonin, 5-HT, and taurine in this model; they report decreased levels of serotonin in the cerebella of offspring at postnatal day 14 but not at day 56 (Winter et al., 2008). Elevated levels of serum serotonin has been reported in a subset of autistic children (Burgess et al., 2006), while low plasma serotonin levels in mothers of autistic children was indicated as a risk factor for autism (Connors et al., 2006). These results indicate that altered serotonin levels may be associated with prenatal immune insult.

The pitfalls of the above-described rodent models are that the growth pattern of the brain differs in humans and rodents. The timing of in utero exposure in these animal models is considered to be still in the early stage of gestation in humans even if in utero challenge occurs in the late pregnancy in rodents. It will be necessary to collect data in pregnant women and outcomes of neuropsychiatric functions in offspring prospectively.

13.4.3.2 Immune Insult in Postnatal Period

It is not well understood whether postnatal immune insult further affects the development/progress of autism. Immune insult can certainly cause oxidative stresses, which may contribute in disease progress in vulnerable individuals after birth as discussed in the previous sections. GI inflammation caused by FA and dysbiosis can also affect the CNS via cytokines, neurotransmitters, and other means. For example, Shultz et al. (2008) reported impaired social behaviors in the rat with the intracerebroventricular injection of propionic acid (PPA), an enteric bacterial metabolic end-product. The brain of the animals injected with PPA revealed astrogliosis—the evidence of neuroinflammation via the activation of CNS innate immune cells (Shultz et al., 2008). The PPA production is likely to increase with the disruption of commensal flora triggered by prolonged antibiosis, severe FA, and viral gastroenteritis. The high frequency of GI symptoms and apparent therapeutic effects of probiotics, vancomycin (Ashwood et al., 2004), and dietary intervention in ASD children (Levy and Hyman, 2005) may support a potential role of PPA in their behavioral symptoms.

In patients with regressive autism, parents often attribute the onset of regression to apparent systemic immune insult such as viral infection and adverse drug reactions. Common viral infection such as influenza causes the systemic activation of innate immunity and the CNS responds to such insults by sensing PAMPS, proinflammatory cytokines, and other mediators as detailed in Section 13.1. In autistic subjects with genetic susceptibility, the activation of the CNS innate immune system could lead to undesirable neuroinflammation and brain dysfunction. Apart from genetic susceptibility associated with neurotransmitter signaling and oxidative stresses as discussed before, are there any primary immune abnormalities or genetic polymorphisms that affect CNS responses to immune insults in ASD children? Given the CNS immune system, such abnormalities, if present, may be likely associated with innate immunity and its key inflammatory mediators. However, so far, no such abnormalities are clearly described in autistic children.

In studying the gene expression of whole peripheral blood from children with autism or ASD, the up-regulation of genes associated with innate immunity has been reported, albeit up-regulation is modest (about twofold) (Gregg et al., 2008). These genes are those expressed by natural killer (NK) cells and many of them belong to the NK cytotoxicity pathways (Gregg et al., 2008). NK cells are one of the major effector cells in innate immunity at the time of viral syndrome. Such findings may support a role of innate immunity in the development of autism. However, such changes were found in both ASD and autism patients (Gregg et al., 2008) and it is unclear whether such changes are more significantly observed in a subset of ASD children with apparent susceptibility to recurrent infection or regression triggered by microbial infection.

Previously, we retrospectively reviewed ASD subjects seen in our clinic for the past 3 years with regard to infection-induced exacerbation. We defined such exacerbation as significant exacerbation in behavioral symptoms as well as the loss of once-acquired cognitive skills documented by caretakers/teachers/therapists independent of parents, excluding initial regression. With such definition, up to 10% of ASD children falls into this category and this does not seem to be associated with atopy or autism sub-types (autism, PDD-NOS, or ASD) (Table 13.2). The diagnosis of primary immunodeficiency such as specific polysaccharide antibody deficiency is not associated with this subset of ASD children. Our findings indicate a more potent role of innate immunity in

TABLE 13.2
Prevalence of Microbial Infection–Induced Exacerbation[b] in ASD Children Evaluated in the Pediatric Allergy/Immunology Clinic

	Infection-Induced Exacerbation
ASD without atopy[a]	
Autism[a]	9/107 (8.4%)
PDD-NOS	6/84 (7.1%)
ASD	2/32 (6.3%)
ASD with atopy	
Autism	4/44 (9.1%)
PDD-NOS	1/43 (2.3%)
ASD	1/11 (9.1%)

[a] Atopy was defined as the presence of atopic disorders (atopic asthma, allergic rhinoconjunctivitis, and atopic dermatitis) with positive skin-test reactivity and/or positive allergen-specific IgE antibodies.

[b] Specific polysaccharide antibody deficiency was diagnosed in a total of 4 ASD children and 2 of them revealed infection-induced exacerbation. No other primary immunodeficiency was diagnosed in this study population.

ASD children with the above-described clinical features and in such children, genetic susceptibility may be defined by altered innate immune responses.

It is also of note that when we tested the effects of the elimination diet in ASD children with NFA (mainly to milk protein), we observed the decline of cellular reactivity to offending food protein, but persistent altered responses to LPS, a TLR4 agonist, in ASD/NFA children but not in non-ASD/NFA children. Such findings may also indicate the presence of aberrant innate immune responses affecting responses to immune insult after birth.

13.5 CONCLUSIONS

No definite evidence exits that the innate immunity affects the development of autism. However, the clinical and laboratory findings described in this chapter appear sufficient to support a role of innate immunity in some autistic children. Further studies in a well-defined subset of ASD children indicative of innate immune abnormalities will help in defining the role of innate immunity in the development/progress of autism.

ACKNOWLEDGMENT

The author is thankful to Dr. L. Huguenin for critically reviewing this chapter.

ABBREVIATIONS

5-HT	5-hydroxyindoleacetic acid
ASD	autism spectrum disorders
Ag	antigen
APC	Ag-presenting cells
BBB	blood brain barrier
BMDM	bone marrow–derived microglial
CAs	catecholamines
CD	Crohn's disease
cf/gf	casein-free, gluten-free
CNS	central nervous system
CSF	cerebrospinal fluid
DCs	dendritic cells
FA	food allergy
GABA	gamma-aminobutyric acid
GABR	GABA receptors
GAD	glutamic acid decarboxylate
GALT	gut-associated lymphoid tissue
GCs	glucocorticoids
GI	gastrointestinal
HPA	hypophysis-pituitary-adrenal
IBD	inflammatory bowel disease
Ig	immunoglobulin

IFN	interferon
IL	interleukin
LNH	lymphoid nodular hyperplasia
LP	lamina propria
LPS	lipopolysaccharide
MCP-1	macrophage chemoattractant protein-1
MHC	major histocompatibility complex
MS	multiple sclerosis
nAChR	nicotinic acetylcholine receptor
NFA	non-IgE-mediated food allergy
NK	natural killer
Nod2	nucleotide oligomerizing domain 2
PAMPs	pathogen associated molecular patterns
PBMCs	peripheral blood mononuclear cells
PGN	proteoglycans
PP	Peyer's patches
PRRs	pattern recognition receptors
SPS	stiff person's syndrome
TGF	transforming growth factor
Th	T-helper
TLR	Toll-like receptors
TNF	tumor necrosis factor
Treg	regulatory T cells
aTreg	adaptive Treg

REFERENCES

Abbott, N.J., Ronnback, L., and Hansson, E. 2006. Astrocyte-endothelial interactions at the blood-brain barrier. *Nat. Rev. Neurosci.* 7:41–53.

Abreu, M.T., Fukata, M., and Arditi, M. 2005. TLR signaling in the gut in health and disease. *J. Immunol.* 174:4453–4460.

Acosta-Rodriguez, E.V., Rivino, L., Geginat, J., Jarrossay, D., Gattorno, M., Lanzavecchia, A., Sallusto, F., and Napolitani, G. 2007. Surface phenotype and antigenic specificity of human interleukin 17-producing T helper memory cells. *Nat. Immunol.* 8:639–646.

Arndt, T.L., Stodgell, C.J., and Rodier, P.M. 2005. The teratology of autism. *Int. J. Dev. Neurosci.* 23:189–199.

Ashley-Koch, A.E., Mei, H., Jaworski, J., Ma, D.Q., Ritchie, M.D., Menold, M.M., Delong, G.R., Abramson, R.K., Wright, H.H., Hussman, J.P., Cuccaro, M.L., Gilbert J.R., Martin E.R., and Pericak-Vance M.A. 2006. An analysis paradigm for investigating multi-locus effects in complex disease: Examination of three GABA receptor subunit genes on 15q11-q13 as risk factors for autistic disorder. *Ann. Hum. Genet.* 70:281–292.

Ashwood, P., Anthony, A., Pellicer, A.A., Torrente, F., Walker-Smith, J.A., and Wakefield, A.J. 2003. Intestinal lymphocyte populations in children with regressive autism: Evidence for extensive mucosal immunopathology. *J. Clin. Immunol.* 23:504–517.

Ashwood, P., Anthony, A., Torrente, F., and Wakefield, A.J. 2004. Spontaneous mucosal lymphocyte cytokine profiles in children with autism and gastrointestinal symptoms: Mucosal immune activation and reduced counter regulatory interleukin-10. *J. Clin. Immunol.* 24:664–673.

Ashwood, P. and Wakefield, A.J. 2006. Immune activation of peripheral blood and mucosal CD3[+] lymphocyte cytokine profiles in children with autism and gastrointestinal symptoms. *J. Neuroimmunol.* 173:126–134.

Ashwood, P., Wills, S., and Van de Water, J. 2006. The immune response in autism: A new frontier for autism research. *J. Leukoc. Biol.* 80:1–15.

Ashwood, P., Kwong, C., Hansen, R., Hertz-Picciotto, I., Croen, L., Krakowiak, P., Walker, W., Pessah, I.N., and Van de Water, J. 2008. Brief report: Plasma leptin levels are elevated in autism: Association with early onset phenotype? *J. Autism Dev. Disord.* 38:169–175.

Astier, A.L. and Hafler, D.A. 2007. Abnormal Tr1 differentiation in multiple sclerosis. *J. Neuroimmunol.* 191:70–78.

Bacchetta, R., Bigler, M., Touraine, J.L., Parkman, R., Tovo, P.A., Abrams, J., de Waal Malefyt, R., de Vries, J.E., and Roncarolo, M.G. 1994. High levels of interleukin 10 production in vivo are associated with tolerance in SCID patients transplanted with HLA mismatched hematopoietic stem cells. *J. Exp. Med.* 179:493–502.

Bakkaloglu, B., Anlar, A.B., Anlar, F.Y., Oktem, F., Pehlivantürk, B., Unal, F., Ozbesler, C., and Gökler, B. 2007. Atopic features in early childhood autism. *Eur. J. Paediatr. Neurol.* 12:476–479.

Bashir, M.E., Louie, S., Shi, H.N., and Nagler-Anderson, C. 2004. Toll-like receptor 4 signaling by intestinal microbes influences susceptibility to food allergy. *J. Immunol.* 172:6978–6987.

Batten, M., Li, J., Yi, S., Kljavin, N.M., Danilenko, D.M., Lucas, S., Lee, J., de Sauvage, F.J., and Ghilardi, N. 2006. Interleukin 27 limits autoimmune encephalomyelitis by suppressing the development of interleukin 17-producing T cells. *Nat. Immunol.* 7:929–936.

Benlounes, N., Candalh, C., Matarazzo, P., Dupont, C., and Heyman, M. 1999. The time-course of milk antigen-induced TNF-alpha secretion differs according to the clinical symptoms in children with cow's milk allergy. *J. Allergy Clin. Immunol.* 104:863–869.

Bettelli, E., Korn, T., and Kuchroo, V.K. 2007. Th17: The third member of the effector T cell trilogy. *Curr. Opin. Immunol.* 19:652–657.

Blotta, M.H., DeKruyff, R.H., and Umetsu, D.T. 1997. Corticosteroids inhibit IL-12 production in human monocytes and enhance their capacity to induce IL-4 synthesis in CD4[+] lymphocytes. *J. Immunol.* 158:5589–5595.

Bode, L., Salvestrini, C., Park, P.W., Li, J.P., Esko, J.D., Yamaguchi, Y., Murch, S., and Freeze, H.H. 2008. Heparan sulfate and syndecan-1 are essential in maintaining murine and human intestinal epithelial barrier function. *J. Clin. Invest.* 118:229–238.

Burgess, N.K., Sweeten, T.L., McMahon, W.M., and Fujinami, R.S. 2006. Hyperserotoninemia and altered immunity in autism. *J. Autism Dev. Disord.* 36:697–704.

Caramalho, I., Lopes-Carvalho, T., Ostler, D., Zelenay, S., Haury, M., and Demengeot, J. 2003. Regulatory T cells selectively express toll-like receptors and are activated by lipopolysaccharide. *J. Exp. Med.* 197:403–411.

Chatila, T.A. 2005. Role of regulatory T cells in human diseases. *J. Allergy Clin. Immunol.* 116:949–959.

Chatila, T.A., Li, N., Garcia-Lloret, M., Kim, H.J., and Nel, A.E. 2008. T-cell effector pathways in allergic diseases: Transcriptional mechanisms and therapeutic targets. *J. Allergy Clin. Immunol.* 121:812–823.

Chauhan, A. and Chauhan, V. 2006. Oxidative stress in autism. *Pathophysiology* 13:171–181.

Chauhan, A., Chauhan, V., Brown, W.T., and Cohen, I. 2004. Oxidative stress in autism: Increased lipid peroxidation and reduced serum levels of ceruloplasmin and transferrin—the antioxidant proteins. *Life Sci.* 75:2539–2549.

Cheslack-Postava, K., Fallin, M.D., Avramopoulos, D., Connors, S.L., Zimmerman, A.W., Eberhart, C.G., and Newschaffer, C.J. 2007. Beta2-Adrenergic receptor gene variants and risk for autism in the AGRE cohort. *Mol. Psychiatry* 12:283–291.

Chez, M.G., Dowling, T., Patel, P.B., Khanna, P., and Kominsky, M. 2007. Elevation of tumor necrosis factor-alpha in cerebrospinal fluid of autistic children. *Pediatr. Neurol.* 36:361–365.

Connors, S.L., Matteson, K.J., Sega, G.A., Lozzio, C.B., Carroll, R.C., and Zimmerman, A.W. 2006. Plasma serotonin in autism. *Pediatr. Neurol.* 35:182–186.

Coombes, J.L., Siddiqui, K.R., Arancibia-Carcamo, C.V., Hall, J., Sun, C.M., Belkaid, Y., and Powrie, F. 2007. A functionally specialized population of mucosal CD103⁺ DCs induces Foxp3⁺ regulatory T cells via a TGF-beta and retinoic acid-dependent mechanism. *J. Exp. Med.* 204:1757–1764.

Corbett, B.A., Mendoza, S., Wegelin, J.A., Carmean, V., and Levine, S. 2008. Variable cortisol circadian rhythms in children with autism and anticipatory stress. *J. Psychiatry Neurosci.* 33:227–234.

Crack, P.J. and Bray, P.J. 2007. Toll-like receptors in the brain and their potential roles in neuropathology. *Immunol. Cell. Biol.* 85:476–480.

Croen, L.A., Braunschweig, D., Haapanen, L., Yoshida, C.K., Fireman, B., Grether, J.K., Kharrazi, M., Hansen, R.L., Ashwood, P., and Van de Water, J. 2008. Maternal mid-pregnancy autoantibodies to fetal brain protein: The early markers for autism study. *Biol. Psychiatry* 64:583–588.

Dai, D., Nanthkumar, N.N., Newburg, D.S., and Walker, W.A. 2000. Role of oligosaccharides and glycoconjugates in intestinal host defense. *J. Pediatr. Gastroenterol. Nutr.* 30(Suppl. 2):S23–S33.

Davoust, N., Vuaillat, C., Androdias, G., and Nataf, S. 2008. From bone marrow to microglia: Barriers and avenues. *Trends Immunol.* 29:227–234.

de Jonge, W.J. and Ulloa, L. 2007. The alpha7 nicotinic acetylcholine receptor as a pharmacological target for inflammation. *Br. J. Pharmacol.* 151:915–929.

de Vries, E., de Bruin-Versteeg, S., Comans-Bitter, W.M., de Groot, R., Hop, W.C., Boerma, G.J., Lotgering, F.K., and van Dongen, J.J. 2000. Longitudinal survey of lymphocyte subpopulations in the first year of life. *Pediatr. Res.* 47:528–537.

Deaglio, S., Dwyer, K.M., Gao, W., Friedman, D., Usheva, A., Erat, A., Chen, J.F., Enjyoji, K., Linden, J., Oukka, M., Kuchroo, V.K., Strom, T.B., and Robson, S.C. 2007. Adenosine generation catalyzed by CD39 and CD73 expressed on regulatory T cells mediates immune suppression. *J. Exp. Med.* 204:1257–1265.

DeFelice, M.L., Ruchelli, E.D., Markowitz, J.E., Strogatz, M., Reddy, K.P., Kadivar, K., Mulberg, A.E., and Brown, K.A. 2003. Intestinal cytokines in children with pervasive developmental disorders. *Am. J. Gastroenterol.* 98:1777–1782.

Denning, T.L., Wang, Y.C., Patel, S.R., Williams, I.R., and Pulendran, B. 2007. Lamina propria macrophages and dendritic cells differentially induce regulatory and interleukin 17-producing T cell responses. *Nat. Immunol.* 8:1086–1094.

Deth, R., Muratore, C., Benzecry, J., Power-Charnitsky, V.A., and Waly, M. 2008. How environmental and genetic factors combine to cause autism: A redox/methylation hypothesis. *Neurotoxicology* 29:190–201.

Di Cristo, G. 2007. Development of cortical GABAergic circuits and its implications for neurodevelopmental disorders. *Clin. Genet.* 72:1–8.

Djukic, M., Mildner, A., Schmidt, H., Czesnik, D., Bruck, W., Priller, J., Nau, R., and Prinz, M. 2006. Circulating monocytes engraft in the brain, differentiate into microglia and contribute to the pathology following meningitis in mice. *Brain* 129:2394–2403.

Dupont, C. and Heyman, M. 2000. Food protein-induced enterocolitis syndrome: Laboratory perspectives. *J. Pediatr. Gastroenterol. Nutr.* 30:S50–S57.

Elder, J.H., Shankar, M., Shuster, J., Theriaque, D., Burns, S., and Sherrill, L. 2006. The gluten-free, casein-free diet in autism: Results of a preliminary double blind clinical trial. *J. Autism Dev. Disord.* 36:413–420.

Elenkov, I.J. 2008. Neurohormonal-cytokine interactions: Implications for inflammation, common human diseases and well-being. *Neurochem. Int.* 52:40–51.

Enstrom, A., Onore, C., Hertz-Picciotto, I., Hansen, R., Croen, L., Van de Water, J., and Ashwood, P. 2008. Detection of IL-17 and IL-23 in plasma samples of children with autism. *Am. J. Biochem. Biotechnol.* (*Special Issue on Autism Spectrum Disorders*) 4:114–120.

Fatemi, S.H., Reutiman, T.J., Folsom, T.D., Huang, H., Oishi, K., Mori, S., Smee, D.F., Pearce, D.A., Winter, C., Sohr, R., and Luckel, G. 2008. Maternal infection leads to abnormal gene regulation and brain atrophy in mouse offspring: implications for genesis of neurodevelopmental disorders. *Schizophr. Res.* 99:56–70.

Fein, D., Dixon, P., Paul, J., and Levin, H. 2005. Brief report: Pervasive developmental disorder can evolve into ADHD: Case illustrations. *J. Autism Dev. Disord.* 35:525–534.

Finegold, S.M., Molitoris, D., Song, Y., Liu, C., Vaisanen, M.L., Bolte, E., McTeague, M., Sandler, R., Wexler, H., Marlowe, E.M., Collins, M.D., Lawson, P.A., Summanen, P., Baysallar, M., Tomzynski, T.J., Read, E., Johnson, E., Rolfe, R., Nasin, P., Shah, H., Haake, D.A., Manning, P., and Kaul, A. 2002. Gastrointestinal microflora studies in late-onset autism. *Clin. Infect. Dis.* 35:S6–S16.

Franchi, L., McDonald, C., Kanneganti, T.D., Amer, A., and Nunez, G. 2006. Nucleotide-binding oligomerization domain-like receptors: Intracellular pattern recognition molecules for pathogen detection and host defense. *J. Immunol.* 177:3507–3513.

Franco, R., Pacheco, R., Lluis, C., Ahern, G.P., and O'Connell, P.J. 2007. The emergence of neurotransmitters as immune modulators. *Trends Immunol.* 28:400–407.

Fu, Y.X. and Chaplin, D.D. 1999. Development and maturation of secondary lymphoid tissues. *Annu. Rev. Immunol.* 17:399–433.

Furlano, R.I., Anthony, A., Day, R., Brown, A., McGarvey, L., Thomson, M.A., Davies, S.E., Berelowitz, M., Forbes, A., Wakefield, A.J., Malker-Smith, J.A., and Murch, S.H. 2001. Colonic CD8 and gamma delta T-cell infiltration with epithelial damage in children with autism. *J. Pediatr.* 138:366–372.

Gladkevich, A., Korf, J., Hakobyan, V.P., and Melkonyan, K.V. 2006. The peripheral GABAergic system as a target in endocrine disorders. *Auton. Neurosci.* 124:1–8.

Glezer, I., Lapointe, A., and Rivest, S. 2006. Innate immunity triggers oligodendrocyte progenitor reactivity and confines damages to brain injuries. *FASEB J.* 20:750–752.

Glezer, I., Simard, A.R., and Rivest, S. 2007. Neuroprotective role of the innate immune system by microglia. *Neuroscience* 147:867–883.

Goeb, J.L., Even, C., Nicolas, G., Gohier, B., Dubas, F., and Garre, J.B. 2006. Psychiatric side effects of interferon-beta in multiple sclerosis. *Eur. Psychiatry* 21:186–193.

Goncharova, L.B. and Tarakanov, A.O. 2007. Molecular networks of brain and immunity. *Brain Res. Rev.* 55:155–166.

Gosselin, D. and Rivest, S. 2007. Role of IL-1 and TNF in the brain: Twenty years of progress on a Dr. Jekyll/Mr. Hyde duality of the innate immune system. *Brain Behav. Immun.* 21:281–289.

Gregg, J.P., Lit, L., Baron, C.A., Hertz-Picciotto, I., Walker, W., Davis, R.A., Croen, L.A., Ozonoff, S., Hansen, R., Pessah, I.N., and Sharp F.R. 2008. Gene expression changes in children with autism. *Genomics* 91:22–29.

Gupta, S., Aggarwal, S., Rashanravan, B., and Lee, T. 1998. Th1- and Th2-like cytokines in $CD4^+$ and $CD8^+$ T cells in autism. *J. Neuroimmunol.* 85:106–109.

Haddad, J.J. 2008. On the mechanisms and putative pathways involving neuroimmune interactions. *Biochem. Biophys. Res. Commun.* 370:531–535.

Harrington, L.E., Hatton, R.D., Mangan, P.R., Turner, H., Murphy, T.L., Murphy, K.M., and Weaver, C.T. 2005. Interleukin 17-producing $CD4^+$ effector T cells develop via a lineage distinct from the T helper type 1 and 2 lineages. *Nat. Immunol.* 6:1123–1132.

Hausmann, M., Kiessling, S., Mestermann, S., Webb, G., Spottl, T., Andus, T., Scholmerich, J., Herfarth, H., Ray, K., Falk, W., and Rogler, G. 2002. Toll-like receptors 2 and 4 are up-regulated during intestinal inflammation. *Gastroenterology* 122:1987–2000.

Hornef, M.W., Frisan, T., Vandewalle, A., Normark, S., and Richter-Dahlfors, A. 2002. Toll-like receptor 4 resides in the Golgi apparatus and colocalizes with internalized lipopolysaccharide in intestinal epithelial cells. *J. Exp. Med.* 195:559–570.

Hornef, M.W., Normark, B.H., Vandewalle, A., and Normark, S. 2003. Intracellular recognition of lipopolysaccharide by toll-like receptor 4 in intestinal epithelial cells. *J. Exp. Med.* 198:1225–1235.

Horvath, K., Papadimitriou, J.C., Rabsztyn, A., Drachenberg, C., and Tildon, J.T. 1999. Gastrointestinal abnormalities in children with autistic disorder. *J. Pediatr.* 135:559–563.

Inohara, N., Ogura, Y., Fontalba, A., Gutierrez, O., Pons, F., Crespo, J., Fukase, K., Inamura, S., Kusumoto, S., Hashimoto, M., Foster, S.L, Moran A.P., Fernandez-Luna, J.L., and Nurez, G. 2003. Host recognition of bacterial muramyl dipeptide mediated through NOD2. Implications for Crohn's disease. *J. Biol. Chem.* 278:5509–5512.

Iwata, M., Hirakiyama, A., Eshima, Y., Kagechika, H., Kato, C., and Song, S.Y. 2004. Retinoic acid imprints gut-homing specificity on T cells. *Immunity* 21:527–538.

James, S.J., Melnyk, S., Jernigan, S., Cleves, M.A., Halsted, C.H., Wong, D.H., Cutler, P., Bock, K., Boris, M., Bradstreet, J.J., Baker, S.M., and Gaylor D.W. 2006. Metabolic endophenotype and related genotypes are associated with oxidative stress in children with autism. *Am. J. Med. Genet. B Neuropsychiatr. Genet.* 141B:947–956.

Jyonouchi H, Geng, L., Ruby, A., and Reddy, C. 2007. Suboptimal responses to dietary intervention in children with autism spectrum disorders and non-IgE mediated food allergy. In *Autism Research Advances*, ed. L. B. Zhao, pp. 169–184. Nova Science Publishers, Inc, Hauppauge, NY.

Jyonouchi, H., Geng, L., Ruby, A., Reddy, C., and Zimmerman-Bier, B. 2005a. Evaluation of an association between gastrointestinal symptoms and cytokine production against common dietary proteins in children with autism spectrum disorders. *J. Pediatr.* 146:605–610.

Jyonouchi, H., Geng, L., Ruby, A., and Zimmerman-Bier, B. 2005b. Dysregulated innate immune responses in young children with autism spectrum disorders: Their relationship to gastrointestinal symptoms and dietary intervention. *Neuropsychobiology* 51:77–85.

Jyonouchi, H., Sun, S., and Itokazu, N. 2002. Innate immunity associated with inflammatory responses and cytokine production against common dietary proteins in patients with autism spectrum disorder. *Neuropsychobiology* 46:76–84.

Kang, S.G., Lim, H.W., Andrisani, O.M., Broxmeyer, H.E., and Kim, C.H. 2007. Vitamin A metabolites induce gut-homing FoxP3+ regulatory T cells. *J. Immunol.* 179:3724–3733.

Karlsson, M.R., Rugtveit, J., and Brandtzaeg, P. 2004. Allergen-responsive CD4+ CD25+ regulatory T cells in children who have outgrown cow's milk allergy. *J. Exp. Med.* 199:1679–1688.

Kelley, E., Paul, J.J., Fein, D., and Naigles, L.R. 2006. Residual language deficits in optimal outcome children with a history of autism. *J. Autism Dev. Disord.* 36:807–828.

Kelly, D., Campbell, J.I., King, T.P., Grant, G., Jansson, E.A., Coutts, A.G., Pettersson, S., and Conway, S. 2004. Commensal anaerobic gut bacteria attenuate inflammation by regulating nuclear-cytoplasmic shuttling of PPAR-gamma and RelA. *Nat. Immunol.* 5:104–112.

Kelly, D., Conway, S., and Aminov, R. 2005. Commensal gut bacteria: Mechanisms of immune modulation. *Trends Immunol.* 26:326–333.

Kleinman, J.M., Ventola, P.E., Pandey, J., Verbalis, A.D., Barton, M., Hodgson, S., Green, J., Dumont-Mathieu, T., Robins, D.L., and Fein, D. 2008. Diagnostic stability in very young children with autism spectrum disorders. *J. Autism Dev. Disord.* 38:606–615.

Knivsberg, A.M., Reichelt, K.L., Hoien, T., and Nodland, M. 2002. A randomised, controlled study of dietary intervention in autistic syndromes. *Nutr. Neurosci.* 5:251–261.

Kohm, A.P., McMahon, J.S., Podojil, J.R., Begolka, W.S., DeGutes, M., Kasprowicz, D.J., Ziegler, S.F., and Miller, S.D. 2006. Cutting edge: Anti-CD25 monoclonal antibody injection results in the functional inactivation, not depletion, of CD4$^+$ CD25$^+$ T regulatory cells. *J. Immunol.* 176:3301–3305.

Korn, T., Reddy, J., Gao, W., Bettelli, E., Awasthi, A., Petersen, T.R., Backstrom, B.T., Sobel, R.A., Wucherpfennig, K.W., Strom, T.B., Oukka M., and Kuchroo V.K. 2007. Myelin-specific regulatory T cells accumulate in the CNS but fail to control autoimmune inflammation. *Nat. Med.* 13:423–431.

Laflamme, N. and Rivest, S. 2001. Toll-like receptor 4: The missing link of the cerebral innate immune response triggered by circulating gram-negative bacterial cell wall components. *FASEB J.* 15:155–163.

Lainhart, J.E., Ozonoff, S., Coon, H., Krasny, L., Dinh, E., Nice, J., and McMahon, W. 2002. Autism, regression, and the broader autism phenotype. *Am. J. Med. Genet.* 113:231–237.

Lala, S., Ogura, Y., Osborne, C., Hor, S.Y., Bromfield, A., Davies, S., Ogunbiyi, O., Nunez, G., and Keshav, S. 2003. Crohn's disease and the NOD2 gene: A role for paneth cells. *Gastroenterology* 125:47–57.

Lee, J., Gonzales-Navajas, J.M., and Raz, E. 2008. The "polarizing-tolerizing" mechanism of intestinal epithelium: Its relevance to colonic homeostasis. *Semin. Immunopathol.* 30:3–9.

Lee, J., Mo, J.H., Shen, C., Rucker, A.N., and Raz, E. 2007. Toll-like receptor signaling in intestinal epithelial cells contributes to colonic homoeostasis. *Curr. Opin. Gastroenterol.* 23, 27–31.

Levy, S.E. and Hyman, S.L. 2005. Novel treatments for autistic spectrum disorders. *Ment. Retard. Dev. Disabil. Res. Rev.* 11:131–142.

Liu, Y., Teige, I., Birnir, B., and Issazadeh-Navikas, S. 2006. Neuron-mediated generation of regulatory T cells from encephalitogenic T cells suppresses EAE. *Nat. Med.* 12:518–525.

Lu, L.F., Lind, E.F., Gondek, D.C., Bennett, K.A., Gleeson, M.W., Pino-Lagos, K., Scott, Z.A., Coyle, A.J., Reed, J.L., and Van Snick, J. 2006. Mast cells are essential intermediaries in regulatory T-cell tolerance. *Nature* 442:997–1002.

Lubick, K., Radke, M., and Jutila, M. 2007. Securinine, a GABAA receptor antagonist, enhances macrophage clearance of phase II C. burnetii: Comparison with TLR agonists. *J. Leukoc. Biol.* 82:1062–1069.

Manel, N., Unutmaz, D., and Littman, D.R. 2008. The differentiation of human T(H)-17 cells requires transforming growth factor-beta and induction of the nuclear receptor RORgammat. *Nat. Immunol.* 9:641–649.

Marin-Teva, J.L., Dusart, I., Colin, C., Gervais, A., van Rooijen, N., and Mallat, M. (2004). Microglia promote the death of developing Purkinje cells. *Neuron* 41:535–547.

Martin-Ruiz, C.M., Lee, M., Perry, R.H., Baumann, M., Court, J.A., and Perry, E.K. 2004. Molecular analysis of nicotinic receptor expression in autism. *Brain Res. Mol. Brain Res.* 123:81–90.

McGeachy, M.J. and Cua, D.J. 2008. Th17 cell differentiation: The long and winding road. *Immunity* 28:445–453.

Meyer, U., Nyffeler, M., Schwendener, S., Knuesel, I., Yee, B.K., and Feldon, J. 2008a. Relative prenatal and postnatal maternal contributions to schizophrenia-related neurochemical dysfunction after in utero immune challenge. *Neuropsychopharmacology* 33:441–456.

Meyer, U., Nyffeler, M., Yee, B.K., Knuesel, I., and Feldon, J. 2008b. Adult brain and behavioral pathological markers of prenatal immune challenge during early/middle and late fetal development in mice. *Brain Behav. Immun.* 22:469–486.

Meylan, E., Tschopp, J., and Karin, M. 2006. Intracellular pattern recognition receptors in the host response. *Nature* 442:39–44.

Molloy, C.A., Morrow, A.L., Meinzen-Derr, J., Schleifer, K., Dienger, K., Manning-Courtney, P., Altaye, M., and Wills-Karp, M. 2006. Elevated cytokine levels in children with autism spectrum disorder. *J. Neuroimmunol.* 172:198–205.

Mouridsen, S.E., Rich, B., Isager, T., and Nedergaard, N.J. 2007. Autoimmune diseases in parents of children with infantile autism: A case-control study. *Dev. Med. Child Neurol.* 49:429–432.

Mucida, D., Park, Y., Kim, G., Turovskaya, O., Scott, I., Kronenberg, M., and Cheroutre, H. 2007. Reciprocal TH17 and regulatory T cell differentiation mediated by retinoic acid. *Science* 317:256–260.

Murch, S.H., Winyard, P.J., Koletzko, S., Wehner, B., Cheema, H.A., Risdon, R.A., Phillips, A.D., Meadows, N., Klein, N.J., and Walker-Smith, J.A. 1996. Congenital enterocyte heparan sulphate deficiency with massive albumin loss, secretory diarrhoea, and malnutrition. *Lancet* 347:1299–1301.

Neish, A.S., Gewirtz, A.T., Zeng, H., Young, A.N., Hobert, M.E., Karmali, V., Rao, A.S., and Madara, J.L. 2000. Prokaryotic regulation of epithelial responses by inhibition of IkappaB-alpha ubiquitination. *Science* 289:1560–1563.

Ni, L., Acevedo, G., Muralidharan, B., Padala, N., To, J., and Jonakait, G.M. 2007. Toll-like receptor ligands and CD154 stimulate microglia to produce a factor(s) that promotes excess cholinergic differentiation in the developing rat basal forebrain: Implications for neurodevelopmental disorders. *Pediatr. Res.* 61:15–20.

O'Connor, R.A. and Anderton, S.M. 2008. Foxp3+ regulatory T cells in the control of experimental CNS autoimmune disease. *J. Neuroimmunol.* 193:1–11.

O'Connor, R.A., Malpass, K.H., and Anderton, S.M. 2007. The inflamed central nervous system drives the activation and rapid proliferation of Foxp3+ regulatory T cells. *J. Immunol.* 179:958–966.

Ogura, Y., Bonen, D.K., Inohara, N., Nicolae, D.L., Chen, F.F., Ramos, R., Britton, H., Moran, T., Karaliuskas, R., Duerr, R.H., Achkar, J.P., Brant, S.P., Hanauer, S.P., Nunez, G., and Cho, J.H. 2001. A frameshift mutation in NOD2 associated with susceptibility to Crohn's disease. *Nature* 411:603–606.

Oliveira, G., Ataide, A., Marques, C., Miguel, T.S., Coutinho, A.M., Mota-Vieira, L., Goncalves, E., Lopes, N.M., Rodrigues, V., Carmona da Mota, H., and Vincente, A.M. 2007. Epidemiology of autism spectrum disorder in Portugal: Prevalence, clinical characterization, and medical conditions. *Dev. Med. Child Neurol.* 49:726–733.

Olson, J.K. and Miller, S.D. 2004. Microglia initiate central nervous system innate and adaptive immune responses through multiple TLRs. *J. Immunol.* 173:3916–3924.

Otte, J.M., Cario, E., and Podolsky, D.K. 2004. Mechanisms of cross hyporesponsiveness to Toll-like receptor bacterial ligands in intestinal epithelial cells. *Gastroenterology* 126:1054–1070.

Pardo, C.A. and Eberhart, C.G. 2007. The neurobiology of autism. *Brain Pathol.* 17:434–447.

Pardo, C.A., Vargas, D.L., and Zimmerman, A.W. 2005. Immunity, neuroglia and neuroinflammation in autism. *Int. Rev. Psychiatry* 17:485–495.

Parracho, H.M., Bingham, M.O., Gibson, G.R., and McCartney, A.L. 2005. Differences between the gut microflora of children with autistic spectrum disorders and that of healthy children. *J. Med. Microbiol.* 54:987–991.

Pessah, I.N., Seegal, R.F., Lein, P.J., LaSalle, J., Yee, B.K., Van De Water, J., and Berman, R.F. 2008. Immunologic and neurodevelopmental susceptibilities of autism. *Neurotoxicology* 29:532–545.

Pickering, M. and O'Connor, J.J. 2007. Pro-inflammatory cytokines and their effects in the dentate gyrus. *Prog. Brain Res.* 163:339–354.

Poling, J.S., Frye, R.E., Shoffner, J., and Zimmerman, A.W. 2006. Developmental regression and mitochondrial dysfunction in a child with autism. *J. Child Neurol.* 21:170–172.

Porter, E.M., Bevins, C.L., Ghosh, D., and Ganz, T. 2002. The multifaceted Paneth cell. *Cell. Mol. Life Sci.* 59:156–170.

Raju, R., Rakocevic, G., Chen, Z., Hoehn, G., Semino-Mora, C., Shi, W., Olsen, R., and Dalakas, M.C. 2006. Autoimmunity to GABAA-receptor-associated protein in stiff-person syndrome. *Brain* 129:3270–3276.

Robertson, M.A., Sigalet, D.L., Holst, J.J., Meddings, J.B., Wood, J., and Sharkey, K.A. 2008. Intestinal permeability and glucagon-like peptide-2 in children with autism: A controlled pilot study. *J. Autism Dev. Disord.* 38:1066–1071.

Rodriguez, M., Alvarez-Erviti, L., Blesa, F.J., Rodriguez-Oroz, M.C., Arina, A., Melero, I., Ramos, L.I., and Obeso, J.A. 2007. Bone-marrow-derived cell differentiation into microglia: A study in a progressive mouse model of Parkinson's disease. *Neurobiol. Dis.* 28:316–325.

Rodriguez-Bores, L., Fonseca, G.C., Villeda, M.A., and Yamamoto-Furusho, J.K. 2007. Novel genetic markers in inflammatory bowel disease. *World J. Gastroenterol.* 13:5560–5570.

Rosenstiel, P., Fantini, M., Brautigam, K., Kuhbacher, T., Waetzig, G.H., Seegert, D., and Schreiber, S. 2003. TNF-alpha and IFN-gamma regulate the expression of the NOD2 (CARD15) gene in human intestinal epithelial cells. *Gastroenterology* 124:1001–1009.

Roumier, A., Bechade, C., Poncer, J.C., Smalla, K.H., Tomasello, E., Vivier, E., Gundelfinger, E.D., Triller, A., and Bessis, A. 2004. Impaired synaptic function in the microglial KARAP/DAP12-deficient mouse. *J. Neurosci.* 24:11421–11428.

Sajdel-Sulkowska, E.M., Lipinski, L.B., Windom, H., Audhya, T., and McGinnis, W. 2008. Oxidative stress in autism: Elevated cerebellar 3-nitrotyrosine levels. *Am. J. Biochem. Biotechnol. (Special Issue on Autism Spectrum Disorders)* 4:73–84.

Sandler, R.H., Finegold, S.M., Bolte, E.R., Buchanan, C.P., Maxwell, A.P., Vaisanen, M.L., Nelson, M.N., and Wexler, H.M. 2000. Short-term benefit from oral vancomycin treatment of regressive-onset autism. *J. Child Neurol.* 15:429–435.

Schmidt-Weber, C.B., Akdis, M., and Akdis, C.A. 2007. TH17 cells in the big picture of immunology. *J. Allergy Clin. Immunol.* 120:247–254.

Shimizu, H., Watanabe, E., Hiyama, T.Y., Nagakura, A., Fujikawa, A., Okado, H., Yanagawa, Y., Obata, K., and Noda, M. 2007. Glial Nax channels control lactate signaling to neurons for brain [Na⁺] sensing. *Neuron* 54:59–72.

Shultz, S.R., MacFabe, D.F., Ossenkopp, K.P., Scratch, S., Whelan, J., Taylor, R., and Cain, D.P. 2008. Intracerebroventricular injection of propionic acid, an enteric bacterial metabolic end-product, impairs social behavior in the rat: Implications for an animal model of autism. *Neuropharmacology* 54:901–911.

Simard, A.R., Soulet, D., Gowing, G., Julien, J.P., and Rivest, S. 2006. Bone marrow-derived microglia play a critical role in restricting senile plaque formation in Alzheimer's disease. *Neuron* 49:489–502.

Singer, H.S., Morris, C.M., Gause, C.D., Gillin, P.K., Crawford, S., and Zimmerman, A.W. 2008. Antibodies against fetal brain in sera of mothers with autistic children. *J. Neuroimmunol.* 194:165–172.

Singer, H.S., Morris, C.M., Williams, P.N., Yoon, D.Y., Hong, J.J., and Zimmerman, A.W. 2006. Antibrain antibodies in children with autism and their unaffected siblings. *J. Neuroimmunol.* 178:149–155.

Sitkovsky, M., Lukashev, D., Deaglio, S., Dwyer, K., Robson, S.C., and Ohta, A. 2008. Adenosine A2A receptor antagonists: Blockade of adenosinergic effects and T regulatory cells. *Br. J. Pharmacol.* 153(Suppl. 1):S457–S464.

Smith, D.W. and Nagler-Anderson, C. 2005. Preventing intolerance: The induction of non-responsiveness to dietary and microbial antigens in the intestinal mucosa. *J. Immunol.* 174:3851–3857.

Smith, P.D., Smythies, L.E., Mosteller-Barnum, M., Sibley, D.A., Russell, M.W., Merger, M., Sellers, M.T., Orenstein, J.M., Shimada, T., Graham, M.F., and Kubagawa, H. 2001. Intestinal macrophages lack CD14 and CD89 and consequently are down-regulated for LPS- and IgA-mediated activities. *J. Immunol.* 167:2651–2656.

Smith, S.E., Li, J., Garbett, K., Mirnics, K., and Patterson, P.H. 2007. Maternal immune activation alters fetal brain development through interleukin-6. *J. Neurosci.* 27:10695–10702.

Splawski, I., Timothy, K.W., Sharpe, L.M., Decher, N., Kumar, P., Bloise, R., Napolitano, C., Schwartz, P.J., Joseph, R.M., Condouris, K., Tager-Flusberg, H., Driori, S.G., Sanguinetti, M.D., and Keating, M.T. 2004. Ca(V)1.2 calcium channel dysfunction causes a multi-system disorder including arrhythmia and autism. *Cell* 119:19–31.

Streit, W.J., Walter, S.A., and Pennell, N.A. 1999. Reactive microgliosis. *Prog. Neurobiol.* 57:563–581.

Stumhofer, J.S., Laurence, A., Wilson, E.H., Huang, E., Tato, C.M., Johnson, L.M., Villarino, A.V., Huang, Q., Yoshimura, A., Sehy, D., Saris, C.J., O'Shea, J.J., Henninghausen, L., Ernst, M., and Hunter, C.A. 2006. Interleukin 27 negatively regulates the development of inter-leukin 17-producing T helper cells during chronic inflammation of the central nervous system. *Nat. Immunol.* 7:937–945.

Sun, C.M., Hall, J.A., Blank, R.B., Bouladoux, N., Oukka, M., Mora, J.R., and Belkaid, Y. 2007. Small intestine lamina propria dendritic cells promote de novo generation of Foxp3 T reg cells via retinoic acid. *J. Exp. Med.* 204:1775–1785.

Sutera, S., Pandey, J., Esser, E.L., Rosenthal, M.A., Wilson, L.B., Barton, M., Green, J., Hodgson, S., Robins, D.L., Dumont-Mathieu, T., and Fein, D. 2007. Predictors of optimal outcome in toddlers diagnosed with autism spectrum disorders. *J. Autism Dev. Disord.* 37:98–107.

Sweeten, T.L., Bowyer, S.L., Posey, D.J., Halberstadt, G.M., and McDougle, C.J. 2003a. Increased prevalence of familial autoimmunity in probands with pervasive developmen-tal disorders. *Pediatrics* 112:e420.

Sweeten, T.L., Posey, D.J., and McDougle, C.J. 2003b. High blood monocyte counts and neop-terin levels in children with autistic disorder. *Am. J Psychiatry* 160:1691–1693.

Sweeten, T.L., Posey, D.J., Shankar, S., and McDougle, C.J. 2004. High nitric oxide pro-duction in autistic disorder: A possible role for interferon-gamma. *Biol. Psychiatry* 55:434–437.

Teitelbaum, J.E. and Allan Walker, W. 2005. The development of mucosal immunity. *Eur. J. Gastroenterol. Hepatol.* 17:1273–1278.

Thompson, W.W., Price, C., Goodson, B., Shay, D.K., Benson, P., Hinrichsen, V.L., Lewis, E., Eriksen, E., Ray, P., Marcy, S.M., Dunn, J., Jackson, L.A., Lieu, T.A., Black, S., Weintraub, E.S., Davis, R.L., and DeStefano, F. 2007. Early thimerosal exposure and neuropsychological outcomes at 7 to 10 years. *N. Engl. J. Med.* 357:1281–1292.

Tochigi, M., Kato, C., Koishi, S., Kawakubo, Y., Yamamoto, K., Matsumoto, H., Hashimoto, O., Kim, S.Y., Watanabe, K., Kano, Y., Nanba, E., Kato, N., and Sasaki, T. 2007. No evidence for significant association between GABA receptor genes in chromosome 15q11-q13 and autism in a Japanese population. *J. Hum. Genet.* 52:985–989.

Torgerson, T.R. and Ochs, H.D. 2007. Immune dysregulation, polyendocrinopathy, enteropathy, X-linked: Forkhead box protein 3 mutations and lack of regulatory T cells. *J. Allergy Clin. Immunol.* 120:744–750.

Torrente, F., Ashwood, P., Day, R., Machado, N., Furlano, R.I., Anthony, A., Davies, S.E., Wakefield, A.J., Thomson, M.A., Walker-Smith, J.A., and Murch, S.H. 2002. Small intestinal enteropathy with epithelial IgG and complement deposition in children with regressive autism. *Mol. Psychiatry* 7:375–382.

Vargas, D.L., Nascimbene, C., Krishnan, C., Zimmerman, A.W., and Pardo, C.A. 2005. Neuroglial activation and neuroinflammation in the brain of patients with autism. *Ann. Neurol.* 57:67–81.

Venken, K., Hellings, N., Broekmans, T., Hensen, K., Rummens, J.L., and Stinissen, P. 2008. Natural naive CD4+ CD25+ CD127low regulatory T cell (Treg) development and func-tion are disturbed in multiple sclerosis patients: recovery of memory Treg homeostasis during disease progression. *J. Immunol.* 180:6411–6420.

Vesce, S., Rossi, D., Brambilla, L., and Volterra, A. 2007. Glutamate release from astrocytes in physiological conditions and in neurodegenerative disorders characterized by neuroin-flammation. *Int. Rev. Neurobiol.* 82:57–71.

Vincent, J.B., Horike, S.I., Choufani, S., Paterson, A.D., Roberts, W., Szatmari, P., Weksberg, R., Fernandez, B., and Scherer, S.W. 2006. An inversion inv(4)(p12-p15.3) in autistic siblings implicates the 4p GABA receptor gene cluster. *J. Med. Genet.* 43:429–434.

Wakefield, A.J., Anthony, A., Murch, S.H., Thomson, M., Montgomery, S.M., Davies, S., O'Leary, J.J., Berelowitz, M., and Walker-Smith, J.A. 2000. Enterocolitis in children with developmental disorders. *Am. J. Gastroenterol.* 95:2285–2295.

Wakefield, A.J., Ashwood, P., Limb, K., and Anthony, A. 2005. The significance of ileo-colonic lymphoid nodular hyperplasia in children with autistic spectrum disorder. *Eur. J. Gastroenterol. Hepatol.* 17:827–836.

Wannemuehler, M.J., Kiyono, H., Babb, J.L., Michalek, S.M., and McGhee, J.R. 1982. Lipopolysaccharide (LPS) regulation of the immune response: LPS converts germfree mice to sensitivity to oral tolerance induction. *J. Immunol.* 129:959–965.

Wark, P.A., Johnston, S.L., Bucchieri, F., Powell, R., Puddicombe, S., Laza-Stanca, V., Holgate, S.T., and Davies, D.E. 2005. Asthmatic bronchial epithelial cells have a deficient innate immune response to infection with rhinovirus. *J. Exp. Med.* 201:937–947.

Wershil, B.K. and Furuta, G.T. 2008. Gastrointestinal mucosal immunity. *J. Allergy Clin. Immunol.* 121:S380–S383.

Westphal, V., Murch, S., Kim, S., Srikrishna, G., Winchester, B., Day, R., and Freeze, H.H. 2000. Reduced heparan sulfate accumulation in enterocytes contributes to protein-losing enteropathy in a congenital disorder of glycosylation. *Am. J. Pathol.* 157: 1917–1925.

White, J.F. 2003. Intestinal pathophysiology in autism. *Exp. Biol. Med. (Maywood)* 228:639–649.

Wildin, R.S., Ramsdell, F., Peake, J., Faravelli, F., Casanova, J.L., Buist, N., Levy-Lahad, E., Mazzella, M., Goulet, O., Perroni, L., Bricarelli, F.D., Byrne, G., McRuen, M., Proll, S., Appleby, H., and Brunkow, M.E. 2001. X-linked neonatal diabetes mellitus, enteropathy and endocrinopathy syndrome is the human equivalent of mouse scurfy. *Nat. Genet.* 27:18–20.

Winter, C., Reutiman, T.J., Folsom, T.D., Sohr, R., Wolf, R.J., Juckel, G., and Fatemi, S.H. 2008. Dopamine and serotonin levels following prenatal viral infection in mouse-Implications for psychiatric disorders such as schizophrenia and autism. *Eur. Neuropsychopharmacol.* 18:712–716.

Zedler, S. and Faist, E. 2006. The impact of endogenous triggers on trauma-associated inflammation. *Curr. Opin. Crit. Care* 12:595–601.

Zerrate, M.C., Pletnikov, M., Connors, S.L., Vargas, D.L., Seidler, F.J., Zimmerman, A.W., Slotkin, T.A., and Pardo, C.A. 2007. Neuroinflammation and behavioral abnormalities after neonatal terbutaline treatment in rats: Implications for autism. *J. Pharmacol. Exp. Ther.* 322:16–22.

Zhu, C.B., Blakely, R.D., and Hewlett, W.A. 2006. The proinflammatory cytokines interleukin-1beta and tumor necrosis factor-alpha activate serotonin transporters. *Neuropsychopharmacology* 31:2121–2131.

Zimmerman, A.W., Connors, S.L., Matteson, K.J., Lee, L.C., Singer, H.S., Castaneda, J.A., and Pearce, D.A. 2007. Maternal antibrain antibodies in autism. *Brain Behav. Immun.* 21:351–357.

Zimmerman, A.W., Jyonouchi, H., Comi, A.M., Connors, S.L., Milstien, S., Varsou, A., and Heyes, M.P. 2005. Cerebrospinal fluid and serum markers of inflammation in autism. *Pediatr. Neurol.* 33:195–201.

Zlokovic, B.V. 2008. The blood-brain barrier in health and chronic neurodegenerative disorders. *Neuron* 57:178–201.

14 Autism, Gastrointestinal Disturbance, and Immune Dysfunction: What Is the Link?

Paul Ashwood,[1,3],* Amanda Enstrom,[1,3] and Judy Van de Water[2,3]

[1]Department of Medical Microbiology and Immunology, [2]Division of Rheumatology, Allergy and Clinical Immunology, Department of Internal Medicine, and [3]M.I.N.D. Institute, University of California at Davis, Davis, CA 95616, USA

CONTENTS

Autism spectrum disorders (ASD) are complex debilitating neurodevelopmental disorders. Despite diagnostic advances and a broader awareness, its causes and underlying pathology remain largely a mystery. Studies have suggested both genetic and environmental components in its etiology, and much attention has been drawn toward a possible role for immune dysfunction. Indications of an increased incidence of chronic gastrointestinal (GI) disturbance in some children with ASD have also generated interest in GI dysfunction as a contributing factor to certain aspects or symptoms and even behavioral characteristics in ASD. Endoscopic, histologic, and

* Corresponding author: Tel.: +1-916-703-0405; fax: +1-916-703-0367 e-mail: pashwood@ucdavis.edu

immunohistochemical analyses of the GI tract in children with ASD who present with GI symptoms have revealed chronic inflammatory changes throughout the gut, including extensive immune cell infiltration of the gut wall and increased pro-inflammatory responses in mucosal T-lymphocyte cells. In addition, some of the changes observed suggest the potential involvement of an autoimmune response that is directed toward the epithelial barrier surrounding the gut lumen. Here, we review evidence supporting a potential role of GI dysfunction in some cases of ASD, the potential link between immune dysfunction and gut inflammation, and the hypotheses regarding the relationship between autistic behaviors and GI-related immune dysfunction.

14.1   INTRODUCTION

Autism, or autistic disorder, is now recognized in the DSM-IV-TR as a heterogeneous syndrome, belonging to a group of neurodevelopmental disorders known as the autism spectrum disorders (ASD) (APA, 2000) that include other specific diagnostic subtypes such as Asperger's disorder and Rett's disorder.

The etiology of autism is largely unknown, although ASD are highly heritable. The evidence for a genetic link came initially from twin studies, where the concordance rate for autism was 60%–90% in monozygotic twins compared with 3%–5% in dizygotic twins (Bailey et al., 1995; Folstein and Rutter, 1977). More recent studies have also produced evidence that twinning is a risk factor for developing autism (Taniai et al., 2008). Betancur, Leboyer, and Gillberg (2002) reported the proportion of twins with autistic sibling pairs was 10%, compared to the expected twinning rate based on the normal population of 2.4%. There is also an indication of fourfold increased autism prevalence among dizygotic twins (Greenberg et al., 2001). Autism has also been associated with single-gene defects such as tuberous sclerosis complex, 15 q duplications, and fragile X syndrome, but these account for only a small percentage of cases (Muhle, Trentacoste, and Rapin, 2004). While these studies yield evidence that there are genes that strongly impact the likelihood of developing autism, no definitive pattern of genes has been identified and a multitude of different and varied candidate genes have been implicated in autism (Muhle, Trentacoste, and Rapin, 2004). Moreover, the replication of these data has been inconsistent, probably due in part to the heterogeneity of the phenotypes within the autism spectrum. However, several studies have linked autism with immune-based genes, such as human leukocyte antigen (HLA)-DRB1*04, interleukin (IL)-4 receptor, and complement C4B null allele (Lee et al., 2006; Torres et al., 2006; Warren et al., 1992, 1995). These data are supported by findings showing the higher prevalence of autoimmune disease in the primary and secondary family members of autistic children when compared to families with no history of autism (Comi et al., 1999; Money, Bobrow, and Clarke, 1971; Mouridsen et al., 2007). These data suggest that alterations in the genes that control the immune system/immune function may act as susceptibility factors for the development of autism. The role of autoimmunity and immune dysfunction in autism is discussed in detail in Section 14.2.1.

It is most likely that the vast majority of the cases of autism are caused by the combination of environmental factors and multiple susceptibility genes (Cederlund and Gillberg, 2004; Glasson et al., 2004). Environmental factors such as congenital rubella infection have previously been reported to be associated with autism; 7% of 250 children with congenital rubella later developed autism (Chess, 1971). However, due to immunization programs, rubella likely accounts for only 0.75% of cases (Fombonne, 1999). Pre- and perinatal *Haemophilus influenzae* and cytomegalovirus infections may also cause autism through significant damage to the immature brain (Gillberg and Coleman, 2000). Thalidomide (Rodier), an anticonvulsant taken during pregnancy, and perinatal hypoxia have also been linked with ASD (Baird et al., 2003). More recently, associations between increased infection early in life and later autism diagnosis have been documented (Niehus and Lord, 2006; Rosen, Yoshida, and Croen, 2007). To date, however, these all remain as mere associations, and no clear causally linked environmental factors have been established.

14.2   AUTISM AND IMMUNE DYSFUNCTION

As our understanding of the immune system increases, it has become more apparent that extensive cross talk between the immune and neurological systems exists. Many of the components of the immune system are capable of directly altering neurological pathways and can affect mood and behaviors. In turn, certain neurotransmitters can modulate the immune response. There have been a number of hypotheses that discuss the links between the immune system and autism. Indeed, altered immune function has been described in autism for almost 40 years (Money, Bobrow, and Clarke, 1971). Alterations of the immune system at the cellular level in autistic individuals include changes in the number and activation status of B cells, T cells, natural killer (NK) cells, and monocytes (Denney, Frei, and Gaffney, 1996; Enstrom et al., 2009; Fiumara et al., 1999; Stubbs and Crawford, 1977; Sweeten, Posey, and McDougle, 2003; Warren, Foster, and Margaretten, 1987). Autism also appears to be associated with a shift in the balance of T-helper type 1 (T_H1) and T_H2 responses, and associated with autoimmune and atopic diseases (Gupta et al., 1998; Molloy et al., 2006; Singh, 1996; Singh, Mehrotra, and Agarwal, 1999). As well as possible shifts in cytokines associated with T_H1/T_H2 balance, there are also reports of abnormalities in proinflammatory and anti-inflammatory cytokine profiles, such as increased IL-1, IL-6, and TNFα (Croonenberghs et al., 2002; Jyonouchi, Sun, and Le, 2001; Vargas et al., 2005).

14.2.1   Autoimmunity and Autism

In the last several years, there have been a number of reports of the increased history of autoimmune disease in families of individuals with ASD (Comi et al., 1999; Mouridsen et al., 2007; Sweeten et al., 2003). One study found that amongst mothers and first-degree relatives of autistic children, there was a 16%–21% incidence of autoimmunity compared with 2%–4% of control families (Comi et al., 1999). In this study, type I diabetes, rheumatoid arthritis (RA), hypothyroidism, and systemic lupus erythematosus were the most common autoimmune diseases. Among the families reporting autoimmune disease, RA was the most common. However, in a similar study, Molloy and colleagues (2006) reported 70% (108/155) of children with regressive autism had a family history (first- or second-degree relatives) of autoimmune disease versus 55% (81/144) of autistic children with no regression. When considering only the families reporting autoimmune disease, 36% in the regressive group and 34% of the non-regressive group reported the family history of RA, which are similar to the results of the study conducted by Comi et al. (1999). The study by the Molloy group, however, does not include a control population and relied on the memory and the accuracy of the caregiver in assessing the autoimmune status of second-degree relatives (Molloy et al., 2006). The study by Comi et al. (1999) also relied on recall by family members, which could introduce significant bias into the study. These factors may mean that the high reports of a familial history of autoimmune disease need further verification. Sweeten et al. (2003) also identified an increased frequency of the familial history of autoimmune disease amongst children with autism and Asperger's disorder when compared with children who had an autoimmune disease and with healthy children. In this study, the most frequent autoimmune disease reported was hypothyroidism. This compares with the findings of the Molloy group, in which regressive-type autism was associated with thyroid disease (41% in regressive type versus 27% in non-regressive autism) (Molloy et al., 2006). Furthermore, in a large study of medical charts of 420 ASD children and 2100 children without the history of developmental delay, an association between the maternal diagnosis of psoriasis, an autoimmune condition, and the ASD was found (Croen et al., 2005). Moreover, in mothers diagnosed with allergy or asthma in the second trimester of pregnancy, there was a two-fold increase in the diagnosis of ASD in the offspring suggesting that immune disorders or immune dysregulation may be a common feature during pregnancy in mothers of children who later develop ASD. It must be noted that although there may be significant bias in family interviews as compared to chart reviews, in turn, chart reviews rely on doctor reports, which may underreport some cases of autoimmunity. However, the role of familial autoimmunity in the etiology of ASD is at present unclear.

Recently, there is growing evidence to suggest that, in some cases, potential alterations in neurodevelopment could be caused by the placental transfer of maternal antibodies that interfere with the development of the fetal brain (Braunschweig et al., 2008; Dalton et al., 2003; Martin et al., 2008; Singer et al., 2008). In a study by Dalton et al. (2003), blood serum was taken from a 38-year old mother of three children. She was the "test mother" of the study, as her first child was a boy with typical development (9 years), her second child was a girl (8 years) with high-functioning ASD and no history of regression, and her third child was a boy (6 years) with a severe language-specific disorder (not autism) after regression at 18 months. For controls, they took serum from four parous women, each of whom had between one and four typically developing children. When brain tissue from adult rats and neonatal mice was exposed to serum samples from the five different mothers, immunohistochemical analysis showed that antibodies to neuronal antigens from the test mother bound more strongly to cerebellar Purkinje cells compared with serum from the control mothers (Dalton et al., 2003). In addition, the investigators injected serum samples from the test mother and two of the control mothers into pregnant mice during several days of gestation. Subsequent assessment of the mouse offspring showed behavioral impairment (e.g., reduced exploratory behavior and impaired righting reflex) and neurochemical changes in the cerebellum in those mice exposed *in utero* to serum from the test mother compared with those mice exposed *in utero* to serum from the control mothers. Recently, purified IgG isolated from sera of mothers of children with autism and from sera of control mothers with typically developing children were injected into pregnant rhesus macaques. The offspring of macaques injected with IgG from mothers of children with autism displayed significant whole body stereotypies and behavioral changes that were strikingly reminiscent of autism and were not present in the offspring of macaques treated with IgG from mothers of typically developing children (Martin et al., 2008).

In addition to potentially increased familial autoimmunity in relatives of subjects with ASD, there are an increasing number of reports that show direct indications of autoimmunity in children with ASD (Cabanlit et al., 2007; Connolly et al., 1999, 2006; Singer et al., 2006; Todd et al., 1988; Weizman et al., 1982; Wills et al., 2007). The presence of self-reactive antibodies has been extensively reported in autistic children. In one study, 27% of ASD children had self-reactive IgG autoantibodies compared with 2% of control children; 36% had self-reactive IgM, compared with none in the control group (Connolly et al., 1999). Specifically of interest, autoantibodies have been detected toward many components of the central nervous system (CNS) in some individuals with autism. These include antibodies toward neuron-axon filament proteins (Singh et al., 1997), myelin basic protein (MBP; Singh et al., 1993), serotonin receptors (Singh, Singh, and Warren, 1997), brain-derived neurotrophic factor (Connolly et al., 2006), nerve growth factor (Kozlovskaia et al., 2000), and brain endothelial cells (Connolly et al., 1999). Although these autoantibodies are not detectable in all individuals with autism, the number of individuals with autism who have one or more of these antibodies is significant. In one study of 68 children with autism, 49% had autoantibodies that were reactive against the caudate nucleus and 18% had antibodies against the cerebral cortex (Singh and Rivas, 2004). In separate studies, Singh et al. (1993, 1997) found 55%–70% of sera collected from children with autism were positive for antibodies against MBP and brain-derived neurofilament protein. However, it is unclear whether these autoantibodies are directly involved in the induction of autistic behavior or secondary to the innate CNS pathology.

14.2.2 Cell-Mediated Immune Response in Autism

Cell-mediated immunity is a host defense system controlled by several different cellular subsets that act in concert with each other and the humoral immune system, in an effort to orchestrate an appropriate immune response to pathogenic insult. Current literature concerning immunological aberrations in ASD has provided valuable insights into potentially dysfunctional cellular subsets. These include a decrease in total lymphocyte numbers (Ashwood et al., 2003), a reduced frequency of CD4$^+$ T cells (Ashwood et al., 2003; Ferrante et al., 2003; Yonk et al., 1990), a decrease in suppressor T cells (Warren et al., 1990), an increase in circulating monocytes (Sweeten et al., 2004), and an altered frequency of NK cells (Fiumara et al., 1999; Enstrom et al., 2009). In addition to reports of quantitative differences in immune function between autistic children and typically developing controls, there have also been reports of qualitative differences. Lymphocytes, in general, have shown a decreased responsiveness when challenged with mitogenic stimulation (Stubbs and Crawford, 1977). In T-cell subsets, there have been reports of partial activation, evinced by an increase in cell surface HLA-DR without the expression of the IL-2 receptor (Plioplys et al., 1994; Warren et al., 1995). NK cells from autistic children also have reduced lytic activity compared to controls (Enstrom et al., 2009; Warren, Foster, and Margaretten, 1987). These studies have provided valuable information on the immune status of autistic children and implicate several cellular subsets as potential antagonists. However, many of these studies were conducted under steady state or nonspecific mitogenic conditions at singular time points in the child's development. At a steady state, i.e., non-challenged milieu, immune cells may only slightly differ from neurotypical controls, but when challenged there may be an altered or inappropriate immune response and corresponding cytokine profile in autism compared with the controls.

14.2.2.1 Cytokines in Autism

It has been hypothesized that neuro-immune factors such as proinflammatory cytokine secretion and CNS-directed antibodies directly contribute to the behavioral changes seen in autoimmune diseases and vice versa immune changes seen in psychiatric disorders. The direct evidence of increased proinflammatory cytokines profiles in the brain specimens of individuals with autism can be difficult to assay due to the limited availability of appropriately preserved brain tissue. However, one study collected human brain tissue and cerebrospinal fluid (CSF) from 11 individuals with autism (ranging in age from 5 to 45 years old) and 6 control individuals (5 to 46 years old) (Vargas et al., 2005). Microglial and astroglial activations present in the brain tissue from individuals with autism were consistent with ongoing inflammatory processes. Furthermore, significant numbers of infiltrating macrophages and monocytes were present in the inflammatory sites. The brain specimens from individuals with autism also showed significant proinflammatory cytokine reactions, including the presence of high levels of transforming growth factor $\beta1$ (TGF-$\beta1$), monocyte chemoattractant protein (MCP)-1, MCP-3, thymus and activation-regulated chemokine, IL-6, IL-10, and eotaxin, among others. Based on the immunohistochemical staining of the tissue, astrocytes and microglia were the primary source of cytokine release. The authors also examined CSF samples of both the control and autism groups and found a 200-fold increase in interferon-γ (IFNγ), a 30-fold increase of TGF$\beta2$, and a 12-fold increase in MCP-1 present in the subjects with autism. While some of these features, such as increased IL-6 and IL-10, may suggest a T_H2 response, overall the findings are more consistent with proinflammatory responses. Others researchers have also reported increases in proinflammatory cytokine profiles in the blood of individuals with autism (Croonenberghs et al., 2002; Jyonouchi, Sun, and Le, 2001; Molloy et al., 2006; Singh, 1996). The increased production of cytokines, especially in the brain and CSF, points to an immune system involvement in autism that may be relevant to the pathophysiology of autism.

14.3 GASTROINTESTINAL DYSFUNCTION IN AUTISM

Although no prospectively designed epidemiological trials have been conducted, there is a growing body of clinical evidence that suggests that a subgroup of children with ASD is prone to persistent gastrointestinal (GI) problems. The prevalence of GI dysfunction in children with ASD reported by different studies varies greatly, with existing data putting the overall rate anywhere between 18% and 91% (Afzal et al., 2003; Horvath and Perman, 2002b; Horvath et al., 1999; Lightdale et al., 2001; Ming et al., 2008; Molloy and Manning-Courtney, 2003; Niehus and Lord, 2006; Parracho et al., 2005; Valicenti-McDermott et al., 2006). Although it has been suggested that GI dysfunction is a more common complaint in children with ASD compared with typically developing children, few studies have utilized adequate controls, making it challenging to come to a definitive conclusion as to the true extent of GI dysfunction in ASD (Erickson et al., 2005; Kuddo and Nelson, 2003; Levy et al., 2007). Despite this, however, it is clear that a substantial proportion of children with autism present with abnormal GI function. Symptoms of GI dysfunction include persistent diarrhea, chronic constipation, alternating bowel habits, vomiting, gaseousness and bloating, abdominal distention, and pain, with the latter symptom often being severe. In a retrospective evaluation of non-referred children with autism or ASD ($n = 137$), 24% had ≥ 1 GI symptom; diarrhea was the most commonly reported symptom (12%, $n = 17$) (Molloy and Manning-Courtney, 2003). In another study, the incidence of GI symptoms in 385 children with pervasive developmental disorders (PDD) was compared with the incidence in 48 non-ASD siblings and 102 unrelated controls (Melmed et al., 2000). Chronic GI symptoms were reported in 46% of children with PDD: 19% had chronic diarrhea, 19% had chronic constipation, and the remaining 8% alternated between diarrhea and constipation. In contrast, only 8% of healthy siblings and 5% of unrelated controls had chronic diarrhea, and 10% of healthy siblings and 5% of controls had chronic constipation. In a recent study of 150 children, the lifetime prevalence of GI symptoms in ASD was 70% compared with 42% of children with developmental delay but not ASD, and compared with 28% of typically developing children (Valicenti-McDermott et al., 2006). The high rates of GI symptoms reported in this group may likely be due to a recording of both previous and current GI symptoms. However, the analysis of more specific symptoms reported was similar to those seen for other studies. For instance, 22% of children with ASD and 8% of typically developing children reported chronic constipation, which were similar to the frequency seen in the study by Melmed et al. (2000).

Children with ASD and GI symptoms are more likely to experience sleep disturbance, sudden irritability, unexplained crying, and aggressive behavior than children with ASD but no GI symptoms (Horvath and Perman, 2002a). In their study, Horvath and colleagues reported disturbed sleep and night-time wake up in 51% of children with ASD who had GI symptoms, compared with 14% of children with autism but no GI symptoms, and compared with only 7% of healthy siblings. The same research team reported that 15.5% of children with ASD had reflux esophagitis, and that nearly two-thirds of these children experienced sleep disturbances (Horvath and Perman, 2002b). They also reported that 43% of children who had abnormal esophageal histology had episodes of unexplained daytime irritability compared with 13% of children with ASD who had normal esophageal histology. Observations that GI symptoms may peak before and are relieved following bowel movements suggest that some autism behaviors may be exacerbated due to GI dysfunction (Ashwood et al., 2003; Wakefield, 2002). However, the significance of the relationship between more severe autistic behaviors and the presence of GI symptoms in ASD requires further investigation.

Studies have focused on assessing the underlying pathology of GI dysfunction in children with ASD. Initial research reported low α-1-antitrypsin concentrations in children with ASD, suggestive of intestinal protein loss (Walker-Smith and Andrews, 1972). More recent endoscopic, histologic, and immunohistochemical analyses of the GI tract in children with ASD who have GI complaints has revealed the presence of a subtle diffuse inflammation of the intestinal tract. For example, in a study of 36 children with autism and GI disturbance, Horvath et al. (1999) reported reflux esophagitis in 69% of children, chronic gastritis in 42%, and chronic duodenitis in 67%. However, this study did not include a group of control patients for comparison. In another study, Wakefield et al. (2000) performed ileocolonoscopies and biopsies on 60 children with developmental disorders (50 diagnosed with ASD) and GI complaints, and 37 developmentally normal controls who were being investigated for possible inflammatory bowel disease (IBD). Significantly increased ileal and colonic lymphoid nodular hyperplasia (LNH) and enterocolitis were reported in ASD children compared with controls. There is the general impression that ileocolonic LNH is a normal finding in children with GI complaints, and that age is a critical factor in presentation (i.e., that LNH is more frequent in younger children) (reviewed in Wakefield et al., 2005). Therefore, it might be regarded that LNH does not represent a significant pathologic finding in autism. In order to address this issue, Wakefield et al. (2005) assessed the prevalence of ileocolonic LNH in a large group of patients with ASD (n = 148) and GI symptoms versus developmentally normal controls with GI symptoms, with or without colonic pathology. The different groups of patients assessed were well balanced, with equivalent median age and gender split. The study found that ileocolonic LNH was more prevalent in children with ASD compared with controls, regardless of whether or not the controls displayed colonic inflammation. Furthermore, there was no correlation between the presence of LNH in children with ASD and the age at which the ileocolonoscopy was performed.

In addition to an increased prevalence of LNH, histology, immunohistochemistry, and flow cytometry studies have consistently shown a subtle pan-enteric infiltration of immune cells such as lymphocytes, NK cells, and eosinophils into the walls of the GI tract in children with ASD, compared with typically developing children who had GI symptoms but no GI pathology. These studies also showed differences in immunopathology in ASD children with GI symptoms compared with typically developing children diagnosed with other GI diseases such as Crohn's disease and ulcerative colitis (Ashwood et al., 2003; Furlano et al., 2001; Torrente et al., 2002, 2004). Furthermore, increased intestinal lymphocyte-mediated proinflammatory response (e.g., increased CD3$^+$ TNF-α^+ cells and CD3$^+$ IFN-γ^+ cells) and reduced regulatory response (e.g., decreased CD3$^+$ IL-10$^+$ cells) were demonstrated in children with ASD and GI symptoms compared with developmentally normal controls (Ashwood and Wakefield, 2006; Ashwood et al., 2004). This data suggests that the infiltrating immune cells may be activated and could contribute to inflammatory processes within the GI tract. Interestingly, in addition to showing the increased immune cell infiltration of the gut mucosa in children with autism, Torrente et al. (2004) have shown a co-localization of immunoglobulin G/complement C1q deposition on the surface epithelium of the GI tract, which not only indicates chronic inflammation but also suggests an autoimmune component to the inflammatory response seen.

These studies, therefore, seem to demonstrate the presence of an underlying subtle chronic inflammatory process in children with autism and GI disturbance, characterized by LNH and enterocolitis, and the mucosal infiltration of immune cells along the length of the GI tract. It is also clear from these studies that endoscopy and histological studies alone may not be sufficient to detect these subtle changes and that more sophisticated and sensitive immunohistochemistry or flow cytometry methods are needed.

14.4 DISCUSSION: POSSIBLE LINKS BETWEEN IMMUNE DYSFUNCTION, GASTROINTESTINAL DYSFUNCTION AND AUTISM

The GI tract represents one of the primary gateways between the internal and external environments, allowing nutrients to enter the body. Likewise, it must also provide a robust barrier against pathogens. A compromise in the integrity of this physical and immunologic barrier can have major consequences. Increased intestinal permeability (sometimes referred to as "leaky gut") may result from impairment in the integrity of the mucosal barrier. D'Eufemia et al. (1996) reported increased intestinal permeability in almost half the children with ASD enrolled in their study compared with no change in healthy controls, despite deliberately excluding from enrollment any child with autism showing clinical signs of GI disease. This suggested damage to the gut mucosa in children with autism with no obvious signs of GI disease. An increase in GI permeability shown in some children with autism has provided support for the "opioid excess" theory, a theory based on an observation that some symptoms of ASD (such as social withdrawal, insensitivity to pain, and repetitive, and stereotyped behaviors) are similar to those found in morphine addicts (Kalat, 1978; Panksepp, 1979). It has been proposed that exogenous opioids from foods may contribute to behavioral and communicative dysfunctions in ASD, and gliadiomorphins and β-casomorphins derived from gluten and casein have been put forward as potential candidates (White, 2003). Although there are reports, mostly anecdotal, of improved behavioral effects following the elimination of gluten and casein from the diet, it has not been rigorously assessed as a therapy (Hyman and Levy, 2005). While only a limited number of trials have been completed, gluten and casein–elimination trials have been reviewed (Christison and Ivany, 2006; Millward et al., 2008), and while the authors noted serious design flaws of the studies, the majority of the studies reported positive behavioral effects from the diets. The most difficult aspects of the rigorous scientific validation of these diets include placebo controls and caregiver bias. To reduce this bias, new studies examining child scores on standardized tests of cognitive function and behavioral assessment should be utilized rather than relying extensively on caregiver perceptions of behavioral changes. The most controlled study to date was performed by Knivsberg, Reichelt, and Nodland (2001), which followed children matched for age and cognitive function who were placed on regular or elimination diets for 1 year. The major advance of this study was that the subjects were assessed by standardized testing at the end of the study period, and the testers were blind to the treatment group of the subject. While they found no benefit to verbal functioning, they reported significant improvements within the diet group in total impairment, including attention, nonverbal cognition, motor skills, and overall behavior. Furthermore, a preliminary study was reported that attempted a double-blinded clinical trial to assess the efficacy of the gluten and casein–free diet (Elder et al., 2006). Food was prepared by a dietician to eliminate caregivers and researchers from identifying the study group each child was in. The children were either placed on a regular diet or modified diet for 6 weeks and then switched. Unfortunately, only 13 children completed the study, so results were statistically insignificant. However, it was noted that there were some children whose verbal communication skills appeared to improve on the diet and regress off the diet. These results are promising in that they show the viability of a double-blind trial of this diet; however, it is unlikely that a short 6 week diet would result in the marked improvement of cognitive and motor functioning. Another factor that must be considered is whether changing to any structured well-balanced diet would have a positive effect in these children. Indeed, it has previously been shown that dietary modification including but not exclusively gluten and casein–free diets resulted in improvement in GI inflammation (Ashwood et al., 2003). These studies need to be replicated to see whether a specific dietary change or a more global shift to a well-balanced diet would be beneficial in addressing GI immunopathology and behavior in children with ASD and GI symptoms.

The lining of the GI tract contains a host of components important for a normal immune response (T-lymphocytes, B-lymphocytes, macrophages, neutrophils, antibodies, etc.), in close proximity to the gut lumen. Increased GI permeability could trigger an adverse immune response and inflammation in the gut, which in turn might trigger a change in behavior. Furthermore, an impaired gut barrier may explain the highly activated immune profiles seen in the GI tract of children with ASD (Ashwood and Wakefield, 2006; Ashwood et al., 2004). In one study, comparing the intracellular cytokine staining of peripheral blood T cells from healthy controls, children with ASD, and children with Crohn's disease, increases in the inflammatory cytokines IFN-γ and TNF-α, pre- and poststimulation, were observed in children with ASD who had GI symptoms compared with controls (Ashwood and Wakefield, 2006). Similar findings in children with ASD have been reported elsewhere (Jyonouchi, Sun, and Le, 2001; Jyonouchi et al., 2005). Although the T-cell cytokine profiles seen in ASD children were different from typically developing noninflamed normal controls, they were not the same as those seen for established IBDs such as Crohn's disease. This is important as the data suggest that the cytokine profiles observed in ASD may be unique. Moreover, these findings suggest that there may be intrinsic defects of the immune response in ASD children with GI symptoms that are not seen in developmentally normal children without GI symptoms. It is plausible that increased intestinal permeability in some children with autism, as shown by D'Eufemia et al. (1996), may result in increased exposure to normally innocuous antigens (e.g., food proteins and typical gut microflora), which may result in increased immune activity leading to inflammation that could affect behavior. Using a rodent model of intestinal bowel disease, Welch et al. (2005) reported increased activity in certain brain areas that are abnormally active in patients with autism following the induction of GI inflammation, and may suggest that the initiation of GI symptoms could affect behaviors

Although GI disturbance may be a comorbidity of autism, such findings have led to growing interest in the hypothesis that GI dysfunction may have an integral role in the etiology of ASD, especially in the regressive phenotype (Wakefield, 2002). Although symptoms such as irritability, aggressive behavior, and sleep disturbance are not part of the DSM-IV criteria for autistic disorder, they are common in children with ASD and GI symptoms (Horvath and Perman, 2002b), and the parental reporting of behavioral changes and GI symptoms may occur at approximately similar times (Lightdale et al., 2001). Additional support for a hypothesis linking neurodevelopmental abnormalities and GI dysfunction in autism comes from analogous findings of behavioral and neurological problems in other diseases characterized by GI dysfunction. For example, an untreated celiac disease is the result of an overt immune response to dietary gluten and is associated with the inflammation of the intestinal mucosa. Asperger (1961) reported that children with celiac disease also often exhibited psychological problems. Anxiety and depression have also been reported in adult patients with celiac disease (Hallert and Derefeldt, 1982). Cooke and Smith (1966) reported on the neurological disorders found in adult patients with celiac disease; these included severe progressive neuropathy, gait ataxia, and limb ataxia. Postmortem analysis revealed extensive inflammatory changes in the CNS, with a notable loss of Purkinje cells and gliosis in the cerebellum. A review of reports from 1964 to 2000 showed that peripheral neuropathy and ataxia were the most common neurological disorders, with other less common manifestations including myelopathy and dementia (Hadjivassiliou, Grunewald, and Davies-Jones, 2002). There is evidence that disturbances such as ataxia, epilepsy, and depression are also associated with celiac disease in children and adolescents (Fasano and Catassi, 2005). It has also been reported that patients with disorders such as irritable bowel syndrome (IBS) and Crohn's disease often have psychiatric symptoms (Ringel and Drossman, 2001, 2002). Research suggests that the symptoms of IBS are caused or maintained by an activated immune system. Increased gut permeability, increased numbers of T-lymphocytes, and enteroendocrine cells in the mucosa are reported in patients with IBS following gut infection (Spiller et al., 2000). There are also reports of elevated intestinal permeability in other diseases characterized by intestinal inflammation and/or abnormal immune response, such as celiac disease (Bjarnason, Peters, and Veall, 1983; Cummins et al., 1991).

In addition, a number of disorders involving the CNS have been associated with immune dysfunction. For example, immune responses to some tumor-derived antigens can trigger rare neurological syndromes (i.e., paraneoplastic syndromes). The antibodies raised against the tumor are thought to cross-react with neuronal antigens in the CNS causing neurological dysfunction (Lang, Dale, and Vincent, 2003). Some patients with lung cancer experience paraneoplastic degeneration of the cerebellum; in a large proportion of these patients, raised levels of antibodies to voltage-gated calcium channels have been found (Graus et al., 2002). Another example is Rasmussen's encephalitis, a progressive inflammatory childhood disease affecting the cerebral cortex, causing intractable seizures, hemiparesis, and decreased motor and cognitive function. It has been suggested that this disease might be autoimmune in origin, as antibodies to the ionotropic glutamate receptor type 3 have been demonstrated in some patients (Rogers et al., 1994). Stiff person syndrome (SPS) is also a disease that displays an autoimmune pathology. This disease is characterized by severe progressive muscle stiffness and spasms triggered by external stimuli. Depression and anxiety are common comorbidities, and psychiatrists are often the first to recognize the disease following a referral for psychiatric evaluation (Murinson and Vincent, 2001). Highly specific autoantibodies to the enzyme glutamic acid decarboxylase are found in most SPS patients, and it is believed that these inhibit the synthesis of GABA. Plasma exchange and intravenous immunoglobulin treatment improve symptoms in patients receiving them (Murinson and Vincent, 2001). There is also some circumstantial evidence that anti-basal ganglia antibodies may be involved in the pathogenesis of tics (e.g., Tourette's disorder) and pediatric obsessive-compulsive disorder. Bacterial infection as a potential cause of this autoimmunity has been hypothesized, and is implicated in pediatric autoimmune disorders associated with streptococcal infections (reviewed by Hoekstra and Minderaa, 2005). However, the precise involvement of autoimmunity in these motor and psychiatric disturbances remains open to debate and further research is needed. Although there is much that remains unknown in this area, such examples suggest that immune dysfunction can have profound effects on the CNS/brain function and may impact the patient's behavior.

The cause of the abnormal GI dysfunction in children with ASD is unknown. However, interest has been raised in the potential role of zonulin, a protein, which is likely to be involved in the regulation of gut permeability (Fasano and Shea-Donohue, 2005; Fasano et al., 2000; Wang et al., 2000). The epithelial cells of the intestinal wall form a semipermeable barrier, and their function is to regulate the passage of molecules from the lumen into the body. The sites at which the epithelial cells adjoin each other form "tight junctions," which act as a gateway allowing molecules to pass through (Fasano and Shea-Donohue, 2005; Liu, Li, and Neu, 2005). The study by D'Eufemia et al. (1996) indicated that increased GI permeability in children with ASD occurred through the paracellular pathway (i.e., increased passage of molecules between the epithelial cells). Tight junctions are formed by a meshwork of proteins; it is thought that zonulin may induce the disassembly of these proteins, allowing increased permeability (Fasano, 2001; Fasano and Shea-Donohue, 2005). Interestingly, zonulin expression is raised in intestinal tissue during the acute phase of celiac disease (Fasano et al., 2000). In addition, a recent study in diabetic-prone rats suggests that the zonulin-mediated loss of intestinal barrier function may be involved in the pathogenesis of type I diabetes (Watts et al., 2005). It is possible, therefore, that some intrinsic defect in the normal functioning of zonulin may be a contributory factor in the increased permeability of the GI tract in some individuals with ASD. However, this remains to be proven.

Another theory as to the role of GI inflammation and neurological inflammation involves increased serotonin levels seen in the blood of approximately 30% of ASD patients (Anderson, 1987; Stahl, 1977). Serotonin, also referred to as 5-hydroxytryptamine (5-HT), is a neurotransmitter, as well as an immunomodulator. Certain forms of 5-HT are stored and released from enterochromaffin cells of the gut epithelium, an action important for the nerve cells lining the small and large intestines. Increased levels of 5-HT in the periphery have been associated with IBD, and use of serotonin reuptake inhibitors result in the alleviation of GI symptoms in many

IBD patients. A correlation between high serum 5-HT and decreased 5-HT receptor sensitivity with the extended HLA haplotype B44-DR4, as well as complement C4B null allele, has been reported in ASD (Warren, 1996). Furthermore self-reactive antibodies to 5-HT receptors were identified in the serum of ASD patients (Cook and Leventhal, 1996; Todd and Ciaranello, 1985). This is consistent with findings of 80% loss of 5-HT binding in mice upon the addition of sera from ASD patients (Singh, Singh, and Warren, 1997). Genetic disequilibrium at the 5-HT transporter gene (SLC6A4) has also been reported in ASD individuals in two separate studies (Cook et al., 1990; Kim et al., 2002). In healthy individuals, approximately 95% of peripheral 5-HT is produced in the GI tract with the rest produced in the brain. Increased levels of 5-HT in the brain have been associated with increased levels of destructive and aggressive behaviors, while increased levels in the GI tract are associated with IBD. Furthermore, the usage of 5-HT reuptake inhibitors risperidone, clomipramine, and fluvoxamine has been shown to decrease certain aberrant behaviors, such as anger, compulsive behavior, and ritualized behavior, in ASD individuals (Gordon et al., 1993; Hellings et al., 1996, 2006; McDougle et al., 1998). The possible links between GI tract inflammation resulting in, or being caused by, increased local 5-HT are compelling based on the connection between serotonin, the immune system, and the nervous system. However, 5-HT in ASD with GI symptoms has not been extensively studied.

How might increased GI permeability, abnormal immune response, and GI inflammation trigger behaviors associated with ASD? Perhaps the most plausible factor may be that of cytokine action. Cytokines and their receptors are distributed throughout the brain and are known to influence neural development, synaptic transmission, and behavioral traits, and have been implicated in autism as well as schizophrenia (Dunn, 2006; Larson, 2002; Licinio, Kling, and Hauser, 1998; Meyer et al., 2006; Muller and Ackenheil, 1998; Nawa, Takahashi, and Patterson, 2000; Smith et al., 2007; Tohmi et al., 2004; Vargas et al., 2005; Vereker, O'Donnell, and Lynch, 2000; Yamada et al., 2000). Importantly, the immunocytochemical analysis of brain tissue from patients with autism showed the marked activation of microglia and astroglia, most notably in the cerebellum. Cytokine profiling indicated that MCP-1 and TGF-β1, derived from neuroglia, were the most prevalent cytokines in brain tissues (Vargas et al., 2005). The authors suggested that the activation of the CNS innate immune system leading to cytokine release may play a role in the pathogenesis of the disease. It is possible that altered levels of peripheral cytokines occur as a result of immune dysregulation in the GI tract. These altered peripheral cytokine levels may subsequently act directly on neurons within the CNS or may trigger a CNS-mediated inflammatory response via glial cells. These actions could in turn affect neurodevelopment and/or elicit behaviors associated with ASD.

Autoimmune responses may also be important in impairing GI function in ASD and may be another mechanism relevant to ASD pathophysiology. It is possible that antibodies toward neuronal tissue seen in some patients with ASD may be generated as a result of secondary inflammation in the CNS. However, it is not known whether these autoantibodies are pathogenic and are involved in the generation of behaviors associated with ASD. Vojdani et al. (2002) demonstrated that antibodies against many neuronal proteins in ASD individuals also cross-react with butyrophilin,

Chlamydia pneumoniae peptide, and *Streptococcus* M proteins. This is interesting as some evidence of autoimmune etiology for many neurologic diseases (e.g., multiple sclerosis and myasthenia gravis) have suggested that "molecular mimicry" may be a key component. Molecular mimicry is defined as immunologic cross-reactivity between foreign and self-antigens. Furthermore, in multiple sclerosis, cross-reactivity has been shown between antibodies against the neuronal peptide myelin oligodendrocyte glycoprotein and butyrophilin, a protein found in milk (Guggenmos et al., 2004). Similarly, the potential mechanisms for how molecular mimicry might result in neuronal damage and/or behavioral effects have been reviewed in more detail elsewhere (Ercolini and Miller, 2005). One plausible mechanism is that B cells may be found in gut lymphoid tissues that recognize neuronal self-antigens (not normally present outside the CNS). These cells form part of a neuroprotective mechanism, designed to deal with antigens released following neuronal damage. Increased GI permeability may lead to the increased exposure of these cells to foreign antigens that share structural homology with self-antigens. This in turn may result in B cells recognizing foreign antigens and generating cross-reactive antibodies. Although antibodies do not normally cross the blood-brain barrier (BBB), there is evidence that inflammatory cytokines may compromise the integrity of the BBB, allowing the antibodies to cross into the CNS (Ercolini and Miller, 2005). Once within the CNS, these antibodies may bind directly to the target tissue and disrupt normal function; alternatively, they may activate macrophages, which could release mediators that in turn could alter the function of the neuronal tissue. It should be noted that Vargas et al. (2005) showed no deposition of IgG, IgA, or IgM immunoglobulins in neuronal or neuroglial cell populations in specimens from brains of individuals with autism. However, the GI status of these patients is not known, and one might assume that the patients included in this study did not have GI inflammation. Therefore, it is not possible to rule out the action of autoantibodies in patients with autism and GI dysfunction. Another potential mechanism is the activation of auto-reactive T cells in the inflamed GI tract of children with ASD. Antigen presenting cells in the gut mucosal tissue may present sequence-homologous antigen to T cells, which in turn recognize both the foreign peptide and "self" neuronal peptide. These T cells may upregulate adhesion molecules, allowing them to cross the BBB. Thus, T cells (including cytotoxic T cells) could then target neuronal tissue expressing the "self" tissue, resulting in damage to the CNS tissue. In addition, T cells may release inflammatory cytokines within the target tissue; in turn, these cytokines may damage neuronal tissue directly or activate further "self-reactive" immune cells to infiltrate the brain and potentially attack it. The resulting damage to self-tissue from the actions of T cells and other immune cells, directly or indirectly, could release further self antigen, thus instigating a self-perpetuating cycle of autoimmune-mediated tissue damage (Figure 14.1).

In conclusion, although the etiology of ASD is not known in the majority of cases, there appears to be a strong link between immune dysfunction and ASD in many individuals; whether the immune dysfunction has a causal relationship to ASD is currently only speculative. However, in other diseases, neurological abnormalities and immune dysfunction are closely linked. Furthermore, the association between ASD and GI dysfunction in many children has been documented. It is not known whether a genetic susceptibility leading to increased GI dysfunction or leading toward altered

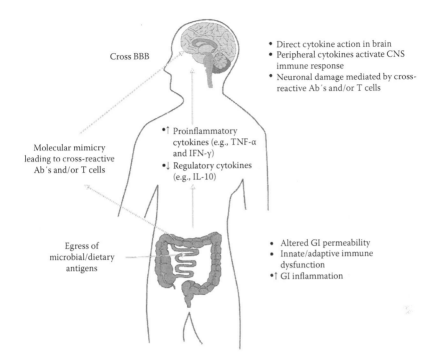

FIGURE 14.1 **(See color insert following page 200.)** Possible mechanism by which GI dysfunction may trigger autistic behaviors in children with autism and GI disturbance.

immune responses, or indeed both, may be important etiologic factors in a sub-group of children with ASD. The role of immune factors and potential mechanisms influencing both GI dysfunction and neurodevelopment, including the onset of autistic behaviors, needs to be studied further. However, research findings to date suggest that therapies, which could improve GI dysfunction and/or immune dysfunction in patients with ASD, may have a beneficial effect. Further investigation to explore and to better understand the underlying immune mechanisms in ASD are warranted.

REFERENCES

Afzal, N., S. Murch, K. Thirrupathy, L. Berger, A. Fagbemi, and R. Heuschkel. 2003. Constipation with acquired megarectum in children with autism. *Pediatrics* 112:939–942.

Anderson, G. M. 1987. Monoamines in autism: An update of neurochemical research on a pervasive developmental disorder. *Med. Biol.* 65:67–74.

APA. 2000. *Diagnostic and Statistical Manual of Mental Disorders*, 4th edition, text revision (DMS-IV-TR), Ed. APA. Arlington, VA: American Psychiatric Association Publishing, Inc.

Ashwood, P. and A. J. Wakefield. 2006. Immune activation of peripheral blood and mucosal CD3+ lymphocyte cytokine profiles in children with autism and gastrointestinal symptoms. *J. Neuroimmunol.* 173:126–134.

Ashwood, P., A. Anthony, A. A. Pellicer, F. Torrente, J. A. Walker-Smith, and A. J. Wakefield. 2003. Intestinal lymphocyte populations in children with regressive autism: Evidence for extensive mucosal immunopathology. *J. Clin. Immunol.* 23:504–517.

292 Autism: Oxidative Stress, Inflammation, and Immune Abnormalities

Ashwood, P., A. Anthony, F. Torrente, and A. J. Wakefield. 2004. Spontaneous mucosal lymphocyte cytokine profiles in children with autism and gastrointestinal symptoms: mucosal immune activation and reduced counter regulatory interleukin-10. *J. Clin. Immunol.* 24:664–673.

Asperger, H. 1961. Psychopathology of children with coeliac disease. *Ann. Paediatr.* 197:346–351.

Bailey, A., A. Le Couteur, I. Gottesman, P. Bolton, E. Simonoff, E. Yuzda, and M. Rutter. 1995. Autism as a strongly genetic disorder: Evidence from a British twin study. *Psychol. Med.* 25:63–77.

Baird, G., H. Cass, and V. Slonims. 2003. Diagnosis of autism. *BMJ* 327:488–493.

Betancur, C., M. Leboyer, and C. Gillberg. 2002. Increased rate of twins among affected sibling pairs with autism. *Am. J. Hum. Genet.* 70:1381–1383.

Bjarnason, I., T. J. Peters, and N. Veall. 1983. Intestinal permeability defect in coeliac disease. *Lancet* 1:1284–1285.

Braunschweig, D., P. Ashwood, P. Krakowiak, I. Hertz-Picciotto, R. Hansen, L. A. Croen, I. N. Pessah, and J. Van de Water. 2008. Autism: Maternally derived antibodies specific for fetal brain proteins. *Neurotoxicology* 29:226–231.

Cabanlit, M., S. Wills, P. Goines, P. Ashwood, and J. Van de Water. 2007. Brain-specific autoantibodies in the plasma of subjects with autistic spectrum disorder. *Ann. N.Y. Acad. Sci.* 1107:92–103.

Cederlund, M. and C. Gillberg. 2004. One hundred males with Asperger syndrome: A clinical study of background and associated factors. *Dev. Med. Child Neurol.* 46:652–660.

Chess, S. 1971. Autism in children with congenital rubella. *J. Autism Child Schizophr.* 1:33–47.

Christison, G. W. and K. Ivany. 2006. Elimination diets in autism spectrum disorders: Any wheat amidst the chaff? *J. Dev. Behav. Pediatr.* 27:S162–171.

Comi, A. M., A. W. Zimmerman, V. H. Frye, P. A. Law, and J. N. Peeden. 1999. Familial clustering of autoimmune disorders and evaluation of medical risk factors in autism. *J. Child Neurol.* 14:388–394.

Connolly, A. M., M. G. Chez, A. Pestronk, S. T. Arnold, S. Mehta, and R. K. Deuel. 1999. Serum autoantibodies to brain in Landau-Kleffner variant, autism, and other neurologic disorders. *J. Pediatr.* 134:607–613.

Connolly, A. M., M. Chez, E. M. Streif, R. M. Keeling, P. T. Golumbek, J. M. Kwon, J. J. Riviello, R. G. Robinson, R. J. Neuman, and R. M. Deuel. 2006. Brain-derived neurotrophic factor and autoantibodies to neural antigens in sera of children with autistic spectrum disorders, Landau-Kleffner syndrome, and epilepsy. *Biol. Psychiatry* 59:354–363.

Cook, E. H. and B. L. Leventhal. 1996. The serotonin system in autism. *Curr. Opin. Pediatr.* 8:348–354.

Cook, E. H., Jr., B. L. Leventhal, W. Heller, J. Metz, M. Wainwright, and D. X. Freedman. 1990. Autistic children and their first-degree relatives: Relationships between serotonin and norepinephrine levels and intelligence. *J. Neuropsychiatry Clin. Neurosci.* 2:268–274.

Cooke, W. T. and W. T. Smith. 1966. Neurological disorders associated with adult coeliac disease. *Brain* 89:683–722.

Croen, L. A., J. K. Grether, C. K. Yoshida, R. Odouli, and J. Van de Water. 2005. Maternal autoimmune diseases, asthma and allergies, and childhood autism spectrum disorders: A case-control study. *Arch. Pediatr. Adolesc. Med.* 159:151–157.

Croonenberghs, J., E. Bosmans, D. Deboutte, G. Kenis, and M. Maes. 2002. Activation of the inflammatory response system in autism. *Neuropsychobiology* 45:1–6.

Cummins, A. G., I. A. Penttila, J. T. Labrooy, T. A. Robb, and G. P. Davidson. 1991. Recovery of the small intestine in coeliac disease on a gluten-free diet: Changes in intestinal permeability, small bowel morphology and T-cell activity. *J. Gastroenterol. Hepatol.* 6:53–57.

D'Eufemia, P., M. Celli, R. Finocchiaro, L. Pacifico, L. Viozzi, M. Zaccagnini, E. Cardi, and O. Giardini. 1996. Abnormal intestinal permeability in children with autism. *Acta Paediatr.* 85:1076–1079.

Dalton, P., R. Deacon, A. Blamire, M. Pike, I. McKinlay, J. Stein, P. Styles, and A. Vincent. 2003. Maternal neuronal antibodies associated with autism and a language disorder. *Ann. Neurol.* 53:533–537.

Denney, D. R., B. W. Frei, and G. R. Gaffney. 1996. Lymphocyte subsets and interleukin-2 receptors in autistic children. *J. Autism Dev. Disord.* 26:87–97.

Dunn, A. J. 2006. Effects of cytokines and infections on brain neurochemistry. *Clin. Neurosci. Res.* 6:52–68.

Elder, J. H., M. Shankar, J. Shuster, D. Theriaque, S. Burns, and L. Sherrill. 2006. The gluten-free, casein-free diet in autism: Results of a preliminary double blind clinical trial. *J. Autism Dev. Disord.* 36:413–420.

Enstrom, A. M., L. Lit, C. E. Onore, J. P. Gregg, R. Hansen, I. N. Pessah, I. Hertz-Picciotto, J. A. Van de Water, F. R. Sharp, and P. Ashwood. 2009. Altered gene expression and function of peripheral blood natural killer cells in children with autism. *Brain Behav. Immun.* 23(1):124–133.

Ercolini, A. M. and S. D. Miller. 2005. Role of immunologic cross-reactivity in neurological diseases. *Neurol. Res.* 27:726–733.

Erickson, C. A., K. A. Stigler, M. R. Corkins, D. J. Posey, J. F. Fitzgerald, and C. J. McDougle. 2005. Gastrointestinal factors in autistic disorder: A critical review. *J. Autism Dev. Disord.* 35:713–727.

Fasano, A. 2001. Intestinal zonulin: Open sesame! *Gut* 49:159–162.

Fasano, A. and C. Catassi. 2005. Coeliac disease in children. *Best Pract. Res. Clin. Gastroenterol.* 19:467–478.

Fasano, A. and T. Shea-Donohue. 2005. Mechanisms of disease: The role of intestinal barrier function in the pathogenesis of gastrointestinal autoimmune diseases. *Nat. Clin. Pract. Gastroenterol. Hepatol.* 2:416–422.

Fasano, A., T. Not, W. Wang, S. Uzzau, I. Berti, A. Tommasini, and S. E. Goldblum. 2000. Zonulin, a newly discovered modulator of intestinal permeability, and its expression in coeliac disease. *Lancet* 355:1518–1519.

Ferrante, P., M. Saresella, F. R. Guerini, M. Marzorati, M. C. Musetti, and A. G. Cazzullo. 2003. Significant association of HLA A2-DR11 with CD4 naive decrease in autistic children. *Biomed. Pharmacother.* 57:372–374.

Fiumara, A., A. Sciotto, R. Barone, G. D'Asero, S. Munda, E. Parano, and L. Pavone. 1999. Peripheral lymphocyte subsets and other immune aspects in Rett syndrome. *Pediatr. Neurol.* 21:619–621.

Folstein, S. and M. Rutter. 1977. Infantile autism: A genetic study of 21 twin pairs. *J. Child Psychol. Psychiatry* 18:297–321.

Fombonne, E. 1999. Are measles infections or measles immunizations linked to autism? *J. Autism Dev. Disord.* 29:349–350.

Furlano, R. I., A. Anthony, R. Day, A. Brown, L. McGarvey, M. A. Thomson, S. E. Davies, M. Berelowitz, A. Forbes, A. J. Wakefield, J. A. Walker-Smith, and S. H. Murch. 2001. Colonic CD8 and gamma delta T-cell infiltration with epithelial damage in children with autism. *J. Pediatr.* 138:366–372.

Gillberg, C. and M. Coleman. 2000. *The Biology of Autistic Syndromes*, 3rd edition. London, U.K.: Mac Keith Press distributed by Cambridge University Press.

Glasson, E. J., C. Bower, B. Petterson, N. de Klerk, G. Chaney, and J. F. Hallmayer. 2004. Perinatal factors and the development of autism: A population study. *Arch. Gen. Psychiatry* 61:618–627.

Gordon, C. T., R. C. State, J. E. Nelson, S. D. Hamburger, and J. L. Rapoport. 1993. A double-blind comparison of clomipramine, desipramine, and placebo in the treatment of autistic disorder. *Arch. Gen. Psychiatry* 50:441–447.

Graus, F., B. Lang, P. Pozo-Rosich, A. Saiz, R. Casamitjana, and A. Vincent. 2002. P/Q type calcium-channel antibodies in paraneoplastic cerebellar degeneration with lung cancer. *Neurology* 59:764–766.

Greenberg, D. A., S. E. Hodge, J. Sowinski, and D. Nicoll. 2001. Excess of twins among affected sibling pairs with autism: Implications for the etiology of autism. *Am. J. Hum. Genet.* 69:1062–1067.

Guggenmos, J., A. S. Schubart, S. Ogg, M. Andersson, T. Olsson, I. H. Mather, and C. Linington. 2004. Antibody cross-reactivity between myelin oligodendrocyte glycoprotein and the milk protein butyrophilin in multiple sclerosis. *J. Immunol.* 172:661–668.

Gupta, S., S. Aggarwal, B. Rashanravan, and T. Lee. 1998. Th1- and Th2-like cytokines in CD4+ and CD8+ T cells in autism. *J. Neuroimmunol.* 85:106–109.

Hadjivassiliou, M., R. A. Grunewald, and G. A. Davies-Jones. 2002. Gluten sensitivity as a neurological illness. *J. Neurol. Neurosurg. Psychiatry* 72:560–563.

Hallert, C. and T. Derefeldt. 1982. Psychic disturbances in adult coeliac disease. I. Clinical observations. *Scand. J. Gastroenterol.* 17:17–19.

Hellings, J. A., L. A. Kelley, W. F. Gabrielli, E. Kilgore, and P. Shah. 1996. Sertraline response in adults with mental retardation and autistic disorder. *J. Clin. Psychiatry* 57:333–336.

Hellings, J. A., J. R. Zarcone, R. M. Reese, M. G. Valdovinos, J. G. Marquis, K. K. Fleming, and S. R. Schroeder. 2006. A crossover study of risperidone in children, adolescents and adults with mental retardation. *J. Autism Dev. Disord.* 36:401–411.

Hoekstra, P. J. and R. B. Minderaa. 2005. Tic disorders and obsessive-compulsive disorder: Is autoimmunity involved? *Int. Rev. Psychiatry* 17:497–502.

Horvath, K. and J. A. Perman. 2002a. Autism and gastrointestinal symptoms. *Curr. Gastroenterol. Rep.* 4:251–258.

Horvath, K. and J. A. Perman. 2002b. Autistic disorder and gastrointestinal disease. *Curr. Opin. Pediatr.* 14:583–587.

Horvath, K., J. C. Papadimitriou, A. Rabsztyn, C. Drachenberg, and J. T. Tildon. 1999. Gastrointestinal abnormalities in children with autistic disorder. *J. Pediatr.* 135:559–563.

Hyman, S. L. and S. E. Levy. 2005. Introduction: Novel therapies in developmental disabilities— hope, reason, and evidence. *Ment. Retard. Dev. Disabil. Res. Rev.* 11:107–109.

Jyonouchi, H., S. Sun, and H. Le. 2001. Proinflammatory and regulatory cytokine production associated with innate and adaptive immune responses in children with autism spectrum disorders and developmental regression. *J. Neuroimmunol.* 120:170–179.

Jyonouchi, H., L. Geng, A. Ruby, and B. Zimmerman-Bier. 2005. Dysregulated innate immune responses in young children with autism spectrum disorders: Their relationship to gastrointestinal symptoms and dietary intervention. *Neuropsychobiology* 51:77–85.

Kalat, J. W. 1978. Speculations on similarities between autism and opiate addiction. *J. Autism Child Schizophr.* 8:477–479.

Kim, S. J., N. Cox, R. Courchesne, C. Lord, C. Corsello, N. Akshoomoff, S. Guter, B. L. Leventhal, E. Courchesne, and E. H. Cook, Jr. 2002. Transmission disequilibrium mapping at the serotonin transporter gene (SLC6A4) region in autistic disorder. *Mol. Psychiatry* 7:278–288.

Knivsberg, A. M., K. L. Reichelt, and M. Nodland. 2001. Reports on dietary intervention in autistic disorders. *Nutr. Neurosci.* 4:25–37.

Kozlovskaia, G. V., T. P. Kliushnik, A. V. Goriunova, I. L. Turkova, M. A. Kalinina, and N. S. Sergienko. 2000. Nerve growth factor auto-antibodies in children with various forms of mental dysontogenesis and in schizophrenia high risk group. *Zh. Nevrol. Psikhiatr. Im. S. S. Korsakova* 100:50–52.

Kuddo, T. and K. B. Nelson. 2003. How common are gastrointestinal disorders in children with autism? *Curr. Opin. Pediatr.* 15:339–343.

Lang, B., R. C. Dale, and A. Vincent. 2003. New autoantibody mediated disorders of the central nervous system. *Curr. Opin. Neurol.* 16:351–357.

Larson, S. J. 2002. Behavioral and motivational effects of immune-system activation. *J. Gen. Psychol.* 129:401–414.

Lee, L. C., A. A. Zachary, M. S. Leffell, C. J. Newschaffer, K. J. Matteson, J. D. Tyler, and A. W. Zimmerman. 2006. HLA-DR4 in families with autism. *Pediatr. Neurol.* 35:303–307.

Levy, S. E., M. C. Souders, R. F. Ittenbach, E. Giarelli, A. E. Mulberg, and J. A. Pinto-Martin. 2007. Relationship of dietary intake to gastrointestinal symptoms in children with autistic spectrum disorders. *Biol. Psychiatry* 61:492–497.

Licinio, J., M. A. Kling, and P. Hauser. 1998. Cytokines and brain function: Relevance to interferon-alpha-induced mood and cognitive changes. *Semin. Oncol.* 25:30–38.

Lightdale, J. R., C. Hayer, A. Duer, C. Lind-White, S. Jenkins, B. Siegel, G. R. Elliott, and M. B. Heyman. 2001. Effects of intravenous secretin on language and behavior of children with autism and gastrointestinal symptoms: A single-blinded, open-label pilot study. *Pediatrics* 108:E90.

Liu, Z., N. Li, and J. Neu. 2005. Tight junctions, leaky intestines, and pediatric diseases. *Acta Paediatr.* 94:386–393.

Martin, L. A., P. Ashwood, D. Braunschweig, M. Cabanlit, J. Van de Water, and D. G. Amaral. 2008. Stereotypies and hyperactivity in rhesus monkeys exposed to IgG from mothers of children with autism. *Brain Behav. Immun.* 22:806–816.

McDougle, C. J., J. P. Holmes, D. C. Carlson, G. H. Pelton, D. J. Cohen, and L. H. Price. 1998. A double-blind, placebo-controlled study of risperidone in adults with autistic disorder and other pervasive developmental disorders. *Arch. Gen. Psychiatry* 55:633–641.

Melmed, R.D., C.K. Schneider, R.A. Fabes, J. Phillips, and K. Reichelt. 2000. Metabolic markers and gastrointestinal symptoms in children with autism and related disorders. *J. Pediatr. Gastroenterol. Nutr.* 31:S31–S32.

Meyer, U., M. Nyffeler, A. Engler, A. Urwyler, M. Schedlowski, I. Knuesel, B. K. Yee, and J. Feldon. 2006. The time of prenatal immune challenge determines the specificity of inflammation-mediated brain and behavioral pathology. *J. Neurosci.* 26:4752–4762.

Millward, C., M. Ferriter, S. Calver, and G. Connell-Jones. 2008. Gluten- and casein-free diets for autistic spectrum disorder. *Cochrane Database Syst. Rev.* CD003498.

Ming, X., M. Brimacombe, J. Chaaban, B. Zimmerman-Bier, and G. C. Wagner. 2008. Autism spectrum disorders: Concurrent clinical disorders. *J. Child Neurol.* 23:6–13.

Molloy, C. A. and P. Manning-Courtney. 2003. Prevalence of chronic gastrointestinal symptoms in children with autism and autistic spectrum disorders. *Autism* 7:165–171.

Molloy, C. A., A. L. Morrow, J. Meinzen-Derr, K. Schleifer, K. Dienger, P. Manning-Courtney, M. Altaye, and M. Wills-Karp. 2006. Elevated cytokine levels in children with autism spectrum disorder. *J. Neuroimmunol.* 172:198–205.

Money, J., N. A. Bobrow, and F. C. Clarke. 1971. Autism and autoimmune disease: A family study. *J. Autism Child Schizophr.* 1:146–160.

Mouridsen, S. E., B. Rich, T. Isager, and N. J. Nedergaard. 2007. Autoimmune diseases in parents of children with infantile autism: A case-control study. *Dev. Med. Child Neurol.* 49:429–432.

Muhle, R., S. V. Trentacoste, and I. Rapin. 2004. The genetics of autism. *Pediatrics* 113: e472–e486.

Muller, N. and M. Ackenheil. 1998. Psychoneuroimmunology and the cytokine action in the CNS: Implications for psychiatric disorders. *Prog. Neuropsychopharmacol. Biol. Psychiatry* 22:1–33.

Murinson, B. B. and A. Vincent. 2001. Stiff-person syndrome: Autoimmunity and the central nervous system. *CNS Spectr.* 6:427–433.

Nawa, H., M. Takahashi, and P. H. Patterson. 2000. Cytokine and growth factor involvement in schizophrenia: Support for the developmental model. *Mol. Psychiatry* 5:594–603.

Niehus, R. and C. Lord. 2006. Early medical history of children with autism spectrum disorders. *J. Dev. Behav. Pediatr.* 27:S120–S127.

Panksepp, J. 1979. Neurochemical theory of autism. *Trends Neurosci.* 2:174–177.

Parracho, H. M., M. O. Bingham, G. R. Gibson, and A. L. McCartney. 2005. Differences between the gut microflora of children with autistic spectrum disorders and that of healthy children. *J. Med. Microbiol.* 54:987–991.

Plioplys, A. V., A. Greaves, K. Kazemi, and E. Silverman. 1994. Lymphocyte function in autism and Rett syndrome. *Neuropsychobiology* 29:12–16.

Ringel, Y. and D. A. Drossman. 2001. Psychosocial aspects of Crohn's disease. *Surg. Clin. North Am.* 81:231–252.

Ringel, Y. and D. A. Drossman. 2002. Irritable bowel syndrome: Classification and conceptualization. *J. Clin. Gastroenterol.* 35:S7–S10.

Rogers, S. W., P. I. Andrews, L. C. Gahring, T. Whisenand, K. Cauley, B. Crain, T. E. Hughes, S. F. Heinemann, and J. O. McNamara. 1994. Autoantibodies to glutamate receptor GluR3 in Rasmussen's encephalitis. *Science* 265:648–651.

Rosen, N. J., C. K. Yoshida, and L. A. Croen. 2007. Infection in the first 2 years of life and autism spectrum disorders. *Pediatrics* 119:61–69.

Singer, H. S., C. M. Morris, P. N. Williams, D. Y. Yoon, J. J. Hong, and A. W. Zimmerman. 2006. Antibrain antibodies in children with autism and their unaffected siblings. *J. Neuroimmunol.* 178:149–155.

Singer, H. S., C. M. Morris, C. D. Gause, P. K. Gillin, S. Crawford, and A. W. Zimmerman. 2008. Antibodies against fetal brain in sera of mothers with autistic children. *J. Neuroimmunol.* 194:165–172.

Singh, V. K. 1996. Plasma increase of interleukin-12 and interferon-gamma. Pathological significance in autism. *J. Neuroimmunol.* 66:143–145.

Singh, V. K. and W. H. Rivas. 2004. Prevalence of serum antibodies to caudate nucleus in autistic children. *Neurosci. Lett.* 355:53–56.

Singh, V. K., E. A. Singh, and R. P. Warren. 1997. Hyperserotoninemia and serotonin receptor antibodies in children with autism but not mental retardation. *Biol. Psychiatry* 41:753–755.

Singh, V. K., S. Mehrotra, and S. S. Agarwal. 1999. The paradigm of Th1 and Th2 cytokines: its relevance to autoimmunity and allergy. *Immunol. Res.* 20:147–161.

Singh, V. K., R. P. Warren, J. D. Odell, W. L. Warren, and P. Cole. 1993. Antibodies to myelin basic protein in children with autistic behavior. *Brain Behav. Immun.* 7:97–103.

Singh, V. K., R. Warren, R. Averett, and M. Ghaziuddin. 1997. Circulating autoantibodies to neuronal and glial filament proteins in autism. *Pediatr. Neurol.* 17:88–90.

Smith, S. E., J. Li, K. Garbett, K. Mirnics, and P. H. Patterson. 2007. Maternal immune activation alters fetal brain development through interleukin-6. *J. Neurosci.* 27:10695–10702.

Spiller, R. C., D. Jenkins, J. P. Thornley, J. M. Hebden, T. Wright, M. Skinner, and K. R. Neal. 2000. Increased rectal mucosal enteroendocrine cells, T lymphocytes, and increased gut permeability following acute *Campylobacter enteritis* and in post-dysenteric irritable bowel syndrome. *Gut* 47:804–811.

Stahl, S. M. 1977. The human platelet. A diagnostic and research tool for the study of biogenic amines in psychiatric and neurologic disorders. *Arch. Gen. Psychiatry* 34:509–516.

Stubbs, E. G. and M. L. Crawford. 1977. Depressed lymphocyte responsiveness in autistic children. *J. Autism Child Schizophr.* 7:49–55.

Sweeten, T. L., D. J. Posey, and C. J. McDougle. 2003. High blood monocyte counts and neopterin levels in children with autistic disorder. *Am. J. Psychiatry* 160:1691–1693.

Sweeten, T. L., S. L. Bowyer, D. J. Posey, G. M. Halberstadt, and C. J. McDougle. 2003. Increased prevalence of familial autoimmunity in probands with pervasive developmental disorders. *Pediatrics* 112:e420.

Sweeten, T. L., D. J. Posey, S. Shankar, and C. J. McDougle. 2004. High nitric oxide production in autistic disorder: A possible role for interferon-gamma. *Biol. Psychiatry* 55:434–437.

Taniai, H., T. Nishiyama, T. Miyachi, M. Imaeda, and S. Sumi. 2008. Genetic influences on the broad spectrum of autism: Study of proband-ascertained twins. *Am. J. Med. Genet. B. Neuropsychiatr. Genet.* 147B:844–849.

Todd, R. D. and R. D. Ciaranello. 1985. Demonstration of inter- and intraspecies differences in serotonin binding sites by antibodies from an autistic child. *Proc. Natl. Acad. Sci. U.S.A.* 82:612–616.

Todd, R. D., J. M. Hickok, G. M. Anderson, and D. J. Cohen. 1988. Antibrain antibodies in infantile autism. *Biol. Psychiatry* 23:644–647.

Tohmi, M., N. Tsuda, Y. Watanabe, A. Kakita, and H. Nawa. 2004. Perinatal inflammatory cytokine challenge results in distinct neurobehavioral alterations in rats: Implication in psychiatric disorders of developmental origin. *Neurosci. Res.* 50:67–75.

Torrente, F., P. Ashwood, R. Day, N. Machado, R. I. Furlano, A. Anthony, S. E. Davies, A. J. Wakefield, M. A. Thomson, J. A. Walker-Smith, and S. H. Murch. 2002. Small intestinal enteropathy with epithelial IgG and complement deposition in children with regressive autism. *Mol. Psychiatry* 7:375–382, 334.

Torrente, F., A. Anthony, R. B. Heuschkel, M. A. Thomson, P. Ashwood, and S. H. Murch. 2004. Focal-enhanced gastritis in regressive autism with features distinct from Crohn's and Helicobacter pylori gastritis. *Am. J. Gastroenterol.* 99:598–605.

Torres, A. R., T. L. Sweeten, A. Cutler, B. J. Bedke, M. Fillmore, E. G. Stubbs, and D. Odell. 2006. The association and linkage of the HLA-A2 class I allele with autism. *Hum. Immunol.* 67:346–351.

Valicenti-McDermott, M., K. McVicar, I. Rapin, B. K. Wershil, H. Cohen, and S. Shinnar. 2006. Frequency of gastrointestinal symptoms in children with autistic spectrum disorders and association with family history of autoimmune disease. *J. Dev. Behav. Pediatr.* 27:S128–S136.

Vargas, D. L., C. Nascimbene, C. Krishnan, A. W. Zimmerman, and C. A. Pardo. 2005. Neuroglial activation and neuroinflammation in the brain of patients with autism. *Ann. Neurol.* 57:67–81.

Vereker, E., E. O'Donnell, and M. A. Lynch. 2000. The inhibitory effect of interleukin-1beta on long-term potentiation is coupled with increased activity of stress-activated protein kinases. *J. Neurosci.* 20:6811–6819.

Vojdani, A., A. W. Campbell, E. Anyanwu, A. Kashanian, K. Bock, and E. Vojdani. 2002. Antibodies to neuron-specific antigens in children with autism: Possible cross-reaction with encephalitogenic proteins from milk, *Chlamydia pneumoniae* and *Streptococcus* group A. *J. Neuroimmunol.* 129:168–177.

Wakefield, A. J. 2002. The gut-brain axis in childhood developmental disorders. *J. Pediatr. Gastroenterol. Nutr.* 34(Suppl. 1):S14–S17.

Wakefield, A. J., A. Anthony, S. H. Murch, M. Thomson, S. M. Montgomery, S. Davies, J. J. O'Leary, M. Berelowitz, and J. A. Walker-Smith. 2000. Enterocolitis in children with developmental disorders. *Am. J. Gastroenterol.* 95:2285–2295.

Wakefield, A.J., P. Ashwood, K. Limb, and A. Anthony. 2005. The significance of ileo-colonic lymphoid nodular hyperplasia in children with autistic spectrum disorder. *Eur. J. Gastroenterol.* 17:827–836.

Walker-Smith J. and J. Andrews. 1972. Alpha-1-antitrypsin, autism, and coeliac disease. *Lancet* 2:883–884.

Wang, W., S. Uzzau, S. E. Goldblum, and A. Fasano. 2000. Human zonulin, a potential modulator of intestinal tight junctions. *J. Cell. Sci.* 113 (Pt. 24):4435–4440.

Warren, R. P., A. Foster, and N. C. Margaretten. 1987. Reduced natural killer cell activity in autism. *J. Am. Acad. Child Adolesc. Psychiatry* 26:333–335.

Warren, R. P., J. D. Odell, W. L. Warren, R. A. Burger, A. Maciulius, W. W. Daniels, and A. R. Torres. 1996. Strong association of the third hypervariable region of HLA-DR beta 1 with autism. *J. Neuroimmunol.* 67:259–274.

Warren, R. P., L. J. Yonk, R. A. Burger, P. Cole, J. D. Odell, W. L. Warren, E. White, and V. K. Singh. 1990. Deficiency of suppressor-inducer (CD4+ CD45RA+) T cells in autism. *Immunol. Invest.* 19:245–251.

Warren, R. P., V. K. Singh, P. Cole, J. D. Odell, C. B. Pingree, W. L. Warren, C. W. DeWitt, and M. McCullough. 1992. Possible association of the extended MHC haplotype B44-SC30-DR4 with autism. *Immunogenetics* 36:203–207.

Warren, R. P., J. Yonk, R. W. Burger, D. Odell, and W. L. Warren. 1995. DR-positive T cells in autism: Association with decreased plasma levels of the complement C4B protein. *Neuropsychobiology* 31:53–57.

Watts, T., I. Berti, A. Sapone, T. Gerarduzzi, T. Not, R. Zielke, and A. Fasano. 2005. Role of the intestinal tight junction modulator zonulin in the pathogenesis of type I diabetes in BB diabetic-prone rats. *Proc. Natl. Acad. Sci. U.S.A.* 102:2916–2921.

Weizman, A., R. Weizman, G. A. Szekely, H. Wijsenbeek, and E. Livni. 1982. Abnormal immune response to brain tissue antigen in the syndrome of autism. *Am. J. Psychiatry* 139:1462–1465.

Welch, M. G., T. B. Welch-Horan, M. Anwar, N. Anwar, R. J. Ludwig, and D. A. Ruggiero. 2005. Brain effects of chronic IBD in areas abnormal in autism and treatment by single neuropeptides secretin and oxytocin. *J. Mol. Neurosci.* 25:259–274.

White, J. F. 2003. Intestinal pathophysiology in autism. *Exp. Biol. Med.* 228:639–649.

Wills, S., M. Cabanlit, J. Bennett, P. Ashwood, D. Amaral, and J. Van de Water. 2007. Autoantibodies in autism spectrum disorders (ASD). *Ann. N.Y. Acad. Sci.* 1107:79–91.

Yamada, K., R. Iida, Y. Miyamoto, K. Saito, K. Sekikawa, M. Seishima, and T. Nabeshima. 2000. Neurobehavioral alterations in mice with a targeted deletion of the tumor necrosis factor-alpha gene: Implications for emotional behavior. *J. Neuroimmunol.* 111:131–138.

Yonk, L. J., R. P. Warren, R. A. Burger, P. Cole, J. D. Odell, W. L. Warren, E. White, and V. K. Singh. 1990. CD4+ helper T cell depression in autism. *Immunol. Lett.* 25:341–345.

15 Possible Mechanism Involving Intestinal Oxytocin, Oxidative Stress, and Signaling Pathways in a Subset of Autism with Gut Symptoms

Martha G. Welch[1,2]* and Benjamin Y. Klein[1,2]

[1]Division of Developmental Neuroscience, Department of Psychiatry and [2]Department of Pathology and Cell Biology, Columbia University Medical Center, New York, NY 10032, USA

CONTENTS

* Corresponding author: Tel.: +1-212-543-5101; fax: +1-212-253-4234; e-mail: mgw13@columbia.edu

15.1 INTRODUCTION

The working hypothesis of our laboratory is that developmental disorders such as autism arise from the dysregulation of a unified gut/brain system, rather than originating in the brain alone. Indeed, 70% of autistic children suffer from at least one chronic gastrointestinal (GI) symptom (Horvath et al., 1999), potentially sorting this group as a subset of autism.

The question of oxytocin (OT) deficiency as a contributing factor in autism was raised over 15 years ago (Modahl et al., 1992). Recent findings have established OT's importance in modulating stress and predict its importance to gut/brain development. OT's antistress (Uvnas-Moberg and Petersson, 2005) and anti-inflammatory properties (Iseri et al., 2005; Petersson et al., 2001) are well known. OT is present in mother's milk. There is an early exposure of the GI tract to this peptide (Stefanidis et al., 2008). OT antagonists alter gut motility (Monstein et al., 2004). To understand how OT deficiency might contribute to the development of autism, one must almost certainly examine stress physiology in the gut. At the cellular level, this means oxidative stress.

Oxidative stress is defined as an imbalance between the generation of reactive oxygen species (ROS) and the decreased antioxidant defense systems. We hypothesize that autism stems from physiological stress, including oxidative stress, which if unmodulated triggers a cascade of adverse interrelated autonomic, endocrinological, neurological, and immunological reactions.

This chapter examines how the deficiency of OT combined with oxidative stress in the gut might dysregulate a unified gut/brain network. It reviews evidence that OT levels and signaling pathways downstream of the oxytocin receptor (OTR) may be involved in the excitatory drive of gut/brain signaling and thereby in the pathogenesis of a subset of autism. It discusses the role of oxidative stress in autism and the possible contribution of differential responses to hypoxia in preterm and full-term infants. Finally, it presents a theoretical framework and cellular mechanism for the modulation of gut/brain signaling by OT and discusses possible implications for the treatment of autism and developmental disorders, specifically those with comorbid GI symptoms and/or inflammation.

15.2 OT SYNTHESIS

Initially, the site of OT synthesis was considered to be restricted to the hypothalamus, where it is synthesized as a preprohormone (Brownstein, 1983). The preprohormone is subsequently cleaved into two bioactive peptides: OT close to the N-terminus and neurophysin from the C-terminus (Gainer et al., 1977a). The OT and neurophysin precursors are converted into bioactive peptides during axonal translocation to the neurohypophysis (Gainer et al., 1977b). Like several other neuropeptides, OT becomes bioactive and resistant to degradation by having its C-terminus amidated (Prigge et al., 1997). Additional tissues have been reported as sites of synthesis and secretion of OT. The mRNA and OT peptide were found in vasculature (Jankowski et al., 2000) and cardiac myocytes consistent with its involvement in the control of vessel tonus and the secretion of atrial natriuretic peptide (Gutkowska et al., 2000).

OT transcription has been detected in the chorio-decidual tissue, increasing threefold during labor (Chibbar et al., 1993). OT is also synthesized in the uterus during pregnancy (Mitchell et al., 1998). This peptide synthesis occurs under estrogen/ progesterone control in two forms, one with an extended C-terminus and very low receptor binding activity, and the other with an amidated C-terminus, which is fully active. Such amidation results in improved stability and receptor binding (Blankenfeldt et al., 1996; Fuhlendorff et al., 1990). During synthesis in the uterus, OT is not coupled to neurophysin as it is in the hypothalamus (Fuhlendorff et al., 1990). OT is also synthesized in myoepithelial and mammary epithelial cells along with OTR (Cassoni et al., 2006). OT and OTR in the mammary gland are active in milk letdown and in the trafficking of milk proteins to the Golgi compartment during lactation (Lollivier et al., 2006). OT is thus present in the milk and could potentially affect intestinal epithelium immediately after birth, when OTR becomes expressed in the GI tract. OTR mRNA is expressed by the cells in human amniotic fluid (Stefanidis et al., 2008) and since OT expression in humans has been detected in the chorion, in the amnion, and weakly in the placenta (Chibbar et al., 1993), one could expect that during fetal life, the GI epithelial OTR gene is already being primed for expression by exposure to amniotic OT. The presence of OT in meconium (Leake et al., 1981) further suggests early GI exposure to the hormone.

Whether OT synthesis occurs in human embryonic gut is yet to be determined. In adult humans, biopsies taken from intact GI tract tissue showed immunoreactivity of OT in myenteric and submucosal nerve cells (Ohlsson et al., 2006). These biopsies showed the presence of OT mRNA by polymerase chain reaction (PCR) and northern blots (Monstein et al., 2004). This suggests that at least the GI and/or adjacent tissues express the OT gene. These studies were done on GI tissue from aging humans (seventh to ninth decades). However, if the newborn GI tract responds to OT, then OTR is expected to be expressed in the enterocytes.

15.3 EXPRESSION AND ACTIVATION OF OTR

OTR is a seven transmembrane G protein-coupled receptor. The OTR gene promoter contains a variety of cis elements responsive to estrogen receptor, cyclic adenosine monophosphate (AMP) binding protein, and activator protein transcription factors (Bale and Dorsa, 1998). The gene itself responds to interleukins and is under epigenetic regulation by methylation and histone acetylation (Kusui et al., 2001). OTR is expressed in tissues targeted by OT, for example, in mammary gland cells (Cassoni et al., 2006), in cardiovascular tissue (Jankowski et al., 2000), and in the uterus (Mitchell et al., 1998). Although transcripts of OTR have been identified in elderly adult GI tissue (Monstein et al., 2004), its protein has not been detected in intestinal epithelium by immunoreagents (Ohlsson et al., 2006). Thus, it is not clear in which GI tract compartment the OTR is expressed in elderly humans. It should also be noted that no data are available for the expression of OTR in human neonates and young adults.

OTR activation by OT inhibits the growth of cells derived from neural, breast epithelium, endometrium, and bone tissues (Cassoni et al., 2001a). In contrast,

OT induces growth in trophoblasts (Cassoni et al., 2001b) and small lung cancer cells (Pequeux et al., 2004). The growth inhibition mediated by OTR was shown to be transduced via cyclic AMP and protein kinase A, whereas growth stimulation was transduced via Ca^{2+} flux and protein kinase C (Cassoni et al., 2001a). This dual activity of OT could also be due to the differential activation of OTR at varying concentrations of OT.

OT concentrations in breast milk increase above those in serum several days postpartum (Leake et al., 1981). Therefore, one would expect the upper GI tract epithelium of the normal breastfed neonate would be exposed to exogenous OT and/or its fragments. If the contact between GI epithelium luminal surface and OT has a physiological significance, then OTR could be expressed somewhere along the GI tract, at least during the neonatal period if not during the entire breastfeeding period.

Indeed, our laboratory has recently shown that OTR is expressed in the epithelium of colon, in the small intestinal villi, in the muscularis mucosa, and in the myenteric neuronal cells in rat newborns (Welch et al., 2009). We have also shown that OTR expression is developmentally regulated. In fact, transcripts of both OT and OTR mRNA peak at postnatal day 7 in rat pups. This pattern of OTR expression in the GI tract could be induced either by endogenous OT from the gut or other sources and/or by exogenous OT from breast milk.

We hypothesize from our experiments to date that the pattern of OTR expression in the mucosal smooth muscles and the autonomous neural plexus implies developmental induction. This expression may also imply the conditioning of gut/brain sensory networks and later functional maintenance, for example, of peristaltic intestinal movements. However, the biological functional advantage of OTR expression in the absorptive enterocytes (villus epithelium) is not clear and its elucidation will require further experiments.

The temporal changes of OTR in the villi suggest that OT/OTR is required for a brief time window, perhaps to regulate the villus maturation process. In rodents, villi develop during the first 2 weeks postpartum (Porter et al., 2002). Our data show that after postnatal day 14, OTR gut expression in rat pups appeared in the crypts and at the crypt–villus junctions where the immature precursors of the crypts develop into functioning villus absorptive cells (Welch et al., 2009). Although this distribution is compatible with the possibility that OT/OTR signaling affects or regulates epithelial maturation, other crypt cells that might also be regulated include Paneth cells and secretory cells.

15.4   OXYTOCIN LEVELS AND OXYTOCIN RECEPTOR IN AUTISM

With the rationale that brain functions controlled by OT coincide with those impaired in autism, OT nasal spray was used to treat autism: preliminary data reported improvement in autistic adults' repetitive behavior relative to placebo (Bartz and Hollander, 2008). The tissue target of OT nasal spray is not known. In any case, there is no indication that OT has acted via GI OTR. Still in question is whether OT acts as mediator between gut and brain regarding specific features of autism. Whatever the target tissue, it is evident that OT plays a role in autism.

There is additional evidence that OT is broadly important in development. OT levels and OTR distribution have been found to correlate with long-term bonding between monogamous and polygamous animals (Hammock and Young, 2006). Single nucleotide polymorphism in the OTR gene ass ociated with autism supports the importance of OT in the pathology of this syndrome (Wu et al., 2005). Interestingly, abnormal newborn delivery may be associated with anomalies in OT secretion. For example, delivery under local anesthesia (Krehbiel et al., 1987) or general anesthesia during cesarean section (Marchini et al., 1988) is associated with low OT. These modern in-hospital obstetric and pediatric procedures interfere with infant suckling responses (Ransjo-Arvidson et al., 2001) and maternal milk let down (Matthiesen et al., 2001), both of which are related to OT release. These challenges to perinatal OT release could add to the risk of developmental disorders including autism.

15.5   AUTISM AND OXIDATIVE STRESS

The mechanisms underlying autism are yet to be defined. Autism is diagnosed based upon various behavioral criteria such as impaired social interaction and communication, and repetitive behaviors. Current autism research is largely focused on identifying genetic and biochemical abnormalities that will serve as diagnostic markers. Such markers are needed to facilitate the highly complicated diagnosis of this disorder and may also lead to understanding its etiology. Several genetic mutations have been associated with autism spectrum disorders (Sebat et al., 2007), suggesting that these behaviorally defined diseases share a disruption of a biological process rather than a single mutation.

Oxidative stress can be identified in a subset of autistic children (Oliveira et al., 2005). Numerous oxidative stress markers in autism were comprehensively reviewed by Chauhan and Chauhan (2006) and McGinnis (2004). Lactic acidemia suggested defects in mitochondrial oxidative phosphorylation and electron transfer complexes (Filipek et al., 2003; Lombard, 1998). Other investigators found decreases in the ratio of reduced/oxidized glutathione in the circulation, with abnormal methionine trans-methylation and transsulfuration pathways (James et al., 2004, 2006). These reveal a susceptibility to chronic oxidative stress in autistic children. Interestingly, parents who lack the autistic phenotype have been shown to exhibit markers of susceptibility to oxidative stress that are similar to their autistic children (James et al., 2008). These findings suggest that metabolic susceptibility to oxidative stress may be either a contributor to autism or part of its mechanism. However, they are per se insufficient to cause clinical manifestations specific to autism.

The presence of ROS and the lack of molecular scavengers that underlies susceptibility to oxidative stress are nonspecific to any single disease. Therefore, one should search for anomalies specific to autism that associate with oxidative stress. One such anomaly is the progressive increase of brain volume in autistic infants (Courchesne et al., 2003; Hardan et al., 2001), presumably resulting from cell packing in the cortex. The histological basis of this phenomenon has been named "mini columns," referring to augmented connections between the neurons in cortical stratifications (Casanova et al., 2006). In addition, brain blood perfusion is diminished in regions important for the development of language capability (Ohnishi et al., 2000; Wilcox et al., 2002). This finding raises the possibility that the hyper-connectivity between neurons in the cortex associated with cell packing, together with reduced blood perfusion, may result in hyperactive neurons on one hand and lower oxygenation on the other. Such partial hypoxia could induce oxidative stress, forming ROS in mitochondria. This sequence could exemplify a nonspecific marker resulting from an autism-specific mini-column phenomenon.

A possible anomaly that could connect autism to oxidative stress is a disruption of the secretion of OT hormone by the newborn hypophysis during labor. Areas in the newborn brain undergo aglycemia and hypoxia during labor, which can lead to neuronal death (Carbillon, 2007). Normally, neuronal death is inhibited by OT-induced switch-off of neuronal firing by gamma aminobutyric acid (GABA) in the brain (Cossart et al., 2006; Tyzio et al., 2006). However, a shortage of OT or the dysfunction of its receptor might contribute to oxidative stress. Of interest to our laboratory is whether the OT/OTR signaling system has a comparable cell-survival function in peripheral organs, particularly the gut, which might be compromised during episodes of perinatal hypoxia when blood flow may be preferentially distributed to the brain (Dyess et al., 1998). Also of great interest is the origin of OT regulating the brain GABA switch. OT was shown to be of maternal origin (Khazipov et al., 2008; Tyzio et al., 2008), but evidence suggests that endogenous fetal OT may be induced by perinatal hypoxia (Carbillon, 2007).

It is logical to assume that the excitatory-to-inhibitory switch in GABA receptor responses to stimulation may not occur by the time of birth in premature infants, inasmuch as this process is normally completed near the time of full-term delivery (Tyzio et al., 2008). Given the effects of OT on mechanisms regulating concentrations of intracellular chloride, which in turn moves the GABA receptor bias toward inhibition (Khazipov et al., 2008), we speculate that the up-regulation of the premature infant OT system through high nurture may promote the maturation of this important neurophysiologic process. If so, we would expect to find this evidence in markers of neural function that would include the normalization of patterns of electroencephalogram development as well as behavior.

15.6 POSSIBLE CONTRIBUTION OF OXIDATIVE STRESS TO GI ASPECTS OF AUTISM

Several factors involving oxidative stress, such as low glutathione, prematurity, and gut inflammation, could individually or collectively predispose an infant to developmental disorders such as autism. One major finding in autistic patients is low glutathione levels in the circulation (James et al., 2004, 2006), which is a reflection of its synthetic biochemical pathway. Glutathione is an important scavenger of ROS, which is generated in excess by complex III of the mitochondrial electron transfer chain under hypoxic conditions (Klimova and Chandel, 2008). Hypoxia during the prenatal period could result in oxidative stress to the gut when cerebral and cardiac blood flow is increased and small-intestinal blood flow is decreased.

During hypoxic stress in a premature animal model, critical brain and heart perfusion is maintained by the redistribution of blood flow away from skin, muscle, and viscera including the gut. While small-intestinal perfusion returns to 97% of baseline after hypoxia in full-term neonates, perfusion returns to only 50% in preterm piglets; this differential gut response to hypoxia in full-term versus preterm animals suggests a mechanism for increased risk of intestinal ischemic disease in preterm human neonates (Dyess et al., 1998). Perinatal hypoxia also suggests a mechanism that could contribute to the increased risk of autism with or without diagnosed GI involvement in a vulnerable preterm population (Limperopoulos et al., 2008).

In addition to premature birth, inflammatory bowel disease can cause hypoxia to the intestine (Hauser et al., 1988). Since OT has a protective effect against hypoxia in the brain (Carbillon, 2007), one could reasonably predict its protective effect against hypoxia in the gut. In such cases, the abnormally low levels of gut OT could lead to chronic inflammation in gut colitis. Indeed, evidence supporting this hypothesis may be provided in an organ system that synthesizes OT and OTR. In a rat model of renal ischemia/reperfusion injury, OT protects against oxidative stress (Biyikli et al., 2006).

Further evidence supporting the role of OT in colitis is provided by findings in our laboratory. We have shown that experimental induction of colitis (oxidative stress) by means of trinitrobenzene sulfonic acid elicited inflammation-related early gene responses in central nervous system nuclei (Welch et al., 2005). Gut/brain signaling measured by c-*fos* activation was inhibited by combined OT/secretin treatment (Welch, unpublished results) in brain areas known to be abnormal in autism (Bauman and Kemper, 1985, 2003; Buchsbaum et al., 2001; Chugani et al., 1997; Rumsey and Ernst, 2000; Sparks et al., 2002; Vargas et al., 2005). Since intestinal inflammation is associated with ROS production in the gut (Ardite et al., 2000), these findings suggest that abnormal gut/brain interactions might be involved in the mechanisms underlying autism.

15.7 PROPOSED CELLULAR MECHANISM IN GUT/BRAIN SIGNALING

ROS has been shown to negatively regulate the Wnt-dependent β-catenin signaling pathway by increasing neuroredoxin (Funato and Miki, 2007). Wnt-dependent β-catenin signaling pathway is a major player in the control of enterocyte proliferation and differentiation. After birth, Wnt, which activates Tcf4-induced transcription (Pinto and Clevers, 2005a), maintains a constant stem cell reservoir at the crypt–villus junction. Thus, epithelial proliferation induced by Wnt provides a constant supply of new absorptive enterocytes that migrate to the tip of the villi where they undergo apoptosis every 3–4 days (Pinto and Clevers, 2005b). Concurrently, Paneth cells migrate in the opposite direction to the bottom of the crypts.

The Wnt-dependent β-catenin pathway is balanced by the bone morphogenetic proteins (BMPs). BMPs, secreted by intravillus mesenchymal cells, activate small mother against decapentaplegic (SMAD) nuclear factors in the epithelium to attenuate epithelial proliferation (Haramis et al., 2004). Remarkably, during crypt development, intensities of crypt OTR expression coincide with crypt BMP4 expression found by others (Haramis et al., 2004). Given the dual effects of OT in activating or inhibiting cell proliferation (Cassoni et al., 2001a), it is possible that OT is cooperating with BMP4 in the regulation of Wnt signaling in perinatal structural and functional development of intestinal villi. Interestingly, BMP4 positively controls the clustering of enteric neurons during development via the induction of extracellular matrix protein–specific sialylation (Faure et al., 2007). This BMP4 activity occurs contemporaneously with OTR protein expression detected in the enteric neurons of newborn rats (Welch et al., 2009).

In addition to the absorptive enterocytes that line the villus surface, equally relevant to our hypothesis are the Paneth cells that line the crypts. Biopsies show that Paneth cells are larger and more numerous in autistic children than in normal controls (Horvath et al., 1999). Paneth cells are part of the innate local immune system. Like macrophages and granulocytes (Ganz and Lehrer, 1994), they provide defense against microbes in the small intestine. When exposed to bacteria or bacterial antigens, Paneth cells secrete a number of antimicrobial molecules into the lumen of the crypt, thereby contributing to the maintenance of the GI barrier. Specifically, Paneth cells contain granules that store precursors of bactericidal peptides, which upon trypsin cleavage secrete defensins into the lumen to kill pathogenic microorganisms (Ghosh et al., 2002). Defensins are even present in Paneth cells of germ-free animals and therefore may have additional functions besides killing pathogens (Putsep et al., 2000). According to Putsep et al (2000): "it is possible that on the crypt level, the release of enteric defensins is induced by bacteria and bacterial components, whereas on the organism level, neural or hormonal signaling could add additional levels of regulation of defensin-producing Paneth cells." We suspect that defensins may have a central nervous system (CNS)-protective role during gut inflammatory-induced oxidative stress, based on an in vitro defensin interaction with ganglionic neurons (Plakhova et al., 2002), as discussed below.

Under conditions of hypoxia, Paneth cells could undergo the inhibition of degranulation and the accumulation of defensin precursors, due to decreased matrix metalloproteinase-7 (MMP7). The MMP-7 gene is a transcription target of β-catenin/Tcf-1 transacting complex factors (Brabletz et al., 1999). This relationship is reflected by its over-expression in colon cancer (Ougolkov et al., 2002), where it co-localizes with β-catenin accumulation in the nuclei of dark crypt precancerous cells (Lu et al., 2008). MMP-7 has been shown to induce defensin secretion in Paneth cells (Satchell et al., 2003), where it cleaves the active defensin from its precursor (Weeks et al., 2006). It is interesting to note that autistic children with GI inflammation have 50% more Paneth cells, that are also larger in volume, than do controls (Horvath et al., 1999). Perhaps not coincidental is the fact that Paneth cells in cases of necrotizing enterocolitis (NEC) in premature infants are also increased twofold in number; despite an increase in human defensin 5 (HD5) mRNA, the intracellular levels of HD5 peptide appeared constant, consistent with the possibility that defensin mRNA translation is inhibited (Salzman et al., 1998). Additionally, as we will postulate in autism (vide infra), it is possible that prodefensin is not being cleaved to defensin. It would be important to examine the data from the cohort of 91 premature infants reported to meet diagnostic criteria for autism spectrum disorders at age 2 (26%) (Limperopoulos et al., 2008) to correlate the relationship, if any, between NEC and later autism spectrum disorder in that premature population.

It is not known how a change in defensin levels could be connected to the disease mechanism and associated oxidative stress. However, an intriguing recent observation may provide a clue. It has been shown in rat dorsal ganglion neuronal culture that sodium currents are attenuated by defensin interaction with the channel protein (Plakhova et al., 2002). During chronic gut inflammation and associated oxidative stress, one can postulate that the augmented firing of ganglionic afferent currents could strongly stimulate nuclei in the brain. If such stimuli occur immediately after birth under conditions that inhibit the attenuation of neuronal sodium currents, noxious stimuli may persist chronically and greatly affect neuronal centers in the brain. The "readout" or imprinting of such chronic and unattenuated intense stimuli could induce epigenetic patterns of gene expression that result in an autistic epigenetically induced phenotype.

15.8 PROPOSED ROLE OF LOW OXYTOCIN IN THE GENERATION OF AN AUTISM PHENOTYPE

Hypothetically, it is possible that in association with hypoxic oxidative stress of GI inflammation, defensin diffusion to ganglion neural cells is greatly diminished because low MMP7 expression reduces the processing of defensin precursors to become active peptides. This could presumably inhibit the release of defensin, which functions to attenuate the afferent noxious stimuli via ganglionic neuronal channels (Figure 15.1) in addition to its canonical function as an antimicrobial peptide.

Two pathways could negatively regulate defensins. The first is BMP over-expression and the second is dysregulated OT levels. BMP4 restricts enteric neuronal numbers and negatively regulates the Wnt pathway in GI epithelium during villus/crypt

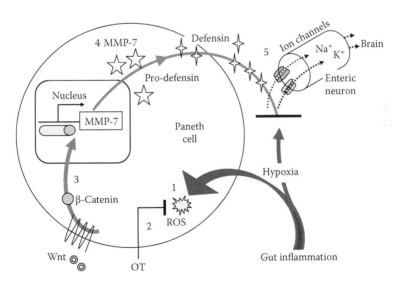

FIGURE 15.1 Possible mechanism in Paneth cell for the modulation of gut inflammation by OT in normal newborns. Hypoxia from gut inflammation stimulates the production of ROS within Paneth cell (1). OT inhibits ROS and/or its effect (2), enabling a Wnt-dependent β-catenin pathway (3). β-catenin in the nucleus transcribes MMP-7, which is then translocated to the cytosol where it catalyzes the cleavage of prodefensin to activate α-defensin (4). The active α-defensin theoretically permeates to enteric neurons to attenuate currents through various ion channels (Na^+ and K^+), thus dampening signaling of hypoxia-induced noxious stimuli to the brain (5).

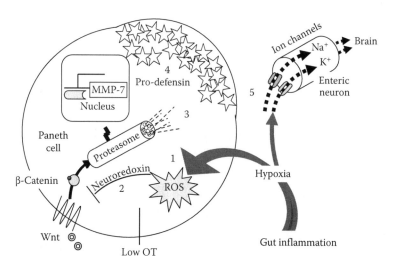

FIGURE 15.2   Possible mechanism in Paneth cell for the dysregulation of gut/brain signaling under the condition of low OT levels in newborns at risk for autism. Hypoxia from gut inflammation stimulates the production of ROS within Paneth cell (1). If OT level is inadequate to counter ROS production, ROS induces neuroredoxin, which in turn inhibits Wnt pathway (2). As a result, β-catenin transcription factor becomes tagged by phosphorylation (small red dot) and degraded by the proteasome (3). Without β-catenin in nucleus, MMP-7 gene is not expressed and defensin precursor peptide granulations (large stars) accumulate within the cell (4). Without the attenuation provided by defensin, hypoxia-induced excitation of ion channels in enteric neurons may drive noxious gut/brain signaling pathways (5).

development (Chalazonitis et al., 2008). Over-expression of BMP could inhibit Wnt and result in intensive afferent stimuli that target brain areas abnormal in autism. Hypothetically, if unchecked, this pattern of hyperstimulation could provide the basis for an autistic phenotype with gut symptoms.

Alternatively, in the absence of the adequate OT inhibition of ROS, gut inflammation-induced oxidative stress could lead to the same outcome as above; although in this case, it would occur via the inhibition of the Wnt pathway by the ROS up-regulation of neuroredoxin and then to a similar decrease in defensin expression with failure to inhibit the excitation of ion channels in enteric neurons that drive afferent stimulation to the brain (Figure 15.2). Moreover, the combined effects of abnormal BMP expression together with impaired OT/OTR signaling in the presence of ROS from gut inflammation or hypoxia could set the stage for gut/brain dysregulation in a subset of autism with gut symptoms.

15.9   POSSIBLE IMPLICATIONS FOR THE TREATMENT OF AUTISM AND DEVELOPMENTAL DISORDERS

The hypothesized role of oxidative stress and OT in the regulation of gut/brain signaling pathways and in the generation of autism and developmental disorders raises interesting questions about possible early interventions that could be effective in the prevention of the diseases. Epigenetic imprinting by nurture might contribute to the regulation of OT levels through activities that are known to stimulate the synthesis and release of OT, such as breastfeeding, holding, and touching (Howard et al., 2006; Uvnas-Moberg, 1996).

This idea is supported by animal models of nurture. Nurturing activities in humans may be analogous to intense licking and grooming (L/G) in animal models: L/G of pups by their high nurture mothers provides stress-attenuating afferent sensory stimuli by demethylation of the steroid hormone receptor gene in an experimental behavioral animal model of epigenetic imprinting (Champagne and Curley, 2009; Champagne et al., 2006; Weaver et al., 2007). The offspring of high licking mothers showed reduced stress profiles, which continued into adulthood.

If gut symptoms in autism are a precursor or marker of the disorder, then it is logical to propose early interventions aimed at the OT-related mechanism postulated in this chapter. Such OT-related interventions would most certainly target activities that are known to regulate OT levels in the newborn infant, for example, natural childbirth without anesthesia (Krehbiel et al., 1987), mother/infant holding, breastfeeding, and nurture (Howard et al., 2006; Uvnas-Moberg, 1996). Interestingly, the literature supports the idea that the absence of these activities of mother/infant nurture is associated with a high incidence of autism. For example, preterm infants are by necessity socially isolated because of the life-sustaining controlled environment of neonatal intensive care. Though a causal connection between such low nurture and autism is yet to be proven, a high incidence (26%) of autism spectrum disorders has been reported in preterm infants, as compared to normal children (0.7%) (Limperopoulos et al., 2008). Yet another population suffering from very low nurture—Romanian orphans from the 1980s and 1990s—is similarly associated with a high incidence (one third) of developmental disorders including autism (Hoksbergen et al., 2005). Future studies must confirm or refute our hypothesis. However, given the extent of the autism burden we are facing, we believe there is sufficient evidence at this time to justify further investigation of the interrelated roles of oxidative stress, OT, and autism with GI involvement.

REFERENCES

Ardite E., M. Sans, J. Panes, F. J. Romero, J. M. Pique, and J. C. Fernandez-Checa. 2000. Replenishment of glutathione levels improves mucosal function in experimental acute colitis. *Lab. Invest.* 80:735–744.

Bale T. L. and D. M. Dorsa. 1998. NGF, cyclic AMP, and phorbol esters regulate oxytocin receptor gene transcription in SK-N-SH and MCF7 cells. *Brain Res. Mol. Brain Res.* 53:130–137.

Bartz J. A. and E. Hollander. 2008. Oxytocin and experimental therapeutics in autism spectrum disorders. *Prog. Brain Res.* 170:451–462.

Bauman M. L. and T. L. Kemper. 1985. Histoanatomic observations of the brain in early infantile autism. *Neurology* 35:866–874.

Bauman M. L. and T. L. Kemper. 2003. The neuropathology of the autism spectrum disorders: What have we learned? *Novartis Found. Symp.* 251:112–122.

Biyikli N. K., H. Tugtepe, G. Sener, A. Velioglu-Ogunc, S. Cetinel, S. Midillioglu, N. Gedik, and B. C. Yegen. 2006. Oxytocin alleviates oxidative renal injury in pyelonephritic rats via a neutrophil-dependent mechanism. *Peptides* 27:2249–2257.

Blankenfeldt W., K. Nokihara, S. Naruse, U. Lessel, D. Schomburg, and V. Wray. 1996. NMR spectroscopic evidence that helodermin, unlike other members of the secretin/VIP family of peptides, is substantially structured in water. *Biochemistry* 35:5955–5962.

Brabletz T., A. Jung, S. Dag, F. Hlubek, and T. Kirchner. 1999. Beta-catenin regulates the expression of the matrix metalloproteinase-7 in human colorectal cancer. *Am. J. Pathol.* 155:1033–1038.

Brownstein M. J. 1983. Biosynthesis of vasopressin and oxytocin. *Annu. Rev. Physiol.* 45:129–135.

Buchsbaum M. S., E. Hollander, M. M. Haznedar, C. Tang, J. Spiegel-Cohen, T. C. Wei, A. Solimando, B. R. Buchsbaum, D. Robins, C. Bienstock, C. Cartwright, and S. Mosovich. 2001. Effect of fluoxetine on regional cerebral metabolism in autistic spectrum disorders: A pilot study. *Int. J. Neuropsychopharmacol.* 4:119–125.

Carbillon L. 2007. Comment on Maternal oxytocin triggers a transient inhibitory switch in GABA signaling in the fetal brain during delivery. *Science* 317:197.

Casanova M. F., I. A. van Kooten, A. E. Switala, H. van Engeland, H. Heinsen, H. W. Steinbusch, P. R. Hof, J. Trippe, J. Stone, and C. Schmitz. 2006. Minicolumnar abnormalities in autism. *Acta Neuropathol.* 112:287–303.

Cassoni P., T. Marrocco, S. Deaglio, A. Sapino, and G. Bussolati. 2001a. Biological relevance of oxytocin and oxytocin receptors in cancer cells and primary tumors. *Ann. Oncol.* 12(Suppl. 2):S37–S39.

Cassoni P., T. Marrocco, A. Sapino, E. Allia, and G. Bussolati. 2006. Oxytocin synthesis within the normal and neoplastic breast: First evidence. *Int. J. Oncol.* 28:1263–1268.

Cassoni P., A. Sapino, L. Munaron, S. Deaglio, B. Chini, A. Graziani, A. Ahmed, and G. Bussolati. 2001b. Activation of functional oxytocin receptors stimulates cell proliferation in human trophoblast and choriocarcinoma cell lines. *Endocrinology* 142:1130–1136.

Chalazonitis A., T. D. Pham, Z. Li, D. Roman, U. Guha, W. Gomes, L. Kan, J. A. Kessler, and M. D. Gershon. 2008. Bone morphogenetic protein regulation of enteric neuronal phenotypic diversity: Relationship to timing of cell cycle exit. *J. Comp. Neurol.* 509:474–492.

Champagne F. A. and J. P. Curley. 2009. Epigenetic mechanisms mediating the long-term effects of maternal care on development. *Neurosci. Biobehav. Rev.* 33:593–600.

Champagne F. A., I. C. Weaver, J. Diorio, S. Dymov, M. Szyf, and M. J. Meaney. 2006. Maternal care associated with methylation of the estrogen receptor-alpha1b promoter and estrogen receptor-alpha expression in the medial preoptic area of female offspring. *Endocrinology* 147:2909–2915.

Chauhan A. and V. Chauhan. 2006. Oxidative stress in autism. *Pathophysiology* 13:171–181.

Chibbar R., F. D. Miller, and B. F. Mitchell. 1993. Synthesis of oxytocin in amnion, chorion, and decidua may influence the timing of human parturition. *J. Clin. Invest.* 91:185–192.

Chugani D. C., O. Muzik, R. Rothermel, M. Behen, P. Chakraborty, T. Mangner, E. A. da Silva, and H. T. Chugani. 1997. Altered serotonin synthesis in the dentatothalamocortical pathway in autistic boys. *Ann. Neurol.* 42:666–669.

Cossart R., Z. Petanjek, D. Dumitriu, J. C. Hirsch, Y. Ben-Ari, M. Esclapez, and C. Bernard. 2006. Interneurons targeting similar layers receive synaptic inputs with similar kinetics. *Hippocampus* 16:408–420.

Courchesne E., R. Carper, and N. Akshoomoff. 2003. Evidence of brain overgrowth in the first year of life in autism. *JAMA* 290:337–344.

Dyess D. L., D. P. Christenberry, G. L. Peeples, J. N. Collins, J. L. Ardell, W. S. Roberts, E. J. Tacchi, and R. W. Powell. 1998. Organ blood flow redistribution in response to hypoxemia in neonatal piglets. *J. Invest. Surg.* 11:381–392.

Faure C., A. Chalazonitis, C. Rheaume, G. Bouchard, S. G. Sampathkumar, K. J. Yarema, and M. D. Gershon. 2007. Gangliogenesis in the enteric nervous system: Roles of the polysialylation of the neural cell adhesion molecule and its regulation by bone morphogenetic protein-4. *Dev. Dyn.* 236:44–59.

Filipek P. A., J. Juranek, M. Smith, L. Z. Mays, E. R. Ramos, M. Bocian, D. Masser-Frye, T. M. Laulhere, C. Modahl, M. A. Spence, and J. J. Gargus. 2003. Mitochondrial dysfunction in autistic patients with 15q inverted duplication. *Ann. Neurol.* 53:801–804.

Fuhlendorff J., N. L. Johansen, S. G. Melberg, H. Thogersen, and T. W. Schwartz. 1990. The antiparallel pancreatic polypeptide fold in the binding of neuropeptide Y to Y1 and Y2 receptors. *J. Biol. Chem.* 265:11706–11712.

Funato Y. and H. Miki. 2007. Nucleoredoxin, a novel thioredoxin family member involved in cell growth and differentiation. *Antioxid. Redox. Signal* 9:1035–1057.

Gainer H., Y. Sarne, and M. J. Brownstein. 1977a. Biosynthesis and axonal transport of rat neurohypophysial proteins and peptides. *J. Cell. Biol.* 73:366–381.

Gainer H., Y. Sarne, and M. J. Brownstein. 1977b. Neurophysin biosynthesis: Conversion of a putative precursor during axonal transport. *Science* 195:1354–1356.

Ganz T. and R. I. Lehrer. 1994. Defensins. *Curr. Opin. Immunol.* 6:584–589.

Ghosh D., E. Porter, B. Shen, S. K. Lee, D. Wilk, J. Drazba, S. P. Yadav, J. W. Crabb, T. Ganz, and C. L. Bevins. 2002. Paneth cell trypsin is the processing enzyme for human defensin-5. *Nat. Immunol.* 3:583–590.

Gutkowska J., M. Jankowski, S. Mukaddam-Daher, and S. M. McCann. 2000. Oxytocin is a cardiovascular hormone. *Braz. J. Med. Biol. Res.* 33:625–633.

Hammock E. A. and L. J. Young. 2006. Oxytocin, vasopressin and pair bonding: Implications for autism. *Philos. Trans. R. Soc. Lond. B Biol. Sci.* 361:2187–2198.

Haramis A. P., H. Begthel, M. van den Born, J. van Es, S. Jonkheer, G. J. Offerhaus, and H. Clevers. 2004. De novo crypt formation and juvenile polyposis on BMP inhibition in mouse. *Science* 303:1684–1686.

Hardan A. Y., N. J. Minshew, M. Mallikarjuhn, and M. S. Keshavan. 2001. Brain volume in autism. *J. Child. Neurol.* 16:421–424.

Hauser C. J., R. R. Locke, H. W. Kao, J. Patterson, and R. D. Zipser. 1988. Visceral surface oxygen tension in experimental colitis in the rabbit. *J. Lab. Clin. Med.* 112:68–71.

Hoksbergen R., J. ter Laak, K. Rijk, C. van Dijkum, and F. Stoutjesdijk. 2005. Post-institutional autistic syndrome in Romanian adoptees. *J. Autism Dev. Disord.* 35:615–623.

Horvath K., J. C. Papadimitriou, A. Rabsztyn, C. Drachenberg, and J. T. Tildon. 1999. Gastrointestinal abnormalities in children with autistic disorder. *J. Pediatr.* 135:559–563.

Howard C. R., N. Lanphear, B. P. Lanphear, S. Eberly, and R. A. Lawrence. 2006. Parental responses to infant crying and colic: The effect on breastfeeding duration. *Breastfeed. Med.* 1:146–155.

Iseri S. O., G. Sener, B. Saglam, N. Gedik, F. Ercan, and B. C. Yegen. 2005. Oxytocin ameliorates oxidative colonic inflammation by a neutrophil-dependent mechanism. *Peptides* 26:483–491.

James S. J., P. Cutler, S. Melnyk, S. Jernigan, L. Janak, D. W. Gaylor, and J. A. Neubrander. 2004. Metabolic biomarkers of increased oxidative stress and impaired methylation capacity in children with autism. *Am. J. Clin. Nutr.* 80:1611–1617.

James S. J., S. Melnyk, S. Jernigan, M. A. Cleves, C. H. Halsted, D. H. Wong, P. Cutler, K. Bock, M. Boris, J. J. Bradstreet, S. M. Baker, and D. W. Gaylor. 2006. Metabolic endophenotype and related genotypes are associated with oxidative stress in children with autism. *Am. J. Med. Genet. B Neuropsychiatr. Genet.* 141B:947–956.

James S. J., S. Melnyk, S. Jernigan, A. Hubanks, S. Rose, and D. W. Gaylor. 2008. Abnormal transmethylation/transsulfuration metabolism and DNA hypomethylation among parents of children with autism. *J. Autism Dev. Disord.* 38:1966–1975.

Jankowski M., D. Wang, F. Hajjar, S. Mukaddam-Daher, S. M. McCann, and J. Gutkowska. 2000. Oxytocin and its receptors are synthesized in the rat vasculature. *Proc. Natl. Acad. Sci. U.S.A.* 97:6207–6211.

Khazipov R., R. Tyzio, and Y. Ben-Ari. 2008. Effects of oxytocin on GABA signalling in the foetal brain during delivery. *Prog. Brain Res.* 170:243–257.

Klimova T. and N. S. Chandel. 2008. Mitochondrial complex III regulates hypoxic activation of HIF. *Cell Death Differ.* 15:660–666.

Krehbiel D., P. Poindron, F. Levy, and M. J. Prud'Homme. 1987. Peridural anesthesia disturbs maternal behavior in primiparous and multiparous parturient ewes. *Physiol. Behav.* 40:463–472.

Kusui C., T. Kimura, K. Ogita, H. Nakamura, Y. Matsumura, M. Koyama, C. Azuma, and Y. Murata. 2001. DNA methylation of the human oxytocin receptor gene promoter regulates tissue-specific gene suppression. *Biochem. Biophys. Res. Commun.* 289:681–686.

Leake R. D., R. E. Weitzman, and D. A. Fisher. 1981. Oxytocin concentrations during the neonatal period. *Biol. Neonate* 39:127–131.

Limperopoulos C., H. Bassan, N. R. Sullivan, J. S. Soul, R. L. Robertson Jr., M. Moore, S. A. Ringer, J. J. Volpe, and A. J. du Plessis. 2008. Positive screening for autism in ex-preterm infants: prevalence and risk factors. *Pediatrics* 121:758–765.

Lollivier V., P. G. Marnet, S. Delpal, D. Rainteau, C. Achard, A. Rabot, and M. Ollivier-Bousquet. 2006. Oxytocin stimulates secretory processes in lactating rabbit mammary epithelial cells. *J. Physiol.* 570:125–140.

Lombard J. 1998. Autism: A mitochondrial disorder? *Med. Hypotheses* 50:497–500.

Lu Q., B. Jiang, C. Lin, and T. Shan. 2008. Dark aberrant crypt foci with activated Wnt pathway are related to tumorigenesis in the colon of AOM-treated rat. *J. Exp. Clin. Cancer Res.* 27:26.

Marchini G., H. Lagercrantz, J. Winberg, and K. Uvnas-Moberg. 1988. Fetal and maternal plasma levels of gastrin, somatostatin and oxytocin. *Early Hum. Dev.* 18:73–79.

Matthiesen A. S., A. B. Ransjo-Arvidson, E. Nissen, and K. Uvnas-Moberg. 2001. Postpartum maternal oxytocin release by newborns: Effects of infant hand massage and sucking. *Birth* 28:13–19.

McGinnis W. R. 2004. Oxidative stress in autism. *Altern. Ther. Health Med.* 10:22–36.

Mitchell B. F., X. Fang, and S. Wong. 1998. Role of carboxy-extended forms of oxytocin in the rat uterus in the process of parturition. *Biol. Reprod.* 59:1321–1327.

Modahl C., D. Fein, L. Waterhouse, and N. Newton. 1992. Does oxytocin deficiency mediate social deficits in autism? *J. Autism Dev. Disord.* 22:449–451.

Monstein H. J., N. Grahn, M. Truedsson, and B. Ohlsson. 2004. Oxytocin and oxytocin-receptor mRNA expression in the human. *Regul. Pept.* 119:39–44.

Ohlsson B., M. Truedsson, P. Djerf, and F. Sundler. 2006. Oxytocin is expressed throughout the human gastrointestinal tract. *Regul. Pept.* 135:7–11.

Ohnishi T., H. Matsuda, T. Hashimoto, T. Kunihiro, M. Nishikawa, T. Uema, and M. Sasaki. 2000. Abnormal regional cerebral blood flow in childhood autism. *Brain* 123:1838–1844.

Oliveira G., L. Diogo, M. Grazina, P. Garcia, A. Ataide, C. Marques, T. Miguel, L. Borges, A. M. Vicente, and C. R. Oliveira. 2005. Mitochondrial dysfunction in autism spectrum disorders: A population-based study. *Dev. Med. Child Neurol.* 47:185–189.

Ougolkov A. V., K. Yamashita, M. Mai, and T. Minamoto. 2002. Oncogenic beta-catenin and MMP-7 (matrilysin) cosegregate in late-stage clinical colon cancer. *Gastroenterology* 122:60–71.

Pequeux C., B. P. Keegan, M. T. Hagelstein, V. Geenen, J. J. Legros, and W. G. North. 2004. Oxytocin- and vasopressin-induced growth of human small-cell lung cancer is mediated by the mitogen-activated protein kinase pathway. *Endocr. Relat. Cancer* 11:871–885.

Petersson M., U. Wiberg, T. Lundeberg, and K. Uvnas-Moberg. 2001. Oxytocin decreases carrageenan induced inflammation in rats. *Peptides* 22:1479–1484.

Pinto D. and H. Clevers. 2005a. Wnt control of stem cells and differentiation in the intestinal epithelium. *Exp. Cell Res.* 306:357–363.

Pinto D. and H. Clevers. 2005b. Wnt, stem cells and cancer in the intestine. *Biol. Cell* 97:185–196.

Plakhova V. B., B. F. Shchegolev, I. V. Rogachevskii, A. D. Nozdrachev, B. V. Krylov, S. A. Podzorova, and V. N. Kokryakov. 2002. A possible molecular mechanism for the interaction of defensin with the sensory neuron membrane. *Neurosci. Behav. Physiol.* 32:409–415.

Porter E. M., C. L. Bevins, D. Ghosh, and T. Ganz. 2002. The multifaceted Paneth cell. *Cell. Mol. Life Sci.* 59:156–170.

Prigge S. T., A. S. Kolhekar, B. A. Fipper, R. E. Mains, and L. M. Amzel. 1997. Amidation of bioactive peptides: The structure of peptidylglycine alpha-hydroxylating monooxygenase. *Science* 278:1300–1305.

Putsep K., L. G. Axelsson, A. Boman, T. Midtvedt, S. Normark, H. G. Boman, and M. Andersson. 2000. Germ-free and colonized mice generate the same products from enteric prodefensins. *J. Biol. Chem.* 275:40478–40482.

Ransjo-Arvidson A. B., A. S. Matthiesen, G. Lilja, E. Nissen, A. M. Widstrom, and K. Uvnas-Moberg. 2001. Maternal analgesia during labor disturbs newborn behavior: Effects on breastfeeding, temperature, and crying. *Birth* 28:5–12.

Rumsey J. M. and M. Ernst. 2000. Functional neuroimaging of autistic disorders. *Ment. Retard. Dev. Disabil. Res. Rev.* 6:171–179.

Salzman N. H., R. A. Polin, M. C. Harris, E. Ruchelli, A. Hebra, S. Zirin-Butler, A. Jawad, E. M. Porter, and C. L. Bevins. 1998. Enteric defensin expression in necrotizing enterocolitis. *Pediatr. Res.* 44:20–26.

Satchell D. P., T. Sheynis, Y. Shirafuji, S. Kolusheva, A. J. Ouellette, and R. Jelinek. 2003. Interactions of mouse Paneth cell alpha-defensins and alpha-defensin. *J Biol. Chem.* 278:13838–13846.

Sebat J., B. Lakshmi, D. Malhotra, J. Troge, C. Lese-Martin, T. Walsh, B. Yamrom, S. Yoon, A. Krasnitz, J. Kendall, A. Leotta, D. Pai, R. Zhang, Y. H. Lee, J. Hicks, S. J. Spence, A. T. Lee, K. Puura, T. Lehtimaki, D. Ledbetter, P. K. Gregersen, J. Bregman, J. S. Sutcliffe, V. Jobanputra, W. Chung, D. Warburton, M. C. King, D. Skuse, D. H. Geschwind, T. C. Gilliam, K. Ye, and M. Wigler. 2007. Strong association of de novo copy number mutations with autism. *Science* 316:445–449.

Sparks B. F., S. D. Friedman, D. W. Shaw, E. H. Aylward, D. Echelard, A. A. Artru, K. R. Maravilla, J. N. Giedd, J. Munson, G. Dawson, and S. R. Dager. 2002. Brain structural abnormalities in young children with autism spectrum disorder. *Neurology* 59:184–192.

Stefanidis K., D. Loutradis, V. Anastasiadou, R. Bletsa, E. Kiapekou, P. Drakakis, P. Beretsos, E. Elenis, S. Mesogitis, and A. Antsaklis. 2008. Oxytocin receptor- and Oct-4-expressing cells in human amniotic fluid. *Gynecol. Endocrinol.* 24:280–284.

Tyzio R., R. Cossart, I. Khalilov, M. Minlebaev, C. A. Hubner, A. Represa, Y. Ben-Ari, and R. Khazipov. 2006. Maternal oxytocin triggers a transient inhibitory switch in GABA signaling in the fetal brain during delivery. *Science* 314:1788–1792.

Tyzio R., M. Minlebaev, S. Rheims, A. Ivanov, I. Jorquera, G. L. Holmes, Y. Zilberter, Y. Ben-Ari, and R. Khazipov. 2008. Postnatal changes in somatic gamma-aminobutyric acid signalling in the rat hippocampus. *Eur. J. Neurosci.* 27:2515–2528.

Uvnas-Moberg K. 1996. Neuroendocrinology of the mother-child interaction. *Trends Endocrinol. Metab.* 7:126–131.

Uvnas-Moberg K. and M. Petersson. 2005. Oxytocin, a mediator of anti-stress, well-being, social interaction, growth and healing. *Z. Psychosom. Med. Psychother.* 51:57–80.

Vargas D. L., C. Nascimbene, C. Krishnan, A. W. Zimmerman, and C. A. Pardo. 2005. Neuroglial activation and neuroinflammation in the brain of patients with autism. *Ann. Neurol.* 57:67–81.

Weaver I. C., A. C. D'Alessio, S. E. Brown, I. C. Hellstrom, S. Dymov, S. Sharma, M. Szyf, and M. J. Meaney. 2007. The transcription factor nerve growth factor-inducible protein a mediates epigenetic programming: Altering epigenetic marks by immediate-early genes. *J. Neurosci.* 27:1756–1768.

Weeks C. S., H. Tanabe, J. E. Cummings, S. P. Crampton, T. Sheynis, R. Jelinek, T. K. Vanderlick, M. J. Cocco, and A. J. Ouellette. 2006. Matrix metalloproteinase-7 activation of mouse paneth cell. *J. Biol. Chem.* 281:28932–28942.

Welch M. G., H. Tamir, K. J. Gross, M. Anwar, and M. D. Gershon. 2009. Expression and developmental regulation of oxytocin (OT) and oxytocin receptors (OTR) in the enteric nervous system (ENS) and intestinal epithelium. *J. Comp. Neurol.* 512:256–270.

Welch M. G., T. B. Welch-Horan, M. Anwar, N. Anwar, R. J. Ludwig, and D. A. Ruggiero. 2005. Brain effects of chronic IBD in areas abnormal in autism and treatment by single neuropeptides secretin and oxytocin. *J. Mol. Neurosci.* 25:259–274.

Wilcox J., M. T. Tsuang, E. Ledger, J. Algeo, and T. Schnurr. 2002. Brain perfusion in autism varies with age. *Neuropsychobiology* 46:13–16.

Wu S., M. Jia, Y. Ruan, J. Liu, Y. Guo, M. Shuang, X. Gong, Y. Zhang, X. Yang, and D. Zhang. 2005. Positive association of the oxytocin receptor gene (OXTR) with autism in the Chinese Han population. *Biol. Psychiatry* 58:74–77.

16 Cytokine Polymorphisms in Autism: Their Role in Immune Alterations

Fabián Crespo,[1,2,] Rafael Fernandez-Botran,[3] Christopher Tillquist,[2] Lonnie Sears,[4] Meghan Mott,[1] and Manuel Casanova[1]*

Departments of [1]Psychiatry and Behavioral Sciences, [2]Anthropology, [3]Pathology and Laboratory Medicine, [4]Pediatrics, University of Louisville, Louisville, KY 40292, USA

CONTENTS

16.1 CYTOKINE BIOLOGY: A GENERAL INTRODUCTION

Cytokines are a diverse group of soluble regulatory proteins that function as mediators in many physiological processes, including inflammation, immunity, and hemopoiesis. As mediators, they regulate the migration, activation, proliferation, differentiation, and function of the many types of cells involved in inflammatory and immune responses. While essential to maintaining protective immunity, cytokines have been implicated in autoimmune diseases and diseases with a chronic inflammation component (Borish and Steinke, 2003).

* Corresponding author: Tel.: +1-502-852-2427; fax: +1-502-852-4560; e-mail: fabian.crespo@louisville.edu

Cytokines are usually very complex in their activities. Most cytokines are highly pleiotropic and act on many different cell types exerting different effects. Different cytokines can have redundant effects, or their activities can be either synergistic or antagonistic depending on the target cells. Normally, cytokines do not act alone, but are produced in a cascade fashion, and it is their combined effect that determines the type of response. The responsiveness of a cell to a particular cytokine is determined by the expression of specific receptors for that cytokine. The binding of the cytokine to its receptor then triggers the activation of a variety of signaling mechanisms that lead to changes at the level of gene expression, resulting in transient- or chronic-altered cellular proliferation, differentiation, and/or function.

Cytokines play an essential role in the regulation of inflammatory responses and are involved in the regulation of both innate (natural) and acquired immunities. The cytokines that function in innate immunity and inflammation are normally produced by cells of the monocitic and myeloid lineages and several other types of cells in response to microbial, chemical, physical, and other types of inflammatory stimuli. The main goal of the cytokines in these responses is the localization and elimination of the instigating insult, orchestrating the recruitment of both cells and molecules (accomplished through increased vascular permeability and leukocyte infiltration) at the local site and a variety of systemic responses that include fever and acute-phase protein synthesis, and the mobilization of leukocytes from the bone marrow. Among the main cytokines involved in these responses are tumor necrosis factor α (TNFα), interleukin (IL)-1, IL-6, IL-12, type I interferons (IFN; IFNα and IFNβ), and chemokines, a family of cytokines that function to mobilize and attract different types of leukocytes to inflammatory sites. These cytokines are said to have a "proinflammatory" activity. If cytokines are secreted in excess as a result of an overwhelming infection, or in cases where the insult cannot be easily eliminated or the stimulus for cytokine secretion persists, leading to chronic inflammation, these same cytokines can have pathologic effects leading to the damage of healthy cells and tissues. Because of its potentially serious consequences, the immune system has mechanisms to prevent excessive inflammation, including cytokines with "anti-inflammatory" activity. These cytokines include transforming growth factor β (TGFβ) and IL-10, which antagonize many of the effects of the "proinflammatory" cytokines mentioned above. It should be kept in mind, however, that certain cytokines can have both pro- and anti-inflammatory effects depending on different factors such as the cell and tissue type and the kinetics of release.

In the case of specific immunity, cytokines play an equally important role. In general, the type of cytokines produced during an immune response determines the effector mechanisms that predominate and major expression patterns have been characterized (Mosmann and Coffman, 1989). For example, different subsets of helper (CD4$^+$) T cells that differ in both their cytokine secretion patterns and the effector mechanisms that they induce have been identified. Cells belonging to the Th1 subset secrete IFNγ, IL-2, and TNFα/β and are primarily involved in cellular immunity mechanisms and delayed-type hypersensitivity reactions; cells of the Th2 subset secrete IL-4, IL-5, IL-10, and IL-13 and are primarily involved in humoral mechanisms and allergic-type reactions; and cells of the newly described Th17 subset secrete IL-17, IL-22, and a variety of other proinflammatory cytokines (Harrington et al., 2006). Th17 cells are thought to be involved not only in immune responses to extracellular bacteria but also in autoimmune diseases. Th1 and Th2 cells affect one another: Th1 cells trigger macrophage activation using IFNγ, which inhibits the proliferation of Th2 cells, and Th2 cells secrete IL-10, which inhibits the secretion of IFNγ by Th1 cells. In keeping with the need for balance in the immune system, a different subset of T cells exists, namely T-regulatory cells (Treg), which act as negative regulators of the activities of other subsets. These cells act, in part, through the secretion of the "anti-inflammatory" cytokines TGFβ and IL-10 (Bettelli et al., 2006).

Both in inflammation/innate immunity as well as in specific immunity, the maintenance of a balance between pro- and anti-inflammatory cytokines or among the different CD4$^+$ T-cell subsets and their cytokines is essential for homeostasis and the proper function of the immune system. Disruptions in this balance can have pathologic implications resulting in excessive inflammation and tissue damage, increased susceptibility to infectious agents, and/or the emergence of autoimmune conditions (Ollier, 2004). For example, abnormal levels of different cytokines have been described in many diseases, such as autoimmune hepatitis, rheumatoid arthritis, asthma, systemic lupus erythematosus, inflammatory bowel disease, and some brain disorders like schizophrenia and Alzheimer's disease (Kronfol and Remick, 2000; Theoharides et al., 2004; Vitkovic et al., 2000). Given that cytokines are key components in the homeostatic mechanisms regulating the immune system, it is not surprising that variations in their structure at the genetic or protein level (qualitative) or their production level (quantitative) have been found to be associated with disease processes and/or susceptibility to infections.

16.2   CYTOKINE POLYMORPHISMS AND CYTOKINE EXPRESSION

Cytokines and their receptors are often encoded by highly polymorphic genes; and these polymorphisms are responsible for the observed interindividual differences in cytokine production and they likely impact the immune response (Hollegaard and Bidwell, 2006; Keen, 2002a; Warlé et al., 2003). Cytokine genes and their receptor genes are highly conserved in their exon sequences, while the majority of polymorphisms are conserved polymorphisms in the non-translated regions of the gene, located within the promoter, the introns, or the untranslated-3′ regions (Keen, 2002b). Cytokine polymorphisms continue to be discovered as mutation detection techniques improved to map the extent of cytokine polymorphisms. Cytokines that were once thought to be non-polymorphic, such as IL-2, IL-8, and IL-12, are now being shown to have single nucleotide polymorphisms (SNPs), often within the 5′ promoter regions (Keen, 2002a). Promoter region polymorphisms impact the levels of protein expression in several ways. Polymorphisms within the 3′ or 5′ regulatory sequences can affect transcription by altering the structure of the binding sites for the transcription factors. Intronic polymorphisms can affect mRNA splicing or the binding of enhancers and silencers (Keen, 2002a). As the amount of data on cytokine polymorphisms increases and becomes available, there are a growing number of studies that show an effect of cytokine gene polymorphism on immune disease susceptibility, severity, and outcome (Keen, 2002b).

It is not surprising that different cytokine genotypes have been associated with a large number of diseases; however, an important caveat must be noted with respect to these putative associations. The vast majority of these studies analyze individual

SNPs or a series of SNPs in a particular cytokine gene in a relatively small sample cohort and control group. A principal concern with this common study design is that the distribution of genomic variation is a function of population history. The frequency of the SNPs may vary among populations according to the ethnic or ancestry background of the disease and control group (Keen, 2002b). Furthermore, results from the HapMap project and other linkage studies have demonstrated large linkage blocks on chromosomes, and recent SNP-based analyses have demonstrated whole-genome phylogeographic effects (Lao et al., 2008). The effect of geographic/genetic correlation is that any given SNP showing an association with a disease may be one of many associated SNPs—others were not detected because they were not part of the original study design. The implication of this observation is that while there is a true statistical association between the SNP under consideration and the clinical endpoint, there is not necessarily an etiological relationship. This is not a novel observation, and work using high-resolution linkage disequilibrium clarifies the situation. A complementary approach to understanding the contribution of immune alterations to human disease is to consider the immune system as a whole, that is, as a single functional phenotype. Investigating the immune response as a single phenotype requires assaying as many functional polymorphisms as possible within a single cytokine gene (or group of cytokine genes) along with the use of more appropriate control groups (Keen, 2002a; Ollier, 2004). This approach will enable the detection of polymorphisms with significant functional effects on the expression of the immune system, either in response to environmental stimuli or as part of the developmental program.

16.3   CYTOKINES AND THE BRAIN

For many years in clinical research, the brain has been considered an immunologically privileged site, with the assumption that there is a reduced qualitative or different immune response compared to the systemic level. Evidence for this statement includes the brain's absence of appropriate lymphatic channels to capture antigens, the blood-brain barrier protecting the brain from circulating blood, and the failure to demonstrate the early invasion of macrophages and leukocytes. However, recent developments in neuroimmunology have challenged this concept. Current data have shown that the brain can exhibit many of the hallmarks of inflammation in response to stress or injury, including edema, the activation of resident phagocytes, the local invasion of the circulating immune cells, and the production of cytokines (Kronfol and Remick, 2000; Vitkovic et al., 2000). Moreover, several studies have reported associations between psychological stress, psychiatric illness, and cytokines (Theoharides et al., 2004). Most cytokines can be synthesized and released within the central nervous system and the majority is produced by microglia and astroglia; there is also some evidence that neurons also produce cytokines under certain conditions. Although cytokines are usually secreted in response to specific stimuli, the low-level expression of specific cytokines appears to be maintained in blood vessels within the brain (Licinio et al., 1998; Vitkovic et al., 2000).

Considerable progress has been made during the past few years in the understanding of the immunological mechanisms that control the immune surveillance and the inflammation in the brain (Bauer et al., 2001). Cytokines in the brain are also regulated in cascades through feedback loops, and cytokine receptors have been detected in the brain (Kronfol and Remick, 2000). Besides providing communication between neural cells, specific cytokines have a significant role in signaling the brain to produce neurochemical, neuroendocrine, neuroimmune, and behavioral changes (Maes et al., 1995). There is suggestive evidence that this signaling is a part of the comprehensive mechanism to mobilize resources to combat physical and physiological stress in an attempt to maintain relative homeostasis. Because cytokines are associated with central neurotransmitters and cytokine regulation is affected by stress, many studies have investigated the possible role for cytokines in psychiatric disorders. These studies have demonstrated the role of abnormal levels of cytokines in major depression, Alzheimer's disease, and schizophrenia (Hanson and Gottesman, 2005; Hopkins, 2007; Maes et al., 1995; McGeer and McGeer, 2001a,b).

16.4   CYTOKINES AND AUTISM

In the last 10 years, workers have reported that increased levels of some proinflammatory cytokines (TNF-α, IL1-β, IL-2, and IFNγ) are present in the peripheral blood mononuclear cells (PBMC) of children with autism spectrum disorders (ASD), fueling the hypothesis that an abnormal immune response could be another component of this multifactorial disorder (Chez et al., 2007; Cohly and Panja, 2005; Croonenberghs et al., 2002; Gupta et al., 1998; Jyonouchi et al., 2001; Korvatska et al., 2002; Molloy et al., 2006; Stubbs and Crawford, 1977; Vargas et al., 2005). In a cytokine analysis at the systemic level, a specific increase of IFNγ and IL-12 was detected suggesting a shift toward a Th1 lymphocyte response (Singh, 1996). This hypothesis of a shift toward a Th1 lymphocyte-dominated response was reinforced with a recent study where an increase of IFNγ was detected in 29 autistic children (Sweeten et al., 2004). Moreover, the high levels of systemic IFNγ correlated with elevated circulating numbers of monocytes in a separate autistic population (Sweeten et al., 2003). However, in an earlier similar study, no increase in IFNγ was observed (Stubbs and Crawford, 1977). In another study, focusing on CD4$^+$ and CD8 T cells, a shift toward a Th2-like response was found in autistic children (Gupta et al., 1998). An association of ASD and an abnormal immune response has support from data of the increased prevalence of autoimmune disorders among first-degree relatives of children with ASD (Kronfol and Remick, 2000), but this suggests a bias toward a Th17-mediated response. The autoimmune component is likely diverse, varying among autistics depending on genetic predisposition and environmental contingencies (Lee et al., 2006; Vojdani et al., 2003; Wills et al., 2007). At present, it is not possible to definitively ascertain characteristic perturbations in the relative balance between Th1/Th2/Th17 responses. In autistic subjects, it is worth noting that some of the seemingly contradictory evidence is likely the result of an incomplete understanding of the balance between major immune response regimes, as well as methodological issues. With regard to the latter, measures of cytokine expression from PBMCs estimates expression from all Th1, Th2, and Th17 lineages. It does appear that autism has an inflammatory component—and contradictory results may reflect the insufficient classification of autistic endophenotypes of variable etiology, age-disparities between autistics and controls, and drug treatments (Ashwood et al., 2006).

It is not clear, however, whether an abnormal or exacerbated immune response is a contributing factor for autism or simply a symptom of the disease.

16.5   WHY STUDY CYTOKINE POLYMORPHISMS IN AUTISM? THE UNDERLYING GENETIC VARIABILITY HYPOTHESIS

Cytokine promoter polymorphisms affect cytokine expression levels; this has been empirically demonstrated. In the current literature, studies have shown differences in cytokines levels between different autistic populations. One potential reason for those differences could be associated with population studies that compare young ASD patients with adult controls, or populations that have a wide range of ages, within patients and controls groups (Ashwood et al., 2006). But, contradictory results obtained until present regarding cytokine expression in different autistic populations could confirm the presence of different endophenotypes in ASD based on cytokine genotypes. It is reasonable to infer that the combination of these different genotypes may bias a characteristic immune response, constitutively affecting Th1/Th2/Th17 balance. In the context of an acute inflammatory episode, such a bias may tip the balance toward a more vigorous—and potentially deleterious— acute-phase immune response or induce a state of chronic inflammation. At this time, we do not propose that an abnormal immune response due to specific cytokine genotypes is necessarily the cause or one of the causes for autism. Moreover, we do not have enough evidence yet, that an abnormal immune response is a contributing factor for autism or a simple by-product of the disease. However, growing evidence is showing that autism may begin with genetic susceptibility or with specific environmental insults during brain development such as particular infections or particular antigens in the diet; and a proinflammatory scenario associated with an abnormal cytokine production would exacerbate the whole process. It may be useful to hypothesize that there are phenotypes of the immune system predisposed to stronger or weaker inflammatory immune responses or chronic inflammation or autoimmunity, but that these phenotypes can manifest from several different combinations of genotypes of different cytokines genes with variable expression. To the extent that inflammation and autoimmunity are associated with autism, the assaying of cytokine genotypes may permit distinguishing endophenotypes within autistics. The combinations of specific genotypes of multiple cytokines may therefore be useful as markers for specific autistic endophenotypes.

16.6   WHY STUDY MATERNAL CYTOKINE POLYMORPHISMS?

Immune activation during pregnancy can impact the neurodevelopment of offspring with far-reaching behavioral sequelae. It is well known that cytokine levels (IL-1β, IL-6, and TNFα) are altered in human pregnancies complicated with infection (Depino, 2006), and maternally generated cytokines can cross the placenta and enter the fetal circulation (Zaretsky et al., 2004). Thus, it is possible that a maternal abnormal immune response linked to infection or injury during pregnancy may be one factor for altered neurological development in the fetus (Shi et al., 2003). During the last decade, new data have reinforced this hypothesis, leading several researchers to include maternal infection/ injury as another risk factor for brain disorders like autism (Gilmore and Jarskog, 1997;

Juul-Dam et al., 2001; Maimburg and Vaeth, 2006; Patterson, 2002). The immune activation of pregnant mice or rats using either lipopolysaccharide (a proxy for bacterial infection) or polyriboinosinic polyribocytidylic acid (a proxy for viral infection) results in modified cytokine expression in the maternal–fetal tandem pair (Gilmore et al., 2005; Urakubo et al., 2001). Furthermore, the timing of the insult during gestation is important with regard to the ultimate neurological and behavioral impact (Smith et al., 2007).

This may have to do with the nature of the link between maternal and fetal immune systems, and when the fetal immune system is capable of mounting an appropriate response. It may be inferred that the timing and etiological origin of immune activation potentiates different neurological and behavioral fetal impacts. The variability of the effect in both the timing of immune activation and time since activation is likely linked both to the innate development of the fetal immune system and to an altered Th1/Th2 balance in the mother. To our mind, variability due to cytokine expression polymorphisms could either exacerbate or attenuate the degree of both maternal and fetal immune activations.

16.7   DISCUSSION

Several studies demonstrate that an abnormal cytokine production is present in some autistic populations, suggesting a more complex scenario where an abnormal immune response is another component in the patient phenotype. If specific cytokine genotypes associated with abnormal cytokine expression are linked to autism, this could be understood as a genetic predisposition in the patient population. However, we must be careful when trying to understand the meaning of "genetic predisposition" in the development of this complex disease. Beyond the "cause or effect" paradox applied to immune alterations in autism, we propose that specific genetic cytokine makeup could be understood as a risk factor that will exacerbate any immune response that was triggered by the multiple factors leading to the oxidative stress present in this disease (Chauhan and Chauhan, 2006). Moreover, if the abnormal cytokine genetic makeup is also present on the mother, since cytokines can cross the placenta, the convergence of both phenotypes (mother and child) leading to an abnormal immune response could significantly increase the risk—during pregnancy—for the development of autism.

Recent findings indicate that during the development of cortical and neuronal organization, unknown factors influence neuronal and neuroglial cell populations, disturbing neurodevelopment and producing the characteristic neuroanatomical changes seen in autism (Vitkovic et al., 2000). This abnormality is best exemplified in the significantly more narrow cortical minicolumns present in autistic individuals when compared to controls (Casanova et al., 2006). As an effect of heterochronic modifications to their developmental program, many autistic subjects have augmented prefrontal cortices. This over-exuberant expansion of the prefrontal cortex is by the addition of minicolumns. Clearly, there is population variability in cortical size and minicolumnar density, and there are normal individuals with large brains and densely packed minicolumns (and indeed autism has a familial component); so why are some of these individuals autistic and others not? The manifestation of emergent properties is dynamic, and their expression is a function of sufficient metabolic supplies and active controls (Casanova and Tillquist, 2008).

Here, we argue that the crossing of the threshold leading a disruption of active controls and impinging upon long-range neural networks, leading to autism, is maternal and/or fetal immune activation. This may have been a single activation, but we would like to propose the novel idea that maternal and/or fetal immune activation may permanently alter the fetal Th1/Th2/Th17 balance, predisposing the fetus to a lifetime of chronic inflammation (or susceptibility to inflammation) or autoimmunity issues. A major underlying genetic contribution to the balance of Th1/Th2/Th17 populations must be related to the expression of different cytokines involved in the immune cascades generated during immune activation. Given expression polymorphisms in certain key cytokine genes, some overall immune phenotypes will be predisposed for stronger or weaker immune activation, contributing to the etiology or emergence of autism.

16.8   FUTURE DIRECTIONS

1. *Pleiotropism and cytokine network considerations.* Because of the well-established pleiotropic and interactive nature of cytokines, we propose a more comprehensive analysis with increased sample numbers and the consideration of polymorphic haplotypes.
2. *Cytokine expression baseline.* Since cytokines can show a broad range of expression levels affected by different factors as age, gender, ethnicity, and annual seasons, we propose to determine the baseline of cytokine expression levels in our populations for those cytokines showing a particular genotype/haplotype for mothers and/or autistic children.
3. *Paternal influence.* Given behavioral similarities between autistic males and their fathers, paternal genetic contribution is likely important for understanding autism; so we propose to ascertain whether a characteristic paternal contribution can be detected in terms of cytokine polymorphisms.
4. *Global survey of cytokine polymorphism in human populations.* As it has been detected for other genetic polymorphisms, cytokines SNPs show a heterogeneous distribution in human populations; so we propose, and are currently conducting (Crespo et al., 2008), a global survey for cytokine polymorphisms in different human populations.

REFERENCES

Ashwood, P., Wills, S., and Van de Water, J. 2006. The immune response in autism: A new frontier for autism research. *J. Leukoc. Biol.* 80:1–15.

Bauer, J., Rauschka, H., and Lassmann, H. 2001. Inflammation in the nervous system: The human perspective. *Glia* 36:235–243.

Bettelli, E., Carrier, Y., Gao, W., Korn, T., Strom, T.B., Oukka, M., Weiner, H.L., and Kuchroo, V.K. 2006. Reciprocal developmental pathways for the generation of pathogenic effector TH17 and regulatory T cells. *Nature* 441:235–238.

Borish, L.C. and Steinke, J.W. 2003. Cytokines and chemokines. *J. Allergy Clin. Immunol.* 111:S460–S475.

Casanova, M. and Tillquist, C. 2008. Encephalization, emergent properties, and psychiatry: A minicolumnar perspective. *Neuroscientist* 14:101–118.

Casanova, M., van Kooten, I.A., Switala, A.E., van Engeland, H., Heinsen, H., Steinbusch, H.W., Hof, P.R., Trippe, J., Stone, J., and Schmitz, C. 2006. Minicolumnar abnormalities in autism. *Acta Neuropathol.* 112:287–303.

Chauhan, A. and Chauhan, V. 2006. Oxidative stress in autism. *Pathophysiology* 13:171–181.

Chez, M.G., Dowling, T., Patel, P.B., Khanna, P., and Kominsky, M. 2007. Elevation of tumor necrosis factor-alpha in cerebrospinal fluid of autistic children. *Pediatr. Neurol.* 36:361–365.

Cohly, H. and Panja, A. 2005. Immunological findings in autism. *Int. Rev. Neurobiol.* 71:317–341.

Crespo, F., Oberst, R., Fernandez-Botran, R., Casanova, M., and Tillquist, C. 2008. Cytokine expression polymorphism in European human populations. *Am. J. Phys. Anthropol.* 135(Suppl. 46):83–84.

Croonenberghs, J., Bosmans, E., Deboutte, D., Kenis, G., and Maes, M. 2002. Activation of the inflammatory response system in autism. *Neuropsychobiology* 45:1–6.

Depino, A. 2006. Maternal infection and the offspring brain. *J. Neurosci.* 26:7777–7778.

Gilmore, J. and Jarskog, F. 1997. Exposure to infection and brain development: Cytokines in the pathogenesis of schizophrenia. *Schizophr. Res.* 24:365–367.

Gilmore, J., Jarskog, L., and Vadlamudi, S. 2005. Maternal poly I:C exposure during pregnancy regulates TNF alpha, BDNF, and NGF expression in neonatal brain and the maternal-fetal unit of the rat. *J. Neuroimmunol.* 159:106–112.

Gupta, S., Aggarwal, S., Rashanravan, B., and Lee, T. 1998. Th1- and Th2-like cytokines in CD4 and CD8 T cells in autism. *J. Neuroimmunol.* 85:106–109.

Hanson, D. and Gottesman, I. 2005. Theories of schizophrenia: A genetic-inflammatory-vascular synthesis. *BMC Med. Genet.* 6:7.

Harrington, L., Mangan, P., and Weaver, C. 2006. Expanding the effector CD4 T-cell repertoire: The Th17 lineage. *Curr. Opin. Immunol.* 18:349–356.

Hollegaard, M. and Bidwell, J. 2006. Cytokine gene polymorphism in human disease: Online databases, supplement 3. *Genes Immun.* 7:269–276.

Hopkins, S. 2007. Central nervous system recognition of peripheral inflammation: A neural, hormonal collaboration. *Acta Biomed.* 78:231–247.

Juul-Dam, N., Townsend, J., and Courchesne, E. 2001. Prenatal, perinatal, and neonatal factors in autism, pervasive developmental disorder-not otherwise specified, and the general population. *Pediatrics* 107:63–68.

Jyonouchi, H., Sun, S., and Le, H. 2001. Proinflammatory and regulatory cytokine production associated with innate and adaptive immune responses in children with autism spectrum disorders and developmental regression. *J. Neuroimmunol.* 120:170–179.

Keen, L. 2002a. The study of polymorphism in cytokine and cytokine receptor genes. *ASHI Q.* 4:174–176.

Keen, L. 2002b. The extent and analysis of cytokine and cytokine receptor gene polymorphism. *Transpl. Immunol.* 10:143–146.

Korvatska, E., Van de Water, J., Anders, T.F., and Gershwin, M.E. 2002. Genetic and immunologic considerations in autism. *Neurobiol. Dis.* 9:107–125.

Kronfol, Z. and Remick, D. 2000. Cytokines and the brain: Implications for clinical psychiatry. *Am. J. Psychiatry* 157:683–694.

Lao, O., Lu, T.T., Nothnagel, M., Junge, O., Freitag-Wolf, S., Caliebe, A., Balascakova, M., Bertranpetit, J., Bindoff, L.A., Comas, D., Holmlund, G., Kouvatsi, A., Macek, M., Mollet, I., Parson, W., Palo, J., Ploski, R., Sajantila, A., Tagliabracci, A., Gether, U., Werge, T., Rivadeneira, F., Hofman, A., Uitterlinden, A.G., Gieger, C., Wichmann, H.E., Ruther, A., Schreiber, S., Becker, C., Nurnberg, P., Nelson, M.R., Krawczak, M., and Kayser, M. 2008. Correlation between genetic and geographic structure in Europe. *Curr. Biol.* 18:1241–1248.

Lee, L., Zachary, A.A., Leffel, M.S., Newschaffer, C.J., Matteson, K.J., Tyler, J.D., and Zimmerman, A.W. 2006. HLA-DR4 in families with autism. *Pediatr. Neurol.* 35:303–307.

Licinio, J., Kling, M., and Hauser, P. 1998. Cytokines and brain function: Relevance of interferon α-induced mood and cognitive changes. *Semin. Oncol.* 25:30–38.

Maes, M., Meltzer, H.Y., Bosmans, E., Bergmans, R., Vandoolaeghe, E., Ranjan, R., and Desnyder, R. 1995. Increased plasma concentrations of interleukin-6, soluble interleukin-6 receptor, soluble interleukin-2 receptor and transferring receptor in major depression. *J. Affect. Disord.* 34:301–309.

Maimburg, R. and Vaeth, M. 2006. Perinatal risk factors and infantile autism. *Acta Psychiatr. Scand.* 114:257–264.

McGeer, P. and McGeer, E. 2001a. Polymorphisms in inflammatory genes and the risk of Alzheimer disease. *Arch. Neurol.* 58:1790–1792.

McGeer, P. and McGeer, E. 2001b. Inflammation, autotoxicity and Alzheimer disease. *Neurobiol. Aging* 22:799–809.

Molloy, C.A., Morrow, A.L, Meizen-Derr, J., Schleifer, K., Dienger, K., Manning-Courtney, P., Altaye, M., and Wills-Karp, M. 2006. Elevated cytokine levels in children with autism spectrum disorder. *J. Neuroimmunol.* 172:198–205.

Mosmann, T. and Coffman, R. 1989. TH1 and TH2 cells: Difference patterns of lymphokine secretion lead to different functional properties. *Annu. Rev. Immunol.* 7:145–173.

Ollier, W. 2004. Cytokines genes and disease susceptibility. *Cytokine* 28:174–178.

Patterson, P. 2002. Maternal infection: Window on neuroimmune interactions in fetal brain development and mental illness. *Curr. Opin. Neurobiol.* 12:115–118.

Shi, L., Fatemi, S.H., Sidwell, R.W., and Patterson, P.H. 2003. Maternal influenza infection causes marked behavioral and pharmacological changes in the offspring. *J. Neurosci.* 23:297–302.

Singh, V. 1996. Plasma increase of interleukin-12 and interferon-γ. Pathological significance in autism. *J. Neuroimmunol.* 66:143–145.

Smith, S.E., Li, J., Garbett, K., Mirnics, K., and Patterson, P.H. 2007. Maternal immune activation alters fetal brain development through interleukin-6. *J. Neurosci.* 27:10695–10702.

Stubbs, E. and Crawford, M. 1977. Depressed lymphocyte responsiveness in autistic children. *J. Autism Child Schizophr.* 7:49–55.

Sweeten, T.L., Posey, D.J., and McDougle, C.J. 2003. High blood monocyte counts and neopterin levels in children with autistic disorder. *Am. J. Psychiatry* 160:1691–1693.

Sweeten, T.L., Posey, D.J., Shanker, S., and McDougle, C.J. 2004. High nitric oxide production in autistic disorder: Possible role for interferon-γ. *Biol. Psychiatry* 55:434–437.

Theoharides, T., Weinkauf, C., and Conti, P. 2004. Brain cytokines and neuropsychiatric disorders. *J. Clin. Psychopharmacol.* 24:577–581.

Urakubo, A., Jarskog, L.F., Lieberman, J.A., and Gilmore, J.H. 2001. Prenatal exposure to maternal infection alters cytokine expression in the placenta, amniotic fluid, and fetal brain. *Schizophr. Res.* 47:27–36.

Vargas, D.L., Nascimbene, C., Krishnan, C., Zimmerman, A.W., and Pardo, C.A. 2005. Neuroglial activation and neuroinflammation in the brain of patients with autism. *Ann. Neurol.* 57:67–81.

Vitkovic, L., Bockaert, J., and Jacque, C. 2000. Inflammatory cytokines: Neuromodulators in normal brain? *J. Neurochem.* 74:457–471.

Vojdani, A., Pangborn, J.B., Vojdani, E., and Cooper, E.L. 2003. Infections, toxic chemicals and dietary peptides binding to lymphocyte receptors and tissue enzymes are major instigators of autoimmunity in autism. *Int. J. Immunopathol. Pharmacol.* 16:189–199.

Warlé, M.C., Farhan, A., Metselaar, H.J., Hop, W.C., Perrey, C., Zondervan, P.E., Kap, M., Kwekkeboom, J., Ijzermans, J.N., Tilanus, H.W., Pravica, V., Hutchinson, I.V., and Bouma, G.J. 2003. Are cytokine gene polymorphisms related to in vitro cytokine production profiles? *Liver Transpl.* 9:170–181.

Wills, S., Cabanlit, M., Bennett, J., Ashwood, P., Amaral, D., and Van de Water, J. 2007. Autoantibodies in autism spectrum disorders (ASD). *Ann. N.Y. Acad. Sci.* 1107:79–91.

Zaretsky, M.V., Alexander, J.M., Byrd, W., and Bawdon, R.E. 2004. Transfer of inflammatory cytokines across the placenta. *Obstet. Gynecol.* 103:546–550.

17 Autism, Teratogenic Alleles, *HLA-DR4,* and Immune Function

William G. Johnson,[1,3,]* Steven Buyske,[4,5]
Edward S. Stenroos,[1,3] and George H. Lambert[2,3]

Departments of [1]Neurology, [2]Pediatrics, [3]Center
for Childhood Neurotoxicology and Exposure
Assessment, Robert Wood Johnson Medical
School, University of Medicine and Dentistry
of New Jersey, Piscataway, NJ 08854, USA

Departments of [4]Statistics and [5]Genetics, Rutgers University,
New Brunswick, NJ 08854, USA

CONTENTS

---

* Corresponding author: Tel.: +1-732-235-4508; fax: +1-732-235-5295; e-mail: wjohnson@umdnj.edu

17.1 TERATOGENIC ALLELES IN NEURODEVELOPMENTAL DISORDERS

Neurodevelopmental disorders are complex disorders in which multiple genes contribute to the clinical phenotype and their effect is modified by environmental factors. Genes contributing to neurodevelopmental disorders are usually thought of as acting in the affected individual, i.e., the child or adult with the neurodevelopmental disorder. In the gene–teratogen model, an additional class of genes is considered, maternal genes that act in the mother to contribute to the phenotype of their affected offspring. The alleles of maternal genes that act in this way are termed "teratogenic alleles" because their effect is in some ways similar to ingested maternal teratogens that affect fetal development. Teratogenic alleles most likely act in the mother during pregnancy to modify the development of the embryo or fetus, e.g., brain development in the affected children, although action on the ovum or in the ovum before conception is also possible. These maternal genes may interact with fetal genes and with environmental factors. These fetal genes are termed "modifying or specificity alleles" in the gene–teratogen model since they may modify the severity of the phenotype in the fetus or determine which organ is affected. At present, at least 34 reports of teratogenic alleles have been published (Johnson et al., 2008, Table 17.1; Johnson et al., 2009).

TABLE 17.1
Reports of Teratogenic Alleles

Teratogenic Allele Report	Disease	Analysis By	References
Maternal TDT			
1. MTR^*2756G	NTD/spina bifida	Mat TDT, log-linear	Doolin et al. (2002)
2. $MTRR^*66G$	NTD/spina bifida	Mat TDT, log-linear	Doolin et al. (2002)
3. $GSTP1^*val105$	Autism	Mat TDT	van Beynum et al. (2006)
Maternal TDT-equivalent			
4. Rh d	Erythroblastosis fetalis	Mat TDT equivalent	Westgren et al. (1995)
5. PAH mutations	Maternal phenylketonuria	Mat TDT equivalent	Rouse and Azen (2004)
6. Rh d	Schizophrenia	Mat TDT equivalent, log-linear	Hollister, Laing, and Mednick (1996), Palmer et al. (2002)
Case–parent log-linear analysis without maternal TDT or equivalent			
7. $MTHFD1^*653Q$	Spina bifida	Log-linear	Brody et al. (2002)
8. $CYP1A1^*6235C$	Low birthweight	Log-linear	Chen et al. (2005)
9. $NAT1$ composite genotypes	NTD/spina bifida	Log-linear	Jensen et al. (2006b)
10. $CCL-2^*2518AA$	NTD/spina bifida	Log-linear	Jensen et al. (2006a)

TABLE 17.1 (Continued)
Reports of Teratogenic Alleles

Teratogenic Allele Report	Disease	Analysis By	References
Regression analysis			
11. *APOE***E2*	Lower LDL-C, apoB, higher HDL-C, and apoA1 in newborns	Forward stepwise regression analysis	Descamps et al. (2004)
12. *APOC3***S2*	Lower newborn LDL-C, apoB, HDL-C, and apoA1	Forward stepwise regression analysis	Descamps et al. (2004)
13. *LPL***S447X*	Lower newborn LDL-C, apoB, and TG	Forward stepwise regression analysis	Descamps et al. (2004)
14. *GSTP1***Val105,* **Val114*	Asthma	Multiple linear regression	Carroll et al. (2005)
Case–control plus case TDT			
15. *MTHFR***677T,* *CT, TT*	Oral-facial clefting, cleft lip ± cleft palate	Case–control, case TDT negative	Martinelli et al. (2001)
16. *MTHFR 677T*	Congenital heart disease	Case–control, case TDT negative	van Beynum et al. (2006)
17. *MTHFR***677TT*	Down syndrome	Case–control, case TDT negative	Rai et al. (2006)
18. *HLA-DR***4*	Autism	Case–control, case TDT negative	Lee et al. (2006)
Case–control			
19. *C4B***0*	Autism	Case–control	Warren et al. (1991)
20. *HLA-DR4*	Autism	Case–control	Warren et al. (1996)
21. *GSTP1–1b*	Recurrent early pregnancy loss	Case–control	Zusterzeel et al. (2000)
22. *MTHFR***1298C*	NTD/spina bifida	Case–control	De Marco et al. (2001)
23. *MTRR***66G* **GG*	Down syndrome	Case–control	O'Leary et al. (2002)
24. *MTHFR***677T/* *MTRR***66GG*	Down syndrome	Case–control	O'Leary et al. (2002)
25. *GSTT1***0*	Oral-facial clefting	Case–control	van Rooij et al. (2001)
26. *MTHFR***1298C*	NTD/spina bifida	Case–control	Gonzalez-Herrera et al. (2002)
27. *GSTM1***0*	Recurrent pregnancy loss	Case–control	Sata et al. (2003)
28. *DHFR***19bp* *deletion*	Spina bifida	Case–control	Johnson et al. (2004)
29. *CYP1A1***2A*	Recurrent pregnancy loss	Case–control	Suryanarayana, Deenadayal, and Singh (2004)

(continued)

TABLE 17.1 (Continued)
Reports of Teratogenic Alleles

Teratogenic Allele Report	Disease	Analysis By	References
30. *DHFR*19bp deletion*	Preterm delivery	Case–control	Johnson et al. (2005)
31. *MTHFR*1298C, CC*	Down syndrome	Case–control	Rai et al. (2006)
32. *MTHFR*1298C, CC*	Down syndrome	Case–control	Scala et al. (2006)
33. *RFC1*A80G, GG*	Down syndrome	Case–control	Scala et al. (2006)

Source: Adapted and reprinted from Johnson, W.G. et al., Teratogenic alleles in autism and other neurodevelopmental disorders, in *Autism: Current Theories and Evidence*, ed. Zimmerman, A., Humana Press, Totowa, NJ, 2008. With permission.

Notes: Reports of teratogenic alleles are listed: (1) according to the method of analysis used and (2) according to the date of the report beginning with the earliest. The specific teratogenic allele is listed on the left, next the specific disease or disorder studied, next the study design, and finally, the literature reference. The specific teratogenic allele is given in the nomenclature: gene symbol*allele designation. The names of the genes corresponding to the gene symbol are given in the text and correspond to the designation in *Online Mendelian Inheritance in Man*. Gene symbols are given in uppercase letters and italicized while the corresponding protein symbol is given in the same uppercase letters but not italicized. Sometimes a genotype is given, as in #31 and 32, where "*MTHFR*1298C*" refers to the C-allele at position 1298 of the gene "*MTHFR*" and *CC*, the genotype, refers to a double dose of the C-allele, i.e., homozygosity. Human genes are given in uppercase italics, corresponding proteins in the same uppercase letters that are not italicized. *MTR*, methionine synthase gene; *MTRR*, methionine synthase reductase gene; *GSTP1*, glutathione S-transferase P1 gene; NTD, neural tube defect; *PAH*, phenylalanine hydroxylase gene; Rh, Rhesus factor, a protein that is either present or absent on the surface of human red blood cells; *MTHFD1*, methylenetetrahydrofolate dehydrogenase gene; *CYP1A1*, cytochrome P450 1A1 gene; *NAT1*, N-acetyltransferase gene; *CCL*, monocyte chemoattractant protein gene; APOE, apolipoprotein E; APOC3, apolipoprotein C3; LPL, lipoprotein lipase; *MTHFR*, methylenetetrahydrofolate reductase gene; HLA, human leukocyte antigen system; OFC, oral-facial clefting; CHD, congenital heart defect; C4B, complement component 4B, a blood group antigen; *GSTT1*, glutathione S-transferase T1 gene; *GSTM1*, glutathione S-transferase M1 gene; *DHFR*, dihydrofolate reductase gene; and *RFC1*, reduced folate carrier 1 gene.

Nearly all of these reports of teratogenic alleles involved neurodevelopmental disorders. Their number has more than doubled since the topic was last reviewed in 2003 (Johnson, 2003). It is possible that teratogenic alleles are a specific and even the defining feature of neurodevelopmental disorders, but too little work has been done so far to clarify their impact. Since only 34 reports of teratogenic alleles are known at present, it is possible that these are rare compared with genes acting in affected individuals themselves and have little overall impact. On the other hand, since the number of reports of teratogenic alleles has more than doubled in the last 5 years, it is possible that they are numerous and their ultimate impact may turn out to be quite large. Clearly, more work needs to be done to assess their importance. In order to identify more teratogenic alleles, this concept needs to be incorporated into study designs at the beginning of a project.

17.2   STUDY DESIGNS THAT SUGGEST OR DOCUMENT ACTION OF A TERATOGENIC ALLELE

To identify a candidate gene for a "modifying or specificity allele," i.e., the genes that act in the fetus in the gene–teratogen model, is straightforward because the ordinary methods of linkage mapping are suitable and well developed, e.g., the lod score method, sib pair methods, or standard case–parent methods. For this reason, genes for neurodevelopmental disorders identified by these methods are likely to be of this type.

However, identifying a candidate gene for a teratogenic allele is not straightforward since it is the mother of the proband with the neurodevelopmental disorder who is the one that is affected, i.e., the "genetic patient" for a teratogenic allele. Pedigrees collected for use with the lod score method often do not contain the right individuals for study if the pedigree is simply re-coded so that the individuals with the neurodevelopmental disorder are now "unaffected" and their mothers are "affected." Sib pair methods are also problematic for the study of a teratogenic locus, even if parents are included, because a sib pair contains only one "affected" individual, the mother. Likewise, in the standard transmission/disequilibrium test (TDT), carried out with neurodevelopmental probands and their parents, the only affected individuals in the family are the mothers.

The presence of a teratogenic allele may be first suspected when the examination of a dataset that contains probands, mothers, and fathers for a neurodevelopmental disorder in a case–control study of allelic association shows a significantly increased frequency for an allele of interest among mothers but not fathers compared to controls. Increased frequency in probands of an allele-of-interest is also to be expected because the probands will often inherit an allele from the mother simply by descent, whether or not the allele acts also in the probands. For a teratogenic allele, the expected disease allele frequencies in family members are from highest to lowest mothers > neurodevelopmental probands > fathers = controls. However, allelic association studies are problematic since the allele may be subject to population stratification. In that situation, the case families may not be matched to the controls and the study may be invalid. Since there may be no data on population stratification for that allele, it may not be realized that the study is invalid.

If maternal allele frequencies are increased and TDT analysis shows the increased frequency of transmissions to probands from mothers but not fathers, then genomic imprinting or mitochondrial transmission is likely; the allele should be investigated to determine if it is subject to imprinting or if the gene is a mitochondrial gene. However, if no increased frequency of transmissions is found, then the action of a teratogenic allele is probable.

There are at present three major approaches for documenting the action of a suspected teratogenic allele. One is to use TDT analysis for transmissions from maternal grandparents to mothers as we and others have suggested (Johnson, 1999; Mitchell, 1997). Since the mother is the genetic patient for a teratogenic locus, the expectation is that such transmission disequilibrium will occur. This approach has been successful in a study of spina bifida (Doolin et al., 2002) (Table 17.1, #1 and 2) and a study of autism (Williams et al., 2007b) (Table 17.1, #3). This approach works best for disorders where the individuals with the neurodevelopmental disorder are young, since living maternal grandparents can more readily be found. This approach is direct and strongly supports the action of a teratogenic allele, but it does not address the interaction between maternal and fetal genes.

A second approach is to use the case–parent log-linear method (Starr, Hsu, and Schwartz, 2005; Weinberg, 1999; Weinberg and Wilcox, 1999; Weinberg et al., 1998; Wilcox, Weinberg, and Lie, 1998). Since this method requires only the trio consisting of the individual with the neurodevelopmental disorder and the two parents, it may be the most suitable approach if living maternal grandparents are difficult to find. It also addresses the question of the interaction between maternal and fetal genes. With this method, the data is stratified by parental mating type and a modeling term is included for maternal genotype. For example, a mother with AA genotype and father with aa genotype represent the same mating type as a mother with aa and father with AA, but the observation that the former pair occurs more often in parents of affected offspring constitutes evidence that the AA genotype in mothers is a risk genotype for offspring. There are reasons to believe that the case–parent log-linear method may have less power than maternal TDT for the same number of families studied based upon the one report that used both methods on the same dataset (Doolin et al., 2002) (Table 17.1, #1 and 2).

A third approach uses "pents," i.e., families with neurodevelopmental proband, parents, and maternal grandparents (five individuals per family) (Mitchell and Weinberg, 2005). The pent approach has the advantage of estimating both maternal and offspring genetic effects, and offers increased power, per proband, compared with the log-linear approaches. Since DNA from maternal grandparents is required, as a practical matter, it will work best for early onset disorders.

These three analytical approaches are not the only possible ones. Other approaches have also been presented (Mitchell et al., 2005). Interestingly, some of the genes identified in affected individuals by conventional approaches, especially allelic association studies, and thought to act in affected individuals may in fact be teratogenic alleles. This is because these affected individuals frequently receive the teratogenic alleles from their mothers simply by descent. These affected individuals will thus themselves have an increased frequency of the teratogenic allele, as discussed earlier, despite the fact that the allele acts in the mothers not in the affected individuals themselves to contribute the phenotype of the affected individuals.

17.3   EARLY EXAMPLES OF TERATOGENIC ALLELES

Two neurodevelopmental disorders, Rh-incompatibility and maternal phenylketonuria (maternal PKU), are perhaps the earliest disorders shown to result from the action of teratogenic alleles, although the concept of teratogenic alleles was not recognized at that time.

17.3.1   Rh Incompatibility

For Rh incompatibility to occur (Table 17.1, #4), the mother must lack the RhD antigen on the surface of her erythrocytes and thus be Rh negative (RhD negative); i.e., she must be a homozygote for the Rh d allele with the d/d genotype. Also the fetus must carry an Rh *D* allele that can only be of paternal origin (father is RhD positive). During the pregnancy, the Rh *d/d* mother is exposed to the RhD antigen produced by the fetus. Since the mother lacks this antigen, she makes antibodies to RhD antigen as the pregnancy progresses. During a subsequent pregnancy with an RhD positive fetus, maternal antibodies are again produced but in greater amount and in an accelerated fashion. With further RhD positive fetuses, the mother mounts an immunological attack upon the fetus who may develop erythroblastosis fetalis and a developmental disorder. This developmental disorder consists of three clinical syndromes in the fetus and neonate: anemia of the newborn; neonatal jaundice that can lead to the severe fetal encephalopathy of kernicterus; and the generalized neonatal edema of hydrops fetalis with massive anasarca, pleural effusions, and ascites. The teratogenic allele here is Rh *d*, for which the mother is a homozygote. Each of her . parents carries an Rh *d* allele and has transmitted an Rh *d* allele to her. Thus, transmission disequilibrium is present. The mechanisms of fetal damage are unclear, but cytokine abnormalities have been observed (Westgren et al., 1995).

Rh incompatibility has also been recently linked to another neurodevelopmental disorder, schizophrenia (Table 17.1, #6). An increased incidence of schizophrenia has been found in the offspring of pregnancies with Rh incompatibility (Hollister, Laing, and Mednick, 1996) compared to control pregnancies. This effect was not demonstrated for autism in a similar study (Zandi et al., 2006).

17.3.2 MATERNAL PHENYLKETONURIA

Maternal PKU results from the major intrauterine effect on fetuses of mothers with PKU. PKU itself is a recessive postnatal disorder. Untreated homozygous PKU mothers and fathers both have elevated blood phenylalanine. However, the heterozygous offspring of untreated PKU mothers may develop maternal PKU, a disorder different from PKU, that has an abnormal developmental and neurodevelopmental phenotype (Abadie et al., 1996; Allen et al., 1994; Koch et al., 1994). Nearly all cases of PKU and hence maternal PKU are known to result from mutations in the *phenylalanine hydroxylase (PAH)* gene. Thus, the mutations in the maternal *(PAH)* gene, through the resulting elevation of maternal blood phenylalanine or other metabolite(s) in the untreated PKU mother, act during pregnancy as teratogenic alleles for the fetus (Table 17.1, #5).

Infants with PKU (Menkes, 1990) are normal at birth and develop a progressive metabolic disorder of postnatal onset characterized by vomiting, eczema, mental retardation, and infantile spasms with hypsarrythmia on the electroencephalogram. In contrast, infants with maternal PKU (Menkes, 1990) have a congenital nonprogressive disorder of fetal onset characterized by microcephaly, abnormal facies, mental retardation, congenital heart disease, and prenatal and postnatal growth retardations. The teratogenic effect in maternal PKU is not dependent upon the fetal genotype, although the fetus is an obligate heterozygote since the mother is a homozygote for PKU and the father (usually) has the normal genotype.

Since PKU mothers of maternal PKU offspring are homozygotes for *PAH* mutations, each maternal grandparent is a heterozygote who has transmitted the mutant allele to the mother. Thus, if a maternal TDT was carried out in these maternal trios (maternal PKU, mothers, and their parents), it would show transmission disequilibrium. However, since the maternal PKU mothers have PKU and are thus known to be homozygotes for *PAH* mutations, such a TDT is now unnecessary. Thus, this documentation of the action of a teratogenic allele in maternal PKU is, in a sense, the equivalent of a maternal TDT.

17.4 A RATIONALE FOR FINDING TERATOGENIC ALLELES IN AUTISM

Children with autism have a change in the normal developmental pattern with impaired social interactions and communication, restricted interests, and repetitive, stereotyped patterns of behaviour that can be observed before 36 months of age (American Psychiatric Association, 1994; Rapin, 1997). Clinical genetic studies suggest the presence of multiple gene loci that interact with each other (Muhle, Trentacoste, and Rapin, 2004; Szatmari, 2003) and possibly with environmental and epigenetic factors (Lawler et al., 2004; Szatmari, 2003) that may contribute to autism. Some of these contributing factors appear to be immune abnormalities.

Neuropathological studies (Rodier et al., 1996; Stromland et al., 1994), cytoarchitectonic studies (Piven and O'Leary, 1999), and minicolumn studies (Casanova et al., 2002; Casanova, Buxhoeveden, and Gomez, 2003) all support the prenatal origin of certain brain abnormalities in autism. Consequently, it is possible that maternal genes, acting during pregnancy, could contribute to the autism phenotype in the fetus.

17.5 *HLA-DR4* AND AUTISM

17.5.1 MAJOR HISTOCOMPATIBILITY COMPLEX

The major histocompatibility complex (MHC) is a major collection of immune-related genes, the largest collection in the genome. The human MHC region contains over 200 genes that have been grouped as class I, class II, and class III genes. Class I loci include *HLA-A* (*human leukocyte antigen-A*), *HLA-B*, and *HLA-C*. Class II loci include *HLA-DR*, *HLA-DQ*, and *HLA-DP* genes. Class III loci include certain complement-related genes, e.g., *C4A* and *C4B*. These genes are polymorphic, many of them highly polymorphic. The region has limited recombination in most areas except for a few recombination hot spots. Since recombination is limited in most areas of the MHC, linkage disequilibrium is seen over long distances leading to the presence of MHC-extended haplotypes. Reed Warren's group studied a number of MHC genes including the class II gene *HLA-DR*, particularly the highly polymorphic β-chain gene, *HLA-DRβ1* (Daniels et al., 1995; Warren et al., 1992, 1996).

17.5.2 CASE–CONTROL STUDIES OF *HLA-DR* AND AUTISM

Early studies in autism by Warren et al. (1996) found that certain polymorphic alleles in the MHC on chromosome 6, including *HLA-DR4*, were increased in frequency in mothers of individuals with autism. As an explanation of their striking maternal findings, Warren et al. raised the question of whether a gene acting in the mother during pregnancy might contribute to autism in her fetus (Warren et al., 1996) (Table 17.1, #20).

Warren and coauthors studied the frequency of an MHC-extended haplotype that contains *HLA-DR4* in a case–control design. This haplotype, *B44-S30-DR4*, is composed of *HLA-B44*, the *S* allele of the *BF* gene, the *3* allele of *C4A*, the *0* or *null* allele of *C4B*, and the *DR4* allele. Compared with controls, *B44-SC30-DR4* was significantly increased in both cases and in mothers but not in fathers of individuals with autism (Warren et al., 1992). Daniels et al. (1995) confirmed this finding in a subsequent case–control study. Subsequently, Warren et al. (1996) found that certain alleles of the third hypervariable region of *HLA-DRβ1* had very strong association with children with autism especially alleles within *HLA-DR4* (Table 17.1, #20).

Torres et al. (2002) carried out a case–control study with individuals with autism spectrum disorder (ASD) compared with control Caucasian allele frequencies from the National Marrow Donor Program and found that *HLA-DR4* occurred more frequently in children with ASD than control subjects.

Recently, Lee et al. (2006) carried out a case–control study of *HLA-DR4* in autism in families from eastern Tennessee and families from the AGRE repository that were selected to be from all parts of the United States and in which multiple males had the diagnosis of autism, and compared them with a control group of healthy unrelated adults (Table 17.1, #18). Compared with controls, children with autism in the east Tennessee group and their mothers but not their fathers had a significantly higher frequency of *HLA-DR4* alleles than did control subjects. The mothers were 5.54 times (95% confidence interval [CI] 1.74, 18.67) and their children with autism 4.20 times (95% CI 1.37, 13.27) more likely to have *HLA-DR4* than control individuals (Lee et al., 2006). However, *HLA-DR4* frequencies of the children with autism from the autism genetic resource exchange (AGRE) repository, their mothers, and their fathers were not significantly different from controls (Lee et al., 2006). The authors interpreted their findings in the eastern Tennessee group as consistent with a hypothesis that maternal–fetal immune interaction *in utero* could affect fetal brain development; such an immune interaction could conceivably involve both HLA and related genes in both genetic and epigenetic mechanisms.

Although these studies suggested a maternal effect of *HLA-DR4* for autism, all of them compared mothers with controls in case–control study designs, and none of them carried out a more direct test such as the maternal TDT that could document the presence of a maternal allele acting during pregnancy to contribute to the autism phenotype (Doolin et al., 2002; Johnson, 1999, 2003; Johnson et al., 2008; Mitchell, 1997).

Case–control studies are powerful and highly useful, but also have certain limitations. One major limitation is that the cases and controls may not be ascertained in the same way and hence may not be identical. The case–control design presumes that controls are drawn from the same population as the cases, or from a population equally at risk. Important as this presumption is, it is often not achieved in practice. Other study designs, e.g., case–parent designs often used with the TDT, use internal controls, e.g., by comparing the genotype of the affected child with the untransmitted parental alleles. Hence, population stratification is not a major limitation for TDT studies. A case–control study is an excellent first step to suggest the action of a teratogenic allele in a dataset, but such studies need to be confirmed with more direct method, e.g., one of the study designs discussed earlier: the maternal TDT, the log-linear method, the method of pentets, or another such design.

The finding of the increased frequency of a polymorphic allele in mothers but not fathers of affected individuals is an interesting one because it may help identify a factor that contributes to the disease. There are several possible explanations of this pattern of increased allele frequency. The known possible reasons for the increased frequency of an allele observed in mothers of affected individuals include the following:

1. The allele is a teratogenic allele.
2. The allele acts by imprinting and is imprinted in the mother.
3. The allele acts in the affected individual and hence will have increased frequency in the parents—sometimes, by chance the allele will have increased frequency in mothers but not fathers.
4. The allele is a mitochondrial allele and hence is transmitted only by mothers to affected individuals and therefore has increased frequency in mothers.

17.5.3 CASE–PARENT STUDY OF AUTISM

A recent study of autism used a case–parent study design to document *HLA-DR4* as a teratogenic allele for autism (Johnson et al., 2009). The study used the maternal TDT method (Johnson, 1999; Mitchell, 1997) in which transmissions from maternal grandparents to mothers of individuals with autism were studied for transmission disequilibrium. *HLA-DR4* was transmitted significantly more frequently than was expected by chance ($p = 0.008$), documenting the action of *HLA-DR4* in mothers of affected individuals, i.e., action as a teratogenic allele. This appeared to explain the elevated frequency of *HLA-DR4* in mothers of individuals with autism. However, as a secondary study, other causes of the elevated frequency of *HLA-DR4* in mothers of cases were considered: transmission disequilibrium was not found for transmissions from mothers to individuals with autism excluding action of *HLA-DR4* in the individual with autism. Two tests of genomic imprinting were negative. *HLA-DR4* is known not to be a mitochondrial gene. Thus, the other possible explanations for the elevated allele frequency of *HLA-DR4* in mothers of individuals with autism, discussed in Section 17.5.2, were not supported.

17.6 POSSIBLE MODES OF ACTION BY WHICH *HLA-DR4* MIGHT CONTRIBUTE TO AUTISM

It is unknown how *HLA-DR4* could act in mothers to influence the brain development of their affected offspring. A number of possible mechanisms are suggested by the work so far that could lead to further studies. Maternal *DR4* could contribute to a subset of autism cases possibly interacting with other risk alleles for autism and with environmental factors to perturb pathways affecting brain development in autism. A possible environmental factor could be the maternal infections during pregnancy (urinary tract, respiratory, and vaginal) reported previously as more common in autism mothers compared with controls, although that increase was not statistically significant (Comi et al., 1999). *HLA-DR4* (along with *DR3*) is a risk allele for type I diabetes mellitus and appears to modulate the humoral immune response to enterovirus antigens (Sadeharju et al., 2003).

Interestingly, in mice, maternal immune stimulation during gestation may affect developmental outcome in offspring. For example, maternal immune stimulation reportedly ameliorated malformations induced by chemical teratogens (Holladay et al., 2002), perhaps through the maternal immune regulation of fetal gene expression, including cell cycle/apoptotic genes (Sharova et al., 2000). Maternal stimulation with IFN-γ (interferon-gamma) decreased the severity of fetal cleft and palate caused by urethane, while stimulation with Freund's complete adjuvant reduced both the incidence and the severity of the lesion (Holladay et al., 2000). Maternal immune stimulation inducing inflammation increased fetal brain cytokine response, decreased the number of reelin-immunoreactive cells in certain areas of postnatal brain of offspring, and altered behavior in adult offspring (Meyer et al., 2006). Reelin gene polymorphisms have been associated with autism (Serajee, Zhong, and Huq, 2006; Skaar et al., 2005) and reelin protein levels are decreased in autism in blood (Fatemi, Stary, and Egan, 2002) and cerebellum (Fatemi et al., 2001).

17.6.1 Oxidative Stress

It is thought that a state of elevated inflammation is a part of normal pregnancy, involving both the mother and the placenta; if this inflammation is increased, e.g., during maternal infection, this could increase the risk of autism (Patterson et al., 2008). Since the immune system can be a major generator of oxidative stress, e.g., during an infection, it is possible that *HLA-DR4* could act to increase maternal oxidative stress and thereby alter fetal brain development, thus contributing to autism in the fetus. Moreover, alterations of proteins that normally diminish oxidative stress by clearing inducers of oxidative stress and products of oxidative stress could potentiate this effect; such polymorphic mutations have been reportedly associated with autism, e.g., paraoxonase (Serajee et al., 2004), glutathione *S*-transferase-P1 (*GSTP1*) (Williams et al., 2007a), and *GSTM1* (Buyske et al., 2006). A resulting increase in oxidative stress could perturb mechanisms of brain development in the fetus and in the neonate.

A number of biochemical changes support this idea (reviewed in Chauhan and Chauhan, 2006): total glutathione was observed to be significantly decreased and oxidized glutathione significantly increased in autism (James et al., 2004). Also, standard markers of oxidative stress, such as malondialdehyde, a lipid peroxidation marker in plasma (Chauhan et al., 2004), and 8-isoprostane in urine (Ming et al., 2005), were found to be significantly increased in individuals with autism.

Ling et al. (2007) recently demonstrated that a rheumatoid arthritis shared epitope (SE) acts as a signaling ligand that activates a nitric oxide–mediated pro-oxidative pathway and blocks a cyclic adenosine monophosphate (cAMP)-mediated antioxidative pathway, leading to increased vulnerability to oxidative damage. The SE consists of alleles encoding certain amino acid sequences in positions 70–74 of the *HLA-DRβ* chain, many of them corresponding to subtypes of *HLA-DR4*, including the most common *DR4* subtypes. This action of the SE, leading to increased vulnerability to oxidative damage, could be of relevance to brain development in autism.

A number of studies support the idea that oxidative stress could play a role in autism (reviewed in Chauhan and Chauhan, 2006). For example, elevated cytokine levels have been reported in children with ASD (Molloy et al., 2006). Interestingly increased *HLA-DR* homozygosity both in pre-eclamptic women and in their partners has been strongly associated with pre-eclampsia (de Luca Brunori et al., 2000), a disorder in which oxidative stress plays a role. A number of possible mechanisms exist by which maternal inflammation during pregnancy can affect neuronal development (Jonakait, 2007). The neuropoietic cytokine family appears to play an important role in nervous system development as well as in affecting neuronal plasticity (Bauer, Kerr, and Patterson, 2007). In a rat model using lipopolysaccharide (LPS) to initiate maternal inflammation and induce maternal infection during pregnancy, it has been demonstrated that cytokines may mediate effects of prenatal infection on the fetus, a finding that has implications for neurodevelopmental disorder such as schizophrenia (Ashdown et al., 2006) and autism. Another approach to inducing maternal infection used maternal poly I:C exposure to cause maternal inflammation without an infectious agent and found that this regulates tumor necrosis factor-α, brain-derived neurotrophic factor, and nerve growth factor expressions in neonatal brain and the maternal–fetal unit of the rat (Gilmore, Jarskog, and Vadlamudi, 2005). In a rat model, the inflammatory/cytokine response from the maternal injection of LPS affected both placenta and fetal brain (Bell, Hallenbeck, and Gallo, 2004). In another report using a rat model, prenatal exposure to maternal inflammation induced by LPS mimicking maternal infection, altered cytokine expression in placenta, amniotic fluid, and fetal brain (Urakubo et al., 2001).

17.6.2   Synaptic Pruning and the MHC

An interesting alternative to the oxidative stress mechanism is that *HLA-DR4* could play a role in brain development through neural pruning. It has recently been reported that the immune system plays a role in brain development through synaptic pruning during development; the classical complement cascade appears to mediate the elimination of synapses in the central nervous system (Stevens et al., 2007). Thus, it is possible that the immune system may contribute to marking, which synapses are to be eliminated and to pruning them. Since this mechanism involves the complement system, it is not clear how *HLA-DR4* might contribute. However, portions of the complement system, class III markers, are in linkage disequilibrium with *HLA-DR4*. Moreover, this mechanism has so far been shown to involve only genes acting in the fetus.

Genes of proteins of the postsynaptic density (PSD) have been shown to be associated with autism supporting the idea that synaptic abnormalities contribute to autism. MHC class I protein co-localizes with PSD-95 postsynaptically in dendrites and appears to contribute to the regulation of synaptic function during development, at least in experimental animals (Goddard, Butts, and Shatz, 2007). MHC class I or Ib antigens are required for the regulation of synaptic pruning on neuronal bodies undergoing retrograde degeneration after axonal transection (Wekerle, 2005). Again, it is not clear how *HLA-DR4*, a class II molecule, might contribute. However, there is strong linkage disequilibrium between *HLA-DR* and class I markers. In an experimental animal model, MHC class I molecules were involved in the stripping off of synapses after an axonal lesion (Thams, Oliveira, and Cullheim, 2008).

17.6.3 *HLA-DR4* AND HIGH RELATIVE BIRTHWEIGHT

Autism is associated with growth abnormalities in the brain, e.g., a striking increase in brain growth after the first year of life. The fetal haplotype *HLA-DR4_DQB1*0302*, the haplotype conferring the highest risk for type I diabetes mellitus, is reportedly associated with intrauterine growth alteration, i.e., increased relative birthweight, in normal pregnancies (Larsson et al., 2005) as well as in pregnancies of mothers with type I diabetes (Hummel et al., 2007), an effect that was aggravated by gestational infections, e.g., gestational fever, gastroenteritis, or both (Larsson et al., 2007).

17.6.4 MATERNAL ANTIBODIES AND AUTISM

Autoantibodies to human fetal brain proteins have been identified in the maternal circulation during pregnancy and may persist for over a year, more frequently in mothers of individuals with autism than in control mothers (Braunschweig et al., 2008; Morris et al., 2008). Maternal immunoglobulin G (IgG) is known to cross the placenta and may also enter the fetal circulation. Certain pathogenic maternal antibodies may cause a number of neonatal autoimmune diseases (Heuer, Ashwood, and Van de Water, 2008). It is possible that such transplacental transfer of maternal antibodies could contribute to the perturbation of fetal brain development (Morris et al., 2008; Zimmerman et al., 2007). Again, it is not clear how *HLA-DR4* might contribute to these processes in such a way as to contribute to the autism phenotype.

17.7 FUTURE STUDIES OF *HLA-DR4* IN AUTISM

A larger study is required to confirm the action of *HLA-DR4* in mothers of individuals with autism and also to address the question of whether interaction occurs between maternal and fetal genotypes. Since linkage disequilibrium is present over large areas of the MHC, it is possible that another gene within the MHC or even an extended haplotype is responsible for the association observed with mothers of individuals with autism.

However, studies of the action of the maternal immune system are very much worth pursuing since therapy for immune-related disorders, e.g., autoimmune disorders, is becoming increasingly varied and effective. If *HLA-DR4* acts during pregnancy, this time is also the earliest opportunity for therapy directed toward the prevention and cure of autism. *In utero* therapeutic approaches are actively being developed.

REFERENCES

Abadie, V., E. Depondt, J. P. Farriaux, J. Lepercq, S. Lyonnet, N. Maurin, H. Ogier de Baulny, and M. Vidailhet. 1996. Pregnancy and the child of a mother with phenylketonuria. *Arch. Pediatr.* 3:489–486.

Allen, R. J., J. Brunberg, E. Schwartz, A. M. Schaefer, and G. Jackson. 1994. MRI characterization of cerebral dysgenesis in maternal PKU. *Acta Paediatr. Suppl.* 407:83–85.

American Psychiatric Association. 1994. *Diagnostic and Statistical Manual of Mental Disorders*, 4th ed., Washington D.C.: American Psychiatric Association.

Ashdown, H., Y. Dumont, M. Ng, S. Poole, P. Boksa, and G. N. Luheshi. 2006. The role of cytokines in mediating effects of prenatal infection on the fetus: Implications for schizophrenia. *Mol. Psychiatry* 11:47–55.

Bauer, S., B. J. Kerr, and P. H. Patterson. 2007. The neuropoietic cytokine family in development, plasticity, disease and injury. *Nat. Rev. Neurosci.* 8:221–232.

Bell, M. J., J. M. Hallenbeck, and V. Gallo. 2004. Determining the fetal inflammatory response in an experimental model of intrauterine inflammation in rats. *Pediatr. Res.* 56:541–546.

Braunschweig, D., P. Ashwood, P. Krakowiak, I. Hertz-Picciotto, R. Hansen, L. A. Croen, I. N. Pessah, and J. Van de Water. 2008. Autism: Maternally derived antibodies specific for fetal brain proteins. *Neurotoxicology* 29:226–231.

Brody, L. C., M. Conley, C. Cox, P. N. Kirke, M. P. McKeever, J. L. Mills, A. M. Molloy, V. B. O'Leary, A. Parle-McDermott, J. M. Scott, and D. A. Swanson. 2002. A polymorphism, R653Q, in the trifunctional enzyme methylenetetrahydrofolate dehydrogenase/ methenyltetrahydrofolate cyclohydrolase/formyltetrahydrofolate synthetase is a maternal genetic risk factor for neural tube defects: Report of the Birth Defects Research Group. *Am. J. Hum. Genet.* 71:1207–1215.

Buyske, S., T. A. Williams, A. E. Mars, E. S. Stenroos, S. X. Ming, R. Wang, M. Sreenath, M. F. Factura, C. Reddy, G. H. Lambert, and W. G. Johnson. 2006. Analysis of case-parent trios at a locus with a deletion allele: Association of GSTM1 with autism. *BMC Genet.* 7:8.

Carroll, W. D., W. Lenney, F. Child, R. C. Strange, P. W. Jones, and A. A. Fryer. 2005. Maternal glutathione S-transferase GSTP1 genotype is a specific predictor of phenotype in children with asthma. *Pediatr. Allergy Immunol.* 16:32–39.

Casanova, M. F., D. Buxhoeveden, and J. Gomez. 2003. Disruption in the inhibitory architecture of the cell minicolumn: Implications for autism. *Neuroscientist* 9:496–507.

Casanova, M. F., D. P. Buxhoeveden, A. E. Switala, and E. Roy. 2002. Minicolumnar pathology in autism. *Neurology* 58:428–432.

Chauhan, A. and V. Chauhan. 2006. Oxidative stress in autism. *Pathophysiology* 13:171–181.

Chauhan, A., V. Chauhan, W. T. Brown, and I. Cohen. 2004. Oxidative stress in autism: Increased lipid peroxidation and reduced serum levels of ceruloplasmin and transferrin— the antioxidant proteins. *Life Sci.* 75:2539–2549.

Chen, D., Y. Hu, F. Yang, Z. Li, B. Wu, Z. Fang, J. Li, and L. Wang. 2005. Cytochrome P450 gene polymorphisms and risk of low birth weight. *Genet. Epidemiol.* 28:368–375.

Comi, A. M., A. W. Zimmerman, V. H. Frye, P. A. Law, and J. N. Peeden. 1999. Familial clustering of autoimmune disorders and evaluation of medical risk factors in autism. *J. Child Neurol.* 14:388–394.

Daniels, W. W., R. P. Warren, J. D. Odell, A. Maciulis, R. A. Burger, W. L. Warren, and A. R. Torres. 1995. Increased frequency of the extended or ancestral haplotype B44-SC30-DR4 in autism. *Neuropsychobiology* 32:120–123.

de Luca Brunori, I., L. Battini, M. Simonelli, F. Clemente, E. Brunori, M. L. Mariotti, and A. R. Genazzani. 2000. Increased HLA-DR homozygosity associated with pre-eclampsia. *Hum. Reprod.* 15:1807–1812.

De Marco, P., M. G. Calevo, A. Moroni, L. Arata, E. Merello, A. Cama, R. H. Finnell, L. Andreussi, and V. Capra. 2001. Polymorphisms in genes involved in folate metabolism as risk factors for NTDs. *Eur. J. Pediatr. Surg.* 11(Suppl. 1):S14–S17.

Descamps, O. S., M. Bruniaux, P. F. Guilmot, R. Tonglet, and F. R. Heller. 2004. Lipoprotein concentrations in newborns are associated with allelic variations in their mothers. *Atherosclerosis* 172:287–298.

Doolin, M. T., S. Barbaux, M. McDonnell, K. Hoess, A. S. Whitehead, and L. E. Mitchell. 2002. Maternal genetic effects, exerted by genes involved in homocysteine remethylation, influence the risk of spina bifida. *Am. J. Hum. Genet.* 71:1222–1226.

Fatemi, S. H., J. M. Stary, and E. A. Egan. 2002. Reduced blood levels of reelin as a vulnerability factor in pathophysiology of autistic disorder. *Cell Mol. Neurobiol.* 22:139–152.

Fatemi, S. H., J. M. Stary, A. R. Halt, and G. R. Realmuto. 2001. Dysregulation of reelin and Bcl-2 proteins in autistic cerebellum. *J. Autism Dev. Disord.* 31:529–535.

Gilmore, J. H., L. F. Jarskog, and S. Vadlamudi. 2005. Maternal poly I:C exposure during pregnancy regulates TNF alpha, BDNF, and NGF expression in neonatal brain and the maternal-fetal unit of the rat. *J. Neuroimmunol.* 159:106–112.

Goddard, C. A., D. A. Butts, and C. J. Shatz. 2007. Regulation of CNS synapses by neuronal MHC class I. *Proc. Natl. Acad. Sci. U.S.A.* 104:6828–6833.

Gonzalez-Herrera, L. J., M. P. Flores-Machado, I. C. Castillo-Zapata, M. G. Garcia-Escalante, D. Pinto-Escalante, and A. Gonzalez-Del Angel. 2002. Interaction of C677T and A1298C polymorphisms in the MTHFR gene in association with neural tube defects in the State of Yucatan, Mexico (abst). *Am. J. Hum. Genet.* 71:367.

Heuer, L, P. Ashwood, and J. Van de Water. 2008. The immune system in autism. Is there a connection? In *Autism: Current Theories and Evidence*, ed. A. W. Zimmerman, Totowa, NJ: Humana Press.

Holladay, S. D., L. Sharova, B. J. Smith, R. M. Gogal Jr., D. L. Ward, and B. L. Blaylock. 2000. Nonspecific stimulation of the maternal immune system. I. Effects on teratogen-induced fetal malformations. *Teratology* 62:413–419.

Holladay, S. D., L. V. Sharova, K. Punareewattana, T. C. Hrubec, R. M. Gogal, Jr., M. R. Prater, and A. A. Sharov. 2002. Maternal immune stimulation in mice decreases fetal malformations caused by teratogens. *Int. Immunopharmacol.* 2:325–332.

Hollister, J. M., P. Laing, and S. A. Mednick. 1996. Rhesus incompatibility as a risk factor for schizophrenia in male adults. *Arch. Gen. Psychiatry* 53:19–24.

Hummel, M., S. Marienfeld, M. Huppmann, A. Knopff, M. Voigt, E. Bonifacio, and A. G. Ziegler. 2007. Fetal growth is increased by maternal type 1 diabetes and HLA DR4-related gene interactions. *Diabetologia* 50:850–858.

James, S. J., P. Cutler, S. Melnyk, S. Jernigan, L. Janak, D. W. Gaylor, and J. A. Neubrander. 2004. Metabolic biomarkers of increased oxidative stress and impaired methylation capacity in children with autism. *Am. J. Clin. Nutr.* 80:1611–1617.

Jensen, L. E., A. J. Etheredge, K. S. Brown, L. E. Mitchell, and A. S. Whitehead. 2006a. Maternal genotype for the monocyte chemoattractant protein 1 A(-2518)G promoter polymorphism is associated with the risk of spina bifida in offspring. *Am. J. Med. Genet. A* 140:1114–1118.

Jensen, L. E., K. Hoess, L. E. Mitchell, and A. S. Whitehead. 2006b. Loss of function poly-morphisms in NAT1 protect against spina bifida. *Hum. Genet.* 120:52–57.

Johnson, W. G. 1999. The DNA polymorphism-diet-cofactor-development hypothesis and the gene-teratogen model for schizophrenia and other developmental disorders. *Am. J. Med. Genet.* 88:311–323.

Johnson, W. G. 2003. Teratogenic alleles and neurodevelopmental disorders. *Bioessays* 25:464–477.

Johnson, W. G., E. S. Stenroos, J. Spychala, S. Buyske, S. Chatkupt, and X. Ming. 2004. A new 19 bp deletion polymorphism in intron-1 of dihydrofolate reductase (DHFR): A risk factor for spina bifida acting in mothers during pregnancy? *Am. J. Med. Genet.* 124A: 339–345.

Johnson, W. G., T. O. Scholl, J. R. Spychala, S. Buyske, E. S. Stenroos, and X. Chen. 2005. Common dihydrofolate reductase 19bp deletion allele: A novel risk factor for preterm delivery. *Am. J. Clin. Nutr.* 81:664–668.

Johnson, W. G., M. Sreenath, S. Buyske, and E. S. Stenroos. 2008. Teratogenic alleles in autism and other neurodevelopmental disorders. In *Autism: Current Theories and Evidence*, ed. A. Zimmerman. Totowa, NJ: Humana Press.

Johnson, W. G., S. Buyske, A. E. Mars, S. Sreenath, E. S. Stenroos, T. A. Williams, R. Stein, and G. H. Lambert. 2009. *HLA-DR4* as a risk allele for autism, acting in mothers of probands possibly during pregnancy. *Arch. Pediatr. Adolesc. Med.* 163:542–546.

Jonakait, G. M. 2007. The effects of maternal inflammation on neuronal development: Possible mechanisms. *Int. J. Dev. Neurosci.* 25:415–425.

Koch, R., H. L. Levy, R. Matalon, B. Rouse, W. B. Hanley, F. Trefz, C. Azen, E. G. Friedman, F. De la Cruz, F. Guttler et al. 1994. The international collaborative study of maternal phenylketonuria: Status report 1994. *Acta Paediatr. Suppl.* 407:111–119.

Larsson, H. E., K. Lynch, B. Lernmark, A. Nilsson, G. Hansson, P. Almgren, A. Lernmark, and S. A. Ivarsson. 2005. Diabetes-associated HLA genotypes affect birthweight in the general population. *Diabetologia* 48:1484–1491.

Larsson, H. E., K. Lynch, B. Lernmark, G. Hansson, A. Lernmark, and S. A. Ivarsson. 2007. Relationship between increased relative birthweight and infections during pregnancy in children with a high-risk diabetes HLA genotype. *Diabetologia* 50:1161–1169.

Lawler, C. P., L. A. Croen, J. K. Grether, and J. Van de Water. 2004. Identifying environmental contributions to autism: Provocative clues and false leads. *Ment. Retard. Dev. Disabil. Res. Rev.* 10:292–302.

Lee, L. C., A. A. Zachary, M. S. Leffell, C. J. Newschaffer, K. J. Matteson, J. D. Tyler, and A. W. Zimmerman. 2006. HLA-DR4 in families with autism. *Pediatr. Neurol.* 35:303–307.

Ling, S., Z. Li, O. Borschukova, L. Xiao, P. Pumpens, and J. Holoshitz. 2007. The rheumatoid arthritis shared epitope increases cellular susceptibility to oxidative stress by antagonizing an adenosine-mediated anti-oxidative pathway. *Arthritis Res. Ther.* 9:R5.

Martinelli, M., L. Scapoli, F. Pezzetti, F. Carinci, P. Carinci, G. Stabellini, L. Bisceglia, F. Gombos, and M. Tognon. 2001. C677T variant form at the MTHFR gene and CL/P: A risk factor for mothers? *Am. J. Med. Genet.* 98:357–360.

Menkes, J. H. 1990. *Textbook of Child Neurology*, 4th ed. Philadelphia, PA: Lea and Febiger.

Meyer, U., M. Nyffeler, A. Engler, A. Urwyler, M. Schedlowski, I. Knuesel, B. K. Yee, and J. Feldon. 2006. The time of prenatal immune challenge determines the specificity of inflammation-mediated brain and behavioral pathology. *J. Neurosci.* 26: 4752–4762.

Ming, X., T. P. Stein, M. Brimacombe, W. G. Johnson, G. H. Lambert, and G. C. Wagner. 2005. Increased excretion of a lipid peroxidation biomarker in autism. *Prostaglandins Leukot. Essent. Fatty Acids* 73:379–384.

Mitchell, L. E. 1997. Differentiating between fetal and maternal genotypic effects, using the transmission test for linkage disequilibrium. *Am. J. Hum. Genet.* 60:1006–1007.

Mitchell, L. E. and C. R. Weinberg. 2005. Evaluation of offspring and maternal genetic effects on disease risk using a family-based approach: the "pent" design. *Am. J. Epidemiol.* 162:676–685.

Mitchell, L. E., J. R. Starr, C. R. Weinberg, J. S. Sinsheimer, L. E. Mitchell, and J. C. Murray. 2005. Maternal genetic effects. Invited Sessions I, #14, *American Society of Human Genetics Annual Meeting*, Oct 26, 2005, Salt Lake City, UT.

Molloy, C. A., A. L. Morrow, J. Meinzen-Derr, K. Schleifer, K. Dienger, Manning-Court, M. Altaye, and M. Wills-Karp. 2006. Elevated cytokine levels in children with autism spectrum disorder. *J. Neuroimmunol.* 172:198–205.

Morris, C. M., M Pletnikov, A. W. Zimmerman, and H. S. Singer. 2008. Maternal antibodies and the placental-fetal IgG transfer theory. In *Autism: Current Theories and Evidence*, ed. A. W. Zimmerman, Totowa, NJ: Humana Press.

Muhle, R., S. V. Trentacoste, and I. Rapin. 2004. The genetics of autism. *Pediatrics* 113: e472–e486.

O'Leary, V. B., A. Parle-McDermott, A. M. Molloy, P. N. Kirke, Z. Johnson, M. Conley, J. M. Scott, and J. L. Mills. 2002. MTRR and MTHFR polymorphism: Link to Down syndrome? *Am. J. Med. Genet.* 107:151–155.

Palmer, C. G., J. A. Turunen, J. S. Sinsheimer, S. Minassian, T. Paunio, J. Lonnqvist, L. Peltonen, and J. A. Woodward. 2002. RHD maternal-fetal genotype incompatibility increases schizophrenia susceptibility. *Am. J. Hum. Genet.* 71:1312–1319.

Patterson, P. H., W. Xu, S. E. P. Smith, and B. E. Devarman. 2008. Maternal immune activation, cytokines and autism. In *Autism: Current Theories and Evidence*, ed. A. W. Zimmerman, Totowa, NJ: Humana Press.

Piven, J. and D. O'Leary. 1999. Neuroimaging in autism. *Child Adolesc. Psychiatr. Clin. N. Am.* 6:305–323.

Rai, A. K., S. Singh, S. Mehta, A. Kumar, L. K. Pandey, and R. Raman. 2006. MTHFR C677T and A1298C polymorphisms are risk factors for Down's syndrome in Indian mothers. *J. Hum. Genet.* 51:278–283.

Rapin, I. 1997. Autism. *N. Engl. J. Med.* 337:97–104.

Rodier, P. M., J. L. Ingram, B. Tisdale, S. Nelson, and J. Romano. 1996. Embryological origin for autism: Developmental anomalies of the cranial nerve motor nuclei. *J. Comp. Neurol.* 370:247–261.

Rouse, B. and C. Azen. 2004. Effect of high maternal blood phenylalanine on offspring congenital anomalies and developmental outcome at ages 4 and 6 years: The importance of strict dietary control preconception and throughout pregnancy. *J. Pediatr.* 144:235–239.

Sadeharju, K., M. Knip, M. Hiltunen, H. K. Akerblom, and H. Hyoty. 2003. The HLA-DR phenotype modulates the humoral immune response to enterovirus antigens. *Diabetologia* 46:1100–1105.

Sata, F., H. Yamada, T. Kondo, Y. Gong, S. Tozaki, G. Kobashi, E. H. Kato, S. Fujimoto, and R. Kishi. 2003. Glutathione S-transferase M1 and T1 polymorphisms and the risk of recurrent pregnancy loss. *Mol. Hum. Reprod.* 9:165–169.

Scala, I., B. Granese, M. Sellitto, S. Salome, A. Sammartino, A. Pepe, P. Mastroiacovo, G. Sebastio, and G. Andria. 2006. Analysis of seven maternal polymorphisms of genes involved in homocysteine/folate metabolism and risk of Down syndrome offspring. *Genet. Med.* 8:409–416.

Serajee, F. J., H. Zhong, and A. H. M. Huq. 2006. Association of Reelin gene polymorphisms with autism. *Genomics* 87:75–83.

Serajee, F. J., R. Nabi, H. Zhong, and M. Huq. 2004. Polymorphisms in xenobiotic metabolism genes and autism. *J. Child Neurol.* 19:413–417.

Sharova, L., P. Sura, B. J. Smith, R. M. Gogal, Jr., A. A. Sharov, D. L. Ward, and S. D. Holladay. 2000. Nonspecific stimulation of the maternal immune system. II. Effects on gene expression in the fetus. *Teratology* 62:420–428.

Skaar, D. A., Y. Shao, J. L. Haines, J. E. Stenger, J. Jaworski, E. R. Martin, G. R. DeLong, J. H. Moore, J. L. McCauley, J. S. Sutcliffe, A. E. Ashley-Koch, M. L. Cuccaro, S. E. Folstein, J. R. Gilbert, and M. A. Pericak-Vance. 2005. Analysis of the RELN gene as a genetic risk factor for autism. *Mol. Psychiatry* 10:563–571.

Starr, J. R., L. Hsu, and S. M. Schwartz. 2005. Assessing maternal genetic associations: A comparison of the log-linear approach to case-parent triad data and a case-control approach. *Epidemiology* 16:294–303.

Stevens, B., N. J. Allen, L. E. Vazquez, G. R. Howell, K. S. Christopherson, N. Nouri, K. D. Micheva, A. K. Mehalow, A. D. Huberman, B. Stafford, A. Sher, A. M. Litke, J. D. Lambris, S. J. Smith, S. W. John, and B. A. Barres. 2007. The classical complement cascade mediates CNS synapse elimination. *Cell* 131:1164–1178.

Stromland, K., V. Nordin, M. Miller, B. Akerstrom, and C. Gillberg. 1994. Autism in thalidomide embryopathy: A population study. *Dev. Med. Child Neurol.* 36:351–356.

Suryanarayana, V., M. Deenadayal, and L. Singh. 2004. Association of CYP1A1 gene polymorphism with recurrent pregnancy loss in the South Indian population. *Hum. Reprod.* 19:2648–2652.

Szatmari, P. 2003. The causes of autism spectrum disorders. *Brit. Med. J.* 326:173–174.

Thams, S., A. Oliveira, and S. Cullheim. 2008. MHC class I expression and synaptic plasticity after nerve lesion. *Brain Res. Rev.* 57:265–269.

Torres, A. R., A. Maciulis, E. G. Stubbs, A. Cutler, and D. Odell. 2002. The transmission disequilibrium test suggests that HLA-DR4 and DR13 are linked to autism spectrum disorder. *Hum. Immunol.* 63:311–316.

Urakubo, A., L. F. Jarskog, J. A. Lieberman, and J. H. Gilmore. 2001. Prenatal exposure to maternal infection alters cytokine expression in the placenta, amniotic fluid, and fetal brain. *Schizophr. Res.* 47:27–36.

van Beynum, I. M., L. Kapusta, M. den Heijer, S. H. Vermeulen, M. Kouwenberg, O. Daniels, and H. J. Blom. 2006. Maternal MTHFR 677C > T is a risk factor for congenital heart defects: Effect modification by periconceptional folate supplementation. *Eur. Heart J.* 27:981–987.

van Rooij, I. A., M. J. Wegerif, H. M. Roelofs, W. H. Peters, A. M. Kuijpers-Jagtman, G. A. Zielhuis, H. M. Merkus, and R. P. Steegers-Theunissen. 2001. Smoking, genetic polymorphisms in biotransformation enzymes, and nonsyndromic oral clefting: A gene-environment interaction. *Epidemiology* 12:502–507.

Warren, R. P., V. K. Singh, P. Cole, J. D. Odell, C. B. Pingree, W. L. Warren, and E. White. 1991. Increased frequency of the null allele at the complement C4b locus in autism. *Clin. Exp. Immunol.* 83:438–440.

Warren, R. P., V. K. Singh, P. Cole, J. D. Odell, C. B. Pingree, W. L. Warren, C. W. DeWitt, and M. McCullough. 1992. Possible association of the extended MHC haplotype B44-SC30-DR4 with autism. *Immunogenetics* 36:203–207.

Warren, R. P., J. D. Odell, W. L. Warren, R. A. Burger, A. Maciulis, W. W. Daniels, and A. R. Torres. 1996. Strong association of the third hypervariable region of HLA-DR beta 1 with autism. *J. Neuroimmunol.* 67:97–102.

Weinberg, C. R. 1999. Methods for detection of parent-of-origin effects in genetic studies of case-parents triads. *Am. J. Hum. Genet.* 65:229–235.

Weinberg, C. R. and A. J. Wilcox. 1999. Re: Distinguishing the effects of maternal and off-spring genes through studies of "case-parent triads" and a new method for estimating the risk ratio in studies using case-parental control design. *Am. J. Epidemiol.* 150:428–429.

Weinberg, C. R., A. J. Wilcox, and R. T. Lie. 1998. A log-linear approach to case-parent-triad data: Assessing effects of disease genes that act either directly or through maternal effects and that may be subject to parental imprinting. *Am. J. Hum. Genet.* 62:969–978.

Wekerle, H. 2005. Planting and pruning in the brain: MHC antigens involved in synaptic plasticity? *Proc. Natl. Acad. Sci. U.S.A.* 102:3–4.

Westgren, M., S. Ek, M. Remberger, O. Ringden, and M. Stangenberg. 1995. Cytokines in fetal blood and amniotic fluid in Rh-immunized pregnancies. *Obstet. Gynecol.* 86:209–213.

Wilcox, A. J., C. R. Weinberg, and R. T. Lie. 1998. Distinguishing the effects of maternal and offspring genes through studies of "case-parent triads." *Am. J. Epidemiol.* 148:893–901.

Williams, T. A., A. E. Mars, S. G. Buyske, E. S. Stenroos, R. Wang, M. F. Factura-Santiago, G. H. Lambert, and W. G. Johnson. 2007a. Risk of autistic disorder in affected offspring of mothers with a glutathione S-transferase P1 haplotype. *Arch. Pediatr. Adolesc. Med.* 161:356–361.

Williams, T. A., A. E. Mars, S. G. Buyske, E. S. Stenroos, R. Wang, M. F. Factura-Santiago, G. H. Lambert, and W. G. Johnson. 2007b. Risk of autistic disorder in affected offspring of mothers with a glutathione S-transferase P1 haplotype. *Arch. Pediatr. Adolesc. Med.* 161:356–361.

Zandi, P. P., A. Kalaydjian, D. Avramopoulos, H. Shao, M. D. Fallin, and C. J. Newschaffer. 2006. Rh and ABO maternal-fetal incompatibility and risk of autism. *Am. J. Med. Genet. B Neuropsychiatr. Genet.* 141:643–647.

Zimmerman, A. W., S. L. Connors, K. J. Matteson, L. C. Lee, H. S. Singer, J. A. Castaneda, and D. A. Pearce. 2007. Maternal antibrain antibodies in autism. *Brain Behav. Immun.* 21:351–357.

Zusterzeel, P. L., W. L. Nelen, H. M. Roelofs, W. H. Peters, H. J. Blom, and E. A. Steegers. 2000. Polymorphisms in biotransformation enzymes and the risk for recurrent early pregnancy loss. *Mol. Hum. Reprod.* 6:474–478.

18 Autism: The Centrality of Active Pathophysiology and the Shift from Static to Chronic Dynamic Encephalopathy

*Martha R. Herbert**

Department of Pediatric Neurology, Massachusetts General Hospital, Harvard Medical School, Charlestown, MA 02129, USA

CONTENTS

* Corresponding author: Tel.: +1-617-724-5920 ; fax: +1-617-812-6334; e-mail: mherbert1@partners.org

The purpose of this chapter is to reflect upon the implications of the identification of active pathophysiological processes in autism spectrum disorders (ASD), and to reflect back upon prior findings and formulations in the light of these recent discoveries. This chapter articulates challenges posed by these discoveries to deeply held assumptions about the ASD. These assumptions are embodied in a classical model framing the ASD as a problem of genes, brain, and behavior, i.e., as a genetically determined developmental disorder of the brain whose main manifestation is behavioral alterations based on an indelible static encephalopathy; this model would not have predicted the growing documentation of pathophysiological disturbances. This chapter also describes an emerging pathophysiology-centered model of autism that can subsume genes, brain, and behavior but also includes much more. Prior findings and models are reevaluated to support the framing of the ASD as (1) not only a developmental but also a chronic condition based on active pathophysiology, (2) not only having behavioral but also having somatic and systemic features that are not secondary but rather intrinsic consequences of underlying mechanisms, (3) not only genetic but also environmental, (4) not a static encephalopathy but a dynamic, recalcitrant encephalopathy, and (5) not a set of discrete behavioral features neatly mapping to specific genetic mechanisms but a set of emergent properties dynamically arising from pathophysiological systems whose parameters have been dramatically and interactively perturbed. It is argued that a research program based on this approach will incorporate the strengths of the classical model, will encourage many more routes to investigations with practical and treatment applications, and may be a much more rapid path to provide much-needed help to affected individuals and their families.

18.1   INTRODUCTION

While autism spectrum disorders (ASD) can involve exquisite gifts and unusual qualities of perception and thought, they can also involve a great deal of suffering, for the individual on the spectrum as well as family and community. On this account, a core question in autism work needs to be how to help the most people in the most effective ways as quickly as possible. The goal of making sense of autism and its mechanisms needs to be deeply harnessed to this core purpose. Our aim should be to relieve suffering at multiple levels—from aversive sensory overload, sleep disruption, recurrent infections, and gastrointestinal (GI) troubles to overcoming obstacles to communication; to misunderstanding by the non-autistic people of the experiences of people with autism; to aggression and self-injurious behavior; to the burden of allocating scarce resources to deliver therapies that may not be optimally designed, targeted, or implemented; and to acrimonious debate and fiscal drain. Last but hardly the least, if any part of the impairment of optimal functioning in new cases of autism is not purely genetically determined, the suffering and severity that is therefore neither inevitable nor necessary should be prevented or ameliorated.

If we are to help most quickly and with the broadest and greatest effectiveness, then how do we do so, and how much can we really help? What can we realistically expect to accomplish? The answers we give to these questions are greatly conditioned by what we understand autism to be. The main goal of this chapter is to explain and compare two models of autism that lead to greatly different expectations: (1) a classical model of autism as a genetically determined developmental brain disorder and static encephalopathy and (2) an emerging model of autism centered around active systemic environmentally as well as genetically influenced pathophysiological processes beginning early in life and leading to an chronic persistent encephalopathy with dynamic features. This comparison will show that the emerging dynamic pathophysiological model not only includes the strengths of the classical static model, but also takes account of emerging data that are incommensurable with the older formulations. It will also give support to the argument that the emerging more inclusive model offers more opportunities for constructive investigation and intervention.

18.1.1   CLASSICAL MODEL: BEHAVIORAL SYNDROME DERIVING FROM GENETICALLY DETERMINED STATIC ENCEPHALOPATHY

Autism has until recently been considered to be a developmental disorder originating in faulty genes that skew early brain development and lead to a devastating and incurable static encephalopathy. Since this perspective frames autism as directly deriving from an indelibly fundamental alteration of brain structure and function, its adherents take the logical next step when they assume that there are fundamental profound limitations to the potential efficacy of any current therapies. An additional commonly held assumption of this classical viewpoint is that the core behavioral features of autism are specifically determined at the genetic and molecular levels. From this vantage point, only extremely precise molecular or genetic interventions targeting some critical aberrant pathways have any chance of unlocking neural functioning, but these pathways have yet to be discovered and the molecules to target them are yet to be invented. Therefore, to identify targets and develop effective and safe interventions, an extensive, expensive, and long-term research strategy is necessary in order even to begin to relieve suffering in any serious way.

The recent framing of autism as heterogeneous, or "autisms" (plural), modifies this model by suggesting that "autism" is really a collection of different "autisms," each with its own mechanism and perhaps even its own gene(s). The research program derived from this framing would still look for distinctive mechanisms, but now may implicitly propose multiple parallel searches for mechanisms. If this is not accompanied by seeking final common pathways that may bridge across these distinct "autisms" and provide routes of intervention that could be beneficial more broadly than to any one small subgroup, then the road ahead is even longer.

18.1.2 Emerging Understanding of Active Persistent Pathophysiology

Clearly some kind of atypical brain functions must be going on in ASD in order for its atypical behaviors to be produced. The very high prevalence of sensory and sleep problems (Leekam et al. 2007, Tomchek and Dunn 2007) and the high rate of epilepsy in ASD (Canitano 2007) also support this. Critical questions for which we have enticing clues but no clearly worked out answers include (1) what are the mechanisms underlying the altered brain function and (2) what are the causes? Within the classical model, a common phrase heard is "genes–brain–behavior." This suggests that the genetic alteration of the brain causes autistic behavior, and it also implies that researching this specific chain of levels and their relationships is sufficient for understanding ASD.

The trouble with the "genes–brain–behavior" framework is that it promotes oversimplified thinking about the way genes alter brain and the way brain alters behavior. Even to use the three words in a string is a problem, because (1) genes themselves do not directly impact brain but shape other processes that alter brain, (2) these processes that alter brain are impacted by other things in addition to genes, (3) the combination of genes and these other processes alter not only brain but also the rest of the body including systemic molecular and cellular mechanisms that are not organ specific, (4) there is not unidirectionality but bidirectionality—indeed Web-line network interconnections—in that the consequences of all of these dynamical alterations can feed back and alter gene expression, and (5) the outputs of all of this complexity are not limited to behavior but also include phenomena at many other levels (Herbert 2002, Noble 2008). Therefore, to say "genes–brain–behavior" leaves unspecified many intermediary levels that need to be explicitly spelled out and investigated.

One formulation more inclusive than "genes–brain–behavior" is "input–pathophysiology–output" (Herbert 2005a). *Input* can include genes and also a range of environmental factors. *Pathophysiology* can not only include prenatal processes with early impacts on brain development that modulate fundamental features of brain, but also processes and impacts at other time points that have other types of effects on both brain and body. *Outputs* can include not only behaviors but also medical illnesses and a host of other functions.

Critical findings in ASD at the level of active, ongoing pathophysiology that inspire the present volume would not have been predicted by the classical genes–brain–behavior model. Particularly of note are the phenomena of oxidative stress, mitochondrial dysfunction, and inflammation that have been identified in a growing number of studies in a substantial number of individuals with ASD. Evidence of these processes has been identified in somatic tissue samples with the measurement of alterations in a variety of substances including in membrane phospholipids (Bu et al. 2006, Chauhan et al. 2004, Vancassel et al. 2001), antioxidant enzymes, and metabolites in the glutathione synthesis pathway (Chauhan and Chauhan, 2006, James et al. 2006); and the documentation of both oxidative stress (Evans et al. 2008, Pardo et al. 2008, Vargas et al. 2006) and neuroinflammation (Li et al. 2009, Vargas et al. 2005) as well as rapid membrane turnover (Minshew et al. 1993) and altered energy metabolism (Chugani et al. 1999) in brain has also been produced. Much more is reviewed extensively in this volume.

These phenomena are active, ongoing pathophysiological abnormalities. While their chronic impacts can be stubbornly persistent, and while they can cause damage that is more stable, their primary mechanisms act on the timescale of hours and days or even less. They cannot be attributed to genetic errors or early insults in a simple or straightforward fashion, although those could contribute vulnerability or get these processes started. It needs to be emphasized that the identification of active, persistent disturbances of physiological functions, particularly in the brain, is a landmark in the history of autism science because it adds dimensions to the parameters we need to include in considering the condition, and also because it changes the temporality from a playing out of something that happened early on to a process that is continuingly active.

18.1.3 Does Active, Ongoing Pathophysiology Actively Impact Functions Central to ASD?

Even granted the existence of active pathophysiological processes in ASD, a skeptic from the classical model vantage point might question whether they have any significant relevance to ASD. From the classical point of view, it would seem obvious that these sorts of influences could be little more than small bubbles on the surface of the genetically determined ocean of profound brain abnormality. To face this challenge, we need to determine whether the ASD phenotype or any of its components or contributors could be created or substantially aggravated by neural functioning alterations that are chronically and actively maintained.

From a pathophysiology-centered point of view, once the chronic persistence and active character of these processes is recognized, it is not so radical to suggest that perhaps these phenomena might affect synaptic and neural systems *function*. In the literature of neurobiology, there is plenty to suggest that oxidative stress and immune activity can be neuromodulatory. The immune system, energy metabolism, and oxidative stress are abundantly documented as impacting the central nervous system and its function (Lowry et al. 2007, Lozovaya and Miller 2003, Mattson 2007, 2008, Mattson and Liu 2002, Miller, Maletic, and Raison 2009, Wrona 2006). These considerations may be particularly pertinent to the phenomenon of autistic regression, which generally occurs somewhere around the middle of the second year of life. Even if "regression" is preceded by a variety of subtle signs of dysfunction, it is occurring far beyond the most critical periods of brain development and deserves investigation as a new event and in particular, as a shift in functional/metabolic/neurodynamic state and not just as an inevitable playing out of early hard-wired brain alterations.

With chronic-active pathophysiology identified systemically and in brain tissue from individuals with autism, with this active pathophysiology having potential neuromodulatory effects, and with functional changes such as regression needing mechanistic explanation, it becomes necessary to consider the possibility that the biological basis of the autism behavioral phenotype may not be determined "architecturally" once and for all *in utero*, but rather may be actively sustained, possibly even caused or at least substantially aggravated by persistently active pathophysiology (Anderson, Hooker, and Herbert 2008, Zimmerman 2008).

We can imagine a number of possibilities: (1) inputs (e.g., genes and environmental factors) create an indelible alteration in prenatal or early postnatal brain development; 1b) these indelible *in utero* impacts of genes and environmental factors are mediated by pathophysiological processes such as inflammation or oxidative stress; (2) some inputs (e.g., genes, teratogens, infections, or immune responses to infections) increase vulnerability to other inputs that alter early prenatal or early postnatal brain development; (3) some inputs increase vulnerability to other inputs (e.g., excitotoxins) or pathophysiological states (e.g., immune triggers and oxidative stress) that alter neural function postnatally; and (4) chronic, persistent alteration in neural function (e.g., cumulative toxic body burden and/or chronic neuroinflammation having a persistent excitotoxic impact) can in turn lead to changes in brain tissue (e.g., mitochondrial damage → cellular dysfunction → cell death), which in turn may feed back to further affect function.

Once these additional dimensions beyond the genetic determination of altered brain development join the parameters of concern, how do we assess what the type of influence and relative weight may be of each class of contributor? How far can this be pushed? For example, if the excitotoxic modulation of synaptic function is chronic (i.e., from ongoing exposure or chronic inflammation) and/or persistent (i.e., with semipermanent effects from even a transient exposure), can we consider whether it could contribute to a chronic encephalopathy? And could such a chronic encephalopathy potentially in some cases not simply modulate the autism but actually be the autism? Could genetic vulnerability and genetic impacts turn into autism (or more severe autism) with the onset of these pathophysiological processes? We obviously do not know the answer, but this chapter reflects on the question.

Insofar as pathophysiological mechanisms can be affected by environmental input, it is also important to consider potential positive impacts. If there is a formative role for pathophysiology, this suggests that factors like diet, sleep quality, stress, exercise, autonomic arousal, environmental exposures, and medications all could be having substantial short-term impacts on symptom severity and the quality of life. It also suggests that such factors, which include both health-promoting and health-destroying variants, can have substantial effects over time on the level of function and the quality of life. On the scale of years, the "ongoing" nature of pathophysiological activity means that some interventions might be able to provide major long-term benefits as well.

18.1.4 EVIDENCE FOR THE POTENTIAL FOR PLASTICITY AND ITS PERTINENCE

To make a plausible argument that active, persistent pathophysiology might strongly modulate or even create core features of autism, there would need to be evidence of some kind of intraindividual variabilities in the phenotype that occurred in relationship to pathophysiologically pertinent processes. Such variability (e.g., symptom onset, marked worsening, or marked improvement) would suggest that fluctuations in modulatory processes might have significant impact. As it happens, such evidence exists.

The idea that physiological modulation could contribute more than marginally is becoming less far-fetched in the light of published reports of short-term marked improvements in core features of autism. Investigators recently pursued suggestions from clinical case reports that behaviors and core capacities in autism may improve markedly in the setting of fever (Curran et al. 2007)—clinicians were fairly commonly hearing from parents that their affected children could relate better, make more eye contact, and sometimes even talk transiently in the setting of fever—one mother poignantly described her experience during her child's fever to the author of the present review as "visiting with my son." A prospective study was thus performed utilizing the Aberrant Behavior Checklist to rate behavior changes; the study found that fewer aberrant behaviors were recorded for febrile patients on the subscales of irritability, hyperactivity, stereotypy, and inappropriate speech compared with control subjects in a fashion that was not associated with the severity of illness. While lethargy scores were greater during fevers, and all improvements were transient, the behavioral improvements could not be attributed to the lethargy and the results instead suggested a genuine improvement in core functions. An earlier paper investigated 11 children with the history common in ASD of a period of often recurrent infection and antibiotic exposure followed by the development of chronic persistent diarrhea and then the onset of autistic features, or "regression" (Sandler et al. 2000). This common phenomenon has spawned research demonstrating abnormal variants of clostridial bacteria in ASD (Finegold et al. 2002, Parracho et al. 2005, Song, Liu, and Finegold 2004) and animal models showing nervous system and behavioral impacts of propionic acid, a metabolic product of clostridia (MacFabe et al., 2007, Shultz et al. 2008a,b) that are part of a larger ferment of research on the influence of intestinal microecology (the "microbiome") on medical and psychiatric health (Alverdy and Chang 2008, Li et al. 2008, Nicholson, Holmes, and Wilson 2005). This study investigated impact on the behavior of oral vancomycin, which is a potent antibiotic normally given intravenously and minimally absorbed from the intestine but that devastates intestinal microorganisms. They noted significant short-term improvement using multiple pre- and post-therapy evaluations coded by a blinded clinical psychologist, with the transiency presumably due to the regrowth of pathogenic intestinal microorganisms after the cessation of antibiotic dosing. In both of these cases, the improvement was notable, rapid in onset, and short in duration suggesting that the maladaptive physiological setpoint was insufficiently challenged by fever or transiently altered intestinal microbiota to shift to a different semi-stable state.

Some challenges prior to conceptions of developmental disorders have also emerged on the laboratory front. Symptom reversal has recently been reported in mouse models of developmental disorders—fragile X syndrome (Hayashi et al. 2007),

Rett syndrome (Guy et al. 2007), and tuberous sclerosis (Ehninger et al. 2008), all considered genetic and incurable—through molecular intervention, including in older animals. This is striking because it forever undermines the basis for simply taking for granted that neurodevelopmental disorders are incurable or have only a narrow critical window after which intervention is pointless. At the other end of the lifecourse, rapid though transient reduction of Alzheimer's disease symptoms within minutes of the administration of perispinal etanercept suggests that chronic-active and potentially reversible pathophysiology may also contribute to the encephalopathy in this devastatingly progressive disorder (Tobinick and Gross 2008a,b).

With regard to the autism clinical papers discussed above, it is critical to note that fever does not create a permanent alteration of immunologic or neurobiological pathways, and oral vancomycin does not permanently alter intestinal flora, consistent with the changes not being persistent. But it is also critical to note that these supposedly lifelong core features of autism could be altered even in the short term, which itself is inconsistent with a "static encephalopathy" model. All of this challenges us to think outside of the box of irretrievable brain damage in relation to the encephalopathy of ASD (and other conditions as well). The potential mechanisms that come to mind are in the domain of active, dynamic pathophysiology (including but hardly limited to altered gene expression) rather than genetic predetermination, as the genetic mechanisms causing an *in utero* disturbance of brain development would not explain such short-term fluctuations. In the Curran et al. (2007) paper on improvement with fever, the authors speculated that the phenomenon was driven by some mechanisms related to immunologic and neurobiological pathways, intracellular signaling, and synaptic plasticity; in the Sandler et al. (2000) paper, the authors speculated that the oral antibiotic transiently suppressed an enteric microorganism and its production of a neurotoxin-like substance.

If such marked short-term changes are possible, the idea that the encephalopathy in ASD is a dynamic (albeit recalcitrant) "state" rather than a wired-in static "trait" becomes conceivable, and the possibility of identifying the mechanism for and extending the duration of such changes can be framed as a worthwhile and important goal for research.

The implication of this is major: it means that we must consider the possibility that the functional impairments we observe in individuals with autism may be products not so much of innate "deficits" as of the active (and obstinate) pathophysiological *obstruction* of capacities for which brain substrate is still at least partly present. Moreover, given that these processes are known to progressively assault and damage cellular integrity, and given the evidence suggesting progressive changes in brain tissue (cellular changes (Bauman and Kemper 2005) and volume loss (Aylward et al. 2002)), the importance of finding ways to medically intervene to slow or stop this degeneration as early as possible comes into clear focus.

18.1.5 RETHINKING BASIC ASSUMPTIONS

As our understanding of these new dimensions take shape, it starts to seem that the assumptions underlying the classical model of ASD need to be revisited. With these features in mind, it becomes possible and necessary to interrogate prior findings for fresh interpretations. The goal of this chapter is thus to spell out how emerging findings are revealing limitations in the assumptions of the classical view, and to outline some core features of a newer more inclusive view. These emerging findings are elucidating mechanisms suggesting that autism is more than a developmental disorder, that more than genes are etiologically contributory, and that the encephalopathy has dynamic features so that it is not strictly static.

We will develop the argument by posing the following questions, and explaining our rationale for the following responses.

Questions:

1. Is the category of "developmental disorder" adequate for autism?
2. Is autism best or most usefully defined at the behavioral level?
3. Is autism's etiology primarily genetic?
4. Is autism best described as a static encephalopathy?
5. Is autism a unique and distinct syndrome?

Responses:

1. *More than developmental:* Autism is more inclusively framed as a chronic and also dynamical/semi-episodic multisystem condition that begins *in utero* or early in life during a period when developmental processes are greatly sensitive to perturbation and that continues through the lifecourse with persistent, ongoing, active, and dynamic pathophysiology that may contribute critically to phenotypic features.
2. *More than behavioral:* Behavioral criteria alone do not encompass the multisystem features that are increasingly being appreciated in ASD, which are so common in affected individuals as to suggest that they may play central rather than secondary roles and/or reflect shared core underlying pathophysiological processes.
3. *More than genes:* Autism is likely to be the result of a complex interaction of multiple risk factors; neither genes nor environmental agents can *a priori* be assumed to be primary in their contributions, and the interaction of contributors persists beyond early development.
4. *From static to active dynamic:* Within-individual variability in the severity of core features and the emerging awareness of plasticity and improvement in autism, alongside of the relative intactness of neural structures in ASD, suggest that the encephalopathy in autism is recalcitrant but rooted strongly in dynamic processes, and that framing it as static is inaccurate.
5. *From autism as a specific entity with the specific genetic determination of each of its subcomponents to ASD as an emergent property of a neural and somatic system altered by physiological challenges during a sensitive period of early development.* From a systems pathophysiology perspective, autism appears as a complex integration of continuously distributed abnormalities in multileveled features and has substantial physiological overlap with underlying pathophysiology in many other chronic diseases. It may be that we do not

need to target features specific to autism, but that therapies targeting underlying physiological features that are contributory but not unique to ASD could lead to altered emergent properties including altered behaviors.

18.2 INTERROGATION OF EARLIER ASSUMPTIONS AND PRIOR FINDINGS FROM NEWER VANTAGE POINT

18.2.1 Is Autism Purely a Developmental Disorder? Or Are Its Active and Persistent Pathophysiological Features Centrally Important?

The idea that ASD is a developmental disorder seems self-evident. ASD begins in early childhood, with abnormalities in responsiveness sometimes even evident at birth. Brain abnormalities have been documented at the neuropathological level consistent with changes occurring *in utero*. The high heritability and high recurrence rate also support this framing. The characteristic clustering of behavioral features in the ASD phenotype suggests some kind of specific causes.

There are other ways of interpreting the above cluster of phenomena. These features of early onset, neuropathology changes suggestive of *in utero* onset, specific behavioral configuration, and high heritability/high recurrence suggestive of genetic cause can be at least partly decoupled from the inferences with which they have been associated. Certainly important events occur at these early stages of development. The problem arises at the level of drawing implications from these observations about underlying mechanisms. If one assumes *a priori* that this is a "developmental disorder" in the neurobiological or neurogenetic sense, clinical and research observations may be given interpretations consistent with the implications of this assumption, while other potentially valid interpretations consistent with a more chronic model may be neglected.

The notion of a "developmental disorder" has a number of different connotations. From a developmental psychology point of view, it can connote simply that because function and capability change with development, a disorder in childhood will manifest differently at different ages. This is unquestionably true. However, there are other perspectives carrying more severe connotations. From a medical and neurobiological vantage point, "developmental disorder" commonly connotes at least the following four characteristics: (1) that there is a profound, if potentially subtle, alteration in the developmental trajectory of the brain, (2) that the ensuing developmental brain alterations are primary core targets of the etiological agent rather than incidental or secondary, (3) that these alterations directly cause the behavioral phenotype, and (4) that these brain features and the accompanying encephalopathy are indelibly unchangeable. This "developmental disorder" model is derived from observations in neurogenetic syndromes and syndromes of brain malformation where there are clearly observable and classifiable alterations in brain development based upon a fault in some neurochemical or regulatory processes that lead to fairly predictable consequences in affected individuals.

While this framing of developmental disorders is most commonly associated with syndromes having genetic etiologies, the fields of developmental neurotoxicology and teratology have shown that exogenous substances can target early developmental processes and lead in a similar fashion to predictable malformations and developmental syndromes, such as fetal alcohol syndrome, fetal valproate syndrome, and fetal Minamata disease. Similar arguments are also being made about disorders of later onset such as schizophrenia (Arnold 2001, Opler and Susser 2005).

Given the widespread assumption that autism is not only a developmental disorder but also a static encephalopathy, it appears that the stronger and more severe model outlined above has been applied in interpreting the presentation of ASD. But if we carefully examine the support for inferring the four characteristics connoted by the medical-neurobiological framing of "developmental disorder" listed above, it turns out that there are major gaps in our knowledge and more particularly in the evidence basis for the assumptions we have been making. We have certainly (1) identified a range of brain alterations that qualify as profound, often as subtle and sometimes pervasive, including changes in limbic system structures, cerebellum, white and gray matter volume, corpus callosum, subcortical gray matter structures, and asymmetry. But we have not (2) shown for all of them that they are primary targets of an identifiable etiological agent rather than secondary consequences of a pathophysiological process, nor have we (3) conclusively demonstrated that they specifically cause the autism behavioral phenotype (we have merely shown association and have not excluded the possibility that some of these changes may be the downstream of something else that is driving the phenotype), and neither have we (4) proved that they are unchangeable, or that their unchangeability correlates with the functional lack of plasticity—for all of these points our "knowledge" is at the level of plausible narrative, not the empirical elucidation of mechanisms.

18.2.1.1 Reassessing What We Know

In the light of emerging pathophysiological findings, it needs to be considered that the set of phenomena leading people to consider autism a "developmental disorder"—i.e., the brain changes, the early onset, the heritability and recurrence, and the clustering of behavioral features—individually and together may have potential additional and/or alternative interpretations. Below are a series of considerations that cannot be encompassed within the "developmental disease" model as described above. Individually and together, they put autism in the "chronic active disease" category and pose challenging questions about what the interfaces may be between chronic processes that begin very early in life and alterations in development.

1. *Weak Spots in "Developmental Disorder" Inferences from Existing Data*
   a. Brains of autistic individuals are for the most part remarkably normal looking. An MRI scan of the brain of most individuals with ASD would be interpreted by a clinical neuroradiologist as normal (and clinical abnormalities when identified are typically idiosyncratic, possibly incidental, and quite possibly secondary to some other processes), and it is only by careful quantitative analysis that macroanatomical differences from brains of neurotypical subjects can be identified—it takes this level of intensive research-grade measurement because for the most part, changes are too subtle to be identified by the unaided eye (Caviness et al. 1999). Indeed, some neuropathological researchers have held that

since the brains lack major dysmorphology, they are unlikely to have suffered significant insult prior to the late gestational or early postnatal period (Ciaranello, VandenBerg, and Anders 1982, Coleman et al. 1985, Raymond, Bauman, and Kemper 1996). The observation has been made that there is a striking disconnection between the almost indiscernible white matter tract as well as general structural abnormalities and the dramatic functional impairments (Conturo et al. 2008).

b. Suggestions that neurodevelopmental disorders can be triggered by events during the fetal period are supported by a growing body of literature (Connors et al. 2008, Fatemi et al. 2002, Patterson 2002, Shi et al. 2003, Smith et al. 2007). There is a huge literature on developmental neurotoxicity (Slikker and Chang 1998) as well as developmental immune injury (Dietert and Dietert 2008, Hertz-Picciotto et al. 2008). However, while these exposures can now be said to increase the *potential* for neurodevelopmental disorders, there is no support at this time for going further—i.e., such exposures have by no means been shown to be *sufficient* on their own to *cause* postnatally emerging developmental disorders or ASD in particular. Nor have developmental disorders or ASD in particular have been shown to be *necessarily* or in all cases preceded by such events.

c. The model of autism derived from the connectivity literature related to connectivity impairments underlying impairments in complex processing (Just et al. 2004, 2007, Muller 2007) is synchronic—i.e., it can be marshaled to explain the apparent selective impairment of complex processing in individuals with fully developed autism at a particular point in time. It is not a *diachronic* model—i.e., it does not help at all in explaining the phenomenon of the *development* of autism, and particularly the phenomenon of *regression* into autism. We do not understand what changes so that a child who was producing behaviors closely consistent with normal developmental milestones either falters, plateaus, shifts tracks, or in some other ways shifts to slow and/or alter development. If one assumes that autism is inborn, then it is possible to construct a narrative stating that the connectivity problem is innate or prenatal in origin, but does not show itself until critical processes kick in (or fail to occur) postnatally at which point the innately altered wiring becomes a problem. An alternative narrative with a slightly later developmental timepoint is the idea that there is the "failure of the pruning" of excess neural processes. We have no direct evidence to prove either narrative, and in fact imaging evidence as noted in point d below goes against the idea that there has been a pruning failure.

2. *Alternative Interpretations of Prior Findings*

d. The brain findings to date contain many suggestions of prenatal events, but it must be remembered that explaining findings in a fully developed brain of a child past toddlerhood and particularly of an adult is an "archaeological" exercise in reading a developmental history from a snapshot—i.e., it is highly interpretive. At least some of the findings interpreted as supporting a prenatal onset have alternate possible interpretations. Moreover, given the scarcity of postmortem brain specimens from people reliably diagnosed with ASD, most neuropathological observations have been noted in only a small number of cases and the observations have not always been replicated. The following are some examples where alternative explanations have been suggested:

- An observed tight packing of a larger number of smaller cells in limbic structures has been interpreted as indicating a mid-gestational event, but it is also becoming evident that limbic structures are especially sensitive to immune influences and could be altered in their cellular structures through other classes of events than the early developmental events initially considered—with these other classes of events conceivably occurring at somewhat later times (Buller and Day 2002, Buller, Hamlin, and Osborne 2005, Nyffeler et al. 2006).

- Minicolumnar alterations have been interpreted as occurring fairly early in gestation, but arguments have been advanced for how they could occur later as well (Gustafsson 2004).

- Purkinje cells appear vulnerable but they may not necessarily be lost: while they do not pick up Nissl stain, they do appear when calbinden staining is used. Purkinje cells are highly vulnerable to excitotoxicity and their failure to be detected by Nissl stain may reflect chromatolysis or excitotoxic-induced alterations in their metabolism (Kern 2003).

- Brainstem and inferior olivary findings in ASD earlier interpreted as indicating the prenatal disturbance of development have upon restudy been identified not only in ASD but also in control brain tissue (Thevarkunnel et al. 2004, Whitney et al. 2008), suggesting that interpretations regarding both developmental trajectory and specificity need to be rethought.

- Brain enlargement was early on attributed to a "failure of pruning" (i.e., a failure to eliminate the super-abundance of neurons produced early in brain development), but magnetic resonance spectroscopy (MRS) studies have shown reduced (DeVito et al. 2007, Endo et al. 2007, Friedman et al. 2003, 2006, Kleinhans et al. 2007) or unchanged (Vasconcelos et al. 2008, Zeegers et al. 2007) rather than increased n-acetylaspartate (NAA) not consistent with neuronal increase.

- Moreover, while NAA is often considered to be a measure of cell density, it can also be construed as measures of cellular and even mitochondrial functions, and its reduction may be an indicator not so much of neuronal loss as of neuronal dysfunction, particularly given the reversibility of NAA decrements in contralateral tissue following the surgical resection of epileptic foci (Hugg et al. 1996, Pan et al. 2008, Serles et al. 2001).

- White matter enlargement has been identified in T1-weighted scans that offer only macroanatomic measures but no resolution at the scale of cellular changes; the distribution of this enlargement suggested an increase in short-cortico-cortical fiber density consistent with local hyperconnectivity and long-distance under-connectivity (Courchesne and Pierce 2005), although there was no neuropathological data on the tissue composition of this enlargement. But as results from diffusion tensor MRI imaging (pertinent to assessing white matter integrity) and MRS imaging (pertinent to measuring metabolites) are appearing, this inference is being contradicted by evidence suggesting that the expanded volume cannot be explained by increased fiber density and in fact may be due to altered water properties in the tissue more consistent with alternative pathophysiology such as neuroinflammation (Hendry et al. 2006, Sundaram et al. 2008, Zimmerman 2008).

The overall point here is not to argue that we have a clear-cut case in every respect for postnatal or pathophysiology/dynamical-influenced events in ASD brain development, but simply to say that there remains a fair amount of ambiguity in the limited data presently available to us.

3. *The Restrictive Impact of Poor Communication between Silos of Hyperspecialization and across Disciplinary Boundaries*

e. Functional imaging methods including fMRI (functional magnetic resonance imaging), EEG (electroencephalography), MEG (magneto-encephalography), PET (positron emission tomography), and SPECT (single photon emission computed tomography) have shown alterations in regional interconnectivity by various methods (e.g., connectivity, coherence, and covariation) (Herbert 2005b, Muller 2007, Herbert and Caviness 2006). Some investigators have inferred that this interconnectivity alteration might be linked to structural alterations in white matter. But demonstrating such a relationship would require coregistering functional data such as fMRI or MEG or PET with anatomical data such as diffusion tensor imaging or MRS, to see whether alterations in white matter integrity occur in a fashion that relates in any consistent manner with alterations in functional connectivity; while such work is in progress, few results have been reported to date (Kleinhans et al. 2007, Just et al. 2007) and so we actually have little evidence-based idea what tissue changes might be causing alterations in functional connectivity, EEG/MEG coherence, or interregional covariation. The possibility has not been tested that an alteration of synaptic function secondary to the excitotoxic effects of chronic tissue pathophysiology could have systems impacts on the patterning of neurodynamic activity that could contribute to altered functional connectivity. In fact, the investigators studying brain connectivity hardly even mention the emerging pathophysiology findings—the silo effect where groups of narrowly specialized investigators fail to cross-fertilize outside their own small circles and the cognitive dissonance effect are both apparently very strong, and the cross-fertilization between the levels of investigation is quite weak.

f. Several neuropathological investigations of brain tissue in ASD have found evidence of neuroinflammation and oxidative stress (Evans et al.

2008, Li et al. 2009, Sajdel-Sulkowska et al. 2008, Vargas et al. 2005, 2006). In addition, some neuropathological investigations into the nature of white matter enlargement are beginning to suggest that there is astroglial activation in the enlarged outer, radiate part of the white matter that is not present in the deeper, non-enlarged white matter, along with microglial activation that is present particularly in the cerebral cortex (Pardo et al. 2008). These early findings point toward fresh ways of making sense of both altered synaptic activity and brain hypoperfusion in ASD.

- Regarding synaptic function, an emerging field of literature relates to the active roles played by glial cells (astroglial, microglial, and oligodendroglial cells) in signal transmission in the brain (Fields 2006, 2008). These cells are being promoted in our understanding from handmaidens of neurons to active players in a much more complicated collaborative endeavor; the importance of these cells has prompted some to say that we should change the name of the field of study from "neurobiology" to neurogliobiology" (Peschanski 1991). Astroglial cells participate in a "tripartite synapse" (Halassa, Fellin, and Haydon 2007) as they wrap themselves around the ends of two synapsing neurons and neurochemically modulate the synaptic activity between these two cells. In two different specialized silos of the research world, it is known that (1) immune-activated astroglial cells behave quite differently neurochemically and (2) astroglial cells are exquisitely sensitive to toxicant exposures, which can also put them into an activated state. Apparently however, the impact of activation of glial cells on their function in the tripartite synapse has not yet been researched—i.e., the silos of glial-immune and glial-toxin specialists are still not communicating and synergizing with the silo of glial-synapse specialists. So some basic science that we would need to understand the functional impact of either white matter enlargement or glial activation simply has not been performed.

- Regarding brain hypoperfusion, it is also known that astroglial cells become larger when they are activated, and since they encircle small vessels, this enlargement can reduce capillary diameter by as much as 50% (Aschner et al. 1999); such a reduction is consistent with (though such consistency does not prove it is the cause of) measures of brain perfusion in ASD, where the several papers report perfusion reduced blood perfusion, albeit in different distributions (Herbert 2005b, Herbert and Caviness 2006). Other possible pathophysiological contributors to hypoperfusion worth investigating include the modulation of vasoconstriction and platelet activation and aggregation by oxidative stress (Yao et al. 2006) and the impact of the activation of microglia encircling cerebral microvasculature (Vargas et al. 2005). Interestingly, the papers reporting hypoperfusion in ASD to date are almost entirely mute on the subject of the tissue biology or the pathophysiology of this hypoperfusion, with the interpretations in the discussion sections of the papers focusing on the psychological significance of the localization of the hypoperfusion with an unstated assumption that this phenomenon is stable, static, and persistent. Here the silo of pathophysiology specialists is not linked with the silo of psychology specialists.

The point of all of these examples is to give a taste of various ways that the introduction of pathophysiological variables can point to rather different interpretations of existing brain findings. It also serves to illustrate how much of what we think we know about the brain in autism is actually a morass of fragments of data being extrapolated to support inferences based on *a priori* assumptions. By showing that when we augment the conceptual input parameters to include chronic pathophysiology and not just genetics and brain development, we get as output a substantially different set of interpretations, I hope I have at least begun to demonstrate how tenuous are the established interpretations. On this basis, I would argue that we have no solid grounds for excluding or dismissing a research program based on a different set of assumptions than "developmental disorder of prenatal onset." On the contrary, there are many reasons for arguing that it is very important that we pursue a research program based on these different assumptions, as well as communication and synergy across specialized silos, and do so aggressively.

18.2.1.2 Probable Centrality of Glial Cells in ASD

The role of glial cell activation in brain dysfunction in autism needs more attention at the functional as well as at the neuropathological levels (Coyle and Schwarcz 2000, Giaume et al. 2007). Glial cell activation can be set off by a myriad of triggers, and many of the downstream consequences are not specific to the initiating agents. While pathophysiologically oriented investigators have been greatly influenced by the identification of activated microglia and astroglia in brain tissue from individuals with autism (Vargas et al. 2005), adherents of the classical "developmental disorder" model often refuse even to discuss it, some arguing insufficient replication. Since the publication of the Vargas et al. (2005) paper that identified activated microglia and astroglia in all 11 of the brains studied, the group has collected at least another 9 brains, one from someone with Asperger's syndrome, and all of these subsequent brains also showed this activation, including the one with Asperger's syndrome, considered to be a milder condition (Zimmerman 2008). And now, as mentioned, another group has also identified central nervous system immune activation in ASD (Li et al. 2009).

Microglia comprise about 10% of the cells in the brain and perform important functions in both the resting and the activated states. They appear to release trophic factors during development, some of which have been measured as having different levels in infants who later develop autism (Nelson et al. 2001). When activated, microglia synthesize and secrete a range of pro-inflammatory cytokines (Hanisch 2002), several of which are neurotoxic, and in this activated state, they also promote astroglial overactivation and dysfunction, as well as edema (Orellana et al. 2009). Astroglia are multipurpose cells that not only support neurons but also perform metabolic and signaling functions (Aschner et al. 1999, Fields 2006, Halassa, Fellin, and Haydon 2007); astrocytes are highly networked into a syncytium through gap junctions (Theis et al. 2005) through which depolarization and calcium waves spread rapidly and interact with neuronal activity; and they are centrally involved in regulating neurovascular coupling (Koehler, Gebremedhin, and Harder 2006). It is increasingly appreciated that astrocytes are influenced by inflammation in a variety of disease states (Kielian 2008); the activation of astroglial and microglial cells have a wide variety of effects that are arguably consistent with many observed features of ASD. Microglia activation is associated with vasogenic and cytotoxic edema associated with hypoperfusion; activated microglia release glutamate that induces astrocyte edema (Han et al. 2004, Liang et al. 2008). Microglial activation can occur rapidly in response to insults; when it persists, its neurotoxic impact progressively increases over time. The astroglial support of neuron chemistry and the secretion of neuromodulators are altered in the activated state (Aschner, Sonnewald, and Tan 2002). Astroglia maintain the redox potential including through the production of glutathione, which they transfer to neurons. In their resting state, astrocyte networks prevent glutamate excitotoxicity in the brain (Schousboe and Waagepetersen 2005). In the setting of acute inflammation, these functions are compromised, leading to increased neuronal vulnerability (Orellana et al. 2009, Tilleux and Hermans 2007). This might lead to a runaway self-reinforcing vicious cycle, with microglial activation releasing glutamate and activating astroglia, and the activation of astroglia reducing their ability to perform their multiple metabolic and signaling functions. In summary, the activation of these classes of glial cells leads to a series of pathophysiological phenomena that can be self-perpetuating and also progressively more excitotoxic and neurotoxic.

Given how insensitive existing *in vivo* imaging is to neuroinflammation and how few clinical measures collected to date pertain to these processes, we have no way of knowing how pervasive these processes are among people with ASD, how they interact with contributory genes, whether the above cascade of cellular and molecular changes is either sufficient or necessary to produce ASD, or whether genetic vulnerability is required. But all of the above raises the possibility that dysfunction in these cells could be central to ASD pathophysiology and functional impairment, prominently triggered by noxious environmental influences, and only subordinately related to genetic influence. These mechanisms suggest that there are substantial complexities beyond the boundaries implied by the assumption that ASD is simply a "developmental disorder."

18.2.1.3 From "Developmental Disorder" to "Chronic Dynamic Encephalopathy"

I would argue that an alternative to the "developmental disorder" model is that we are dealing at the core with an *alteration of neural function*. It would follow from this that the brain structural changes we observe might very well be to a significant extent a *consequence* of the underlying pathophysiology that alters *function* either in addition to or rather than being the structural *basis* for the functional alterations. In terms of this model, an alteration of cellular function would lead to gradual decrements; at some point, there would be a "tipping point" with a shift from quantity to quality leading to qualitative alterations in neurodynamics (i.e., interregional connectivity, patterns of oscillation and synchronization, etc). This shift would manifest itself at the brain systems level as "underconnectivity" and at the level of behavior as a "regression" process.

What is being offered here is a model of *chronic dynamic encephalopathy*. It is different from the classical model in the critical respect of being able to accommodate a number of features including the relative gross anatomical normality of most brains of people with ASD; and in particular, the phenomenon of transient improvements that is increasingly being appreciated. It also can accommodate the highly common sensory and sleep problems and common epilepsy. It can accommodate somatic features. It can even accommodate the high intraindividual variability in many individuals at the level of the intensity of their reactivity. And finally, it can accommodate autistic regression.

18.2.1.4 Sample Scenario of Pathophysiology-Based Narrative of Autistic Regression

Many scenarios have been advanced in the literature of how prenatal influences could set the stage for ASD; many of these are useful, but will not be repeated here.* We will instead present an example of a scenario that links existing data into a chronic pathophysiology-based narrative of autistic regression, since such a discussion is harder to find in the existing literature.

- *In utero* events (infection, toxicants, radiation, stress, maternal metabolic, or immune factors), possibly but not necessarily in the setting of genetic vulnerabilities, have epigenetic effects that increase the responsivity of the organism to subsequent immune, metabolic, and infectious stressors.
- The infant has a series of exposures or experiences that challenge the system at the points of vulnerability. These could include infections that the immune system cannot handle well; antibiotic exposure that disrupts GI micro-ecology; and the immune and metabolic functions played by this complex intestinal microbiome, food allergens, toxic exposures, and other stressors. These exposures alter physiological function, and some of the alterations have neuromodulatory impact. Repeated exposures may lead to hypersensitivity and maladaptive responses at lower doses.
- Metabolic resiliency is cumulatively challenged: for example, every input that promotes the development of a pro-inflammatory cytokine profile and/ or the depletion of glutathione and reduction of ability to buffer pro-oxidant stress and that is not followed by a recovery of a more normal cytokine profile, the repletion of glutathione, etc. increases the infant's vulnerability to subsequent challenging inputs. The weakening of metabolic resiliency may also be accompanied by subtle signs of impairment of higher cortical functions as well as by various medical symptoms.
- At some point, the ability of astrocytes to continue to maintain their local and syncitial support for neuronal function and their appropriate release of neuromodulatory "gliotransmitters" and glutathione is overcome by immune activation and toxic and redox challenges. At this point (which may have gradual or sudden onset), optimal neural systems connectivity can no longer be maintained. A functional consequence is the sharp curbing

---

* Table 2 in Herbert and Anderson (2008) schematically lays out other possibilities.

of the ability for engagement in activities requiring exquisitely timed and coordinated mental processing (such as the core behavioral domains of ASD—sensitivity to social nuance in communication and the ability to be flexible in the face of transitions). Mitochondrial function, a component of these physiological networks, is also challenged, which is a major problem given the enormous energy demands of brain activity; this further undermines neural systems integration and increases brain irritability and hypersensitivity. Cerebral microvascular regulation is altered. The system enters into a self-propelling pathogenic feedback loop that is difficult to interrupt and leads to a maladaptive "stable state." The whole process has many commonalities with mechanisms operative in neurodegenerative disorders (Standridge 2006).

- Impacts are widespread, including altered neural networks; altered perfusion patterns; neurotransmitter alterations; and a pattern of potentially progressive inflammation and oxidative stress in the brain causing a chronic state of excitotoxicity, hyperreactivity, and increased excitation/inhibition ratio, with consequent electrophysiological disturbances causing the disruption of sleep and sensory processing, motor tone and coordination decrements, and the increased onset of seizures with time and exposure to further stressors (e.g., pubertal hormonal shifts). With all of these system challenges and breakdowns of optimal neural systems activity and coordination, the child withdraws from the social universe and seeks a manageable sameness.
- Cellular function in other systems, e.g., GI barrier function, is challenged by the same mechanisms that are challenging the function of gap junction and redox buffering in astrocyte syncitial networks, with resultant somatic symptoms as a consequence. This may be either due to problems with glial cells or analogs in extra-CNS sites like the GI tract (Ruhl 2005), or to related physiological vulnerabilities and cascades.

While the details of this scenario could be modified at various places along the way, and while many linkages have not been tested, the starting points and subsequent features for each step of the narrative are taken from existing literature. The point of presenting this sample narrative is to show that aberrant pathophysiology, with or perhaps even without genetic vulnerability, could lead to a systems shift in state that would cause altered brain function that could plausibly produce outputs including autistic behaviors.

Another very important point is that much of what has been identified in autism neuropathology and imaging could potentially be *caused by* rather than the cause of this cascade. Purkinje cell loss or dysfunction could be due to excitotoxicity (Blaylock and Strunecka 2009, Kern 2003, Yip, Soghomonian, and Blatt 2008). White matter enlargement could be due to inflammation (Hendry et al. 2006, Pardo et al. 2008, Dager et al. 2008). Limbic structure enlargement could also be due to inflammatory processes particularly given some evidences that these structures have greater immune sensitivity and vulnerability(Buller and Day 2002, Churchill et al. 2006, Kim et al. 2000). Altered connectivity could be due to an interaction of factors including reduced perfusion, gap junction closure, mitochondrial dysfunction, and altered astrocyte metabolic activity as discussed above. Impairment in complex processing could be a result of the inability of a system whose cellular infrastructure is energetically and metabolically compromised to optimally coordinate information required to pull the components of complexity together in a timely and useful fashion (Anderson, Hooker, and Herbert 2008).

This chronic dynamic encephalopathy model could in particular accommodate the way that systemic alterations at the level of pathophysiology (e.g., oxidative stress, mitochondrial dysfunction, and inflammation) could impact brain *function* not only on an ongoing basis but also in a fashion that is malleable—which is potentially consistent with reports of the level of functioning that is *dynamic*—i.e., that *changes* with physiological alterations whether naturalistically or therapeutically induced (e.g., fever and metabolic treatment). That is, if cells in the CNS can be supported so that their degree of energetic and metabolic compromise is reduced or eliminated and damage from chronic persistence of the pathological state is not too far advanced, the neurodynamic state of the system may be able to qualitatively shift and allow marked improvements in coordination and integrative function.

I think that this model needs to be built out into a detailed research program that in particular links cognitive neuroscience questions with pathophysiological considerations, and also includes a systematic re-interrogation of existing data in a fashion I could only begin to sketch here. Some further suggestions of what this could involve will appear in later sections below. This chronic dynamic encephalopathy model can not only incorporate developmental contributors to vulnerability, but it can also accommodate the interaction of such risk factors with subsequent environmental triggers, something that the "developmental disorder" approach does less well.

If we sit in the "developmental disorder" model and assume that specific genetically based developmental mechanisms are in there messing up brain development but we just have not found them yet, we will intensively orient our research program to seeking these mechanisms and arguing for the causal linkage of candidate mechanisms when we find them with core components of the behavioral phenotype before we have elucidated the intermediary mechanisms through all the levels that these candidate mechanisms must traverse to impact brain and behavior. The above arguments support a different approach, a pathophysiologically centered neurodynamic research program that incorporates etiological inputs and behavioral outputs, but that focuses on core pathophysiological mechanisms and on their potential for dynamic change. The outcome can be cooperative and collaborative, since this approach does not lose the strengths of the classical model, but rather reincorporates those strengths into a more inclusive framework. More strongly, this dynamical model not only accommodates the observed metastability, variability, and plasticity in ASD but also allows the investigation of intervention strategies that can be implemented in the short term with potential substantial reduction severity and suffering.

18.2.2   Is Autism Best or Most Usefully Defined at the Behavioral Level? Multisystem and Multileveled Complexity in Autism

Autism was initially identified by a psychiatrist (Kanner 1943); and with its prominent behavioral manifestations, it has been studied first as a psychiatric syndrome and for the last few decades with the accumulation of evidence of brain and ner-vous system abnormalities as a neuropsychiatric, neurodevelopmental syndrome (Tuchman and Rapin 2006). At the same time, there has long been a more whole-body physiological strand in autism research and treatment. Although several early scattered papers appeared describing measurable changes in somatic and systemic physiological features, these insights have not been integrated or assimilated into the dominant model of autism.

There are several reasons for this lack of integration of physiological and behav-ioral understanding:

1. Many of the physiological studies have been weak: small sample size, meth-odological problems, and inconsistency of results between studies have contributed to keeping these findings marginalized.
2. The immaturity of methods of investigation has limited the strength of such findings and hindered their ability to engender serious interest.
3. The behavioral definition of ASD has made it seem necessary or at least important to map physiological findings to specific behavioral features of this syndrome in order to support their significance to the condition, but attempts to do this have produced weak results, probably because the systems pathophysiology is unlikely to lead to this kind of specific mecha-nism-to-behavior mapping.
4. The heterogeneity of ASD is only recently being appreciated, so that most studies to date have not been designed to tease out distinctive subgroups. The problem of subgroups is particularly pertinent here: a pathophysiology-centered approach would emphasize that subgroups may be effectively distinguished at the physiological level; but at the same time, there is no guarantee of discerning any one specific measure at the metabolic or immune level that is present in the majority of a cohort. Thus, physiological insights, particularly those that could be pertinent to such subgroups, have not been clearly identified.

In recent years, multisystem and systemic features of autism have been getting more attention, in part because of research (Herbert 2005a) and also because of the experiences of patients and the insistence of many such patients and their families that these are major issues and should not be ignored. Most commonly appreciated at this point are the GI symptoms (such as chronic constipation, diarrhea, and gas-troesophageal reflux) (Afzal et al. 2003, Torrente et al. 2002, Valicenti-McDermott et al. 2006) and the immune abnormalities (such as recurrent infections and chronic allergies) (Ashwood and Van de Water 2004a,b, Ashwood, Wills, and Van de Water 2006), both of which appear to have high prevalence in individuals with ASD and sometimes in their family members (Croen et al. 2005). Less widely known but sup-ported by a growing body of literature are the underlying abnormalities in oxidative metabolism and sulfur metabolism already discussed above (Chauhan and Chauhan 2006, James et al. 2006). There are also various nervous system manifestations that are highly prevalent but that fall outside the triad of behaviors that define autism; these include sensory abnormalities (present in as many as 95% of individuals with autism) (Tomchek and Dunn 2007), sleep disturbances (Malow 2004, Malow et al. 2006), abnormal autonomic reactivity (Goodwin et al. 2006, Groden et al. 2005, Ming et al. 2004), epilepsy (Canitano 2007), and various motor and neuromuscular abnormalities. In parallel with these developments in the ASD literature, there are analogous developments in other neuropsychiatric fields where the interest is expanding beyond behaviors to include pathophysiology and systemic biomarkers (Schwarz and Bahn 2008).

18.2.2.1 Are Systemic and Somatic Features Really "Secondary"?

From the vantage point of framing of autism as a genetically based neurodevelopmental syndrome, it is logical to assume that the brain problems come first, that developmentally rooted alterations in brain structure and function lead to the behaviors we observe and use to define autism, and that while we may find other features in large subsets of autistic individuals, they are secondary and not directly related to the core brain-based behavioral features. Even so, a growing number of people holding this classical point of view are acknowledging somatic/systemic features in ASD; how do they explain the frequent occurrence of these features?

Within the framework of a primarily genetic and developmental neurobiological model of ASD, there are two main distinct but non-mutually exclusive explanations for this co-occurrence or "comorbidity" of somatic and neurological problems. One of them relates to the noxious impacts of physical discomfort: this is the idea that physical symptoms may create problem behaviors or reduce the level of function; for example, pain (e.g., from esophageal reflux or constipation) may contribute to aggression or self-injurious behavior, while sleep dysregulation may reduce attention and cognitive function (Bauman 2006). The second goes deeper and touches on cause: this is the important insight that genes may express in multiple systems, so that genes that impact the brain may also impact the gut or the immune system.

Both of these explanations seem substantially true and important. But they do not exhaust what needs to be said about the issue of the so-called "comorbidities." The pain argument takes for granted that the somatic features are secondary and not mechanistically related to brain alterations, while the "genes express in multiple systems" argument assumes that genes are the main effect and ignores environmental influences and gene–environment interactions (Rutter 2008). Neither explanation promotes reflection about other mechanisms of brain–body interaction that may be in play, either developmentally or chronically. Both explanations leave much unexplained.

What if the pathophysiology leading to pain is part of the same disturbance that is also altering brain function—either developmentally, chronically, or both? And what if genes are contributory but not the main effect? Both of these are reasonable questions. If the answer to either is in any way positive, then the above two explanations for the comorbidity of brain and somatic/systemic features must be considered incomplete.

Because of the notion that autism is a genetically caused brain-based syndrome, the important clinical insight described above, that physical symptoms may aggravate behavioral problems or reduce levels of function, is often accompanied by an additional comment or implicit assumption: "but this has nothing to do with the core autism." First of all, it needs to be asked, "How do you *know* it has nothing to do with the core autism? Where are the documented *specific* mechanisms proving that your framing of autism as not only specifically neurobiological but also nothing more than a genetically caused brain-based syndrome is actually the best framing? Do we have enough multidisciplinary systems biological phenomic research to prove that there are really cases of 'pure autism' with absolutely no features other than the three core behaviors? Where are the systematic studies conducting sufficient appropriately sensitive measures in people with apparently nonsystemic, non-somatic presentations to exclude all implicated dysregulated physiology? Can anyone point to a literature reporting the systematic investigation and exclusion of the possibility that there may indeed be a relationship between brain and body features in affected individuals?"

In fact, from the vantage point of a pathophysiology-centered approach to autism, there are many reasons to expect that there is a vital linkage between body and brain, and strong reason to disagree with the idea that the somatic and systemic features are simply secondary to "the autism." In truth, as mentioned in the introduction, there are many mechanisms by which brain and body may very well be related in autism (and in many other settings), and in particular, by which body may significantly influence brain, and there are many papers in the non-autism peer-reviewed literature showing immune–brain and gut–brain relationships via mechanisms that may very well also be operating in autism. We do not need to remind people that the notions that such mechanisms are irrelevant or of minimal effect because the brain is immune-privileged and/or the blood-brain barrier is fully protective are obsolete (Carson et al. 2006). Particularly pertinent are that both brain and body are known to be affected by oxidative stress, mitochondrial abnormalities, and inflammation, mechanisms that growing evidence implicates in autism.

18.2.2.2   Beyond a Behavior-Centered Definition of Autism

Because systematic and phenomic studies of ASD are just beginning, it is premature to propose a rigorous definition of ASD that includes biological features. But it is time to treat the behavioral definition with a great deal of circumspection. With a high prevalence of a range of somatic/systemic features, the behavioral definition of autism can be appreciated as a starting point that gives some uniformity to subject characterization in research studies. But it should not be assumed that it is directly and specifically caused by the core underlying biology. This argument was made some years ago by Morton and Frith (1995), who diagrammed the complex pathways leading from genes (consistent with dominant genetic determinist biases they did not discuss environmental influences, but the argument about complex multileveled interacting cascades of influences would be the same for how any pathogenic factor leads to an impact on phenotype) to brain tissue changes to brain system changes to behaviors where the connections were much more likely to be circuitous and interactive than simple, straight, and direct. In the meantime, systematic work needs to be done to tackle the question of somatic/systemic–brain–behavior relationships directly.

18.2.2.3   Research Questions for a Whole-Body Approach to ASD

Three of the core challenges facing a pathophysiology-centered approach to autism are

1. To develop study designs that have the capacity to concretely address and elucidate brain–body–systemic relationships in autism itself, and not merely by inference from other domains

2. To develop research methods and identify measures optimally sensitive to the changes at the brain level that may be associated with changes at the somatic/systemic level in ASD
3. To develop treatment research programs that utilized these sensitive measures in whole-body, whole person treatment research, and treatment efficacy tracking (Herbert 2007)

To achieve these goals, we need to work across silos of narrow specialization so that pathophysiology-centered studies incorporate brain function measures and cognitive neuroscience studies incorporate somatic and systemic measures. We also need a network of collaborating researchers and infrastructure to pool our data. All of this requires infrastructure capable of supporting these cross-silo integrative collaborations.

18.2.2.4   Characterizing the Relationship between Brain and Somatic/Systemic Features

A number of key questions need to be addressed now that somatic/systemic features are on the table in ASD.

- Are systemic features really secondary? To study this problem, we will need not only to look for the presence of systemic and somatic features in individuals with autism, but also to assess what kinds of relationship these features may have to the brain. Is there any kind of correlation of somatic with brain features? Is there any covariation of measures of somatic or systemic symptom severity with the severity of behavior or neurocognitive impairment?
- Does any kind of treatment of somatic systems measurably alter brain function?
- In comparing biomedical treatments, is there a difference in measurable brain impact between treating somatic symptoms as compared with treating systemic/metabolic root causes? For practitioners holding the classical "developmental disorder" model, the goal is to relieve symptoms in order to achieve the reduction of discomfort and improved function by virtue of the absence of pain, sleeplessness, etc.; there is no goal of achieving change in the autistic encephalopathy itself. On the other hand, for practitioners with a pathophysiology orientation, targets further upstream would be sought, with the idea that correcting systemic pathophysiology would make possible reconfiguring of systems to healthier adaptation in body and brain together. To test whether it matters how far upstream treatments are targeted, outcomes could be compared between upstream and symptomatic approaches. For example, for diarrhea, stopping symptoms by medicating to reduce gut motility would not treat a mechanism that could drive both body and brain involvement, while treating an inflammatory process at an upstream point or removing an inflammatory trigger (such as by treating and eliminating a chronic infection) might have a more widespread effect; can this theoretical difference be demonstrated in practical studies?

- What domains of brain structure or function might be most sensitive to pathophysiological disturbances and to modulating these disturbances therapeutically? What neurobiological-dependent variables that can be measured noninvasively in a living individual (from coherence to sensory and motor to social and emotional, from auditory to language, and more) might be most useful to include in brain–body and treatment research in ASD? It would seem that if we are talking about chronic alterations of synaptic function, then measures sensitive to activity at the timescale of synaptic transmission, such as EEG and MEG that have millisecond temporal resolution, would probably be more sensitive than measures looking at brain activation in anatomical space, such as functional MRI, which has excellent spatial but poor temporal resolutions.
- What are the implications of tissue pathophysiology for cognitive neuroscience? Here are some questions that have hardly even been posed, let alone answered:
  - Is there any correlation between particular pathophysiological features and particular behavioral features?
  - Are language, communication, and theory of mind impairments a manifestation of the psychologically based lack of motivation or of a physiologically based inability to mobilize cellular activity to drive these functional systems? That is, are the core "impairments" we see in ASD the consequence of a "deficit" or of a pathophysiology-based heavily reinforced *obstruction* of a capacity that is potentially still at least partly present?
  - What kinds of vulnerabilities are created by oxidative stress, neuroinflammation, and immune dysfunction at the levels of neuronal and glial functioning, synaptic functioning, and connectivity? Sensory processing and sleep? Is there any specificity or preferential impact?
- Is autism a cluster of coexisting, comorbid distinct endophenotypic components? Or are there underlying mechanistic interconnections between apparently specific behavioral and somatic/systemic domains? This is a question that has received significant attention at the level of behavioral phenotype (Happe and Ronald 2008, Happe, Ronald, and Plomin 2006), and could also receive fruitful further attention with the inclusion of somatic and systemic features of autism. The investigation of pathophysiological mechanisms and their response to treatment, when accompanied by the careful documentation of neurocognitive response, could help address whether change happens in modules or systemically, or somewhere in between.

Addressing the above research questions will lay the foundation for incorporating somatic/systemic features into phenotyping and defining autism spectrum disorders, and help us develop a coordinated research and clinical approach that integrates somatic and systemic features with brain, behavior, and genetic factors.

18.2.2.5 Somatic/Systemic Autism Animal Models

Alongside human studies, it is possible to utilize a somatic/systemic pathophysiological approach in constructing animal models. A particularly comprehensive approach to implementing this has been performed by MacFabe, using a propionic acid environmental stimulus. Propionate as mentioned in the introduction is a short-chain fatty acid produced by clostridial bacteria, abnormal varieties of which have been documented in stool samples from children with ASD (Finegold et al. 2002, Parracho et al. 2005, Song, Liu, and Finegold 2004). Propionate is also used as a food preservative. MacFabe injected this substance into the ventricles of mice, and induced features spanning the levels of autism manifestations, ranging from stereotypies and social isolation behaviors through electrophysiological spiking to neuroinflammation and oxidative stress in brain tissue to the upregulation of genes such as neurexin and neuregulin that have been identified as candidate genes by genetics researchers (MacFabe et al. 2007, Shultz et al. 2008a,b). This model also includes reversibility, as the effects of the injection wear off over weeks; on the other hand, it includes a kindling effect—repeated injections result in prolonged abnormalities and slower recovery.

The complex multilevel-integrated model MacFabe has constructed could be repeated for a variety of other environmental stimuli, and would probably again show the unification of features across the range of complexity characterizing ASD. It could also be used as a treatment research platform, testing the multisystem effects and efficacy of treatment interventions.

18.2.3 Is Autism's Etiology Primarily Genetic? Genes, Environment, and Epigenetics in Autism

There is nothing in the formal *DSM-IV* (*Diagnostic and Statistical Manual*, 4th edition) definition of autism relating to etiology except for one thing: to qualify for a diagnosis of childhood autism, the disturbance cannot be better accounted for by Rett's syndrome or childhood disintegrative disorder. Beyond this, there is no exclusion for any specific genetic etiology or for that matter, for any biological etiology whatsoever. The disorder is defined simply by a constellation of behavioral symptoms. This clustering of behavioral symptoms into a diagnosis not unique to ASD but is standard procedure in the *DSM* (American Psychiatric Association 1994).

In the early literature, some papers noted that a high proportion of parents of individuals with autism had occupations that would expose them to potentially toxic chemicals (Coleman 1979, Felicetti 1981, Rosenberger-Debiesse and Coleman 1986). But for decades, the emphasis in thinking about etiology has been on genetics. More recently, there has been increasing openness to considering environmental influences and gene—environment interactions (Campbell et al. 2006, 2008, D'Amelio et al. 2005, Newschaffer et al. 2007, Persico and Bourgeron 2006, Tsuang et al. 2004). By now, there are fewer who would maintain that autism is purely genetic, but still many who would expect that genetic influence is primary and greater, while environmental influence is lesser and of much smaller effect.

While a variety of genes have been implicated as associated with autism, no gene identified to date has both high impact and high prevalence. Even developmental or neurogenetic disorders associated with high rates of ASD, such as fragile X or tuberous sclerosis, do not have anything near a 100% prevalence of ASD amongst affected individuals (Belmonte and Bourgeron 2006), suggesting that the genetic alterations underlying these conditions would be better construed as conferring high risk, rather than being called causal.

The basis for privileging genetics is largely inference from indirect evidence rather than a solid knowledge of which specific genes are implicated and in what ways they lead to what we call ASD, since such knowledge does not exist. As with the discussion of prior points, the issue becomes examining whether the indirect evidence makes a strong case for a uniquely primary genetic contribution, or whether it is also consistent with a significant contribution from nongenetic factors.

A full discussion of these issues is beyond the scope of this chapter, and good coverage of much of this is available elsewhere (Corrales and Herbert in press). The discussion here focuses on what is most pertinent in the setting of articulating a pathophysiology-centered approach to autism.

Two key pieces of indirect evidence for a strong or primary role for genetics are the high monozygotic-twin concordance rates and the high sibling-recurrence rates. However, a number of factors could contribute to at least somewhat altered interpretations of these numbers:

1. High heritability is often overinterpreted as being exclusive of genetic influences, whereas in fact, high-genetic contributions can coexist with high-environmental contributions—i.e., the total percentage can add up to much more than 100% (Rothman and Greenland 1998, Visscher, Hill, and Wray 2008).

2. Intriguingly, it has been found that when monozygotic twins are distinguished by whether they shared a placenta (were monochorionic) versus whether they each had their own (were dichorionic), the monozygotic monochorionic twins averaged 60% concordance for schizophrenia, whereas for the dichorionic monozygotic twins the concordance was only 10.7% (Davis, Phelps, and Bracha 1995). The investigators suggested that this implies an infection, probably viral; it could also be due to perfusion differential imposed between placentas; notably oxidative stress modulates vascular reactivity (Yao et al. 2006) and there is a particular sensitivity to this problem later in gestation during periods of rapid growth (McGinnis 2007). To date, a comparison of monochorionic with dichorionic monozygotic twins has not been performed in ASD research in spite of some efforts, due to the obstacle of poor delivery-room record-keeping regarding placenta characteristics in US hospitals (Hallmayr 2008).

3. Some recent as yet unpublished twin studies are showing high-dizygotic concordance rates, one interpretation of which is that shared uterine environment is pertinent. Fetal impacts are being approached in a variety of ways in the ASD field by a number of investigators (Braunschweig et al. 2008, Connors et al. 2008, James et al. 2008, Smith et al. 2007).

4. It is not clear at all how to quantitate the potential impact of epigenetics that could be an enormous confound, potentially reflecting environmental influences over several generations and not just in the current individual.

5. The identification of copy number variant genetic alterations in singleton children but not in their parents, as well as the increase in autism incidence with increasing paternal age suggest that environmental influence could destabilize gene replication or mutate genes (Corrales and Herbert in press).

6. Arguments that increase in ASD prevalence are due to greater awareness or earlier diagnosis and looser criteria are being challenged by recent empirical epidemiological studies suggesting a strong role for environment (Hertz-Picciotto and Delwiche 2009).

In addition, various pathophysiological abnormalities identified in ASD can result from environmental and not just (or perhaps even more than) genetic contributors. Some examples are as follows:

- Some studies have identified mitochondrial abnormalities in a significant fraction of individuals with ASD (Correia et al. 2006, Filipek et al. 2004, Oliveira et al. 2005). This has raised the question of whether the abnormality in mitochondria is associated with disease entities (presumably genetically based and rare) or whether it is a dysfunction that is more common (Rossignol and Bradstreet 2008). Our appreciation of the complexity of mitochondrial disease and dysfunction has increased enormously in recent years. But it has been known for some time that mitochondria are exquisitely sensitive to dysfunction resulting from the impact of exogenous substances whether pharmaceutical or xenobiotic—thousands of which target various phases of mitochondrial metabolism (Wallace and Starkov 2000). Recent work by Holtzman (2008) identified mitochondrial dysfunction, most commonly in Complex I of the electronic transport chain, in 12 out of 12 cell cultures of individuals with autism as compared with their unaffected siblings. It is quite unlikely that all of these unrelated individuals carried the same mitochondrial genes; it is much more conceivable that Complex I as well as potentially other parts of mitochondrial metabolism are targets for a diverse array of influences and hence highly vulnerable.
- The activation of microglia and astroglia is well known to be associated with a large range of environmental influences, including, but not limited to infections, ultrafine particulate matter, heavy metals, and other pollutants (Calderon-Garciduenas et al. 2008a,b). The identification of significant numbers of these activated glial cells in the brains of individuals with autism suggests an environmental influence.
- Many xenobiotics are known to impact aspects of synaptic development and activity (Slikker and Chang 1998), although this is not often mentioned in discussions of "autism as a disorder of the synapse" (Zoghbi 2003). These impacts could interact with underlying genetic vulnerability and exert their effects at lower dosage or with more severe effects (Pessah and Lein 2008). The identification of genes associated with autism being regulated by neuronal activity (Morrow et al. 2008) raises the question of how the environmental (and particularly xenobiotic) modulation of this neuronal activity might interact with such genes to lead to the amplification of impact on the phenotype.

In reviewing psychiatric gene–environment interaction literature, Rutter (2008) notes the apparent contradiction between high heritability and the miniscule effects of individual genes as assessed through molecular genetic investigation. He comments

> The GxE findings raise the possibility that the mistake has been to assume that all genetic effects are "main" effects independent of the environment. The truth may be that there is much more gene–environment interdependence than has been appreciated up until now (see Caspi and Moffitt 2006, Rutter 2007). Also, it is very striking that the GxE effects that have been found are of moderate size and by no means are as small as the main effects of single genes considered independently of the environment (Rutter 2008).

The chronic features of autism, the fact that environmental triggers are known more broadly to be associated with much of the pathophysiology identified in ASD (even if specific linkages have not yet been established in this context) as well as the other above arguments all point toward the need for a framework that includes environment as well as genes.

18.2.4 Is Autism a Static Encephalopathy? Plasticity in Autism

There is nothing in the formal definition of autism that specifies prognosis. A person simply has to meet behavioral criteria at a particular point of time. For a diagnosis of autism disorder, a child has to meet these criteria fully and before the age of 3. If some criteria are missing or if not all become evident before 3 years of age, there are variants of spectrum diagnoses available. But there is nothing to say that a person who meets these criteria at one point and no longer meets them later in life did not "really" meet them in the first place. Yet it is generally, though not universally, assumed that autism involves lifelong and irreversible impairment.

It also needs to be remembered that autism is not at all universally accompanied by mental retardation. The IQs of individuals with ASD range from mentally retarded to highly gifted. The alterations leading to the "autism" are not a function of intelligence.

The impact of any belief system is to focus attention toward information and questions consistent with belief, and to filter out the perception of features not pertinent or contradictory to the belief system or conceptualization. In the field of ASD research and treatment, because the improvement or loss of diagnosis has not been considered conceivable, most outcome studies in autism have not collected data pertinent to documenting and discriminating the details of such positive outcomes. In some questionnaires, a child who started as nonverbal and then becomes verbal will produce a score that goes down (implying worsening), presumably due to the lack of anticipation of this outcome in the design of the measure. Reports of improvement have often been met with dismissive and even indignant assertions that the individual "could not have been really autistic in the first place," generally without an acknowledgment that making such a statement goes beyond either the definition of autism (which does not include prognosis) or the evidence of published outcomes (which has not been sensitive to the loss of diagnosis).

This dismissive attitude has not made recovery stories go away. A substantial number of anecdotal reports are circulating that describe transient improvement under conditions of stress, intense emotion, clear fluid diet in preparation for colonoscopy/endoscopy, and after anesthesia. In addition, the Internet and YouTube abound in narrative and video documentations and parent testimonials about recovered autistic children. But for decades, there has also been a small amount of the academic documentation of improvement, the loss of diagnosis, and recovery. Early reports of improved outcome include the Case #1 in the 1943 paper by Kanner in which autism was first described and named. This individual appeared severely affected through childhood—his parents were in fact told that there was nothing to be done for him and were advised to let him live with a caring family elsewhere and get on with their lives. In late adolescence after a severe illness diagnosed as juvenile rheumatoid arthritis, for which gold salts treatment was administered, he experienced a remission not only of the arthritis but also of the autistic symptoms, and went on to earn a bachelor's degree, live independently, hold down a job, and travel widely (Kanner 1968, 1971, Olmsted 2005). Early documentation of improvement and recovery also includes papers coauthored by Rutter, Greenfeld, and Lockyer (1967), Rutter and Lockyer (1967), Gajzago and Prior (1974), DeMyer, Hingtgen, and Jackson (1981), and Lovaas (1987). Fein and colleagues have produced a further review of outcome studies and the notion of autism recovery (Helt et al. 2008). Recent reports of the loss of diagnosis in children rigorously diagnosed with autism according to current diagnostic standards suggest that the loss of diagnosis is likely to be accompanied by residual neurodevelopmental impairments such as attention deficit disorder or language impairment, and that good motor functioning is predictive of optimal outcome (Fein et al. 2005, Kelley et al. 2006, Sutera et al. 2007). In addition to recoveries, there are also the transient improvements (e.g., fever or oral antibiotic associated) and animal model reversals of developmental disorders already reviewed in the introduction.

The loss of diagnosis and the cases of transient improvement in core features—as well as the fairly common short-term fluctuation between more lucid days and days of being more severely "zoned out" that parents can find maddening—raise intriguing questions about what kinds of underlying neurobiological basic features and changes could enable such variability and improvement to occur (Herbert and Anderson 2008). The transient improvements add further intrigue by suggesting that changes occurring over a very short timescale can lead to significant observable improvements in the level of functioning, further honing the questions posed by these phenomena—what kinds of neurobiological mechanisms could be amenable to such rapid change?

An interesting potentially related phenomenon is an increasing recognition of an often substantial discrepancy between expressive and receptive language impairments. Many clinicians and parents are observing signs of receptive language abilities in some individuals with autism far in advance of their expressive language capabilities. Some such individuals test extremely well on IQ tests and can read and use keyboards to express themselves (sometimes showing great creativity and nuance), but not produce speech. Some attribute this discrepancy to oro-motor apraxia and others focus on sensory-processing issues; increasing research attention is being paid to this phenomenon, which supports the importance of remembering that mental retardation is not coupled with ASD, and that individuals with ASD can have great potential. It again suggests that the brain changes causing the autism may not be about deficit but could be about the difference or alteration or perhaps obstruction of a potentiality for which brain capacity is present but whose utilization or expression is heavily obstructed in some fashion.

There are various further clinical findings and ASD-pertinent pathophysiological phenomena that suggest either the presence of plasticity or pathophysiological mechanisms that would be consistent with plasticity potential:

- Certain metabolic disorders that are frequently accompanied by autism are amenable to treatment where resulting improvement in the metabolic conditions is sometimes accompanied by improvement in autistic features such as the lessening of severity (Page 2000). Autistic symptoms are reduced in phenylketonuria by a low phenylanlanine diet (Gillberg and Coleman 2000), in hyperuricosuric autism by a low purine diet with or without allopurinol (Coleman 1989, Gillberg and Coleman 2000, Page and Moseley 2002), in patients with low cerebrospinal fluid (CSF) biopterin by biopterin supplementation (Fernell et al. 1997), in some hypocalcinuric autistic patients by calcium supplementation (Coleman 1989), in some patients with lactic acidemia by thiamine and/or ketogenic diet (Coleman 1989), in cerebral folate deficiency by folinic acid supplementation (Bauman 2006, Moretti et al. 2005), and in Smith-Lemli-Opitz syndrome by cholesterol treatments (Natowicz 2004). Some clinicians use vitamin cocktails to treat mitochondrial disease and report that when this is done with autistic children, some show significant improvement in function and reduction in the severity of autistic-like behaviors (Gold and Cohen 2001).
- Many individuals with ASD and other neurodevelopmental disorders are noted to have sub-epileptic electrophysiological disturbances on their EEGs. In addition, some children with autism experience improvement in core symptoms when treated with antiepileptic medications, even if they do not have epilepsy. This raises intriguing questions of the extent to which language impairment, emotional information processing, sensory disturbances, and sleep problems may be on a continuous electrophysiological distribution with seizures and epilepsy. This may well be the level at which metabolic disturbances and neurophysiological disturbances interact to produce what is here being labeled "chronic dynamic encephalopathy." This issue cannot be addressed by the current standard neurological evaluation for seizures, which does not include an evaluation for other nervous system functions governed by brain electrophysiological activity. While the clinical evaluation of EEG studies is generally done by visual inspection only, the contemporary computational analysis of electrophysiological tracings has great potential for identifying patterns of disturbance not apparent to the unaided eye, and their utilization in probing studies of the neurophysiology of sleep and sensory processing in ASD appear to be on a path to contributing insight beyond seizure diagnosis and expanding the clinical

utility of electrophysiological assessment. This clinical research ferment is an example of a shift from a disease model (i.e., seizures vs. no seizures) to a functional pathophysiology model at the level of brain signaling (i.e., the examination of the clinical impact of more subtle electrophysiological disturbances).

- Findings from an MRS study documenting the recovery of reduced NAA discussed under question #1 in item #4 suggest both that cells are alive rather than missing and that function can potentially be restored if the irritant is removed. It also raises intriguing research questions, such as what the impact might be on the cortical connectivity of cellular dysfunction sufficient to lower NAA, and whether both of these measures might be expected to improve coordinately in improvement associated with pertinent pathophysiological change. This is a question that, to be entertained most appropriately, requires an integration of measures sensitive to pathophysiology with sophisticated cognitive neuroscience.

- The administration of lipopolysaccharide, a bacterial cell membrane component to wild-type mice and elicited an elevation of tumor necrosis factor-α that subsided in the serum within 9 h and in the liver within a week but persisted in the brain for 10 months (Qin et al. 2007); a variety of other pro-inflammatory brain factors also showed increased expression. This suggests that many triggers of brain inflammation, even if sporadic, can lead to a chronic inflammatory state. With any kind of reexposure to triggers, this state can become unremitting and even self-propelling due to its long persistence. For all intents and purposes, this persistence will create the impression of a static trait, even though there is an underlying dynamic, active component.

- The excitotoxic impact of glial activation as well as its impact on gap junctions, which in turn could substantially impact electrophysiology and have further downstream impacts on electrophysiologically mediated functions such as sleep, sensory processing, and seizures, suggest that dysfunction in all of these downstream areas is dynamic rather than static.

- The modulation of glial activation as well as the opening and closing of gap junctions modulated among other things by glial activation can occur on a short timescale commensurate with the timescale of the transient improvements reported in Curran et al.'s paper (2007) on improvement with fever and Sandler et al.'s paper (2000) on improvement with oral antibiotic discussed in the introduction.

- The dietary depletion of tryptophan, which is a precursor of serotonin (very frequently documented as abnormal in ASD), has been shown to exacerbate autistic behaviors (McDougle et al. 1996); tryptophan can also be depleted by neuroinflammation, which upregulates the tryptophan-dependent synthesis of kynurenin, thereby depleting the tryptophan available for the synthesis of brain serotonin (Maes et al. 1997).

- A provocative recent theoretical paper hypothesizes that the strikingly improved behavior and enhanced communication manifested in some individuals with ASD during fever suggests the involvement of a pervasive neural system that can affect relatively rapid changes in the functional activity of widespread neural networks involved in the core features of ASD (Mehler and Purpura 2009). The authors specifically suggest that fever might transiently restore normal function to a dysregulated locus ceruleus–noradrenergic system (LC/NA). This system is capable of facilitating rapid and widespread neural network remodeling to behavioral adaptations to environmental challenges. The authors note that their hypothesis is in keeping with studies that have failed to find substantive neuropathological lesions in the cerebral cortex and other brain sites. Both their specific hypothesis about LC/NA and the more general notion that a mechanism performing the rapid regulation of functional remodeling is likely to be operative are intriguing and will undoubtedly trigger further research on mechanisms of plasticity and interventions for enhancing it.

Each of these examples suggests in its own way that if some of the pathophysiology or dysfunction can be reduced, there is a potential for clinical improvement that would not be predicted in the classical "developmental disorder" framing of ASD. These insights come from a pathophysiology-centered approach to autism which, not being bound by the model of static encephalopathy, can orient us to a range of possible mechanisms that could contribute to transient and sustained improvement. Such an orientation is better suited than a central focus on genetic alterations of brain development for studying these changeable features that are more suggestive of dynamic than static encephalopathy. The possibility that we are not dealing with a developmentally based *deficit* but with potentially partly or fully functional domains whose dysfunction is not only or even necessarily structurally base but also has a significant contribution from *obstruction* by pathophysiological dysfunction can be considered in this fresh framework; this can open a greater range of approaches to potentially helpful treatments. Moreover even if there *is* a developmentally based alteration of brain development, that in itself is not sufficient reason to exclude the possibilities of (1) brain plasticity and (2) clinically significant improvement via the amelioration of exacerbating contributors such as metabolic and energetic dysfunctions.

Finally, investigating dynamic features of autism could contribute to our understanding of underlying mechanisms. The treatment of pathophysiological maladaptation (e.g., remediation of inflammation or oxidative stress) could be an interesting cognitive neuroscience probe. If these treatments have any efficacy in improving behavioral function, it would be most interesting to document the nature and distribution of the functional and structural neural systems impacts, and ask some important questions: Does functional improvement occur one domain at a time or in an across the board fashion? Might some treatments (e.g., the treatment of disrupted gut microbiology) more specifically target repetitive behaviors, obsessions, and stereotypies while other treatments (e.g., the reduction of oxidative stress) have more general effects? The answers would tell us a lot about underlying brain mechanisms; but to get these answers, a real partnership in research and treatment between pathophysiology and cognitive neuroscience is necessary.

18.2.5 How Does Specificity in Autism Relate to Many of the Pathophysiological Features That Are Not Unique to Autism? Non-Specificity of Important Pathophysiological Features in Autism and Its Implications

Neither genetics nor environmental research has to date found any one factor that seems clearly and dominantly causal in ASD. On the other hand, some of the physiological (including metabolic) changes being identified relate to vulnerability to a multiplicity of agents and stressors. Methylation and transsulfuration pathways are vulnerable to a myriad of environmental agents; mitochondria are exquisitely vulnerable to an enormous number of pharmaceuticals and xenobiotics; and the immune system shifts being identified are potentially both caused and perpetuated by a wide range of triggers. In addition, these features are not unique to ASD; very similar underlying physiological alterations are being identified in an impressive range of other contemporary chronic illnesses.

Meanwhile, we know that there have been perpetrated an exponentially increasing number of technological innovations leading to an evolutionarily unprecedented increase in the range of new-to-nature exposures (Goldman and Koduru 2000, Grandjean and Landrigan 2006). In effect, a whole panoply of exposures and stressors are converging on a smaller number of physiological pathways, overwhelming them and altering their systems dynamics. One output of this alteration arguably is autistic behaviors.

Thus, from a systems point of view, the "outputs" of the pathophysiological disturbances are "emergent properties" of the system rather than specifically determined by particular inputs, such as a particular gene or a particular toxin. It is perhaps fortunate in an ironic kind of way that there appear to be final common pathways of physiological compromise. This means that interventions might not need to be so specific, and that the support of the vulnerable physiological functions could serve to address harm from many inputs, break out of the gridlocked maladaptive state and allow a resetting of the system into a more adaptive homeostasis (Jones 2005, Rose 2001).

However, our methods for developing and evaluating interventions are based on a more determinist model, where we look for sensitivity and specificity of both biomarkers and targets for pharmacological intervention. From this determinist point of view, it would seem to be an odd notion to use a more generically oriented treatment (e.g., the treatment of inflammation) to treat a much more specific problem. This presents an obstacle to the study of systems-oriented treatment research. As research accumulates to support the systems-oriented active pathophysiological model of autism described above, it is hoped that methodologies will be developed and find acceptance that are suitable to the complexity and individuality of ASD pathophysiology, and to its amenability to a range of physiology-supportive interventions.

18.3 SUMMARY AND CONCLUSIONS

The complex dynamic pathophysiological features of ASD cannot be encompassed within a classical view that formulates the condition as a genetically determined brain-based static encephalopathy. Much information already exists suggesting a more inclusive model formulating ASD behaviors as one of a range of outputs of a set of active, persistent dynamic and interactive pathophysiological disturbances resulting from inputs that include environment as well as genes.

It is important to aggressively pursue approaches to research and treatment based upon this more inclusive model because there are strong reasons to believe that it will deliver palpable help sooner and will open the way to a greater range of constructive approaches. Cooperation and collaboration will allow the knowledge and skill sets of a range of specialists to come together in a synergistic approach to the multileveled challenges posed by autism (as also by other complex chronic conditions). In ASD, well-designed demonstrations of environmental influence, of physiological dimensions, and of physiological interventions regarding whether and how they lead to demonstrable, measurable brain change are probably the most critical leverage points to address in helping to redirect the central force of our efforts toward the helping most effectively.

The identification of pathophysiological disturbances in ASD consistent with environmental contributors, alongside of an increase in the prevalence of the condition, raise concerning questions not only about autism but also about much broader features of our way of life. The need for a transition to a more complex systems pathophysiological approach to autism is paralleled by the need for a transition to more integrative ecological approaches to healthy sustainable production that would reduce the destructive inputs that now appear to be overwhelming physiological (as well as social, psychological, ecological, and biogeochemical) systems. That a dynamic pathophysiological is supported by phenomena consistent with plasticity and malleability is encouraging and should help speed the advance of our models and the delivery of much needed help to affected individuals, and also encourage us to look for critical leverage points in other challenged systems.

REFERENCES

Afzal, N., S. Murch, K. Thirrupathy, L. Berger, A. Fagbemi, and R. Heuschkel. 2003. Constipation with acquired megarectum in children with autism. *Pediatrics* 112:939–942.

Alverdy, J. C. and E. B. Chang. 2008. The re-emerging role of the intestinal microflora in critical illness and inflammation: Why the gut hypothesis of sepsis syndrome will not go away. *J. Leukoc. Biol.* 83:461–466.

American Psychiatric Association. 1994. *Diagnostic and Statistical Manual of Mental Disorders*, 4th ed. (DSM IV). Washington DC: APA.

Anderson, M. P., B. S. Hooker, and M. R. Herbert. 2008. Bridging from cells to cognition in autism pathophysiology: Biological pathways to defective brain function and plasticity. *Am. J. Biochem. Biotechnol. (Special Issue on Autism Spectrum Disorders)* 4:167–176.

Arnold, S. E. 2001. Contributions of neuropathology to understanding schizophrenia in late life. *Harv. Rev. Psychiatry* 9:69–76.

Aschner, M., U. Sonnewald, and K. H. Tan. 2002. Astrocyte modulation of neurotoxic injury. *Brain Pathol.* 12:475–481.

Aschner, M., J. W. Allen, H. K. Kimelberg, R. M. LoPachin, and W. J. Streit. 1999. Glial cells in neurotoxicity development. *Annu. Rev. Pharmacol. Toxicol.* 39:151–173.

Ashwood, P. and J. Van de Water. 2004a. A review of autism and the immune response. *Clin. Dev. Immunol.* 11:165–174.

Ashwood, P. and J. Van de Water. 2004b. Is autism an autoimmune disease? *Autoimmun. Rev.* 3:557–562.

Ashwood, P., S. Wills, and J. Van de Water. 2006. The immune response in autism: A new frontier for autism research. *J. Leukoc. Biol.* 80:1–15.

Aylward, E. H., N. J. Minshew, K. Field, B. F. Sparks, and N. Singh. 2002. Effects of age on brain volume and head circumference in autism. *Neurology* 59:175–183.

Bauman, M. 2006. Beyond behavior: Biomedical diagnoses in autism spectrum disorders. *Autism Advocate* 45:27–29.

Bauman, M. L. and T. L. Kemper. 2005. Neuroanatomic observations of the brain in autism: A review and future directions. *Int. J. Dev. Neurosci.* 23:183–187.

Belmonte, M. K. and T. Bourgeron. 2006. Fragile X syndrome and autism at the intersection of genetic and neural networks. *Nat. Neurosci.* 9:1221–1225.

Blaylock, R. L. and A. Strunecka. 2009. Immune-glutamatergic dysfunction as a central mechanism of the autism spectrum disorders. *Curr. Med. Chem.* 16:157–170.

Braunschweig, D., P. Ashwood, P. Krakowiak, I. Hertz-Picciotto, R. Hansen, L. A. Croen, I. N. Pessah, and J. Van de Water. 2008. Autism: Maternally derived antibodies specific for fetal brain proteins. *Neurotoxicology* 29:226–231.

Bu, B., P. Ashwood, D. Harvey, I. B. King, J. V. Water, and L. W. Jin. 2006. Fatty acid compositions of red blood cell phospholipids in children with autism. *Prostaglandins Leukot. Essent. Fatty Acids* 74:215–221.

Buller, K. M. and T. A. Day. 2002. Systemic administration of interleukin-1beta activates select populations of central amygdala afferents. *J. Comp. Neurol.* 452:288–296.

Buller, K. M., A. S. Hamlin, and P. B. Osborne. 2005. Dissection of peripheral and central endogenous opioid modulation of systemic interleukin-1beta responses using c-fos expression in the rat brain. *Neuropharmacology* 49:230–242.

Calderon-Garciduenas, L., A. Mora-Tiscareno, E. Ontiveros, G. Gomez-Garza, G. Barragan-Mejia, J. Broadway, S. Chapman, G. Valencia-Salazar, V. Jewells, R. R. Maronpot, C. Henriquez-Roldan, B. Perez-Guille, R. Torres-Jardon, L. Herrit, D. Brooks, N. Osnaya-Brizuela, M. E. Monroy, A. Gonzalez-Maciel, R. Reynoso-Robles, R. Villarreal-Calderon, A. C. Solt, and R. W. Engle. 2008a. Air pollution, cognitive deficits and brain abnormalities: A pilot study with children and dogs. *Brain Cogn.* 68:117–127.

Calderon-Garciduenas, L., A. C. Solt, C. Henriquez-Roldan, R. Torres-Jardon, B. Nuse, L. Herritt, R. Villarreal-Calderon, N. Osnaya, I. Stone, R. Garcia, D. M. Brooks, A. Gonzalez-Maciel, R. Reynoso-Robles, R. Delgado-Chavez, and W. Reed. 2008b. Long-term air pollution exposure is associated with neuroinflammation, an altered innate immune response, disruption of the blood-brain barrier, ultrafine particulate deposition, and accumulation of amyloid beta-42 and alpha-synuclein in children and young adults. *Toxicol. Pathol.* 36:289–310.

Campbell, D. B., J. S. Sutcliffe, P. J. Ebert, R. Militerni, C. Bravaccio, S. Trillo, M. Elia, C. Schneider, R. Melmed, S. Sacco, A. M. Persico, and P. Levitt. 2006. A genetic variant that disrupts MET transcription is associated with autism. *Proc. Natl. Acad. Sci. U.S.A.* 103:16834–16839.

Campbell, D. B., C. Li, J. S. Sutcliffe, A. M. Persico, and P. Levitt. 2008. Genetic evidence implicating multiple genes in the MET receptor tyrosine kinase pathway in autism spectrum disorder. *Autism Res.* 1:159–168.

Canitano, R. 2007. Epilepsy in autism spectrum disorders. *Eur. Child Adolesc. Psychiatry* 16:61–66.

Carson, M. J., J. M. Doose, B. Melchior, C. D. Schmid, and C. C. Ploix. 2006. CNS immune privilege: Hiding in plain sight. *Immunol. Rev.* 213:48–65.

Caspi, A. and T. E. Moffitt. 2006. Gene-environment interactions in psychiatry: Joining forces with neuroscience. *Nat. Rev. Neurosci.* 7:583–590.

Caviness, V. S., Jr, N. T. Lange, N. Makris, M. R. Herbert, and D. N. Kennedy. 1999. MRI-based brain volumetrics: Emergence of a developmental brain science. *Brain Dev.* 21:289–295.

Chauhan, A. and V. Chauhan. 2006. Oxidative stress in autism. *Pathophysiology* 13:171–181.

Chauhan, V., A. Chauhan, I. L. Cohen, W. T. Brown, and A. Sheikh. 2004. Alteration in amino-glycerophospholipids levels in the plasma of children with autism: A potential biochemical diagnostic marker. *Life Sci.* 74:1635–1643.

Chugani, D. C., B. S. Sundram, M. Behen, M. L. Lee, and G. J. Moore. 1999. Evidence of altered energy metabolism in autistic children. *Prog. Neuropsychopharmacol. Biol. Psychiatry* 23:635–641.

Churchill, L., P. Taishi, M. Wang, J. Brandt, C. Cearley, A. Rehman, and J. M. Krueger. 2006. Brain distribution of cytokine mRNA induced by systemic administration of interleukin-1beta or tumor necrosis factor alpha. *Brain Res.* 1120:64–73.

Ciaranello, R. D., S. R. VandenBerg, and T. F. Anders. 1982. Intrinsic and extrinsic determinants of neuronal development: Relation to infantile autism. *J. Autism Dev. Disord.* 12:115–145.

Coleman, M. 1979. Studies of the autistic syndromes. In *Congenital and Acquired Cognitive Disorders*, ed. R. Katzman. New York: Raven Press, pp. 265–275.

Coleman, N. 1989. Autism: Nondrug biological treatments. In *Diagnosis and Treatment of Autism*, ed. C. Gillberg. New York: Plenum Press, pp. 219–235.

Coleman, P. D., J. Romano, L. Lapham, and W. Simon. 1985. Cell counts in cerebral cortex of an autistic patient. *J. Autism Dev. Disord.* 15:245–255.

Connors, S. L., P. Levitt, S. G. Matthews, T. A. Slotkin, M. V. Johnston, H. C. Kinney, W. G. Johnson, R. M. Dailey, and A. W. Zimmerman. 2008. Fetal mechanisms in neurodevelopmental disorders. *Pediatr. Neurol.* 38:163–176.

Conturo, T. E., D. L. Williams, C. D. Smith, E. Gultepe, E. Akbudak, and N. J. Minshew. 2008. Neuronal fiber pathway abnormalities in autism: An initial MRI diffusion tensor tracking study of hippocampo-fusiform and amygdalo-fusiform pathways. *J. Int. Neuropsychol. Soc.* 14:933–946.

Corrales, M. and M. Herbert. Autism and environmental genomics: Synergistic systems approaches to autism complexity. In *Autism Spectrum Disorders*, eds. D. Amaral, G, Dawson, and D. Geschwind. New York: Oxford University Press. (in press).

Correia, C., A. M. Coutinho, L. Diogo, M. Grazina, C. Marques, T. Miguel, A. Ataide, J. Almeida, L. Borges, C. Oliveira, G. Oliveira, and A. M. Vicente. 2006. Brief report: High frequency of biochemical markers for mitochondrial dysfunction in autism: No association with the mitochondrial aspartate/glutamate carrier SLC25A12 gene. *J. Autism Dev. Disord.* 36:1137–1140.

Courchesne, E. and K. Pierce. 2005. Why the frontal cortex in autism might be talking only to itself: Local over-connectivity but long-distance disconnection. *Curr. Opin. Neurobiol.* 15:225–230.

Coyle, J. T. and R. Schwarcz. 2000. Mind glue: implications of glial cell biology for psychiatry. *Arch. Gen. Psychiatry* 57:90–93.

Croen, L. A., J. K. Grether, C. K. Yoshida, R. Odouli, and J. Van de Water. 2005. Maternal autoimmune diseases, asthma and allergies, and childhood autism spectrum disorders: A case-control study. *Arch. Pediatr. Adolesc. Med.* 159:151–157.

Curran, L. K., C. J. Newschaffer, L. C. Lee, S. O. Crawford, M. V. Johnston, and A. W. Zimmerman. 2007. Behaviors associated with fever in children with autism spectrum disorders. *Pediatrics* 120:e1386–e1392.

D'Amelio, M., I. Ricci, R. Sacco, X. Liu, L. D'Agruma, L. A. Muscarella, V. Guarnieri, R. Militerni, C. Bravaccio, M. Elia, C. Schneider, R. Melmed, S. Trillo, T. Pascucci, S. Puglisi-Allegra, K. L. Reichelt, F. Macciardi, J. J. Holden, and A. M. Persico.

2005. Paraoxonase gene variants are associated with autism in North America, but not in Italy: Possible regional specificity in gene-environment interactions. *Mol. Psychiatry* 10:1006–1016.

Dager, S. R., S. D. Friedman, H. Pegropoulos, and D. W. W. Shaw. 2008. Imaging evidence for pathological brain development in autism spectrum disorders. In *Autism: Current Theories and Evidence*, ed. A. Zimmerman. Totowa, NJ: Humana Press.

Davis, J. O., J. A. Phelps, and H. S. Bracha. 1995. Prenatal development of monozygotic twins and concordance for schizophrenia. *Schizophr. Bull.* 21:357–366.

DeMyer, M. K., J. N. Hingtgen, and R. K. Jackson. 1981. Infantile autism reviewed: A decade of research. *Schizophr. Bull.* 7:388–451.

DeVito, T. J., D. J. Drost, R. W. Neufeld, N. Rajakumar, W. Pavlosky, P. Williamson, and R. Nicolson. 2007. Evidence for cortical dysfunction in autism: A proton magnetic resonance spectroscopic imaging study. *Biol. Psychiatry* 61:465–473.

Dietert, R. R. and J. M. Dietert. 2008. Potential for early-life immune insult including developmental immunotoxicity in autism and autism spectrum disorders: Focus on critical windows of immune vulnerability. *J. Toxicol. Environ. Health B. Crit. Rev.* 11:660–680.

Ehninger, D., S. Han, C. Shilyansky, Y. Zhou, W. Li, D. J. Kwiatkowski, V. Ramesh, and A. J. Silva. 2008. Reversal of learning deficits in a Tsc2+/− mouse model of tuberous sclerosis. *Nat. Med.* 14:843–848.

Endo, T., T. Shioiri, H. Kitamura, T. Kimura, S. Endo, N. Masuzawa, and T. Someya. 2007. Altered chemical metabolites in the amygdala-hippocampus region contribute to autistic symptoms of autism spectrum disorders. *Biol. Psychiatry* 62:1030–1037.

Evans, T. A., S. L. Siedlak, Lian Lu, X. Fu, Z. Wang, W. R. McGinnis, E. Fakhoury, R. J. Castellanio, S. L. Hazen, W. H. Walsh, A. T. Lewis, R. G. Salomon, M. A. Smith, and G. Zhu X. Perry. 2008. The autistic phenotype exhibits a remarkably localized modification of brain protein by products of free radical-induced lipid oxidation. *Am. J. Biochem. Biotechnol. (Special Issue on Autism Spectrum Disorders)* 4:61–72.

Fatemi, S. H., J. Earle, R. Kanodia, D. Kist, E. S. Emamian, P. H. Patterson, L. Shi, and R. Sidwell. 2002. Prenatal viral infection leads to pyramidal cell atrophy and macro-cephaly in adulthood: Implications for genesis of autism and schizophrenia. *Cell. Mol. Neurobiol.* 22:25–33.

Fein, D., P. Dixon, J. Paul, and H. Levin. 2005. Pervasive developmental disorder can evolve into ADHD: Case illustrations. *J. Autism Dev. Disord.* 35:525–534.

Felicetti, T. 1981. Parents of autistic children: Some notes on the chemical connection. *Milieu Ther.* 1:13–16.

Fernell, E., Y. Watanabe, I. Adolfsson, Y. Tani, M. Bergstrom, P. Hartvig, A. Lilja, A. L. von Knorring, C. Gillberg, and B. Langstrom. 1997. Possible effects of tetrahydrobiopterin treatment in six children with autism—clinical and positron emission tomography data: A pilot study. *Dev. Med. Child Neurol.* 39:313–318.

Fields, R. D. 2006. Advances in understanding neuron-glia interactions. *Neuron Glia Biol.* 2:23–26.

Fields, R. D. 2008. Oligodendrocytes changing the rules: Action potentials in glia and oligodendrocytes controlling action potentials. *Neuroscientist* 14:540–543.

Filipek, P. A., J. Juranek, M. T. Nguyen, C. Cummings, and J. J. Gargus. 2004. Relative carnitine deficiency in autism. *J. Autism Dev. Disord.* 34:615–623.

Finegold, S. M., D. Molitoris, Y. Song, C. Liu, M. L. Vaisanen, E. Bolte, M. McTeague, R. Sandler, H. Wexler, E. M. Marlowe, M. D. Collins, P. A. Lawson, P. Summanen, M. Baysallar, T. J. Tomzynski, E. Read, E. Johnson, R. Rolfe, P. Nasir, H. Shah, D. A. Haake, P. Manning, and A. Kaul. 2002. Gastrointestinal microflora studies in late-onset autism. *Clin. Infect. Dis.* 35:S6–S16.

Friedman, S. D., D. W. Shaw, A. A. Artru, T. L. Richards, J. Gardner, G. Dawson, S. Posse, and S. R. Dager. 2003. Regional brain chemical alterations in young children with autism spectrum disorder. *Neurology* 60:100–107.

Friedman, S. D., D. W. Shaw, A. A. Artru, G. Dawson, H. Petropoulos, and S. R. Dager. 2006. Gray and white matter brain chemistry in young children with autism. *Arch. Gen. Psychiatry* 63:786–794.

Gajzago, G. and M. Prior. 1974. Two cases of "recovery" in Kanner syndrome. *Arch. Gen. Psychiatry*. 31:264–268.

Giaume, C., F. Kirchhoff, C. Matute, A. Reichenbach, and A. Verkhratsky. 2007. Glia: The fulcrum of brain diseases. *Cell Death Differ.* 14:1324–1335.

Gillberg, C. and M. Coleman (eds.). 2000. *The Biology of the Autistic Syndromes (Clinics in Developmental Medicine)*. Cambridge, U.K.: Cambridge University Press.

Gold, D. R. and B. H. Cohen. 2001. Treatment of mitochondrial cytopathies. *Semin. Neurol.* 21:309–325.

Goldman, L. R. and S. Koduru. 2000. Chemicals in the environment and developmental toxicity to children: A public health and policy perspective. *Environ. Health Perspect.* 108(Suppl. 3):443–448.

Goodwin, M. S., J. Groden, W. F. Velicer, L. P. Lipsitt, M. G. Baron, S. G. Hofmann, and G Groden. 2006. Cardiovascular arousal in individuals with autism. *Focus Autism Other Dev. Disabil.* 21:100–123.

Grandjean, P. and P. J. Landrigan. 2006. Developmental neurotoxicity of industrial chemicals. *Lancet* 368:2167–2178.

Groden, J., M. S. Goodwin, M. G. Baron, G. Groden, W. F. Velicer, L. P. Lipsitt, S. G. Hofmann, and B. Plummer. 2005. Assessing cardiovascular responses to stressors in individuals with autism spectrum disorders. *Focus Autism Other Dev. Disabil.* 20:244–252.

Gustafsson, L. 2004. Comment on disruption in the inhibitory architecture of the cell minicolumn: Implications for autism. *Neuroscientist* 10:189–191.

Guy, J., J. Gan, J. Selfridge, S. Cobb, and A. Bird. 2007. Reversal of neurological defects in a mouse model of Rett syndrome. *Science* 315:1143–1147.

Halassa, M. M., T. Fellin, and P. G. Haydon. 2007. The tripartite synapse: Roles for gliotransmission in health and disease. *Trends Mol. Med.* 13:54–63.

Hallmayr, J. 2008. Personal communication.

Han, B. C., S. B. Koh, E. Y. Lee, and Y. H. Seong. 2004. Regional difference of glutamate-induced swelling in cultured rat brain astrocytes. *Life Sci.* 76:573–583.

Hanisch, U. K. 2002. Microglia as a source and target of cytokines. *Glia* 40:140–155.

Happe, F. and A. Ronald. 2008. The fractionable autism triad: A review of evidence from behavioural, genetic, cognitive and neural research. *Neuropsychol. Rev.* 18:287–304.

Happe, F., A. Ronald, and R. Plomin. 2006. Time to give up on a single explanation for autism. *Nat. Neurosci.* 9:1218–1220.

Hayashi, M. L., B. S. Rao, J. S. Seo, H. S. Choi, B. M. Dolan, S. Y. Choi, S. Chattarji, and S. Tonegawa. 2007. Inhibition of p21-activated kinase rescues symptoms of fragile X syndrome in mice. *Proc. Natl. Acad. Sci. U.S.A.* 104:11489–11494.

Helt, M., E. Kelley, M. Kinsbourne, J. Pandey, H. Boorstein, M. Herbert, and D. Fein. 2008. Can children with autism recover? If so, how? *Neuropsychol. Rev.* 18:339–366.

Hendry, J., T. DeVito, N. Gelman, M. Densmore, N. Rajakumar, W. Pavlosky, P. C. Williamson, P. M. Thompson, D. J. Drost, and R. Nicolson. 2006. White matter abnormalities in autism detected through transverse relaxation time imaging. *Neuroimage* 29:1049–1057.

Herbert, M. 2007. Transcending the gaps in autism research. Interview with Martha Herbert, MD by Frank Lampe and Suzanne Snyder. *Altern. Ther. Health Med.* 13:62–73 or http://www.alternative-therapies.com/at/web_pdfs/herbert_long.pdf.

Herbert, M. R. 2002. Genetics finding its place in larger living schemes. *Crit. Pub. Health* 12:221–236.

Herbert, M. R. 2005a. Autism: A brain disorder or a disorder that affects the brain? *Clin. Neuropsychiatry* 2:354–379.

Herbert, M. R. 2005b. Large brains in autism: The challenge of pervasive abnormality. *Neuroscientist* 11:417–440.

Herbert, M. R. and M. P. Anderson. 2008. An expanding spectrum of autism models: From fixed developmental defects to reversible functional impairments. In *Autism: Current Theories and Evidence*, ed. A. Zimmerman. Totowa, NJ: Humana Press, pp. 429–463.

Herbert, M. R. and V. S. Caviness. 2006. Neuroanatomy and imaging studies. In *Autism: A Neurobiological Disorder of Early Brain Development*, eds. R. Tuchman and I. Rapin. London: Mac Keith Press, 115–140.

Hertz-Picciotto, I. and L. Delwiche. 2009. The rise in autism and the role of age at diagnosis. *Epidemiology* 20:84–90.

Hertz-Picciotto, I., H. Y. Park, M. Dostal, A. Kocan, T. Trnovec, and R. Sram. 2008. Prenatal exposures to persistent and non-persistent organic compounds and effects on immune system development. *Basic Clin. Pharmacol. Toxicol.* 102:146–154.

Holtzman, D. 2008. Autistic spectrum disorders and mitochondrial encephalopathies. *Acta Paediatr.* 97:859–860.

Hugg, J. W., R. I. Kuznicky, F. G. Gilliam, R. B. Morawetz, R. E. Fraught, and H. P. Hetherington. 1996. Normalization of contralateral metabolic function following temporal lobectomy demonstrated by 1H magnetic resonance spectroscopic imaging. *Ann. Neurol.* 40:236–239.

James, S. J., S. Melnyk, S. Jernigan, M. A. Cleves, C. H. Halsted, D. H. Wong, P. Cutler, K. Bock, M. Boris, J. J. Bradstreet, S. M. Baker, and D. W. Gaylor. 2006. Metabolic endophenotype and related genotypes are associated with oxidative stress in children with autism. *Am. J. Med. Genet. B Neuropsychiatr. Genet.* 141:947 956.

James, S. J., S. Melnyk, S. Jernigan, A. Hubanks, S. Rose, and D. W. Gaylor. 2008. Abnormal transmethylation/transsulfuration metabolism and DNA hypomethylation among parents of children with autism. *J. Autism Dev. Disord.* 38:1966–1975.

Jones, D. S. 2005. *Textbook of Functional Medicine*. Gig Harbor, WA: Institute for Functional Medicine.

Just, M. A., V. L. Cherkassky, T. A. Keller, and N. J. Minshew. 2004. Cortical activation and synchronization during sentence comprehension in high-functioning autism: Evidence of underconnectivity. *Brain* 127:1811–1821.

Just, M. A., V. L. Cherkassky, T. A. Keller, R. K. Kana, and N. J. Minshew. 2007. Functional and anatomical cortical underconnectivity in autism: Evidence from an FMRI study of an executive function task and corpus callosum morphometry. *Cereb. Cortex* 17:951–961.

Kanner, L. 1943. Autistic disturbances of affective contact. *Nerv. Child* 10:217–250.

Kanner, L. 1968. Early infantile autism revisited. *Psychiatry Dig.* 29:17–28.

Kanner, L. 1971. Follow-up study of eleven autistic children originally reported in 1943. *J. Autism Child Schizophr.* 1:119–145.

Kelley, E., J. J. Paul, D. Fein, and L. R. Naigles. 2006. Residual language deficits in optimal outcome children with a history of autism. *J. Autism Dev. Disord.* 36:807–828.

Kern, J. K. 2003. Purkinje cell vulnerability and autism: A possible etiological connection. *Brain Dev.* 25:377–382.

Kielian, T. 2008. Glial connexins and gap junctions in CNS inflammation and disease. *J. Neurochem.* 106:1000–1016.

Kim, W. G., R. P. Mohney, B. Wilson, G. H. Jeohn, B. Liu, and J. S. Hong. 2000. Regional difference in susceptibility to lipopolysaccharide-induced neurotoxicity in the rat brain: Role of microglia. *J. Neurosci.* 20:6309–6316.

Kleinhans, N. M., B. C. Schweinsburg, D. N. Cohen, R. A. Muller, and E. Courchesne. 2007. N-acetyl aspartate in autism spectrum disorders: Regional effects and relationship to fMRI activation. *Brain Res.* 1162:85–97. [Epub 2007 May 21. 1162:85–97].

Koehler, R. C., D. Gebremedhin, and D. R. Harder. 2006. Role of astrocytes in cerebrovascular regulation. *J. Appl. Physiol.* 100:307–317.

Leekam, S. R., C. Nieto, S. J. Libby, L. Wing, and J. Gould. 2007. Describing the sensory abnormalities of children and adults with autism. *J. Autism Dev. Disord.* 37;894–910.

Li, M., B. Wang, M. Zhang, M. Rantalainen, S. Wang, H. Zhou, Y. Zhang, J. Shen, X. Pang, M. Zhang, H. Wei, Y. Chen, H. Lu, J. Zuo, M. Su, Y. Qiu, W. Jia, C. Xiao, L. M. Smith, S. Yang, E. Holmes, H. Tang, G. Zhao, J. K. Nicholson, L. Li, and L. Zhao. 2008. Symbiotic gut microbes modulate human metabolic phenotypes. *Proc. Natl. Acad. Sci. U.S.A.* 105:2117–2122.

Li, X., A. Chauhan, A. M. Sheikh, S. Patil, V. Chauhan, X. M. Li, L. Ji, T. Brown, and M. Malik. 2009. Elevated immune response in the brain of autistic patients. *J. Neuroimmunol.* 207:111–116.

Liang, J., H. Takeuchi, Y. Doi, J. Kawanokuchi, Y. Sonobe, S. Jin, I. Yawata, H. Li, S. Yasuoka, T. Mizuno, and A. Suzumura. 2008. Excitatory amino acid transporter expression by astrocytes is neuroprotective against microglial excitotoxicity. *Brain Res.* 1210:11–19.

Lovaas, O. I. 1987. Behavioral treatment and normal educational and intellectual functioning in young autistic children. *J. Consult. Clin. Psychol.* 55:3–9.

Lowry, C. A., J. H. Hollis, A. de Vries, B. Pan, L. R. Brunet, J. R. Hunt, J. F. Paton, E. van Kampen, D. M. Knight, A. K. Evans, G. A. Rook, and S. L. Lightman. 2007. Identification of an immune-responsive mesolimbocortical serotonergic system: Potential role in regulation of emotional behavior. *Neuroscience* 146:756–772.

Lozovaya, N. and A. D. Miller. 2003. Chemical neuroimmunology: Health in a nutshell bidirectional communication between immune and stress (limbic-hypothalamic-pituitary-adrenal) systems. *Chembiochem* 4:466–484.

MacFabe, D. F., D. P. Cain, K. Rodriguez-Capote, A. E. Franklin, J. E. Hoffman, F. Boon, A. R. Taylor, M. Kavaliers, and K. P. Ossenkopp. 2007. Neurobiological effects of intra-ventricular propionic acid in rats: Possible role of short chain fatty acids on the pathogenesis and characteristics of autism spectrum disorders. *Behav. Brain Res.* 176:149–169.

Maes, M., R. Verkerk, E. Vandoolaeghe, F. Van Hunsel, H. Neels, A. Wauters, P. Demedts, and S. Scharpe. 1997. Serotonin-immune interactions in major depression: Lower serum tryptophan as a marker of an immune-inflammatory response. *Eur. Arch. Psychiatry Clin. Neurosci.* 247:154–161.

Malow, B. A. 2004. Sleep disorders, epilepsy, and autism. *Ment. Retard. Dev. Disabil. Res. Rev.* 10:122–125.

Malow, B. A., M. L. Marzec, S. G. McGrew, L. Wang, L. M. Henderson, and W. L. Stone. 2006. Characterizing sleep in children with autism spectrum disorders: A multidimensional approach. *Sleep* 29:1563–1571.

Mattson, M. P. 2007. Mitochondrial regulation of neuronal plasticity. *Neurochem. Res.* 32:707–715.

Mattson, M. P. 2008. Glutamate and neurotrophic factors in neuronal plasticity and disease. *Ann. N.Y. Acad. Sci.* 1144:97–112.

Mattson, M. P. and D. Liu. 2002. Energetics and oxidative stress in synaptic plasticity and neurodegenerative disorders. *Neuromolecular Med.* 2:215–231.

McDougle, C. J., S. T. Naylor, D. J. Cohen, G. K. Aghajanian, G. R. Heninger, and L. H. Price. 1996. Effects of tryptophan depletion in drug-free adults with autistic disorder. *Arch. Gen. Psychiatry* 53:993–1000.

McGinnis, W. R. 2007. Could oxidative stress from psychosocial stress affect neurodevelopment in autism? *J. Autism Dev. Disord.* 37:993–994.

Mehler, M. F. and D. P. Purpura. 2009. Autism, fever, epigenetics and the locus coeruleus. *Brain Res. Rev.* 59:388–392.

Miller, A. H., V. Maletic, and C. L. Raison. 2009. Inflammation and its discontents: the role of cytokines in the pathophysiology of major depression. *Biol. Psychiatry* 65:732–741.

Ming, X., P. O. Julu, J. Wark, F. Apartopoulos, and S. Hansen. 2004. Discordant mental and physical efforts in an autistic patient. *Brain Dev.* 26:519–524.

Minshew, N. J., G. Goldstein, S. M. Dombrowski, K. Panchalingam, and J. W. Pettegrew. 1993. A preliminary 31P MRS study of autism: Evidence for undersynthesis and increased degradation of brain membranes. *Biol. Psychiatry* 33:762–773.

Moretti, P., T. Sahoo, K. Hyland, T. Bottiglieri, S. Peters, D. del Gaudio, B. Roa, S. Curry, H. Zhu, R. H. Finnell, J. L. Neul, V. T. Ramaekers, N. Blau, C. A. Bacino, G. Miller, and F. Scaglia. 2005. Cerebral folate deficiency with developmental delay, autism, and response to folinic acid. *Neurology* 64:1088–1090.

Morrow, E. M., S. Y. Yoo, S. W. Flavell, T. K. Kim, Y. Lin, R. S. Hill, N. M. Mukaddes, S. Balkhy, G. Gascon, A. Hashmi, S. Al-Saad, J. Ware, R. M. Joseph, R. Greenblatt, D. Gleason, J. A. Ertelt, K. A. Apse, A. Bodell, J. N. Partlow, B. Barry, H. Yao, K. Markianos, R. J. Ferland, M. E. Greenberg, and C. A. Walsh. 2008. Identifying autism loci and genes by tracing recent shared ancestry. *Science* 321:218–223.

Morton, J. and U. Frith. 1995. Causal modelling: A structural approach to developmental psychopathology. In *Manual of Developmental Psychopathology*, eds. D. Cicchetti and D. J. Cohen. New York: John Wiley, pp. 357–390.

Muller, R. A. 2007. The study of autism as a distributed disorder. *Ment. Retard. Dev. Disabil. Res. Rev.* 13:85–95.

Natowicz, M. 2004. Personal communication.

Nelson, K. B., J. K. Grether, L. A. Croen, J. M. Dambrosia, B. F. Dickens, L. L. Jelliffe, R. L. Hansen, and T. M. Phillips. 2001. Neuropeptides and neurotrophins in neonatal blood of children with autism or mental retardation. *Ann. Neurol.* 49:597–606.

Newschaffer, C. J., L. A. Croen, J. Daniels, E. Giarelli, J. K. Grether, S. E. Levy, D. S. Mandell, L. A. Miller, and J. Pinto-Martin. 2007. The epidemiology of autism spectrum disorders. *Annu. Rev. Pub. Health* 28:235–256.

Nicholson, J. K., E. Holmes, and I. D. Wilson. 2005. Gut microorganisms, mammalian metabolism and personalized health care. *Nat. Rev. Microbiol.* 3:431–438.

Noble, D. 2008. *The Music of Life.* New York: Oxford University Press.

Nyffeler, M., U. Meyer, B. K. Yee, J. Feldon, and I. Knuesel. 2006. Maternal immune activation during pregnancy increases limbic GABAA receptor immunoreactivity in the adult offspring: Implications for schizophrenia. *Neuroscience* 143:51–62.

Oliveira, G., L. Diogo, M. Grazina, P. Garcia, A. Ataide, C. Marques, T. Miguel, L. Borges, A. M. Vicente, and C. R. Oliveira. 2005. Mitochondrial dysfunction in autism spectrum disorders: A population-based study. *Dev. Med. Child Neurol.* 47:185–189.

Olmsted, D. 2005. The age of autism: Case 1 revisited. *American Chronicle.* Available online at http://www.americanchronicle.com/articles/view/1872

Opler, M. G. and E. S. Susser. 2005. Fetal environment and schizophrenia. *Environ. Health Perspect.* 113:1239–1242.

Orellana, J. A., P. J. Saez, K. F. Shoji, K. A. Schalper, N. Palacios-Prado, V. Velarde, C. Giaume, M. V. Bennett, and J. C. Saez. 2009. Modulation of brain hemichannels and gap junction channels by pro-inflammatory agents and their possible role in neurodegeneration. *Antioxid. Redox Signal.* 11:369–399.

Page, T. 2000. Metabolic approaches to the treatment of autism spectrum disorders. *J. Autism Dev. Disord.* 30:463–469.

Page, T. and C. Moseley. 2002. Metabolic treatment of hyperuricosuric autism. *Prog. Neuropsychopharmacol. Biol Psychiatry* 26:397–400.

Pan, J. W., A. Williamson, I. Cavus, H. P. Hetherington, H. Zaveri, O. A. Petroff, and D. D. Spencer. 2008. Neurometabolism in human epilepsy. *Epilepsia* 49(Suppl. 3):31–41.

Pardo, C. A., D. Wheeler, Vargas. D., N. Haughey, and A. Zimmerman. 2008. Abnormalities in cholesterol, ceramides and markers of oxidative stress are revealed by lipidomic analysis of brain tissues in autism. *IMFAR*: Poster #155.13.

Parracho, H. M., M. O. Bingham, G. R. Gibson, and A. L. McCartney. 2005. Differences between the gut microflora of children with autistic spectrum disorders and that of healthy children. *J. Med. Microbiol.* 54:987–991.

Patterson, P. H. 2002. Maternal infection: Window on neuroimmune interactions in fetal brain development and mental illness. *Curr. Opin. Neurobiol.* 12:115–118.

Persico, A. M. and T. Bourgeron. 2006. Searching for ways out of the autism maze: Genetic, epigenetic and environmental clues. *Trends Neurosci.* 29:349–358.

Peschanski, M. 1991. Le temps venu de la "Neurogliobiologie." *Médecine/Sciences* 7:766–767.

Pessah, I. N. and P. J. Lein. 2008. Evidence for environmental susceptibility in autism: What we need to know about gene *x* environment interactions. In *Autism: Current Theories and Models*, ed. A. Zimmerman, Totowa, NJ: Humana Press, pp. 409–428.

Qin, L., X. Wu, M. L. Block, Y. Liu, G. R. Breese, J. S. Hong, D. J. Knapp, and F. T. Crews. 2007. Systemic LPS causes chronic neuroinflammation and progressive neurodegeneration. *Glia* 55:453–462.

Raymond, G. V., M. L. Bauman, and T. L. Kemper. 1996. Hippocampus in autism: A Golgi analysis. *Acta Neuropathol.* 91:117–119.

Rose, G. 2001. Sick individuals and sick populations. *Int. J. Epidemiol.* 30:427–432; discussion 433–434.

Rosenberger-Debiesse, J. and M. Coleman. 1986. Preliminary evidence for multiple etiologies in autism. *J. Autism Dev. Disord.* 16:385–392.

Rossignol, D. A. and J. J. Bradstreet. 2008. Evidence of mitochondrial dysfunction in autism and implications for treatment. Special Issue on Autism Spectrum Disorders, *Am. J. Biochem. Biotechnol.* 4:208–217.

Rothman, K. J. and S. Greenland. 1998. *Modern Epidemiology*. Philadelphia, PA: Lippincott Williams and Wilkins.

Ruhl, A. 2005. Glial cells in the gut. *Neurogastroenterol. Motil.* 17:777–790.

Rutter, M. 2007. Gene-environment interdependence. *Dev. Sci.* 10:12–18.

Rutter, M. 2008. Biological implications of gene-environment interaction. *J. Abnorm. Child Psychol.* 36:969–975.

Rutter, M. and L. Lockyer. 1967. A five to fifteen year follow-up study of infantile psychosis. I. Description of sample. *Br. J. Psychiatry* 113:1169–1182.

Rutter, M., D. Greenfeld, and L. Lockyer. 1967. A five to fifteen year follow-up study of infantile psychosis. II. Social and behavioural outcome. *Br. J. Psychiatry* 113:1183–1199.

Sajdel-Sulkowska, E. M., B. Lipinski, H. Windom, T. Audhya, and W. McGinnis. 2008. Oxidative stress in autism: Elevated cerebellar 3-nitrotyrosine levels. *Am. J. Biochem. Biotechnol. (Special Issue on Autism Spectrum Disorders)* 4:73–84.

Sandler, R. H., S. M. Finegold, E. R. Bolte, C. P. Buchanan, A. P. Maxwell, M. L. Vaisanen, M. N. Nelson, and H. M. Wexler. 2000. Short-term benefit from oral vancomycin treatment of regressive-onset autism. *J. Child Neurol.* 15:429–435.

Schousboe, A. and H. S. Waagepetersen. 2005. Role of astrocytes in glutamate homeostasis: Implications for excitotoxicity. *Neurotox. Res.* 8:221–225.

Schwarz, E. and S. Bahn. 2008. The utility of biomarker discovery approaches for the detection of disease mechanisms in psychiatric disorders. *Br. J. Pharmacol.* 153(Suppl. 1): S133–S136.

Serles, W., L. M. Li, S. B. Antel, F. Cendes, J. Gotman, A. Olivier, F. Andermann, F. Dubeau, and D. L. Arnold. 2001. Time course of postoperative recovery of *N*-acetyl-aspartate in temporal lobe epilepsy. *Epilepsia* 42:190–197.

Shi, L., S. H. Fatemi, R. W. Sidwell, and P. H. Patterson. 2003. Maternal influenza infection causes marked behavioral and pharmacological changes in the offspring. *J. Neurosci.* 23:297–302.

Shultz, S. R., D. F. Macfabe, S. Martin, J. Jackson, R. Taylor, F. Boon, K. P. Ossenkopp, and D. P. Cain. 2009. Intracerebroventricular injections of the enteric bacterial metabolic product propionic acid impair cognition and sensorimotor ability in the Long-Evans rat: Further development of a rodent model of autism. *Behav. Brain Res.* 200: 33–41.

Shultz, S. R., D. F. MacFabe, K. P. Ossenkopp, S. Scratch, J. Whelan, R. Taylor, and D. P. Cain. 2008b. Intracerebroventricular injection of propionic acid, an enteric bacterial metabolic end-product, impairs social behavior in the rat: Implications for an animal model of autism. *Neuropharmacology* 54:901–911.

Slikker, W. and L. W. Chang. 1998. *Handbook of Developmental Neurotoxicology.* San Diego, CA: Academic Press.

Smith, S. E., J. Li, K. Garbett, K. Mirnics, and P. H. Patterson. 2007. Maternal immune activation alters fetal brain development through interleukin-6. *J. Neurosci.* 27:10695–106702.

Song, Y., C. Liu, and S. M. Finegold. 2004. Real-time PCR quantitation of clostridia in feces of autistic children. *Appl. Environ. Microbiol.* 70:6459–6465.

Standridge, J. B. 2006. Vicious cycles within the neuropathophysiologic mechanisms of Alzheimer's disease. *Curr. Alzheimer Res.* 3:95–108.

Sundaram, S. K., A. Kumar, M. I. Makki, M. E. Behen, H. T. Chugani, and D. C. Chugani. 2008. Diffusion tensor imaging of frontal lobe in autism spectrum disorder. *Cereb. Cortex* 18:2659–2665.

Sutera, S., J. Pandey, E. L. Esser, M. A. Rosenthal, L. B. Wilson, M. Barton, J. Green, S. Hodgson, D. L. Robins, T. Dumont-Mathieu, and D. Fein. 2007. Predictors of optimal outcome in toddlers diagnosed with autism spectrum disorders. *J. Autism Dev. Disord.* 37:98–107.

Theis, M., G. Sohl, J. Eiberger, and K. Willecke. 2005. Emerging complexities in identity and function of glial connexins. *Trends Neurosci.* 28:188–195.

Thevarkunnel, S., M. A. Martchek, T. L. Kemper, M. B. Bauman, and G. J. Blatt. 2004. A neuroanatomical study of the brainstem nuclei in autism. *Society for Neuroscience Abstract* 1028.14.

Tilleux, S. and E. Hermans. 2007. Neuroinflammation and regulation of glial glutamate uptake in neurological disorders. *J. Neurosci. Res.* 85:2059–2070.

Tobinick, E. L. and H. Gross. 2008a. Rapid cognitive improvement in Alzheimer's disease following perispinal etanercept administration. *J. Neuroinflammation* 5:2.

Tobinick, E. L. and H. Gross. 2008b. Rapid improvement in verbal fluency and aphasia following perispinal etanercept in Alzheimer's disease. *BMC Neurol.* 8:27.

Tomchek, S. D. and W. Dunn. 2007. Sensory processing in children with and without autism: A comparative study using the short sensory profile. *Am. J. Occup. Ther.* 61:190–200.

Torrente, F., P. Ashwood, R. Day, N. Machado, R. I. Furlano, A. Anthony, S. E. Davies, A. J. Wakefield, M. A. Thomson, J. A. Walker-Smith, and S. H. Murch. 2002. Small intestinal enteropathy with epithelial IgG and complement deposition in children with regressive autism. *Mol. Psychiatry* 7: 334, 375–382.

Tsuang, M. T., J. L. Bar, W. S. Stone, and S. V. Faraone. 2004. Gene-environment interactions in mental disorders. *World Psychiatry* 3:73–83.

Tuchman, R. and I. Rapin. 2006. *Autism: A Neurobiological Disorder of Early Brain Development.* London, U.K.: Mac Keith Press.

Valicenti-McDermott, M., K. McVicar, I. Rapin, B. K. Wershil, H. Cohen, and S. Shinnar. 2006. Frequency of gastrointestinal symptoms in children with autistic spectrum disorders and association with family history of autoimmune disease. *J. Dev. Behav. Pediatr.* 27:S128–S136.

Vancassel, S., G. Durand, C. Barthelemy, B. Lejeune, J. Martineau, D. Guilloteau, C. Andres, and S. Chalon. 2001. Plasma fatty acid levels in autistic children. *Prostaglandins Leukot. Essent. Fatty Acids* 65:1–7.

Vargas, D. L., C. Nascimbene, C. Krishnan, A. W. Zimmerman, and C. A. Pardo. 2005. Neuroglial activation and neuroinflammation in the brain of patients with autism. *Ann. Neurol.* 57:67–81.

Vargas, D. L., V. Bandaru, M. C. Zerrate, A. W. Zimmerman, N. Haughey, and C. A. Pardo. 2006. Oxidative stress in brain tissues from autistic patients: Increased concentration of isoprostanes. *IMFAR*: Poster #PS2.6.

Vasconcelos, M. M., A. R. Brito, R. C. Domingues, L. C. da Cruz, Jr., E. L. Gasparetto, J. Werner, Jr., and J. P. Goncalves. 2008. Proton magnetic resonance spectroscopy in school-aged autistic children. *J. Neuroimaging* 18:288–295.

Visscher, P. M., W. G. Hill, and N. R. Wray. 2008. Heritability in the genomics era: Concepts and misconceptions. *Nat. Rev. Genet.* 9:255–266.

Wallace, K. B. and A. A. Starkov. 2000. Mitochondrial targets of drug toxicity. *Annu. Rev. Pharmacol. Toxicol.* 40:353–388.

Whitney, E. R., T. L. Kemper, M. L. Bauman, D. L. Rosene, and G. J. Blatt. 2008. Cerebellar Purkinje cells are reduced in a subpopulation of autistic brains: A stereological experiment using Calbindin-D28k. *Cerebellum* 7:406–416.

Wrona, D. 2006. Neural-immune interactions: An integrative view of the bidirectional relationship between the brain and immune systems. *J. Neuroimmunol.* 172:38–58.

Yao, Y., W. J. Walsh, W. R. McGinnis, and D. Pratico. 2006. Altered vascular phenotype in autism: Correlation with oxidative stress. *Arch. Neurol.* 63:1161–1164.

Yip, J., J. J. Soghomonian, and G. J. Blatt. 2008. Increased GAD67 mRNA expression in cerebellar interneurons in autism: Implications for Purkinje cell dysfunction. *J. Neurosci. Res.* 86:525–530.

Zeegers, M., J. van der Grond, E. van Daalen, J. Buitelaar, and H. van Engeland. 2007. Proton magnetic resonance spectroscopy in developmentally delayed young boys with or without autism. *J. Neural Transm.* 114:289–295.

Zimmerman, A. 2008. Personal communication.

Zoghbi, H. Y. 2003. Postnatal neurodevelopmental disorders: Meeting at the synapse? *Science* 302:826–830.

19 A Reevaluation of the State of Autism Treatment: The Need for a Biopsychosocial Perspective

Eric London*

Department of Psychology, New York State Institute for Basic Research in Developmental Disabilities, Staten Island, NY 10314, USA

CONTENTS

19.1 INTRODUCTION

An anecdote (take 1): My 21-year-old adult son with autism was taken to a klezmer music concert. The staff of his treatment program reports that it was a wonderful success. He loved the music, so much so that he got up and jumped up and down and waved his arms ecstatically. His joy was infectious and made many of the other

* Corresponding author: Tel.: +1-718-494-3695; fax: +1-718-494-3650; e-mail: naarlondon@gmail.com

concert-goers loosen up and enjoy the concert. His treatment team will look for other concerts, which might also make him that happy.

Anecdote (take 2): My 21-year-old son was taken to a klezmer music concert. The staff of his treatment program reported that this was not a successful outing. He became so excited by the music that he could not sit in his seat; he waved his arms and jumped, which must have disturbed others at the concert. Redirection was ineffective as he was so excited. The plan will be to take him to more concerts but perhaps not as stimulating for him so that he can learn appropriate behavior in a concert setting; however, for the foreseeable future, klezmer music will not be part of his plan.

These two versions of events are composites of a host of true stories that go on every day in the world of autism. Aside from being a tactical decision as to whether or not the treatment team should enforce "appropriate" behavior, the question also speaks to a whole concept of how society and those with the disease of autism should interface with each other. To explore this topic will raise a host of questions as to how the presently established systems, which interface with autism, might be redirected toward revised roles and relationships with each other.

Autism and its related disorders are among the most severe of the chronic child-hood onset illnesses. A diagnosis given to a two-year-old will surely be a life-altering experience. That family will never be the same. Nearly any measure of morbidity can document the severity of this disease and for that reason, there is a pressing need for treatment. In the past 20 years, we have seen great progress in the development of some treatments for autism. These treatments have grown out of existing tech-nologies such as applied behavior analysis (ABA) and psychopharmacology. These techniques have been applied to autism, sometimes with a great deal of success and sometimes not. Looking at the situation broadly however, Howlin et al. (2004) pres-ent a bleak picture. Only 12% of autistic adults were rated as having a very good outcome with 46% poor and another 12% were termed very poor outcomes. Some of the measures used in this report were cognitive, language, social, communication measures, as well as behavioral problems. Few of those individuals lived alone, had close friends, or permanent employment. In another report studying a cohort born in the 1960s through the 1980s, Billstedt et al. (2005) overall outcome was poor in 78% of the cases. It is likely that with more developed and more generally available treatments, the numbers would be better if measured now; however, the overall con-clusion must be that a very significant number of autistic individuals have and will continue to have negative outcomes, which dwarf that of most other diseases.

The great need for treatments has directed the discussion, thinking, and plan-ning about autism to simple questions as to whether these treatments are effective and or whether they have side effects that outweigh their benefits. While even these questions are difficult to answer, there exists little discussion in the literature or at professional meetings as to what the more overarching goals of autism treatment ought to be.

The science of the treatment of autism (and the other developmental disabilities) can reasonably be characterized as being in its infancy. Although the state of the art is disappointing to those who are in dire need of relief, the more optimistic view is that we have an opportunity to conceptualize treatment possibilities in a fresh way.

We can learn from some of the mistakes made in other areas of the medical psychological and social treatments for various diseases and conditions.

The goal of this chapter is to elucidate some of the issues, which have been either totally ignored or received less than adequate attention by the professional and the advocacy community. As this is a broad task, many topics will only be alluded to rather than exhaustively explored. Clearly, there are no simple answers as to the best way to approach the treatment of autism and with a spirit of humility, we must strive to understand our predicament. In doing so, we must evaluate our conceptual models with an attitude of inquiry. Quick fixes and sound bites will only hamper the effort to provide benefit to those who most need it. I will attempt to challenge some prevailing concepts around autism treatment and make a list of action items, which might be used in moving toward a more effective and rational treatment portfolio for autism. These action items will include the creating of a primary care model for autism treatment, the creation of specialized assessment and treatment centers, the formation of collaborations to cross disciplines including both the voluntary sector as well as the government, the recognition and the more explicit treatment of autonomic dysregulation, and the shift in focus of intervening in the environmental factors that have large effects on the outcomes in autism. The central concept that unifies all of these modifications is the application of the biopsychosocial model of treatment delivery.

19.2 BIOPSYCHOSOCIAL MODEL

I would like to propose the utility of the biopsychosocial model. This terminology was introduced and popularized by George Engel (Engel, 1977, 1980, 1992, 1997). It became an important focus of discussion in the 1970s. His papers were largely aimed at the medical community although at this point in the twenty-first century, it appears that his message is relevant for a wider group of readers. As it is likely that many of the readers will be unfamiliar with Engel's body of work, I would like to outline the basic concepts of this model. That will be followed by a description of some proposed ideas of how this model can be applied to autism.

After World War II and into the 1960s and 1970s, the medical field was moving dramatically in a direction toward a more and more biologically based practice. New discoveries and techniques supported the development of more technologically advanced practitioners. This along with a trend to more urban and suburban living at the expense of rural living hastened the decline of the G.P., that is, the general practitioner. Medical students were in greater numbers convinced that to have successful and an up-to-date career, it was necessary to specialize and even to subspecialize. In addition, the 1960s was a time of social upheaval and activism and there was a movement away from disjointed and impersonal health care. The new social consciousnesses lead to the creation of the family practice specialty with its own training programs. This new specialty had to fight for hospital privileges and to be recognized as a legitimate specialty. Family practitioners struggled to have their own departments in medical schools. This movement was largely successful in capturing the support of the public, primarily due to its philosophy of humanizing medicine again. There was also a very clearly stated awareness that medicine had nearly totally focused in the realm of pathology and how to remediate it. Preventive medicine (except for some of the neater technologic fixes such as vaccinations and plumbing to produce clean water) was left in the dust.

In reality, another societal force, the introduction of managed health care and cost containment, helped the family practitioners to prosper at first with the concept of replacing higher priced specialists with lower cost generalists. Perhaps for the same reason, they became the next target of cost containment. In 1998, the number of family practice residencies positions filled by U.S. medical graduates began to fall. This appears not to be inconsistent with a move back to "expert" technically oriented care or in other words, back to what has been called the medical model. Preventive medicine and a more holistic practice continue to be only a minor part of the physician's role.

Engle, in describing his theory of biopsychosocial medicine, draws from general systems theory and outlines a number of interacting "systems." He describes these starting with subatomic particles, and progressing to atoms, molecules, organelles, cells, tissues, organs/organ systems, nervous system, person, two person, family, community, culture/subculture, society/nation, and biosphere. Looking at the above list of systems and conceptualizing them one a linear chart, one can subcategorize that the first few systems from subatomic particles to nervous system are what we usually term basic sciences. These are the foci of the medical model. The next level of person up to the family is usually under the prevue of psychology while the systems of community up to biosphere are generally thought of as social. In our specialized world of medical care, the physician handles medical model, the psychologist handles the psychological issues, and the social worker deals with the social issues. If health problems were to neatly fit into these systems there may be no reason to even do this level of analysis; however, this is not the case. Each of these systems maintains a separate existence and separate boundaries only up to a point. There is always a dynamic interplay between the systems. A molecule, for example, retinoic acid, if ingested, can lead to a depression, which can lead to family problems, or even rise to the level of societal problem if the protagonist is in a central enough position. In the other direction, wars cause emotional trauma, which we now know can alter levels of the molecules made in the brain. Systems interact with each other not only on this vertical level, but also a two-person system can interact with other two-person system. The relationship between an employer and his employee can influence the relationship between that employee and his wife.

The application of a systems model would change the content and certainly the emphasis of the scientific literature associated with clinical issues. Scientific method is inherently reductionist. The more complex the system, the less elegant the science will be to study it. It is no accident that despite a desire to be scientific, there remains very little "good science" to prove the benefits of psychotherapy. The evidence that does exist is largely limited to behavioral therapy and cognitive therapies. Both of these two therapies lend themselves more easily to manualization and therefore standardization. Therapies that call for more spontaneity on the part of the therapist are much more difficult to standardize and study (Frank, 1979). Those therapies with more concrete outcomes are more easily measured. For example, it is easier to measure a behavior than an insight. The more factors one includes in their analysis (as is inevitable in a systems-based approach), the less amenable the therapy becomes to being researched. There is now a general appreciation that often, randomized controlled clinical trials give results that differ from "real-life" population-based studies. This is to say that the studies that take into account the larger or more systemic issues, while being less specific, may offer results closer to the realities of clinical problems. Effectiveness studies, also known as naturalistic, pragmatic, practical, or real-life studies attempt to mimic daily clinical practice but often at the cost of scientific reducibility. Therefore, one could say that clinical studies may suffer if scientific rigor is elevated at the expense of a systemic understanding. It is only recently that "real-life" studies are appearing in the literature and that funding sources are acknowledging their necessity.

What is true for research is all the more of an issue in clinical practice. The patient, who typically identifies a problem (be it on a biological or psychological or social level), generally choose to go to one practitioner. If that practitioner is limited in his or her scope, which nearly all practitioners are, this can lead to inferior care and often to a lack of success in treatment. Despite the wide spread acknowledgment of Engel's work (up until 2002, there were 1419 citations of his science article), it appears that the biopsychosocial model remains on the margins of medicine. Lindau et al. (2003) believes that the biopsychosocial model has failed to replace the biomedical model for two major reasons both of which are conceptual. One is because of our being wedded to a particular model of fighting disease (rather than promoting health) and the second is our existing institutions are historically rooted in the medical model. I would like to add that the failure of this model to be more accepted could also be explained by systems theory itself. Physicians live in multiple systems. Physicians are also humans who desire to make money to support their families. Managed care discourages this model as each physician spends only a few minutes with each patient. If physicians were to delve into the psychological and social spheres with the same zest that they approach the biological issues, it would take much more time. This would be financed directly by reducing the physicians' own income. This is a huge disincentive to broaden ones view of the patient. Medical schools despite giving lip service to the biopsychosocial model, I would suspect, continue to prefer the biomedical model, and therefore, reward students who are more interested in that model. A brief glance at the National Institute of Health funding patterns should convince anyone that the road to an academic career (except in rare cases) is not paved through the biopsychosocial model. Further, with other disciplines staking out their "turf," it seems safer to fall back on the skill that makes the practitioner unique, which for the MD is biological. Despite the psychiatric establishment being sympathetic to the biopsychosocial model, a huge political effort was aroused when psychologists tried to get prescribing privileges thus potentially usurping their biologic role. Despite the ongoing calls of prestigious institutions, the National Research Council and the Institute for Medicine, to embrace this model, it appears that this will require much more effort than one can reasonably expect from our currently empowered institutions.

19.3   SCOPE OF THE TERM "AUTISM"

Over the past few years, very few diseases have gotten the amount of public attention as the autistic disorders. It is also likely that no other disease sparks the levels of controversy that autism does at this time. There could be a host of reasons for this; however, I believe that the heterogeneity of the illness is a major factor. Most clinicians and investigators are in agreement that autism is the syndromic endpoint of an etiologic heterogeneous group of diseases (London, 2007). Further, there is a huge heterogeneity of the phenotype, which may or may not correlate with the etiologic heterogeneity (Happe et al., 2006). Autism is present with a huge range of core symptom and severities. In addition, there is a wide range of associated symptoms with varying severities. Even in a given individual, one can note an ever-changing set of symptoms, which vary and sometimes even disappear with age and development. Nosologic considerations dictate that we continue to use the word "autism" (Miller et al., 2006), yet this leads to a situation characterized by the elephant and the blind-man paradigm, that is, the vantage point that one is looking from and even the time frame of when you look will determine what you see.

With this level of heterogeneity, one might easily understand that the concept of "treatment" for "autism" is a very broad and often a confusing topic. Many treatments, from many theoretical origins, practiced by many different practitioners; with a dearth of literature support are the norm at this point. Despite all of these difficulties, it appears to me that autism could be much better treated, and managed with the application of biopsychosocial principles. Some of the ways we can improve treatment would be by creating specificity about what we are treating, and clearly defining the treatment goals. Through the inclusion more disciplines as part of a broader treatment team and through an optimized treatment delivery system, the lives of autistic individuals and their families can be greatly improved.

19.4   TREATMENT OF AUTISM

At this point in time, the one most proven and accepted treatment for autism is ABA. Although there seems to be little doubt that, ABA is effective for some people and for some reasons, the real benefit of ABA and its superiority to other interventions are not well documented. Foxx (2008) points out that there have been over a thousand peer-reviewed autism articles describing ABA's success and that various impartial agencies such as the New York State health department recommended only ABA. Disturbingly, there seems to be a surprising lack of critical analysis of ABA by its proponents. Reviews of ABA (Foxx, 2008; Green, 1996) at times seem to confuse a lack of research with the proof of the lack of benefit for any other forms of treatment. They conclude that ABA and only ABA should be instituted as treatment, and even combining ABA with other treatments will only detract from the outcome. The motivation for this advocacy of one particular intervention is likely due to the frustration accumulated over many years of parents choosing untested and often dangerous treatments sometimes to the exclusion of treatments with more evidence and a much greater likelihood of success.

Ospina et al. (2008) in a recent review arrived at a very different conclusion. They found that although Lovass therapy showed benefits versus no treatment, they found no evidence suggesting the superiority of that treatment when comparing it to other active interventions. The evidence reviewed showed some support for discrete trial training in terms of motor and functional skills but not for communication skills. They further found some evidence of benefit of a host of other interventions although similar to ABA, there was often a lack of quality studies or adequately sized studies. Their overall conclusion was that based on the lack of hard evidence for ABA as well as other treatments that interventions be guided by individual needs and the availability of resources. In a similar vein, Reichow et al. (2008) motivated by the lack of any treatment (for young autistic individuals) that meets the criterion for evidence-based practice in autism, suggest better methods of evaluating research so that the practitioner can have more informed guidance for their clinical work.

It is clear that ABA has much to offer the autistic individual. However, the quantitation of how much it offers remains less clear. The argument often invoked by behaviorists that unproved treatments could crowd out the better—proven behavioral treatment can be looked upon in a different way. Although the leading treatment at the moment, the history of medicine also shows that conventional treatments eventually yield to other types or treatments. We must be vigilant not to exclude other forms of treatment, which currently have less or no evidence of benefit solely due to a lack of research to document benefit. These facts call for the necessity of the rigorous but also creative study of many types of treatments. A blind adherence to orthodoxy can be almost as dangerous as blind faith in unproven treatments. A case that I had some personal experience with involved an orthodox ABA school that when confronted with an increase in previously well-treated behaviors, resumed behavioral procedures to extinguish these behaviors. A few days later the young man died of a ruptured appendix. The staff was just unaware that not all behaviors should be treated with ABA and only ABA.

Perhaps an even more confusing situation exists for the use of psychopharmaceutical agents in autism. Mandell et al. (2008) in a survey of Medicaid enrolled children with the diagnosis of autism spectrum disorders found that 56% were on at least 1 psychotropic medication and 20% were on 3 or more medications. The use of psychotropics was common even in the <2 age group. These numbers are not out of line with previous estimates (Aman et al., 2005). Similar to behavioral interventions, it seems that there can be little serious doubt that psychopharmacology has much to offer to the autistic population. The specifics, sadly, are again not that clear.

The most established medication for use in autism is risperidone, which has obtained Food and Drug Administration approval for the indication of irritability associated with autism (Parikh et al., 2008). Risperidone and virtually all other medications used in autism target associated rather than the core symptoms of autism. In contrast, there are no drugs that are commonly used or proven effective in the treatment of the core social and communication impairments that are hallmarks of the pervasive developmental disorders (PDDs) (Posey et al., 2008). The lack of a clear understanding of the pathophysiology of the core symptoms of autism makes it difficult to identify drug targets for autism.

Therefore, current medications are targeted at symptoms rather than the disease. It would appear that the attempt to show that a medication can treat as heterogeneous disease as autism might be a conceptual error. The literature almost invariably frames the benefit of the medicine in the context of the disease although nearly all medications in psychiatry cross diagnostic boundaries in their efficacies. Medications that may be very effective at treating one or more associated symptoms in some individuals may be rather ineffective at treating the broad group of patients diagnosed with autism.

Another related conceptual problem is the use of the "dual diagnosis" concept, which has been developed over the years for mental retardation. The concept is that intellectual disability is not the reason for a behavioral syndrome. Therefore, there must be a second diagnosis to explain the behavior. This is based on many assumptions, which are problematic. One is the fact that mental retardation or intellectual disabilities are gross descriptors of a very heterogeneous group. It seems almost certain that some forms of intellectual disability can explain behavior problems on a biological level. A second problem is the imposition of *Diagnostic and Statistical Manuel of Disorders* (*DSM*) diagnoses which were formulated and validated on more "neurotypical" individuals and applying these diagnoses to those who have various types of brain development abnormalities. Is the repetitive behavior observed in autism the same (on a neurobiological level) as obsessive symptoms seen in obsessive compulsive disorder? Are the social difficulties seen in autism the same as that seen in social anxiety disorder? Although there is likely an overlap between a developmentally disabled and a more neurotypical persons with these symptoms, it is also very likely that when the neurobiology is clarified, it will show many fundamental differences despite having similar behavioral endpoints. Again, medications are more likely to be efficiently targeted to specific symptoms, which will cross diagnostic boundaries; however, in many cases, medications may be more specific if the underlying pathophysiology is treated rather than the symptom.

Clinicians treating autism, due to a lack of literature support, generally have to form their own practice styles and call on their clinical experience (which may be of great value or highly skewed). An example of the problems facing the pharmacologically oriented clinician, trying to practice evidence-based medicine is highlighted by a recent publication. Tyrer et al. (2008) compared haloperidol, risperidone, and placebo in 86 nonpsychotic intellectually disabled subjects having aggressive challenging behaviors. Remarkably, the placebo group showed the most benefit in reducing the aggression scale score, with placebo, risperidone, and haloperidol showing 79%, 58%, and 65% improvement, respectively. The author's conclusion was that "antipsychotic drugs should no longer be regarded as an acceptable routine treatment for aggressive challenging behavior in people with intellectual disability." What was meant by an acceptable routine treatment is not clear to me. An interpretation of this conclusion could be that they are contending that this type of patient is being inadequately treated on a non-pharmacologic basis although they do not state that explicitly. In the same issue of *Lancet* (Matson and Wilkens, 2008), there is a comment on that article. These authors point out that in most cases of aggression in people with intellectual disability, there is an environmental component such as escape from demands, attracting one's caregiver, or gaining access to preferred items. They are taking a more biopsychosocial perspective and suggesting that perhaps a behavioral intervention or a combination of treatments would be more effective. Scahill et al. (2008), in response to this study, point out a couple of methodological flaws to the Tyrer article. These include the use of two active comparators with a small sample size and the selection criterion used.

Tyrer et al. (2008) themselves also note that their findings were not concordant with other studies in the literature, which have shown antipsychotics valuable for this population. It seems that Tyrer et al. (2008) as well as Matson and Wilkins (2008) were tying to put forth the argument that a psychosocial intervention should be tried in aggressive persons with intellectual disabilities. The data presented had little to do with that conclusion. Rather instead of clearly promoting a biopsychosocial approach, the impression was left that antipsychotics are no better than placebo in this group that strains credulity. It is striking that a 79% improvement on placebo was not even commented on by the authors. A 79% improvement on placebo, if taken literally, might necessitate that all intellectually impaired subjects with aggression problems be given a trial on placebo despite the ethical issues that might be raised. Another and perhaps the most important lesson from the above discussion might be acknowledging the enormous complexity in conceptualizing benefit in this population.

The lack of a biopsychosocial model and a lack of attention to the limitations of reductionist assumptions that permeate the clinical research field continue to make evidence-based understandings difficult if not impossible for the clinician interested in autism and developmental disorders. A much more interesting and informative publication would have been an analysis of why this study was able to document such a robust placebo effect. The psychopharmacologic literature rarely, if ever, controls or even comments on psychosocial treatments, which the subjects are invariably exposed too (even if only in school). This is true also for the behavioral and educational literature making little comment on the medications being used by their subjects. My own experience includes being an MD prescribing medications to autistic children who were in behavioral (ABA) studies, where the medications were not mentioned in the publications documenting the benefits of ABA. I suppose that I am not alone in having that experience.

It is estimated that as many as 50%–75% of children with autism may be treated with complimentary and alternative medicine (CAM) treatments (Levy and Hyman, 2008). Levy et al. (2003) reported that almost one-third of children referred for evaluation were already being treated with dietary therapies by their parents even before the confirmation of the diagnosis. This should not be surprising in that the National Center for Complimentary and Alternative Medicine reports that over three-fourths of American adults use CAM treatments for disease or to maintain health. It is estimated that 2%–50% of children in the United States are given CAM therapies (Davis and Darden, 2003), and this is likely to be an underestimate. Children with chronic illness such as cancer asthma, rheumatoid arthritis, and developmental disorders are even more likely to be using CAM therapies. Although there are some CAM treatments with evidence to support its use (such as melatonin for sleep), many other treatments have been clearly disproved (e.g., secretin), or are disproportionately dangerous (e.g., chelating agents). The majority of CAM treatments, however, have not been studied and there is scant evidence to support or deny their use. Levy and Hyman (2008) comment on the issue of families even reporting CAM use to their clinicians. Although there may be many reasons for this, I would contend that the lack of a biopsychosocial perspective on the part of the clinician leads the families to disqualify the practitioners as consultants on this topic. The assumption is made that the physician is constricted in their thinking and unable to see past what is an inadequate literature. Often this drives the families into a counterculture of practitioners who are resistant to examining the evidence at all and tout their own treatments. These practitioners sometimes make rather fantastic profits on treatments, which have no medical evidence. A few years ago when the hormone secretin was reputed to be beneficial for autism, there were practitioners charging five figure amounts per injection.

I would also hypothesize that a large part of the reason for the sizable anti-medical and antiscience movements, which have grown around the families of autistic individuals, is related to the lack of the application of the biopsychosocial model. An important article "Needs of parents of mentally retarded children" was written by Murray (1959), a chairperson of the Virginia Association for Mentally Retarded Children (an organization now know as ARC). In this article, she outlined six basic problems that the parents faced. One was "coping with inept, inaccurate, or ill-timed professional advice." Rather than this being rejecting of need for professionals, she goes on to say "The greatest single need of parents of mentally retarded (MR) children is constructive professional counseling at various stages in the child's life which will enable the parents to find the answers to their own individual problems."

There is a feeling of disconnection that the families feel from their practitioners. Parents perceive that practitioners tailor treatments to their own theoretical predispositions, tout their brand of therapy to the exclusion of others, dismiss other forms of therapy, and have little understanding or interest in how the families perceive the problems. Into that vacuum enter other parent advocates, often with little understanding of medicine, psychology, or science but with a great deal of understanding of the problems (often systemic) that they are encountering on a daily basis. The response has been to take the solutions to these problems into their own hands and become their own case managers. There is no shortage of "alternative" practitioners who are willing to lead this overtly angry charge against "conventional" practitioners. A plausible way of framing the issue is that the treatment community, by isolating themselves from the families issues (bio, psychological, and social) have not only facilitated the propagation of an industry of dubious practices, but also the spin-off has been the creation of a dangerous anti-vaccine lobby that is currently threatening the public health both in America and worldwide (Offit, 2008).

19.5 RECOMMENDATIONS FOR AUTISM TREATMENT

Having analyzed the current state of the thinking around autism treatment, I would like to now propose some innovations that if implemented might be beneficial. These will be presented in the context of the biopsychosocial model. Although it is my intent to be specific, each recommendation should be considered as a direction to go in and will undoubtedly be subject to refinement and improvement.

One might rightly ask why autism as a disease would need these special considerations. The answer is that our medical model and our educational model are not good fits for this entity. The medical model is primarily set up around acute illness. It is struggling today to accommodate the chronic diseases, which are becoming more prevalent in our world. Alzheimer's disorder is a good case in point. The services needed for Alzheimer's are heavily loaded toward care giving and nursing. Medicare does not support nursing homes. It does support acute care hospitals and very expensive procedures that are for acute care. Therefore, there has been a cost burden shifted to the families and the states through Medicaid. Medical students are trained primarily in acute care medicine. Autism is a chronic illness. Even more than in Alzheimer's disease, the burden of care giving falls in nontraditional settings, that is, the families and the school systems. Schools have the legal obligation to provide an "appropriate education," a vague term if there ever was one. The educational system has de facto become the major treatment entity for autism. This role has not been fondly embraced. Evidence for this is the microscopic funding that the federal Department of Education spends on autism treatment research, which is at odds with an astronomical budget that school districts pay for the special education of autistic children.

Each of the recommendations made involve major changes conceptualizing how we treat autism. Each one involves multiple systems to be involved in the changes. Again I would hope that these recommendations are looked upon as conceptual directions and that further work will need to go into refining the details of how to facilitate real change and hopefully improvement.

19.5.1 PRIMARY CARE AUTISM PROFESSIONAL

I am calling for the creation of a "primary care autism professional" (PCAP) to serve the patient and their families. This would be modeled after the role most often associated with a primary care physician. Although some physicians or other professionals may be playing this role now, I believe they are rare. It could be debated; however, I would propose that the primary care professional be a nurse practitioner. Perhaps sadly, I do not believe that medical practitioners, as the system exists, now would be able to perform this role adequately. The practitioner will need the time to spend with the families to work on psychosocial issues as well as the medical issues. The medical field over the past 30 years has gone away from the biopsychosocial model despite calls for its implementation as I have outlined earlier. I would doubt that this situation would change any time in the near future.

The PCAP would be the first line of help for the family. That person would have to be fluent with the needs of the early diagnosed, middle childhood, adolescence, and up to geriatric individuals. The goal would be for this person to be in that role for the long term, with that individual and family, again modeled after the concept of the family practitioner.

The role would call for a strong knowledge of autism, which will only occur through the knowledge gained through specialization. The practitioner would need to be trained in many of the disciplines, which are relevant to helping the patients and their families and much like a primary care physician would have to know their limitations and when more specialized care is needed. Postgraduate training programs for this position would need to be created and should exist in universities. Some universities have already developed certificate programs beyond the bachelors or graduate degree that focuses on autism (Swiezy et al., 2008). As these practitioners would specialize in autism, they will likely over time become very sophisticated in recognizing the issues encountered and experienced at solving them. The practitioner would need to be competent in medicine (this is the reason I am recommending a nurse practitioner). This person could do a primary care–type medical visit. Simple problems could be treated, and more complex ones would be referred on to the supervising pediatrician or other physician. Many of the complaints, which will be present in these cases, will be related to autism symptoms but many will not be. The PCAP must have the expertise to make that differentiation. Many problems may cross over. An example might be self-abusive behavior. Although wounds must be tended to on a medical level, the behavior must also be controlled. The PCAP must also have to have a working knowledge of behavioral treatments, including ABA, psychopharmacology, as well as other emerging treatment modalities. The practitioner would need to have the ability to institute some treatments and also a good working understanding of places to refer. The practitioner would also need to be conversant with the educational system and be able to function as a case manager for obtaining the right fit for an educational placement. As the autistic individual ages toward adulthood, the PCAP will help council the family as to their options and help to supervise the transitional planning toward the work world. The PCAP would also function in the role that social workers usually take in geriatrics. That is facilitating the process of obtaining support systems such as respite. The PCAP, by virtue of being "in the middle" of these issues, would be able to perform an advocacy role. They would be fully aware of the services that are not available but badly needed in that community.

People with autism grow up and live roughly normal life spans. It is not a childhood disease when the subject becomes an adult. The practitioner should be equally conversant with the problems encountered in adulthood. The existence of a discipline such as PCAP is more than just a bureaucratic nicety. As the disease of autism is not likely to be eliminated any time in the near future, a host of treatment-based decisions must be made. Bergsma and Engel (1988) discuss this issue in reference to medical decisions, which must be made around the concept of the quality of life (QOL). Some of these decisions entail when and how much palliative care should be instituted especially at the end of life. They outline three different models of the doctor–patient relationship. One is the model of the doctor being authoritative. That is he or she will basically make the decision due to their knowledge and experience.

A second option is the one where the patients make their own decision, and the physician's opinion is only of minor importance. Other sources of information can be used such as getting second opinions, consulting with friends, relatives, and, nowadays, the Internet. This leads to "doctor shopping" or going to different doctors until one is found who takes the position already formulated. Unfortunately, this type of doctor–patient relationship is not uncommon now in those families afflicted with autism. With only specialists to consult with (the behaviorist, the occupational therapist, the psychopharmacologist, etc.) families find themselves with professionals who have only one treatment. Often each one touts his/her own treatment, sometimes to the exclusion of the other. More perniciously, there are many practitioners who predict dire consequences if their treatment is not done exclusively and around the clock. It is no wonder that the families at this point regroup and decide that only they can make the choices. This is often done during times of crisis and under extreme emotional pressure (not unlike the end of life decisions discussed above). Most families are going through this issue for the first time and have little of their own experience to fall back on. In making these decisions, they can be more influenced by those with the slickest message promising the best outcome. Parents bond together using the Internet and advise each other; however, the highly emotionally charged nature of these interactions can readily be seen. All of this often leads to poor choices or worse dangerous ones. The danger appears now to spilling over from the autism cases themselves to the community at large (Offit, 2008).

The third kind of relationship is one characterized by openness and mutual respect. In this relationship, it is possible to have a dialogue and to arrive at a conclusion together. This type of relationship is unfortunately becoming quite rare in our society. It calls for trust, which is formed through a personal relationship. In most cases, this can only be formed through long-term relationships.

Decisions are often multifactorial and often there is no absolute right answer. Sandler and Hulgus (1992) analyze the clinical application of the biopsychosocial model and its applicability in clinical situations. They outline three components to the decision-making process in medicine. The first can be described as having the scientific knowledge and the experience that the clinician can offer in their role. The second is the ethical aspect. In this sphere, decisions need to be made based on values. At times, the values held by the patient or the family might be different than that of the doctor, that is, "I would rather die than have my legs amputated." The biopsychosocially competent practitioner must be able to represent their own values but at the same time be respectful of the patient's values. A dialogue about these values might help the patient (or the doctor) revise their thinking. The third component is the pragmatic aspect. For example, if a behavioral program is recommended and is not available or the finances to pay for it are not available, what should be done? Perhaps a legal consultation is needed or perhaps, an alternative type of therapy should be explored first. Again the clinician might have a great deal to offer in helping the family make the very hard decisions of how to proceed.

I would propose the PCAP could serve in these roles for autism. As one who is knowledgeable about the field as well as the patient and their family, decisions can be informed by the longitudinal history developed over years. The PCAP must be trained in systems theory, to understand that these decisions are often not one-dimensional. If the family needs to hire an attorney to fight for behavioral therapy, will that mean that the sibling cannot go to summer camp that year? This might be the real issue, which the family is facing. How often is a family able to express problem to a clinician? How often does the clinician actually help the family address the issue? Systems theory might suppose that the stress on the family would lead to stress on the autistic individual, which could lead to behavioral acting out. This would lead the psychopharmacologist to suggest a medication. This may have side effects such as sedation or gastrointestinal problems, which could lead to further consultations. This cycle could go on and the only way to get a handle on it is for someone (at this point it is generally the parent) to see the whole chain of events and work with the system to maximize benefits.

19.5.2 ASSESSMENT AND TREATMENT CENTERS

To compliment a primary care model of autism treatment, it is imperative that there also be a cadre of well-qualified specialists and it is equally important that these specialists be accessible to those who are in need of the services. In order to accomplish this, I am proposing the formation of assessment and treatment centers. At the present time, there are many university-based programs, which are fundamentally functioning as assessment and treatment centers. There is no necessity to reinvent the wheel; however, there are several considerations that need to be fulfilled to make this effective. The primary difference between existing programs and these proposed centers is in the methods of delivering the services. Although many university-based programs are excellent, they tend to serve only a small portion of the people in need of services. Further each center at this point might have certain areas of focus rather than being broad based. In the proposed assessment and treatment centers, a goal will be to make the specialty services as accessible as possible. This will be accomplished by a more consultative model rather than being a primary treatment center.

The concept of assessments should not be confused with diagnosis, although diagnosis is one function of an assessment center. Rather, assessments need to be focused on the needs of the patients. Assessments can be done throughout the life span in order to help guide treatment decisions. Assessments currently are mandated by school districts for their own considerations, that is, when this information is needed for educational classification. Assessments could be done when problems arise or decisions need to be made. Examples might include a young autistic subject who is not easily managed at school and more routine efforts and remedying the situation have failed. Another example would be around the beginning of adulthood to help facilitate the transition to adult programming. These assessments would most often be multidisciplinary. The team could include behaviorists, medical generalists or specialists, psychiatrists, speech therapists, educational consultants, physical therapists, etc. The staff of these centers would be specialists in autism and have a great deal of expertise, which is often not easily found in the community. These assessments would yield treatment recommendations, which could be carried out back in the community by the PCAP, teachers, job coaches, pediatricians, etc. The centers should provide ongoing supervision and consultation to the practitioners. This component of the plan is more difficult than it might seem at first glance. The ability to have an active dialogue between these centers and community-based practitioners might seem simple but is rarely accomplished in the real world. There must be a recognized budget for the time spent in this dialogue. Creative funding strategies need to be implemented to accommodate this invaluable communication.

The centers should provide treatments not available in the community. One example would be the treatment of the very highly behaviorally disturbed autistic individuals. At the present time, there is an acute lack of service for this individual. More general psychiatric units are not set up to handle autistic patients. Their treatment modalities used in general psychiatric units such as group therapies are clearly not pertinent to this group. The staff is taught interventions that are more pertinent to other conditions such as schizophrenia and mood disorders, which comprise the overwhelming majority of their patients. There are a very few hospital-based settings that are set up for this group, but they have waiting lists that make delivering acute care impossible. Often families have to live with ongoing violence for weeks or months prior to a bed being available. If these individuals are to be reintegrated in the community, a "step-down" system must be available, with a slowly decreasing amount of support available and an inclusion of the family and the ultimate community service deliverers into the treatment package. This would imply that there also must be a geographic distribution of these assessment and treatment centers to realistically serve the public. Other examples might include medical clinics with medical specialists who are familiar with autism, and perhaps new types of specialists such as environmental specialist who can consult about issues such as noise pollution, which may be having a negative impact on the success of a given individual.

19.5.3 FUNDING, GOVERNMENT, AND COLLABORATION

As a physician, I am not trained nor do I have experience in designing funding issues around health care. Our society has been struggling with issues around funding for some time now with no consensus solutions having been reached. With this disclaimer in place, it appears that without a simultaneous discussion of funding issues on the table, any hope of significant changes in the treatment delivery system is futile. The pragmatic element of what service is available and how to fund that service may be more important to the outcome of a given case than what medication they are on, or what type of therapy is instituted. A significant problem is that perhaps more than any other disease, autism is treated by many players with many different missions, and their own budgets and funding sources.

The first step in the clinical odyssey of a family with autism is to get a diagnosis. This is done generally through a pediatrician and is generally paid for with health care insurance. If diagnosis is done early enough (up to age 2), the next step is an early intervention program, which also is a medical cost. The next stop is generally with the educational establishment. For those age 3 and above, there is preschool and then later the school program, funded largely by the local school district. It is unclear how much treatment the school districts are responsible for and this is often fought in courts. It might be worth noting that the educational establishment might recoil at my even using the word treatment, as they do not see themselves as treatment professionals but rather educators. In reality, whether intentional or not, at this point, I would guess that 80% or the real treatment of autism is going on in the school setting.

Some examples of the interface between education and medicine include such services as speech therapy. Speech therapy, which may or may not be adequately available in the school, could be supplemented by speech therapy after school hours at home. Health insurance often covers only "restorative" therapies. That is, contending that if the child never had language then it is not restorative. Behaviors are also an unclear issue. How much and what type of behavioral and cognitive therapies are needed outside of the interventions done in the school are a source of contention. Adult services also cross boundaries. The educational systems are usually done with their responsibility to this group after age 21. States have agencies, which service the developmentally disabled, and that budget line becomes operative for many of the needs of that individual. Again there is often a lack of clarity in how far that responsibility must go. Housing is sometimes supported by Medicaid (a health care fund), and ironically offices of mental retardation at times directly reimburse physicians for health care. The health care of this group has largely been taken out of the private sector, as most private physicians are not participants in the Medicaid program as the reimbursement is very low. Being a very underemployed group (with health care in our country largely tied into employment), this cohort is in reality served by the government or agencies directly contracting with the government such as Medicaid managed care.

Despite my being a physician serving this group as well as being a parent of an autistic individual, and being interested in the policy issues of the autistic population, I must confess that I am still very confused by the system. Simply stated, if after a couple of decades of trying, I still have trouble explaining the system to anyone, it is just too complex. This complexity, aside from being very frustrating to the community trying to access services, is ripe for abuses, inefficiency, lacks transparency, and makes the system nearly impossible to reform.

At the time that this is being written, there is a deep economic recession in the United States and around the world. For the foreseeable future, it is impractical to think about increasing services through increased budgets. It is equally unthinkable that as we progress in our understanding and capabilities of treating disease, we settle for suboptimal outcomes because we are bogged down in a bureaucratic quagmire. We must be willing to look at the realities of what we have created and make the needed changes.

A conceptual solution to this quagmire also involves the understanding and implementation of systems theory. If the treatment of an autistic individual involves funding from three or four sources, these agencies need to be in communication and budgets should be combined or shared to solve problems. A state government funds their Departments of Education, Office of Developmental Disabilities, and the Department of Health. If these three agencies are not cooperating, we are wasting money. An example of this might be to invest hundreds of thousands of dollars into the education of an autistic individual, train him for a job, and pay for a job coach but not pay for transportation to the job. The individual then sits at home. Do we ask the parents to quit their jobs to stay at home with the individual? I can attest that this is a very real scenario, which I have encountered in my practice many times. Just as the medical institutions need to reward physicians for being biopsychosocial physicians, government agencies that can collaborate for the public good must also be rewarded. The public needs to be aware of the efforts and successes of government agencies and they should not be taken for granted. The public often views the government as a giant pocketbook. As described in Section 19.5.1 in terms of the doctor–patient relationship, a consultative relationship between the government and the public could be formed.

In New York State, we are attempting to create such a partnership. The New York Autism Consortium is being formed. This will comprise all of the elements invested in the treatment and research of autism. Medical centers, schools, agencies, and the advocacy community will be organized to tackle problems. Pilot programs and research can take place with both public and private fundings. This consortium has a seat at a newly formed interagency autism committee, which is comprised of all of the state agencies that have an interest in autism. Having a direct line of communication from government to the private players has enormous potential. A similar concept involving collaboration has already been started in Indiana (Swiezy et al., 2008). If my estimate is correct or even partly correct, and 80% of the treatment of autism is going on in the schools, it would seem unconscionable to fail to acknowledge this and to promote the most efficient and efficacious programs possible. By bridging the silo effect of the medical world and the educational world, there would be a synergistic effect of improving outcome.

Up to this point, this chapter has focused mostly on issues related to service delivery and the systemic roles of the players. There are specific treatment-oriented items in the literature, which have received very little attention, and which would have a large influence on the way autism treatment could be approached.

19.5.4 POSITIVE PSYCHOLOGY

Dykens (2006) in a recent paper proposes the use of positive psychology in the treatment of mental retardation. This would be a radical departure from the current treatment concepts employed in autism. The predominant conceptual guide to the treatment of autism at this time is behavioral treatment. In no way do I propose to devalue the need to do treatments to make autistic individuals fit into the world and enjoy the company of the people in their families and communities. Appropriate behavior makes it possible for autistic individuals to work, go to the movies and restaurants, family gatherings, etc. It could be argued however that all of those accomplishments are vehicles in the effort to produce happiness. Behaviorism rarely if ever asks the question of whether the individual is happy. Happiness is not an easy thing to measure and code. It is highly subjective. It is even more difficult to measure it in an individual with language disability. In the field of intellectual disability, there has been some movement toward a psychology of capitalizing on the strengths and capabilities of this population although this remains somewhat outside of the mainstream of the field and the correlations to happiness and to autism are still lacking (Shogren et al., 2006).

Seligman (2002) states that before World War II, psychology had three distinct missions. These were curing mental illness; making the lives of all people more productive; and fulfilling, identifying, and nurturing high talent. Right after the war, he posits that two major events changed the field of psychology. One was the founding of the Veterans Administration, which had the effect of enticing thousands of psychologists to make a living treating mental illness. In 1947, the National Institute of Mental Health was founded. It was grounded in the disease model and grants were much more available for studying pathology. Seligman acknowledges that this brought about great benefit, in that huge strides were made in the treatment of mental illness. The downside of this was that the other roles of psychology were largely forgotten. He contends that the effect of this extended even to the way we see ourselves. We see ourselves as fixed entities having biological and environmental forces assaulting us and if severe enough, making us ill. Our job was to fight them off, in other words to fix what is wrong. The opposite viewpoint would be to focus and understand what our strengths are and to nurture and work with them. He goes on to trace the reintroduction of the awareness of positive psychology to the 1998 American Psychological Association meeting at which prevention of mental illness was the theme. His contention is that human strengths are the buffers against mental illness and therefore a powerful tool for prevention. Some of the traits associated with these strengths include hope, gratitude, engagement, skill, and the ability to achieve what is termed "flow," happiness and optimism.

Dykens (2006) reviews the history of treatment in mental retardation with its emphasis on "external measures of success and how happiness has been de-emphasized." She reviews four major movements. These movements include the QOL movement, the dual diagnosis movement, the personality motivation movement, and family research.

There have been some efforts to quantify the "QOL" in developmental disabilities, autism, and Aspergers disorder (Fresher-Samways et al., 2003; Gerber et al., 2008; Jennes-Coussens et al., 2006) and in their families (Allik et al., 2006; Mugno et al., 2007). The concept of QOL is in itself an elusive concept (Fresher-Samways et al., 2003) with 44 different definitions found in 47 studies on the topic. The questions asked are highly subjective. With a nonverbal population, the studies have had to rely on proxies to survey (Gerber et al., 2008) with the finding that staff and families have different opinions and the scores are considerably different. QOL includes the following dimensions: (1) emotional well-being, (2) interpersonal relations, (3) material well-being, (4) personal development, (5) physical well-being, (6) self-determination, (7) social inclusion, and (8) rights. Only 1% of the questions in QOL surveys related directly to the concepts of happiness, contentment, enjoyment, and zest for life. It is true that QOL items found in the surveys are likely to be indirectly correlated to happiness; however, caution should be exercised in that we are not projecting a "neurotypical" slant on what makes an autistic person happy. Direct measurement of these factors would be very difficult; nevertheless, strategies need to be developed to accomplish this task. A possible solution will be discussed below under the topic of autonomic functioning.

The issue of psychiatric problems or the "dual diagnosis" movement is Dykens' second area of focus. The 40% of MR population has clinically significant psychiatric problems (Einfeld and Tongue, 1997) and 52% of autistic individuals are on psychotropic medications. The most common issues include self-injury, depression, aggression, anxiety, and stereotypies. It would seem that these behaviors or symptoms would have a profound influence on happiness. There remain questions of how many of these problems are related to biologic or brain-based abnormalities (to be treated largely with medications and biologic treatments) and how many of them are related to environmental issues (to be treated with various psychologically based treatments). A third outlook on the problem and one rarely taken is that the symptoms are a response to a lack of happiness and can be treated by the focus and development on those factors that will increase happiness such as working toward creating a sense of pleasure in ones work.

The third movement is described as the personality-motivation movement. This describes the phenomenon, which aside from the low IQ or brain lesion is causing problems. These secondary problems may be very significant. Often the MR population has a sense of low expectations for success, which leads to a low motivation to master challenge and ultimately a learned helplessness (which has been tied to depression). This issue of motivation might be both in the realm of psychology, that is, learned helplessness, and there is also a biologic overlap, which appears large in autism. There have been studies on "intrinsic motivation" a concept that due to a lack of attention, which might be a very profound deficiency in our understanding of autism. The basis of behavioral treatments in autism is to provide artificial motivators (such as edibles) for children who typically receive intrinsic motivation. An example is in playing with toys. Autistic children in behavioral programs are given edibles to induce them to increase the time they might spend playing with a toy in contrast to the typical child who cannot be kept away from a new toy or in other words have a powerful intrinsic motivation. While the behaviorist focuses on the endpoint of the length of time spent in playing, there has been little or no attention paid to the phenomenon of the intrinsic reward or lack of it, and whether there are ways to improve the intrinsic rewards.

The last movement described is the family research movement. Systemic family therapy has long viewed the system or in this case, the family as the "identified patient." With developmental disabilities and perhaps more so autism, there has been a reluctance to view the family functioning as an object of treatment. The reason for this is likely due to the early history of autism treatment in which Bettelheim (1967) and the psychoanalytic movement introduce the concept of the "refrigerator mother" who was too emotionally cold to raise a healthy child. Autistic children were taken away from their families and placed in inpatient settings. Much of the early advocacy in autism was aimed at reversing this notion. In reality, some families do function better than others and there are correctable systemic issues, which would make the family happier and most likely the individual also. This could be framed in a positive psychology format. The clear message should be that the families functioning did not create the autism but rather the family has the ability to use their discretion to set up systems to problem solve. Research to examine this is just beginning.

Dykens asks us to ponder the applicability of these formulations to mental retardation. She notes that based on the research, little can be said; as there has not been "a shred of research" in mental retardation that speaks to the issues that makes people thrive and be happy. She then proposes that the same features that help people in general to thrive and be happy—positive emotions, gratifications, flow, virtues and strengths—also operate in the context of mental retardation. I agree with Dykins on this concept. It would seem very improbable if there were not a set of properties that would be concordant with producing happiness in the developmentally disabled. It would be hard to argue that producing happiness is not a worthwhile goal. The question that appears to be the more controversial might be whether the field of autism treatment will consciously adopt the happiness of the individual and his systems as a treatment target to be spoken about, planned for, measured, and researched in order to improve the technology for that goal. There is no doubt that behaviorists as well as psychopharmacologists consciously or unconsciously target their treatments toward creating happiness. Many of the competencies built through behaviorism have been shown to be a powerful part of the arsenal of the positive psychologist.

Perhaps a more productive way of framing the debate would be about the balancing of the goals. Referring back to the opening paragraphs of this chapter, let us review the initial question. Should ecstatic jumping and arm waving be encouraged as an integral part of achieving happiness during the music concert, or is the competency of being able to sit appropriately in the concert hall and be an accepted part of the crowd more important. Dykens call to research on this topic is more than an academic exercise. Rather it might speak to the heart of treatment programs for autism.

A new phenomenon that is going to be present in the next few years will be the emergence of an unprecedented numbers of autistic adults. This new demographic group might color the thinking related to these questions. The field has long been dominated by a rehabilitative, learning model to correct what is "wrong" with the autistic individual. I suspect that this will continue to be the model adopted and supported by the parents of young children who are hopeful that the autism will be "cured." As the child ages, an alternative viewpoint would be created by the tacit acknowledgment that these adults are largely going to be who they are now and that the amount of biologic or internal capacity improvement in older teens or adults is likely to be minimal. Instead, the most beneficial treatments of these older groups will be to organize optimal systems around them. The question of how to optimize these systems is first dependent on our clearly prioritizing our goals. If we do clarify our priorities, the development of the systems to optimally create happiness will still be very challenging. I would like to suggest two specific directions that would be important for this goal, although many more ideas need to be created.

19.6 AUTISM, ANXIETY, AND AUTONOMIC REGULATION

Autism is defined by the triad of symptoms including language disturbance, social impairment, and the repetitive need for sameness. It is the rare case however, who has only these three symptoms and no comorbidities. A case can be made to consider that there is a nearly invariant symptom, which might be described as anxiety or perhaps more accurately described as autonomic dysregulation.

The interface of autism and anxiety is a complex topic. Anxiety was described by Kanner in his initial account of autism (Kanner, 1943). The *DSM III* recognized the presence of intense and unusual anxieties in a description of childhood onset PDD (American Psychiatric Association, 1980). Anxiety plays a prominent role in that diagnostic schema with the criteria including a number of emotional regulation symptoms such as sudden excessive anxiety, catastrophic reactions to everyday occurrences, inability to be consoled when upset, unexplained panic attacks, unexplained rage reactions, and extreme mood liability. *DSM IV* lists abnormal reactions such as excessive fearfulness in response to harmless objects as an associated feature of autism (American Psychiatric Association, 1994). It could also be argued that the core symptom of "insistence on sameness" is a reflection of anxiety (Sukhodolsky et al., 2008). Volkmar et al. (1999) made the observation that the interruption of stereotyped behaviors may increase anxiety, tension, and emotional upset in children with PDD. An attractive hypothesis (Bodfish et al., 2000; Hirstein et al., 2001) is that repetitive behaviors may be for the purpose of reducing anxiety. Muris et al. (1998) reported in a series of 44 cases of PDD that as many as 84% of the children had a diagnosis of at least one anxiety disorder. They found that only 9% had a diagnosable panic disorder but 57% had regularly experienced isolated panic attacks. Thus, in addition to its core symptoms, autism may carry a high level of anxiety as an almost invariant symptom.

Gadow et al. (2004) found in their 6–12 year olds, a wide range of different types of anxiety disorders and compared them to regular education students. Generalized anxiety disorder was present in 24% of the sample as opposed to 3% of the controls.

Specific phobias were present in 59% as opposed to 24%, obsessions in 41% as opposed to 18%, and compulsions in 29% compared to 3%. Sukhodolsky et al. (2008) found 43% of their sample had met screening criteria of an anxiety disorder and noted that this was twice as high as the lifetime prevalence of anxiety disorders in the population.

The causes and significance of these findings of high anxiety are largely unknown but raise some interesting questions. It has been speculated that the awareness of social deficits and the legacy of failure may raise the anxiety levels especially in the high functioning with autism. This hypothesis is attractive and clinicians who work with this population often hear the angst of the repeated failures; however, there is no data to support this hypothesis. Chamberlin et al. (2007) contend almost the opposite, by describing an apparent lack of awareness or caring about social failure. Another theory advanced by Sukhodolsky et al. (2008) is that children with autism have weak central coherence and that they might be experiencing everyday situations as chaotic and therefore frightening. This also has intuitive resonance, but another study by Burnette et al. (2005) found no association between weak central coherence and anxiety in a high-functioning group. A third hypothesis concerning the origins of anxiety in this population is a more biologic one with documented abnormalities of the amygdala (Amaral and Corbett, 2003; Baron-Cohen et al., 2000) being responsible for the clinically observed anxiety. Juranek et al. (2006) reported significant correlations between anxiety/depression scores, the total amygdala volume, and the right amygdala volume.

The discussion and literature review presented above concerns anxiety and autism, but it is worthy of consideration that the concept of anxiety may not exactly describe the phenomena observed in autism, especially in lower functioning individuals. The National Library of Medicine defines anxiety with the following three definitions: (1) feelings of distress or apprehension whose source is unknown; (2) a vague, uneasy feeling of discomfort or dread accompanied by and autonomic response: a feeling of apprehension caused by the anticipation of danger. It is an alerting signal that warns of impending danger and enables the individual to take measures to deal with the threat; and (3) apprehension or fear of impending actual or imagined danger, vulnerability, or uncertainty. Anxiety is described as a feeling and is highly subjective. The scales reported on in some of the studies listed above used items such as "has difficulty rating controlling worries" and "is excessively shy with peers." Items like this are hard to interpret in individuals who have little or no language, little social interest, a severe lack of social awareness, and even a lack of self-awareness. It would be more scientifically accurate to call the phenomena observed in autism "anxiety-like." Another descriptor of these phenomena could be termed "autonomic dysregulation."

There is ample evidence that there is autonomic dysregulation in autism (Althous et al., 2004; Graveling and Brooke, 1978; Hirstein et al., 2001; Hutt et al., 1975; Jansen et al., 2006; Ming et al., 2005; Toichi and Kamio, 2003; Zahn et al., 1987). Many of the symptoms found in autism including sleep disturbance, GI disturbance, and immune system abnormalities all can be plausibly explained by autonomic dysregulation (Axelrod et al., 2006; Czura and Tracey, 2005; Powley, 2000). Neuroanatomically, abnormal findings in the amygdala, frontal and temporal cortex, cerebellum, and the brain stem can support a central nervous system hypothesis of autonomic dysregulation (Courchesne, 1997). Abnormalities in the oxytocin systems of the brain in autism (Green et al., 2001; Modahl et al., 1998) and some evidence of symptom improvement with oxytocin (Hollander et al., 2003) would also fit an autonomic dysregulation hypothesis. Oxytocin has been shown to reduce the fear-inducing activation of the amygdala, which via a brain-stem pathway regulates autonomic functioning (Kirsch et al., 2005). These findings are consistent with the polyvagal theory (Porges, 2006), which predicts that there will be pathologic findings in a social engagement system in which vagal functioning is dysregulated.

Studies have shown low cortisol levels in autism or normal levels despite the autonomic hyperactivity and or high adrencorticotropic hormone (ACTH) levels (Curin et al., 2003; Jansen et al., 2003; Tani et al., 2005) with a slow response to ACTH (Marinovic-Curin et al., 2008) leading to the speculation that some of the symptoms seen in autism are a result of the lack of a normal hypothalamic–pituitary–adrenal axis and autonomic physiologic functioning that helps the organism cope with stress.

Despite the substantial amount of evidence that these types of symptoms are very common in autism, and that they likely have a profound impact on behavior, the ability to learn and to adjust to various situations and settings, there has been very little systematic study of the treatment of these problems. Pharmaceuticals have been studied (Findling, 2005) and no doubt have an important role; however, safety and tolerability considerations make this option less than optimal. One successful study of cognitive behavioral therapy with high functioning autism or Aspergers syndrome has been published (Chalfant et al., 2007). The question of how generalized this is to the lower functioning group as well as how many of even the higher functioning group will cooperate with this is unknown. Alternative methods such as relaxation and yoga have been suggested; however, there is little in the literature to document its practicality as a treatment.

A concerted effort would need to be made to monitor the extent of this above discussed phenomena and to prove that treatments are available that could lower the anxiety, with the likely outcome of improving behavior, improving cognition, and perhaps even enhancing happiness.

19.7   TREATING THE ENVIRONMENT

Another form of treatment, which is in line with a biopsychosocial perspective, is that of creating "safe" environments for those with autism or more accurately put, environments that are perceived as safe. Conceptually, rather than having the autistic person learn to cope with the environment (which in some cases is never successful), a form of treatment would involve having the environment meet the autistic individual half way. This is not a new concept and in the 1960s, this concept was very popular in psychiatry. Often called milieu therapy, this concept appears to have only taken hold for the addicted population, although the potential of these concepts should be explored (Karst, 1991). Fifty years ago, the "therapeutic communities" captured the imagination of the psychiatric community. Partly based on the discovery of Thorazine for schizophrenia, the concept of deinstitutionalization took root. This was a very popular concept and the large state-run psychiatric hospitals around America emptied out and many were closed. The identified alternative to the large institutions was to be "community psychiatry," that is, to bring the needed treatments into the communities of the patients and to have them integrated in their community rather than being institutionalized. Very much like the fate of the family practitioner, community psychiatry was never adequately funded and became more of a concept than a viable alternative. This failure to follow through and support the community-based treatment programs lead to the homelessness, which became rampant in the 1970s. Despite the apparent lack of success of these movements, it would be grossly unfair to term the concepts as failures. Rather it appears that the enticement of cutting budget by closing institutions was much more inviting than increasing budget to support new community-based alternatives.

Aside from the public health issues discussed above, there was a rich theoretical basis for milieu therapy, therapeutic community, and community psychiatry. All three concepts were based on the systems approach that the individual is not an island unto himself but rather his success or failure is largely dependent on the milieu or system or community that he or she is part of.

Various arguments might be made against the idea of meeting autistic individuals half way. Young autistic children often tantrum when the environment is not to their liking, and behaviorists often argue that the tantrum is a form of avoidance that if reinforced will lead the autistic individual not to develop coping skills. This is true up to a point. No doubt, there are individuals who if not confronted with a challenge, might never develop coping skills to a particular issue. To use a more physical analogy, one could posit that the use of ramps is not thought of as a way that physically impaired individuals "avoid" stairs and if forced to deal with stairs, they would eventually master them. The fact that we cannot perceive the subjective neurological responses felt by an autistic individual, in no way negates the reality of their limitations. There is little doubt that people with autism perceive the world differently than neurotypical individuals (Grandin, 1991). Anecdotal reports document sensory distortions, which make the individual uncomfortable (Dunne et al., 2002). The habilitative model has been the dominant theoretical force in mental retardation treatment; however, a pertinent question has rarely been asked. When should rehabilitation stop and adjustment to the realities of the condition begin? As we deal with more autistic adults, this will become an important question.

Although it is well known that autistic children can be easily distracted by the environment, there has been little attention paid to the environments that they are actually in. Temple Grandin (1991) discusses the fact that noise and confusion at large gatherings overwhelm her senses and "at times speech reached her brain like the noise of an onrushing freight train." Jeffrey Kittay (2008) presents a discussion in more depth about the ambient sounds that autistic and other handicapped children must cope with and that the field in general has not dealt with. People who live in rural areas are often astounded by the levels of ambient noise, which city dwellers must live with. Those who live in New York City accommodate to sirens and other street noises, which they hear on a constant basis. A question that has not been answered is the extent to which autistic individuals are sensitive to the sounds in their environment and a second question is their abilities to accommodate to those sounds. Some treatment settings have put up sound proofing materials and have anecdotally reported improvements in overall behaviors of the residents. The study of this to prove efficacy is lacking. This might place into question the advisability of the common practice of putting autistic people together as the noises created by one individual might be less tolerable for another autistic individual than it is for a neurotypical peer. Again, the extent that this is a problem especially in the lower functioning nonverbal population is not known. It is possible that attention to these parameters, despite their "low tech" nature, might have treatment effects, which could be profound. These arguments, which were made about sound, can be generalized to many environmental factors including the architectural space, visual stimulation, food, chemical substances in the environment, temperature, and the textures of clothing among others.

Of all the environmental influences that might have an impact on the outcome of an individual, it could be argued that none has as profound an effect as the caring and love that one receives. This is a very difficult topic to address for even social scientists and the vagaries of the concept of love and caring make it even more difficult for the more biological scientist. Yet, there is an emerging science of love (Esch and Stefano, 2005) and there are attempts to analyze love in terms of its effect on neurological biologic systems and neurotransmitter systems involved. This topic is of utmost importance in the understanding of the holistic treatment of autism. There is a voluminous body of work, which over many years has established the value of social affiliation and intimacy bonds to the overall functioning of the organism (Cassidy, 2001). These social functions have wide-ranging effects, including emotional and cognitive functioning as well as the production of general physical well-being resulting in the overall health of the organism. The family is the structural unit responsible for the formation and sustenance of these bonds for the vast majority of children both autistic and otherwise. The attention and support that we give to the caregivers can have a profound effect on the functioning and the beneficial effects, which the family can create. It would seem that supporting the families in many ways might reduce the need for other mental health interventions down the road.

In individuals with autism, except for the very rare exception, the path of formation of intimacy bonds does not follow the typical pattern. Rather than growing and developing slowly with the formation of autonomy and individuation, the autistic person generally remains in a dependent and often childlike position. It is only the very exceptional autistic person who marries and has his or her own family. As the family of origin ages, affiliative bonding will most likely occur with paid staff of work programs or residential programs. Kittay (2001) reviews many of the sociological and philosophical issues around the attitudes of society toward caregiving and the caregivers (both paid and family). She proposes that the most effective advocacy for the one cared for would be to advocate for the caregivers. At this point, caregiving is usually a minimum or close to minimum wage job (Pollack, 2007), with little in the way of professional training and little in the way of career growth possible. These jobs are often a temporary (most direct caregivers stay no more than a few months at a given job) stopping point for those who are more ambitious and unfortunately may be a place where some with their own personal problems may find work sometimes leading to scandalous examples of abuse (Kittay, 2001). Family caregivers likewise face enormous stress; by 2004, there were an estimated 711,000 Americans with intellectual disability living with caregivers over the age of 60 (Pollack, 2007).

The goal of public health (Talley and Crews, 2007) is to promote healthy individuals living in healthy communities, pursuing QOL rather than just the absence of disease. Caregiving has become an issue that affects the QOL for millions of individuals. Scientists and practitioners rarely thought of caregiving as a public health matter. The authors call for the public health systems to understand more about the caregivers themselves and then to design and implement evidence-based interventions to address the identified needs. Research needs to be done to uncover the possible risk factors associated with the endless types of caregiving situations. Of all diseases, progress in this area seems most critical for autism.

19.8   CONCLUSION

To many in society, and even to those in the health professions, autism seems to have placed itself in our consciousness, as if sneaking in from nowhere. This may be because the prevalence is actually on the rise or the more likely explanation is that it is due to redefinition, and the awareness of these symptoms in the population. In practical terms, there is no debate that there must be a new and improved set of interventions for this very hard to treat group. Defying easy classification, autism straddles many systems (i.e., educational and medical) diagnostic entities (psychiatric or intellectual disability) and, to some extent, has led the way to an intensified interest in brain development and early childhood development. It is also true that those searching for answers do have many bases of knowledge to start from. Many medications developed for psychiatric indications work fairly well for autism. Much of the progress in the conceptualization and integration of intellectual disability can be transferred to autism. Models of care, which have been developed and held out much hope such as milieu therapy and the biopsychosocial model of medicine, need to be dusted off and applied more consciously to autism. The new advances in neuroscience hold out great hope for our understanding, leading to treatments and prevention for autism and if added to enhance clinical delivery systems, there is great promise for improvement in the lives of these affected individuals.

REFERENCES

Allik, H., J.O. Larsson, and H. Smedje. 2006. Health-related quality of life in parents of school-age children with Asperger syndrome or high-functioning autism. *Health Qual. Life Outcomes* 4: 1, http://www.hqlo.com/content/4/1/1

Althous, M., A.M. Van Roon, L.J. Mulderm, G. Mulder, C.C. Aarnoudse, and R.B. Minderaa. 2004. Autonomic response patterns observed during performance of an attention-demanding task in two groups of children with autistic-type difficulties in social adjustment. *Psychophysiology* 41: 893–904.

Aman, M.G., K.S. Lam, and M.E. Van Bourgndien. 2005. Medication patterns in patients with autism: Temporal, regional, and demographic influences. *J. Child Adolesc. Psychopharmacol.* 15: 116–126.

Amaral, D.G. and B.A. Corbett. 2003. The amygdala, autism and anxiety. *Novartis Found. Symp.* 251: 177–187.

American Psychiatric Association (1980) *Diagnostic and Statistical Manual of Mental Disorders*, 3rd edition, Washington DC: American Psychiatric Association Press.

American Psychiatric Association (1994) *Diagnostic and Statistical Manual of Mental Disorders*, 4th edition, Washington DC: American Psychiatric Association Press.

Axelrod, F.B., G.C. Chelimsky, and D.E. Weese-Mayer. 2006. Pediatric autonomic disorders. *Pediatrics* 118: 309–321.

Baron-Cohen, S., H.A. Ring, E.T. Bullmore, S. Wheelwright, C. Ashwin, and S.C. Williams. 2000. The amygdala theory of autism. *Neruosci. Biobehav. Rev.* 24: 355–364.

Bergsma, J. and G.L. Engel. 1988. Quality of life: Does measurement help? *Health Policy* 10: 267–279.

Bettelheim, B. 1967. *"The Empty Fortress" Infantile Autism and the Birth of the Self*, New York: The Free Press.

Billstedt, E., I.C. Gillberg, and C. Gillberg. 2005. Autism after adolescence: Population-based 13-22 year follow-up study of 120 individuals with autism diagnosed in childhood. *J. Autism Dev. Disord.* 33: 351–360.

Bodfish, J.W., F.J. Symons, D.E. Parker, and M.H. Lewis. 2000. Varieties of repetitive behavior in autism: Comparisons to mental retardation. *J. Autism Dev. Disord.* 30: 237–243.

Burnette, C.P., P.C. Mundy, J.A. Meyer, S.K. Sutton, A.E. Vaughan, and D. Charak. 2005. Weak central coherence and its relations to theory of mind and anxiety in autism. *J. Autism Dev. Disord.* 35: 63–73.

Cassidy, J. 2001. Truth lies and intimacy: An attachment perspective. *Attach. Hum. Dev.* 3: 121–155.

Chalfant, A.M., R. Rapee, and L. Carroll. 2007. Treating anxiety disorders in children with high functioning autism spectrum disorders: A controlled trial. *J. Autism Dev. Disord.* 37: 1842–1857.

Chamberlin, B., C. Kasar, and E. Rothcram-Fuller. 2007. Involvement or isolation? The social networks of children with autism in regular classrooms. *J. Autism Dev. Disord.* 37: 230–242.

Courchesne, E. 1997. Brainstem, cerebellar and limbic neuroanatomic abnormalities in autism. *Curr. Opin. Neurobiol.* 7: 269–278.

Curin. J.M., J. Terzic, Z.B. Petkovic, L. Zekan, I.M. Terzic, and I.M. Susnjara. 2003. Lower cortisol and higher ACTH levels in individuals with autism. *J. Autism Dev. Disord.* 33: 443–448.

Czura, C.J. and K.J. Tracey. 2005. Autonomic neural regulation of immunity. *J. Intern. Med.* 257: 156–166.

Davis, M.P. and P.M. Darden. 2003. Use of complementary and alternative medicine by children in the United States. *Arch. Pediatr. Adolesc. Med.* 157: 393–396.

Dunne, W., B.S. Myles, and S. Orr. 2002. Sensory processing issues associated with Asperger syndrome: A preliminary investigation. *Am. J. Occup. Ther.* 56: 97–102.

Dykens, E.M. 2006. Toward a positive psychology of mental retardation. *Am. J. Orthopsychiatry* 76: 185–193.

Einfeld, S. and B. Tonge. 1997. Population prevalence of psychopathology in children and adolescents with intellectual disability II: Epidemiologic findings. *J. Intellect. Disabil. Res.* 40: 90–109.

Engel, G.L. 1977. The need for a new medical model: A challenge for biomedicine. *Science* 196: 129–135.

Engel, G.L. 1980. The clinical application of the biopsychosocial model. *Am. J. Psychiatry* 137: 535–544.

Engel, G.L. 1992. How much longer must medicine's science be bound by a seventeenth century world view? *Psychother. Psychosom.* 57: 3–16.

Engel, G.L. 1997. From biomedical to biopsychosocial. *Psychother. Psychosom.* 66: 57–62.

Esch, T. and G.B. Stefano. 2005. The neurobiology of love. *Neuroendocrinol. Lett.* 26: 175–192.

Findling, R. 2005. Pharmacologic treatment of behavioral symptoms in autism and pervasive developmental disorders. *J. Clin. Psychiatry* 66(Suppl. 10): 26–31.

Foxx, R.M. 2008. Applied behavior analysis treatment of autism: The state of the art. *Child Adolesc. Psychiatr. Clin. N. Am.* 17: 821–834.

Frank, J.D. 1979. The present status of outcome studies. *J. Consult. Clin. Psychol.* 47: 310–316.

Fresher-Samways, K., S.E. Roush, K. Choi, Y. Desrosiers, and G. Steel. 2003. Perceived quality of life of adults with developmental and other significant disabilities. *Disabil. Rehabil.* 25: 1097–1105.

Gadow, K.D., C.J. DeVincent, J. Pomeroy, and A. Azizian. 2004. Psychiatric symptoms in preschool children with PDD, clinical and comparisons samples. *J. Autism Dev. Disord.* 34: 379–393.

Gerber, F., M.A. Baud, M. Geroud, and G. Galli Carninati. 2008. Quality of life of adults with pervasive developmental disorders and intellectual disabilities. *J. Autism Dev. Disord.* 38: 1654–1665.

Grandin, T. 1991. *Emergence: Labeled Autistic*, Novato, CA: Arena Press.

Graveling, R.A. and J.D. Brooke. 1978. Hormonal and cardiac response of autistic children to changes in environmental stimulation. *J. Autism Child Schizophr.* 8: 441–455.

Green, G. 1996. Early behavioral intervention for autism: What does research tell us? In *Behavioral Intervention for Young Children with Autism: A Manual for Parents and Professionals*, eds. C. Maurice, G. Green, and S.C. Luce, Austin, TX: Pro-Ed, pp. 29–44.

Green, L., D. Fein, C. Modhal, C. Feinstein, L. Waterhouse, and M. Morris. 2001. Oxytocin and autistic disorder: Alterations in peptide forms. *Biol. Psychiatry* 50: 609–613.

Happe, F., A. Ronald, and R. Plomin. 2006. Time to give up on a single explanation for Autism. *Nat. Neurosci.* 9: 1218–1220.

Hirstein, W., P. Iversen, and V.S. Ramachandran. 2001. Autonomic responses of autistic children to people and objects. *Proc. Biol. Sci.* 268: 1883–1888.

Hollander, E., S. Novotny, M. Hanratty, R. Yaffe, C.M. DeCaria, B.R. Aronowitz, and S. Mosovich. 2003. Oxytocin infusion reduces repetitive behaviors in adults with autistic and Aspergers disorders. *Neuropsychopharmacology* 28: 193–198.

Howlin, P., S. Goode, J. Hutton, and M. Rutter. 2004. Adult outcome for children with autism. *J. Child Psychol. Psychiatry* 54: 212–229.

Hutt, C., S.J. Forrest, and J. Richer. 1975. Cardiac arrhythmia and behaviour in autistic children. *Acta Psychiatr. Scand.* 51: 361–372.

Jansen, L., C.C. Gispen-de Weid, R.J. van der Gaag, and H. van Engeland. 2003. Differentiation between autism and multiple complex developmental disorder in response to psychological stress. *Neuropsychopharmacology* 28: 582–590.

Jansen, L., C.C. Gispen-de Wied, V.M. Wiegant, H.G. Westenberg, B.E. Lahuis, and R.J. van Engeland. 2006. Autonomic and neuroendocrine responses to a psychosocial stressor in adults with autistic spectrum disorder. *J. Autism Dev. Disord.* 36: 891–899.

Jennes-Coussens, M., J. Magill-Evans, and C. Koning. 2006. The quality of life of young men with Asperger syndrome: A brief report. *Autism* 10: 403–414.

Juranek, J., P.A. Fillpek, G.R. Berenji, C. Modahl, K. Osann, and M.A. Spence. 2006. Association between amygdala volume and anxiety level: Magnetic resonance imaging study in autistic children. *J. Child Neurol.* 21: 1051–1058.

Kanner, L. 1943. Autistic disturbances of affective contact. *Nervous Child* 2: 217–250.

Karst, T.O. 1991. Historical rational of the therapeutic community. In *Autistic Adults at Bittersweet Farms*, eds. N.S., Giddan and J.J. Giddan, Binghampton, NY: Haworth Press, pp. 30–52.

Kirsch, P., C. Esslinger, Q. Chen, D. Mier, S. Lis, S. Siddhanti, and H. Gruppe. 2005. Oxytocin modulates neuronal circuitry for social cognition and fear in humans. *J. Neurosci.* 25: 11489–11493.

Kittay, E.F. 2001. When caring is just and justice is caring: Justice and mental retardation. *Public Cult.* 13: 557–580.

Kittay, J. 2008. The sound surround exploring how one might design the everyday soundscape for the truly captive audience. *Nord. J. Music Ther.* 17: 41–54.

Levy, S.E. and S.L. Hyman. 2008. Complementary and alternative medicine treatments for children with autism spectrum disorders. *Child Adolesc. Psychiatr. Clin. N. Am.* 17: 803–820.

Levy, S.E., D.S. Mandell, S. Merhar, R.F. Ittenbach, and J.A. Pinto-Martin. 2003. Use of complementary and alternative medicine among children recently diagnosed with autistic spectrum disorder. *J. Dev. Behav. Pediatr.* 24: 418–423.

Lindau, S.T., E.O. Laumann, W. Levinson, and L.J. Waite. 2003. Synthesis of scientific disciplines in pursuit of health: The interactive biopsychosocial model. *Perspect. Biol. Med.* 46(Suppl. 3): S74–S86.

London, E. 2007. The role of the neurobiologist in redefining the diagnosis of autism. *Brain Pathol.* 17: 408–411.

Mandell, D.S., K.H. Morales, S.C. Marcus, A.C. Stahmer, J. Doshi, and D.E. Polsky. 2008. Psychotropic medication use among medicaid enrolled children with autism spectrum disorders. *Pediatrics* 121: e441–e448.

Marinovic-Curin, J, I. Marinovic-Terzicet, Z. Bujas-Petkovic, L. Zekan, V. Skrabic, Z. Dogas, and J. Terzic. 2008. Slower cortisol response during ACTH stimulation test in autistic children. *Eur. Child Adolesc. Psychiatry* 17: 39–43.

Matson, J.S. and J. Wilkins. 2008. Antipsychotic drugs for aggression in intellectual disability. Comment. *Lancet* 371: 9–10.

Miller, F.A., M.E. Begbie, M. Giacomini, C. Ahern, and E.A. Harvey. 2006. Redefining disease? The nosologic implications of molecular genetic knowledge. *Perspect. Biol. Med.* 49: 99–114.

Ming, X., P.O. Julu, M. Brimacombe, S. Connor, and M.L. Daniels. 2005. Reduced cardiac parasympathetic activity in children with autism. *Brain Dev.* 27: 509–516.

Modahl, C., L. Green, D. Fein, M. Morris, L. Waterhouse, C. Feinstein, and H. Levin. 1998. Plasma oxytocin levels in autistic children. *Biol. Psychiatry* 43: 270–277.

Mugno, D., L. Ruta, V.G. D'Arrigo, and L. Mazzone. 2007. Impairment of quality of life in parents of children and adolescents with pervasive developmental disorder. *Health Qual. Life Outcomes* 5: 22, http://www.hqlo.com/contents/5/1/22

Muris, P., P. Steerneman, H. Meckelbach, I. Holdrinet, and C. Meesters.1998. Comorbid anxiety symptoms in children with pervasive developmental disorders. *J. Anxiety Disord.* 12: 387–393.

Murray, M.A. 1959. Needs of parents of mentally retarded children. *Am. J. Ment. Defic.* 63: 1078–1088.

Offit, P.A. 2008. *Autism's False Prophets: Bad Science, Risky Medicine, and the Search for a Cure*, New York: Columbia University Press.

Ospina, M.B., J. Krebs Seida, B. Clark, M. Karkhaneh, L. Hartling, L. Tjosvold, B. Vandermeer, and V. Smith. 2008. Behavioural and developmental interventions for autism spectrum disorder: A clinical systematic review. *PLOS ONE* 3: e3755.

Parikh, M.S., A. Kolevzon, and E. Hollander. 2008. Psychopharmacology of aggression in children and adolescents with autism: A critical review of efficacy and tolerability. *J. Child Adolesc. Psychopharmacol.* 18: 157–178.

Pollack, H. 2007. Learning to walk slow: America's partial policy success in the arena of intellectual disability. *J. Policy Hist.* 19: 95–112.

Porges, S.W. 2006. The polyvagal perspective. *Biol. Psychol.* 74: 116–143.

Posey, D.J., C.A. Erickson, and C.J. McDougle. 2008. Developing drugs for core social and communication impairment in autism. *Child Adolesc. Psychiatr. Clin. N. Am.* 17: 787–801.

Powley, T.L. 2000. Vagal input to the enteric nervous system. *Gut* 47(Suppl. iv): 30–32.

Reichow, B., F.R. Volkmar, and D.V. Ciccetti. 2008. Development of the evaluative method for evaluating and determining evidence-based practices in autism. *J. Autism Dev. Disord.* 38: 1311 1319.

Sandler, J.Z. and Y.F. Hulgus. 1992. Clinical problem solving and the biopsychosocial model. *Am. J. Psychiatry* 149: 1315–1323.

Scahill, L., M.G. Aman, J.T. McCracken, C.J. McDougle, and B. Vitiello. 2008. Beware of over-interpreting negative trials. *J. Autism Dev. Disord.* 38: 1609–1610.

Seligman, M. 2002. Positive psychology, positive prevention and positive therapy. In *Handbook of Positive Psychology*, eds. C.R. Snyder and S.J. Lopez, New York: Oxford University Press, pp. 3–13.

Shogren, K.A., M.L. Wehmeyer, C.L. Buchanan, and S.J. Lopez. 2006. The application of positive psychology and self-determination to research in intellectual disability: A content analysis of 30 years of literature. *Res. Pract. Pers. Severe Disabil.* 31: 338–345.

Sukhodolsky, D.G., L. Scahill, K.D. Gadow, L.E. Arnold, M.G. Aman, C.J. McDougle, J.T. McCracken, E. Tierney, S. Williams White, L. Lecavalier, and B. Viteillo. 2008. Parent rated anxiety symptoms in children with pervasive developmental disorders: Frequency and association with core autism symptoms and cognitive functioning. *J. Abnorm. Child Psychol.* 36: 117–128.

Swiezy, N., M. Stuart, and P. Korzekwa. 2008. Bridging for success in Autism: Training and collaboration across medical, educational and community systems. *Child Adolesc. Psychiatr. Clin. N. Am.* 17: 907–922.

Talley, R.C. and J.E. Crews. 2007. Framing the public health of caregiving. *Am. J. Public Health* 97: 224–228.

Tani, P., N. Lindberg, V. Matto, B. Appelberg, T. Nieminen-von Wendt, L. von Wendt, and T. Porka-Heiskanen. 2005. Higher plasma ACTH levels in adults with Aspergers syndrome. *J. Psychsom. Res.* 58: 533–536.

Toichi, M. and T. Kamio. 2003. Paradoxical autonomic response to mental tasks in autism. *J. Autism Dev. Disord.* 33: 417–426.

Tyrer, P., P.C. Oliver-Africano, Z. Ahmed, N. Bouras, S. Cooray, S. Deb, D. Murphy, M. Hare, M. Meade, B. Reece, K. Kramo, S. Bhaumik, D. Harley, A. Regan, D. Thomas, B. Rao, B. North, J. Eliahoo, S. Kartela, A. Soni, and M. Crawford. 2008. Risperidone, haloperidol and placebo in the treatment of aggressive challenging behaviour in patients with intellectual disability: A randomized controlled trial. *Lancet* 371: 57–63.

Volkmar, F., E.H. Cook, J. Pomeroy, G. Realmuto, and P. Tanguay. 1999. Practice parameters for the assessment of and treatment of children, adolescents and adults with autism and other pervasive developmental disorders. *J. Am. Acad. Child Adolesc. Psychiatry* 38 (Suppl. 12): 32–54.

Zahn, T.P., J.M. Rumsey, and D.P. Van Kammen. 1987. Autonomic nervous system activity in autistic schizophrenic and normal men: Effects of stimulus significance. *J. Abnorm. Psychol.* 96: 135–144.

Index